MW01202039

MINIMALLY INVASIVE GYNECOLOGIC SURGERY

EVIDENCE-BASED LAPAROSCOPIC, HYSTEROSCOPIC AND ROBOTIC PROCEDURES

MINIMALLY INVASIVE GYNECOLOGIC SURGERY

EVIDENCE-BASED LAPAROSCOPIC, HYSTEROSCOPIC AND ROBOTIC PROCEDURES

Edited by

JON IVAR EINARSSON MD, PhD, MPH
Associate Professor of Obstetrics and Gynecology
Harvard Medical School
Director, Division of Minimally Invasive Gynecologic Surgery
Brigham and Women's Hospital
Boston, Massachusetts
USA

ARNAUD WATTIEZ MD
Professor of Obstetrics and Gynecology
Gynecology Department
University of Strasbourg
Strasbourg
France

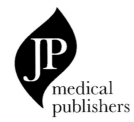

JP
medical
publishers

London • Philadelphia • Panama City • New Delhi

© 2016 JP Medical Ltd.
Published by JP Medical Ltd, 83 Victoria Street, London, SW1H 0HW, UK
Tel: +44 (0)20 3170 8910   Fax: +44 (0)20 3008 6180
Email: info@jpmedpub.com   Web: www.jpmedpub.com

The rights of Jon I Einarsson and Arnaud Wattiez to be identified as editors
of this work have been asserted by them in accordance with the Copyright,
Designs and Patents Act 1988.

All rights reserved. No part of this publication may be reproduced, stored
or transmitted in any form or by any means, electronic, mechanical,
photocopying, recording or otherwise, except as permitted by the UK
Copyright, Designs and Patents Act 1988, without the prior permission in
writing of the publishers. Permissions may be sought directly from JP Medical
Ltd at the address printed above.

All brand names and product names used in this book are trade names,
service marks, trademarks or registered trademarks of their respective owners.
The publisher is not associated with any product or vendor mentioned in this
book.

Medical knowledge and practice change constantly. This book is designed
to provide accurate, authoritative information about the subject matter
in question. However, readers are advised to check the most current
information available on procedures included and check information from the
manufacturer of each product to be administered, to verify the recommended
dose, formula, method and duration of administration, adverse effects
and contraindications. It is the responsibility of the practitioner to take all
appropriate safety precautions. Neither the publisher nor the editors assume
any liability for any injury and/or damage to persons or property arising from
or related to use of material in this book.

This book is sold on the understanding that the publisher is not engaged in
providing professional medical services. If such advice or services are required,
the services of a competent medical professional should be sought.

Every effort has been made where necessary to contact holders of copyright
to obtain permission to reproduce copyright material. If any have been
inadvertently overlooked, the publisher will be pleased to make the necessary
arrangements at the first opportunity.

ISBN: 978-1-909836-09-9

British Library Cataloguing in Publication Data
A catalogue record for this book is available from the British Library

Library of Congress Cataloging in Publication Data
A catalog record for this book is available from the Library of Congress

Publisher: Richard Furn
Associate Publisher: Geoff Greenwood
Development Editor: Gavin Smith
Editorial Assistant: Katie Pattullo
Design: Designers Collective Ltd

Preface

Minimally invasive gynecologic surgery (MIGS) has advanced significantly over the past 20 years and is gradually becoming the standard of care for the surgical treatment of benign and malignant conditions in gynecology. Although the adoption of a minimally invasive approach was slow at first, we have now reached a tipping point where patients and surgeons alike recognize the benefits of offering patients a less invasive surgical option. It is conceivable that in the near future the term 'minimally invasive gynecologic surgery' will be redundant, as this will become the standard in gynecologic surgery.

Nevertheless, several challenges remain for the safe and widespread implementation of MIGS into general practice. Some gynecologists may not have the necessary surgical volume to sustain the learning curve to perform surgical procedures safely and effectively. This has been one of the main barriers in developing and spreading MIGS further. The implementation of MIGS fellowships by the AAGL in 2001 has been instrumental in turning the tide, since these MIGS fellowship graduates have joined surgical practices and academic institutions across the United States and have helped to train others in the specialty. They have also helped to develop centers of excellence for advanced gynecologic surgery and these centers will be vital to further developing our surgical field.

Another important challenge is inadequate training and education. Many surgeons have not received sufficient training in minimally invasive surgery during their residency and may have limited access to credible educational resources. It can be challenging to maintain and develop knowledge, while maintaining a busy clinical practice. A quick and practical guide for the practicing gynecologic surgeon is needed.

We have published *Minimally Invasive Gynecologic Surgery* to address this deficiency. We are fortunate to have assembled the most pre-eminent experts in the field to share their knowledge and expertise. Each chapter stands independently, but the flow of the book is logical, starting with anatomy, laparoscopic exposure and other general topics, such as electrosurgery, suture materials, instrumentation, hysteroscopy, complications, laparoscopy in pregnancy, laparoscopic tissue extraction and single port surgery. The book then covers procedures for benign conditions in detail, enabling the reader to follow the steps of each procedure while the authors share their surgical tips. Each chapter is accompanied by illustrations and clinical photographs for greater clarity.

Robotic surgery has enjoyed a rapid adoption since its FDA approval for gynecologic surgery in 2005. While robotic surgery is essentially laparoscopic surgery, there are several unique challenges and instruments associated with this mode of access. As a result, we have devoted several chapters to robotic surgery, both tips for instrumentation and setup as well as practical procedure – specific information by subject experts in the field.

Minimally Invasive Gynecologic Surgery covers several chapters on laparoscopic procedures for malignant conditions. Just as in benign gynecology, minimally invasive surgery has become the standard for most procedures for malignant conditions. Experts in gynecologic oncology share their knowledge in a number of chapters, covering the most common minimally invasive procedures in gynecologic oncology and including a chapter devoted to the role of minimally invasive surgery in the surgical treatment of advanced gynecologic cancer. Robotic surgery in gynecologic oncology is also covered in a separate chapter.

We sincerely hope this book will be helpful to our readers in their quest for greater proficiency in minimally invasive surgery. While we acknowledge that reading is not enough to acquire surgical competency, we are confident that the content of this book will enable the reader to increase their knowledge of the field and to gain valuable insight into how to perform surgical procedures more safely and effectively. Enjoy and best of luck!

Jon Ivar Einarsson
Arnaud Wattiez
March 2016

Contents

Contributors

Karolina Afors MBBS, BSc, MRCOG
Specialty Registrar in Obstetrics and Gynecology
Kings College Hospital NHS Trust
London
UK

Mobolaji O Ajao MD
Clinical Fellow
Division of Minimally Invasive Gynecologic Surgery
Department of Obstetrics and Gynecology
Brigham and Women's Hospital
Harvard Medical School
Boston, Massachusetts
USA

Geetanjali Agarwal Joshi MS
Consultant Oncosurgeon
Galaxy Care Laparoscopy Institute
Pune
India

Claudia Andrade MD
Gynecologist Obstetrician
Department of Gynecologic Oncology
Centre Oscar Lambret
Lille
France

Shan Biscette MD
Assistant Professor of Obstetrics and Gynecology
Department of Obstetrics and Gynecology
University of Louisville
Louisville, Kentucky
USA

David M Boruta II MD
Associate Professor of Obstetrics, Gynecology, and Reproductive Medicine
Harvard Medical School
Vincent Obstetrics and Gynecology Service
Massachusetts General Hospital
Boston, Massachusetts
USA

Jan Bosteels MD, PhD
Consultant in Obstetrics and Gynaecology
Department of Obstetrics and Gynaecology
Imelda Ziekenhuis
Bonheiden
Belgium

Revaz Botchorishvili MD
Consultant in Obstetrics and Gynecology
Department of Gynecological Surgery
Estaing University Hospital
Clermont-Ferrand
France

Lucie Bresson MD
Gynecologist Obstetrician
Department of Gynecolgic Oncology
Centre Oscar Lambret
Lille
France

Michel Canis MD, PhD
Professor of Obstetrics and Gynaecology
Department of Obstetric and Gynaecology
Centre Hospitalier Universitaire de Clermont Ferrand
Clermont-Ferrand
France

Jesús Castellano Moros MD
Medical Chief of Minimally Invasive Surgery and IVF
Medical Director
Medifem
Zulia
Venezuela
Consultant
IRCAD
Strasbourg
France

Gabriele Centini MD
Researcher in Obstetrics and Gynecology
Department of Molecular and Developmental Medicine
University of Siena
Siena
Italy

Roberto Clarizia MD, PhD
Consultant in Gynecology and Obstetrics
Gynecologic Oncology and Minimally-Invasive Pelvic Surgery
International School of Surgical Anatomy
Sacred Heart Hospital
Verona
Italy

Sarah L Cohen MD, MPH
Director of Research
Assistant Fellowship Program Director
Assistant Professor
Division of Minimally Invasive Gynecologic Surgery
Department of Obstetrics and Gynecology
Brigham and Women's Hospital
Harvard Medical School
Boston, Massachusetts
USA

Marianne de Bennetot–Julien MD
Staff Physician
Department of Obstetrics and Gynaecology
Centre Hospitalier d'Aurillac
Aurillac
France

Marjolein De Cuypere MD
Gynecologic Oncologist
Department of Obstetrics and Gynecology
CHU de Liège
University of Liège
Liège
Belgium

Rudy Leon De Wilde MD, PhD
Professor and Head of Department for Gynecology,
Obstetrics and Gynecological Oncology
Department for Gynecology, Obstetrics and
Gynecological Oncology
University Clinic of Gynecology
Pius Hospital
Carl von Ossietzky University
Oldenburg
Germany

Katty Delbecque MD
Anatomopathologist
Department of Pathology
CHU de Liège
University of Liège
Liège
Belgium

Giuseppe Di Pierro MD
Department of Gynecology and Obstetrics
San Carlo Hospital
Potenza
Italy

Elisabeth J Diver MD
Fellow in Gynecologic Oncology
Department of Obstetrics and Gynecology
Massachusetts General Hospital
Harvard Medical School
Boston, Massachusetts
USA

Jean Doyen MD
Gynecologist
Department of Obstetrics and Gynecology
CHU de Liège
University of Liège
Liège
Belgium

Alfredo Ercoli MD, PhD
Professor of Obstetrics and Gynecology
SCDU Obstetrics and Gynecology Clinic
Azienda Ospedaliero 'Maggiore della Carità' di Novara
Università del Piemonte Orientale
Novara
Italy

Anna Fagotti MD, PhD
Gynecologic Oncologist
Catholic University of the Sacred Heart
Rome
Italy

Francesco Fanfani MD
Professor of Gynecologic Oncology
Department of Medicine and Aging Science
University of Chieti-Pescara
Chieti
Italy

Rodrigo P Fernandes MD
Professor of Gynaecology Oncology and Minimally
Invasive Surgery
Department of Gynaecology Oncology
Institute of Cancer Studies of São Paulo (ICESP)
University of Sao Paulo Faculty of Medicine
São Paulo
Brasil

Hervé Fernandez MD, PhD
Professor of Gynaecology and Obstetrics
Department of Gynaecology and Obstetrics
Hospital Bicêtre (AP-HP)
Le Kremlin Bicêtre
Paris
France

Maria Lucia Gagliardi MD
Gynecologist
Department of Obstetrics and Gynecology
Hospital F. Veneziale
Isernia
Italy

Olivier Garbin MD
Gynecologist
Department of Obstetrics and Gynecology
CMCO, University Hospital
Strasbourg
France

Antonio R Gargiulo MD
Medical Director
Center for Robotic Surgery
Department of Obstetrics and Gynecology
Brigham and Women's Hospital
Assistant Professor of Obstetrics, Gynecology and
Reproductive Biology
Harvard Medical School
Boston, Massachusetts
USA

Amélie Gervaise MD
Adjuncted Professor
McGill University
Montreal
CISSSO Gatineau
Gynecology and Obstetric Department
Quebec
Canada

Ali Ghomi MD
Chief
Robotic Surgery
Director, Female Pelvic Medicine & Reconstructive
Surgery
Sisters of Charity Hospital
New York City, New York
USA

Frederic Goffin MD, PhD
Gynecologic Oncologist
Department of Obstetrics and Gynecology
CHU de Liège
University of Liège
Liège
Belgium

James A Greenberg MD, FACOG
Associate Professor of Obstetrics, Gynecology and
Reproductive Biology
Harvard Medical School
Boston, Massachusetts
USA

Delphine Hudry MD
Gynecologist Obstetrician
Department of Gynecologic Oncology
Centre Oscar Lambret
Lille
France

Keith Isaacson MD
Associate Professor of Obstetrics and Gynecology
Harvard Medical School
Boston, Massachusetts
USA

Olav Istre MD, PhD
Professor in Minimal Invasive Gynecological Surgery
University of Southern Denmark
Aleris-Hamlet Hospitaler
Copenhagen
Denmark

Saurabh N Joshi MS
Consultant Oncosurgeon
Galaxy Care Laparoscopy Institute
Pune
India

Athanasios Kakkos MD
Gynecologic Oncologist
Department of Obstetrics and Gynecology
CHU de Liège
University of Liège
Liège
Belgium

Cara R King DO, MS
Assistant Professor of Obstetrics and Gynecology
Division of Benign Gynecology
Minimally Invasive Gynecologic Surgery
University of Wisconsin-Madison
Madison, Wisconsin
USA

Philippe R Koninckx MD, PhD
Professor of Obstetrics and Gynecology
University of Leuven
Leuven
Belgium
Oxford University
Oxford, UK
Catholic University of the Sacred Heart
Rome
Italy

Frederic Kridelka MD, PhD
Gynecologic Oncologist
Head, Gynecological Oncology Unit
Department of Obstetrics and Gynecology
CHU de Liège
University of Liège
Liège
Belgium

Sanjay Kumar MS
Fellow, Minimal Access Surgery
Galaxy Care Laparoscopy Institute
Pune
India

Demetrio Larrain MD
Gynecologist
Department of Obstetrics and Gynaecology
CHU de Clermont Ferrand
Clermont Ferrand
France

Eric Leblanc MD
Surgeon
Head, Department of Gynaecological Oncology
Oscar Lambret Cancer Center
Lille
France

Ted Lee MD
Director
Minimally Invasive Gynecologic Surgery
University of Pittsburgh Medical Center
Pittsburgh, Pennsylvania
USA

Megan Loring MD
Clinical Instructor of Obstetrics and Gynecology
Harvard Medical School
Boston, Massachusetts
USA

Javier F Magrina MD
Professor of Obstetrics and Gynecology
Department of Gynecologic Surgery
Mayo Clinic Arizona
Phoenix, Arizona
USA

Hubert Manhes MD
Gynecologist
Department of Obstetrics and Gynaecology
Centre Hospitalier Universitaire de Clermont Ferrand
Clermont Ferrand
France

Patricia J Mattingly MD
AAGL Minimally Invasive Gynecologic Surgery Fellow
Department of Obstetrics and Gynecology
Columbia University Medical Center
New York City, New York
USA

Carolina Meza Paul MD
Fellow in Minimally Invasive Gynaecologic Surgery
Department of Gynaecological Surgery
Strasbourg University Hospital
IRCAD
Strasbourg
France

Ignacio Miranda Mendoza PhD
Obstetrician and Gynecologist
Department of Gynecology
Clínica Alemana
University of Desarrollo
Santiago
Chile

Neha Mookim MS
Fellow
Galaxy Care Laparoscopy Institute
Pune
India

Rouba Murtada MD
Gynecologist
Department of Gynecology and Obstetrics
Hôpital Jean Verdier (AP-HP)
Bondy
France

Didier Mutter MD, PhD, FACS
Professor and Chairman of Digestive Surgery
Department of Digestive Surgery
University Hospital of Strasbourg
Strasbourg
France

Fabrice Narducci MD
Gyn-Oncologist
Department of Gynecology Oncology
Centre Oscar Lambret
Lille
France

Marie Fidela R Paraiso MD
Professor of Obstetrics and Gynecology
Center for Urogynecology and Pelvic Reconstructive Surgery
Obstetrics, Gynecology & Women's Health Institute
Cleveland Clinic
Cleveland, Ohio
USA

Maria Laura Pisaturo MD
Gynecologist
Department of Gynecology and Obstetrics
San Carlo Hospital
Potenza
Italy

Jean-Luc Pouly MD, PhD
Professor of Obstetrics and Gynaecology
Unit of Reproductive Medicine
Department of Obstetrics and Gynaecology
Centre Hospitalier Universitaire de Clermont Ferrand
Clermont-Ferrand
France

Marco Puga MD
Gynecologic Oncologist
Gynecological Oncology Unit
National Institute for Cancer
Department of Gynecology
Clinica Alemana
University of Desarrollo
Santiago
Chile

Seema S Puntambaker MS
Consultant Gynaecologist
Galaxy Care Laparoscopy Institute
Pune
India

Shailesh P. Puntambaker MS
Consultant Oncosurgeon
Director
Galaxy Care Laparoscopy Institute
Pune
India

Benoit Rabischong MD, PhD
Professor of Obstetrics and Gynaecology
Unit of Gynaecological Surgery
Department of Obstetrics and Gynaecology
CHU de Clermont Ferrand
Clermont Ferrand
France

Giovanni Roviglione MD
Consultant in Gynecology and Obstetrics
Department of Obstetrics and Gynecology
International School of Surgical Anatomy
Sacred Heart Hospital
Verona
Italy

Giovanni Scambia MD
Director of Department of Gynecology and Obstetrics
Department of Gynecology and Obstetrics
Catholic University (A. Gemelli) Hospital
Rome
Italy

Sergio Schettini MD
Head of Department of Gynecology and Obstetrics
San Carlo Hospital
Potenza
Italy

Jessica A Shepherd MD, MBA
Assistant Professor of Obstetrics and Gynecology
Director of Minimally Invasive Gynecology
University of Illinois at Chicago
Chicago, Illinois
USA

Matthew T Siedhoff MD, MSCR
Assistant Professor
Director
Minimally Invasive Gynecologic Surgery
University of North Carolina at Chapel Hill
Charlotte, North Carolina
USA

Daniela FS Siufi MD
Surgical Oncologist
Hospital Sírio – Libanês
Sao Paulo
Brazil

João Siufi Neto MD
Surgical Oncologist
Hospital Sírio – Libanês
Sao Paulo
Brazil

Craig J Sobolewski MD, FACOG
Chief
Division of Minimally Invasive Gynecologic Surgery
Duke University
Durham, North Carolina
USA

Kevin JE Stepp MD
Program Director
Female Pelvic Medicine and Reconstructive Surgery
Chief
Urogynecology and Minimally Invasive Gynecologic
Surgery
Clinical Associate Professor
Department of Obstetrics and Gynecology
University of North Carolina at Chapel Hill
Charlotte, North Carolina
USA

Sophie Taieb MD
Radiologist
Department of Imaging
Centre Oscar Lambret
Lille
France

Alain Thille MD
Radiologist
Department of Medical Imaging
CHU de Liège, University of Liège
Liège
Belgium

Valerie To MD
Resident
Department of Obstetrics and Gynecology
McGill University
Montreal, Quebec
Canada

Audrey Tsunoda MD, PhD
Surgical Oncologist
Gynecologic Oncology Department
Hospital Erasto Gaertner
Curitiba
Brazil

Togas Tulandi MD, MHCM
Professor of Obstetrics and Gynecology
Milton Leong Chair in Reproductive Medicine
Department of Obstetrics and Gynecology
McGill University
Montreal, Quebec
Canada

Cecile A Unger MD, MPH
Assistant Professor of Obstetrics and Gynecology
Center for Urogynecology and Pelvic Reconstructive Surgery
Obstetrics, Gynecology & Women's Health Institute
Cleveland Clinic
Cleveland, Ohio
USA

Anastasia Ussia MD
Director of Gruppo Italo-Belga
Villa del Rosario Clinic
Rome
Italy

Bruno J van Herendael MD
Professor Emeritus of Gynaecologic Endoscopy
Consultant
Department of Obstetrics and Gynaecology
Division of Endoscopic Surgery
ZNA Stuivenberg – St Erasmus
Antwerp
Belgium

Rahul Vashishth MS
Fellow
Galaxy Care Laparoscopy Institute
Pune
India

Karen C Wang MD
Instructor
Harvard Medical School
Department of Obstetrics and Gynecology
Brigham and Women's Hospital
Boston, Massachusetts
USA

Arnaud Wattiez MD
Professor of Gynecological Surgery
University Hospital of Strasbourg
Strasbourg
France
Head of the Gynecological Department
Latifa Hospital, Dubai Health Authority
Dubai
United Arab Emirates

Morris Wortman MD, FACOG
Director
Center for Menstrual Disorders Rochester
New York, New York
Clinical Associate Professor of Gynecology
University of Rochester Medical Center
Rochester, New York
USA

Errico Zupi MD
Professor of Obstetrics and Gynecology
University of Rome Tor Vergata
Rome
Italy

Jonathan L Zurawin MD
Resident Physician
Department of Urology
Tulane University School of Medicine
New Orleans, Louisiana
USA

Robert K Zurawin MD
Associate Professor
Department of Obstetrics and Gynecology
Baylor College of Medicine
Houston, Texas
USA

Chapter 1 Surgical anatomy of the pelvis

Marcello Ceccaroni, Roberto Clarizia, Giovanni Roviglione, Alfredo Ercoli

INTRODUCTION

The pelvis is a convex funnel-shaped cavity, forming the caudad portion of the abdomen, limited by the pelvic bones and by muscles, covered by a double layer of fascial sheet forming the parietal pelvic fascia (PPF).

MUSCLES

The main portion of the muscular layer of the pelvis is represented by the pelvic floor (pelvic diaphragm) constituted by the levator ani muscle and the coccygeus muscle covered by the PPF (**Figure 1.1**). The levator ani is made of three components (the pubococcygeus, puborectalis, and iliococcygeus muscles). The pelvic floor has two hiatuses (gaps): anteriorly the urogenital hiatus, through which the urethra and vagina pass, and posteriorly the rectal hiatus, through which the anal canal passes. The pelvic cavity of the true pelvis has the pelvic floor as its inferior border (and the pelvic brim as its superior border). The perineum has the pelvic floor as its superior border. The pelvic floor separates the pelvic cavity above from the perineal region (including perineum) below.

The pubococcygeus, the main part of the levator ani muscle, runs along the midline, from the body of the pubic bone to the coccyx and may be damaged during parturition. Some fibers are inserted into the urethra and the vagina.

The right and left puborectalis muscles join behind the anorectal junction to form a muscular sling, arising from the caudad part of the

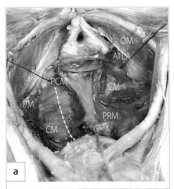
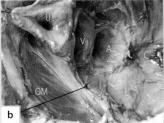

Figure 1.1 The pelvic floor viscera and muscle in a fresh cadaver specimen in a ventro-dorsal view. PM, Piriformis muscle; CM, Coccygeus muscle; PCM, Pubo-coccygeus muscle; PRM, Pubo-rectalis muscle; ICM, Ileo-coccygeus muscle; ATLA, Arcus tendineus levator ani; OM, Obturator muscle; U, Urethra; V, Vagina; A, Anus; C, Coccyx.

pubic symphysis and the urogenital diaphragm. Its fibers form the external anal sphincter.

The iliococcygeus, the most dorsal part of the levator ani, is often poorly developed and it inserts laterally at the level of the obturator muscle forming a fibrous tendon called the 'white line,' representing the tendinous arch of the fascia lata.

The coccygeus muscle is situated dorsally with respect to the levator ani and frequently is equally tendinous as it is muscular, extending from the caudad margin of the ischial spine to the lateral margin of the sacrum and coccyx.

The obturator internus muscle originates from the superior and inferior pubic rami; specifically, it partly originates from the inner surface of the obturator membrane that covers most of the obturator foramen; the widest portion of the muscle originates along the bony back edge of the obturator foramen; finally, the caudad end of the muscle narrows to a tendon that inserts into the middle of the bony surface of the greater trochanter of the femur, the bulbous portion of the upper thigh bone. At the level of the tendinous arch of levator ani, the obturator internus muscle completes the canal for the passage of the obturator vessels and nerve, called the 'obturator canal.' The muscle is innervated by the obturator nerve that originates from L5 and from S1–S2. It is a lateral rotator of the thigh and it assists in holding the head of the femur in the acetabulum.

The pelvis is limited dorsolaterally by the piriformis muscle, a flat pyramidal-shaped muscle originating from the ventral face of the sacrum and from the superior margin of the greater sciatic notch (as well as the sacroiliac joint capsule and the sacrotuberous ligament). The piriformis muscle exits the pelvis through the greater sciatic foramen to insert into the greater trochanter of the femur. The piriformis is a very important landmark in the gluteal region; as it travels through the greater sciatic foramen, it effectively divides the foramen into an inferior and a superior part. This determines the name of the vessels and nerves in this region; the nerve and vessels that emerge superior to the piriformis are the superior gluteal nerve and superior gluteal vessels, respectively. In the same way, the inferior gluteal nerve and vessels, together with the sciatic nerve, caudally cross the piriformis.

FASCIAE

In the pelvis, two different fascial systems may be identified, the PPF and the visceral pelvic fascia (VPF). The PPF covers the osteomuscular structures, which define the pelvic cavity and the contiguous structures (hypogastric vessels and sacral roots). It strongly adheres to the periosteum and to the muscles, and reflects at the level of the urogenital hiatus over the pelvic viscera, covering and fixing them to the pelvic wall and forming the VPF. At the level of the sacral bone, the PPF is called presacral fascia, covering the ventral face of the sacrum and the coccyx. Above the piriformis muscle, the PPF is called hypogastric fascia and covers the sacral roots and the pelvic plexus.

The VPF is an adventitial membrane that is not uniformly distributed. It is thicker in the junctional areas among the pelvic viscera where it forms connective transverse or longitudinal septa, which keep the viscera separated.

The connective tissue lying between the PPF and the VPF represents the so-called extraserous pelvic fascia, which contains the lympho-vascular nervous support to the pelvic viscera and is usually called by the generic term 'parametrium.'

PELVIC SPACES

A virutal or potential space is defined as an anatomical site but created by the surgical dissection of the connective tissue surrounding the viscera (**Figure 1.2**).

The virtual pelvic spaces are represented from ventral to dorsal (**Figure 1.2**) by the retropubic (Retzius') space (RPS), the retroinguinal (Bogros') spaces, the paravesical spaces (PVS), the pararectal spaces (PRS), and the retrorectal (or presacral) space. The iliolumbar spaces, obtained by caudad dissection between the pelvic wall and the external iliac vessels, represent more lateral spaces of the pelvis on both sides.

Two more spaces may be dissected among the pelvic viscera: the vesicovaginal space and rectovaginal space. Each pelvic space is part of the retroperitoneum, and its caudad limit is represented by the pelvic floor.

Retropubic (Retzius') space

It is the most ventral space of the pelvis, obtained by surgical transection of the urachus and caudad blunt dissection of the anterior abdominal wall from the anterior aspects of the bladder and the pubic symphysis. It is completely avascular and its limits are as follows:

- Ventral: pubic symphysis and medial third of the ischiopubic branches
- Dorsal: ventral face of the bladder and pubovesical fascia, vascular stalk of internal iliac vessels with the umbilicoprevesical fascia
- Lateral: Bogros' space, bladder pillars
- Caudad: pubovesical ligament, Santorini's retropubic venous plexus, urethra, pubourethral fascia, and reflection of the superior

fascia of the levator ani muscle: arcus tendineus of pelvic fascia (ATPF) and arcus tendineus of levator ani (ATLA)
- Cranial: peritoneum of the vesical couple and pelvic side wall

Retroinguinal (Bogros') space

It is defined as the lateral extension of the RPS, ventrally limited by the ischiopubic branches and continuing laterally with the PVS.

Paravesical space

It is one of the most important spaces of the pelvis, as it gives initial access to the anterolateral compartment of the pelvis for the performance of pelvic lymphadenectomy, radical hysterectomy, or for the lateral approach to the bladder during the course of ureteroneocystostomy. It can be divided into a medial PVS and a lateral PVS with respect to the obliterated umbilical artery and the umbilical prevesical fascia, which, respectively, represent its lateral and medial limits. The anatomical limits of the PVS on each side are as follows:

- Lateral: PPF, external iliac vein/artery, Bogros' space
- Medial: for the medial PVS, the lateral aspects of the bladder with the bladder pillars and the vesicocervical fascia. For the lateral PVS, the obliterated umbilical artery and the umbilical prevesical fascia
- Ventral: Bogros' retroinguinal space and ischiopubic branches
- Dorsal: Mackenrodt's cardinal ligament (lateral parametrium)
- Cranial: peritoneum of the anterior leaf of the broad ligament
- Caudal: pelvic floor, i.e. iliococcygeus muscle covered by the PPF and its attachment to the obturator muscle (ATPF and ATLA)

Pararectal space

Typically, the medial PRS (Okabayashi's space) is developed between the mesoureter and the rectouterine ligament by opening a space between the posterior leaf of the broad ligament (medial) and the ureter (lateral). In contrast, the lateral PRS (Latzko's space) is developed between the mesoureter and the pelvic wall by opening up the space between the internal iliac artery (lateral) and the ureter (medial). The opening of these spaces is a key step during a radical hysterectomy for cervical carcinoma. To obtain full mobilization of the rectosigmoid and to access the lower mesorectum at the level of the rectal wings (also known as the lateral rectal ligaments), both the medial and lateral PRS are opened. This step also allows an anatomical identification of the posterior and lateral parametrial ligaments (rectovaginal, lateral rectal, and cardinal ligament).

Its anatomical limits are as follows:
- Medial: fascia propria recti, rectal pillars; the ureter for the lateral PRS
- Lateral: PPF, inferior hypogastric plexus with pelvic splanchnic nerves, internal iliac artery, piriform muscle; the ureter for the medial PRS
- Dorsal: presacral fascia, sacrum
- Ventral: Mackenrodt's cardinal ligament (lateral parametrium)
- Caudad: pelvic floor, i.e. ischiococcygeal muscle, branches of the puborectal and pubococcygeal muscle
- Cranial: peritoneum of the posterior leaf of the broad ligament

Retrorectal space

The presacral space is a virtual space limited ventrally by the rectum and the rectal stalks, and dorsally by the sacral bone covered by the presacral fascia. It contains connective and adipous tissue defined by Waldeyer's tela adiposa retrorectalis. Blunt dissection in the retrorectal space is further performed, in the laterocaudal direction, along the

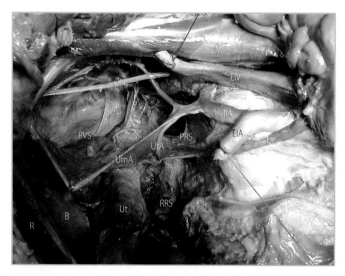

Figure 1.2 Medio-lateral view of the pelvis in a fresh cadaver specimen showing landmarks of the main spaces. R, Retzius space; B, Bladder; Ut, Uterus; RRS, Retrorectal space; PVS, Paravesical space; UmA, Umbilical artery; PRS, pararectal space; Ur, Ureter; EIA, External iliac artery; IIA, Internal iliac artery; EIV, external iliac vein; ON, Obturator nerve; PM, psoas muscle.

sacral bone's concavity, opening down the so-called 'holy plane of Heald' on the midline. Its limits are as follows:

- Dorsal: sacrum covered by the presacral fascia, a portion of the PPF, strictly adherent to the bone, and covering the sacral artery and veins and arteriovenous anastomoses
- Ventral: posterior face of the rectum covered by the fascia propria recti (part of the VPF)
- Lateral: common iliac vessels and the ureters
- Cranial: abdominal retroperitoneum
- Caudad: rectosacral (Waldeyer's) fascia reflecting from presacral fascia to the fascia propria recti; it represents the posterior support of the rectum and maintains the sacrococcygeal angle during defecation

Iliolumbar space

The iliolumbar space is the most lateral space of the pelvis, obtained by medialization of the external iliac artery and vein, and limited laterally by the psoas muscle and, more caudally, by the lateral pelvic wall. It is usually dissected during pelvic lymphadenectomy or as the lateral approach to somatic nerves (**Figure 1.3**). It contains the lumbosacral trunk, the pelvic portion of the obturator nerve, and vessels from their origin to their exit through the obturator foramen, the sciatic nerve, the sacral roots (S2–S4), and the pudendal nerve and vessels. Its limits are as follows:

- Lateral: pelvic wall and medial face of the great psoas muscle
- Medial: external iliac vessels, gluteal vein, hypogastric artery
- Ventral: obturator internus muscle, obturator foramen
- Dorsal: piriformis muscle, and sacral plexus and roots
- Caudal: pelvic floor
- Cranial: pelvic peritoneum

Vesicovaginal space

The vesicovaginal space is made up of two compartments: the vesicocervical and vesicovaginal spaces, which are separated by the vesicocervical ligament, a transverse line of dense adherence between the supratrigonal bladder and the cervicovaginal junction (anterior vaginal fornix). The vesicocervical space lies between the posterior bladder and the cervix; it is covered cranially by the peritoneum of the vesicouterine fold and limited laterally by the vesicouterine ligaments, the most superior portion of the bladder pillars. The vesicovaginal space is limited laterally by the bladder pillars and inferiorly by the urogenital diaphragm; its anterior wall is formed by the bladder, the urethra, and pubourethral ligaments.

Rectovaginal space

The anterolateral rectum is connected to the vagina by two longitudinal rows of fibrovascular tissue, the rectal pillars, which form the posterior parametrium together with the uterosacral and rectovaginal ligaments. Between these parallel structures is the rectovaginal space, which is lined by thickened endopelvic fascia. The anterior layer of this fascia constitutes the rectovaginal septum (Denonvilliers' fascia) that adheres more to the vagina than to the rectum. The posterior layer is the rectal fascia, which can be dissected by the rectum, but injury to the rectum is more likely to occur while dissecting in this plane than if the same is carried out in the rectovaginal space proper. The rectovaginal space has a thin apex as it opens dorsocaudally where adipose tissue lies and permits an easy dissection of the posterior vaginal wall from the anterior middle third of the rectum.

THE OVARIES

The ovaries are macroscopically formed by a pars corticalis (containing the functional parenchyma) and a pars midullaris (containing the vascular and lymphatic in and outflow pathways).

The ovarian surface is not covered by peritoneum (which ends at the meso-ovary at the so-called Farre–Waldeyer line) in order to allow monthly ovulation. Physiologic ovarian vascularization derives from the infundibulopelvic ligament (coming from the aorta on both sides and draining from the so-called plexus pampiniformis in the vena cava on the right side and into the renal vein on the left side). Collateral vascular circles come from the uterine artery via a direct connection or from the utero-ovarian ligament so that if the main ovarian vessels are damaged or interrupted (i.e. during renal transplantation), ovarian flow may completely recover within a 6-month period.

THE FALLOPIAN TUBES

The fallopian tubes are situated within the mesosalpinx, are usually 10–12 cm in length, and are macroscopically divided into four parts: the uterine, the isthmic, the ampullar, and the infundibular. Each tube consists of a mucosa (cylindrical epithelium), a muscularis (internal circular and external longitudinal fibers entangle each other in a spiral manner in order to allow progression of the gametes and zygotes), and a serosa.

THE UTERUS

Physiologic uterus consists of one corpus, one isthmus, and one cervix. Uterine layers consist of a serosa, a muscularis, and a mucosa (the endometrium). The uterine corpus muscles are organized in a subserosal layer (longitudinal and oblique fibers), a supravascular layer (circular fibers), a vascular layer (plexiform fibers surrounding the myometrial vessels), and a submucosal layer (circular fibers).

The endometrium is the most shape-varying and hormone-responsive mucosa in the human body, consisting of a glandular (basal) and a desquamative (superficial) layer.

Anatomic landmarks of the uterus are fundamental for benign and oncologic surgery (**Figure 1.4**).

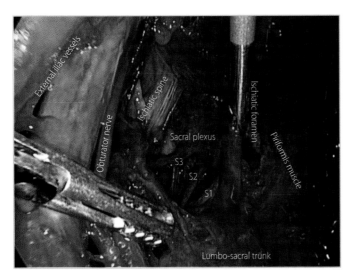

Figure 1.3 Laparoscopic view of the somatic nerves of the pelvis on a fresh cadaver specimen (right hemipelvis). S1–S3= sacral roots 1–3.

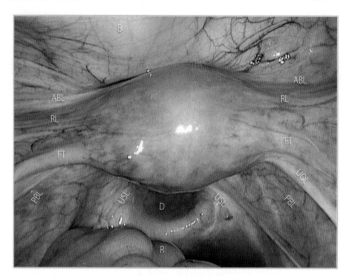

Figure 1.4 In vivo laparoscopic view of the uterus before extrafascial hysterectomy for endometrial cancer. B, Bladder; RL, Round ligament; FT, Fallopian tube; UOL, Utero-ovarian ligament; ABL, Anterior broad ligament; PBL, Posterior broad ligament; USL, Utero-sacral ligament; D, Douglas pouch; R, Rectum

Anteriorly, the vesicouterine septum consists of loose connective tissue separating the supravaginal part of the cervix from the retrotrigonal fossa of the vesical basis. It is laterally limited by the vesicouterine ligaments (or bladder pillars).

The anatomical region situated lateral to the uterus is the so-called parametrium (see below).

Posteriorly, the isthmus and the supravaginal portion of the cervix give rise to the uterosacral ligaments, horizontally marked by a line called torus uterinus. More caudally and dorsally, the rectovaginal septum divides the vagina from the rectum, consists of loose connective tissue, and is laterally limited by the rectovaginal ligament fibers (part of the posterior parametrium).

Uterine ligaments are as follows:

- The round ligaments are essentially composed of myometrial fibers but contain the so-called Samson artery. Their insertion is on the lateral surface of the uterus and directs caudally and laterally through the inguinal channel toward the labia majora
- The vesicouterine ligaments is a peritoneal fold extending from the uterus to the posterior aspect of the bladder
- The uterosacral ligaments are fibrous structures running alongside the lateral surface of the rectum, and directing caudally and dorsally toward the presacral fascia at the level of S2–S4
- The cardinal ligaments (otherwise known as lateral parametrium)
- The rectouterine ligament, which is sometimes referred to as the most distal portion of the uterosacral ligament
- The uterine broad ligament is a double-layered peritoneal lamina classically divided into four parts: mesometrium, mesosalpinx, meso-ovarium, and mesoinfundibulum. It contains in between the two-layer vessels, nerves, embryological remnants, and ligaments

Uterine arteries come from the hypogastric trunk in a variable manner. In 60% of cases, the uterine trunk comes directly from the anterior branch of the internal iliac artery and the obliterated umbilical artery from a separated trunk. In 40% of cases, the uterine artery represents a branch of the umbilical artery itself. More rarely it derives from the obturator artery. It directs medially and caudally, descending at the level of the ischiatic spine, then leading toward the uterus transversally and then ascending along the side of the lateral uterine wall in a typical spiral manner. Once originating as a uterine terminal branch, those arteries ascend in a typical spiral manner in order to allow a 9–10 fold expansion during gestation.

The uterine artery crosses the ureter at about 1.5 cm from the uterine wall. Collateral branches are vesicovaginal (up to five arising laterally to the ureteric cross), ureteric (inconstant), cervicovaginal artery (arising as unique medially to the ureteric cross and dividing into an anterior and a posterior branch), and visceral branches for the cervix and uterine corpus.

Several anastomotic systems might be crossed by the external iliac vessels, internal iliac vessels, aortic circle (i.e. the mesenteric arteries and lumbar vessels) in a complex fashion, so that if one or both uterine arteries is sacrificed during surgical procedures, uterine vascular feeding may completely recover.

Uterine muscle fibers also overgrow during pregnancy and their contraction is not only achieved in labor but also in menstruation and in orgasm itself.

THE PARAMETRIUM

The parametrium is represented by a connective web lying between the PPF and the VPF until the pelvic wall, and containing lymphovascular tissue connecting and draining the pelvic viscera. It is usually divided into lateral, anterior, and posterior parts.

Lateral parametrium

What is commonly termed the 'lateral parametrium' is defined after surgical opening and development of the medial and lateral PVS and PRS (**Figure 1.5**).

It is split into cranial and medial portions and into lateral and caudad portions by the course of the ureter, which, respectively, correspond to the cardinal ligament (or Mackenrodt's ligament) and the paracervix. The cardinal ligament consists of tissue surrounding the uterine artery between the uterine corpus and the pelvic sidewall cranial to the ureter that corresponds to the superficial uterine pedicle (uterine artery and superficial uterine vein) and the related connective and lymphatic tissue. The paracervix consists of a cranial

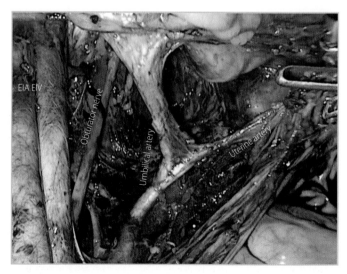

Figure 1.5 Laparoscopic in vivo appearance of the lateral parametrium after systematic pelvic lymphadenectomy, in course of laparoscopic nerve-sparing radical hysterectomy (left hemipelvis). EIA, External iliac artery; EIV, External iliac vein

(anterior, superficial) vascular, connective, and lymphatic aspects and a caudad (posterior, deep) neural component. The deep uterine vein (DUV) is a constant landmark between the two components. Moreover, the structure named by surgeons as the 'paracolpos' or 'paracolpium' is included with the paracervix in the international anatomic nomenclature.

The paracervix may also be divided into two parts: the medial part – a condensation of connective tissue, and the lateral part, which is made of fatty tissue that contains lymph nodes and surrounds vessels and nerves. The most stable anatomical landmark that marks the limit between these two parts is the terminal ureter. Anatomically, the nervous component of the paracervix is the inferior hypogastric plexus that crosses caudally the paracervix. The part of the cardinal ligament that is medial to the ureter is mainly fibrous, whereas the part that is lateral to the ureter is nonfibrous and similar to any area of cellulolymphatic tissue that surrounds nerves and vessels.

Anterior parametrium

This is also termed the 'bladder pillar,' and is defined after surgical opening and development of the vesicouterine septum (vesicocervical and vesicovaginal spaces) and the medial and lateral PVS. The bladder pillar is split into cranial and medial portions and into lateral and caudad portions by the ureter that, respectively, correspond to the vesicouterine ligament and the lateral ligament of the bladder (or the cranial and caudad portions of vesicouterine ligaments).

The anterior parametrium (**Figure 1.6**) is made of fibrous fibers with muscular elements that originate from the lateral parametrium and the lateral border of the cervix.

The portion of anterior parametrium cranial to the ureter corresponds the cranial limit of the so-called ureteral 'tunnel.'

Posterior parametrium

What is commonly called 'posterior parametrium' consists in the joining of three important anatomical structures:
1. The uterosacral ligaments, extending in the cranial proportion of retroperitoneum from the cervicoisthmic dorsal portion of the uterus to the ventral portion of the sacral bone

2. The rectovaginal ligaments, extending in the caudad portion of retroperitoneum from the ventrocaudad portion of the rectum to the dorsal and caudad portion of the vagina, up to the pelvic floor
3. The lateral rectal ligaments (also called rectal stalk, rectal pillars, or 'rectal wings'), extending from the lateral border of the rectum (when mesorectum wraps into the fascia propria recti) to the laterocaudad pelvic wall (from lateral border of S2-S4 segments of sacral bone, to PPF covering the obturator and piriformis muscles). Parasympathetic innervation of pelvic viscera, rectosigmoid, and anal canal is given by the pelvic splanchnic nerves from the anterior rami of sacral roots S2–S4.

THE URINARY BLADDER

The empty bladder is situated in the pelvis, back to the symphysis and the pubis, in front of the uterus and the pelvic diaphragm.

The filled bladder exceeds the pubic symphysis superior border. Fixity structures of the bladder are as follows:
- The vesical fascia covering the vesical fundus (otherwise called the retrovesical fascia and containing the terminal ureter) and the inferolateral surfaces
- The umbilicoprevesical fascia whose superior sheet contains the median umbilical ligament and the umbilical arteries
- The vesical ligaments (the median umbilical ligament, the pubovesical ligaments, the lateral vesical ligaments, the vesicouterine ligaments).
- The bladder has an apex, a base, a superior surface, and two inferolateral surfaces.

The apex of the bladder is directed toward the top of the pubic symphysis; a structure known as the median umbilical ligament (a remnant of the embryologic urachus) directs itself from it up in the anterior abdominal wall to the navel.

The base of the bladder has an inverted triangle shape and faces dorsocaudally. The two ureters enter the bladder through each upper corner of the base, and the urethra drains inferiorly from the lower corner of the base. The triangular area between the openings of the ureters and urethra is known as the trigone.

The inferolateral surfaces of the bladder are cradled between the levator ani muscles and the adjacent obturator internus muscles.

Bladder structure consists of an external tunic (the vesical fascia and the serosa), a median tunic (or the detrusor muscle, with internal longitudinal, median circular, and external longitudinal fibers), and an internal tunic (the urothelium).

Blood supply to the bladder comes from the superior and inferior vesicular arteries, tributaries of the internal iliac arteries.

THE URETER

It represents the upper urinary conduit, from kidney to bladder. It has a median length of 25 cm. Topographically, it is divided into an abdominal part of 12 cm, an iliac part of 3 cm, and a pelvic part of 10 cm in length.

Classically, a lumbar fuse and a pelvic fuse are described in three curves – the iuxta-renal and the pelvic on the frontal plane and the marginal flexure on the sagittal plane.

With regard to the peritoneal covering, we can say that the lumbar and iliac ureter are retroperitoneal, whereas the pelvic ureter may be considered as mid-peritoneal, as it finds its pathway within the PRS (dividing the medial from the lateral peritoneal sheath).

Fixation is guaranteed by a proper mesoureter only in the lumbar region, based on renal pedicle; in the pelvic region fixity is guaranteed only by peritoneum.

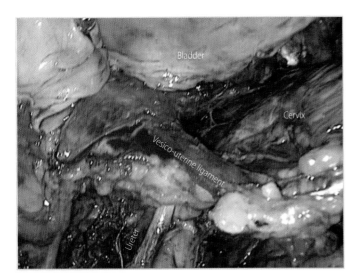

Figure 1.6 Laparoscopic in vivo appearance of the anterior parametrium in course of laparoscopic nerve-sparing radical hysterectomy for cervical cancer (left hemipelvis).

Vascularization of the ureter derives from the long ureteral arteries (originating from the renal arteries and the hypogastric arteries) and the short ureteral arteries (originating from the ovarian arteries).

Innervation to the ureter is given by superior and inferior hypogastric plexa (with prevalence of afferent fibers), where ureteral peristalsis appears, under physiologic conditions, only to be myogenic.

SIGMOID COLON

This is the distal portion of the colon that begins in the iliac fossa lateral to the common iliac vessels and terminates in front of the third sacral vertebra. It is S-shaped and is intraperitoneal, has a variable mobility and length (usually about 40 cm), and is often covered by many appendices epiploicae.

The anatomical distal limit of the sigmoid is generally defined as the sacral promontorium; however, the general area of change from sigmoid colon to rectum is commonly referred to as rectosigmoid.

The mesosigmoid completely surrounds the colon and it does not fix dorsally to the abdominopelvic wall, thus maintaining a relative mobility; at this level, Toldt's fascia is not present. The mesosigmoid contains the inferior mesenteric vessels, the inferior mesenteric plexus, the superior hypogastric plexus, and nerves and lymphatic structures. The opening of the so-called 'mesocolic or mesosigmoid window' represents a fundamental surgical step in course of laparoscopic colorectal surgery.

Features indicating the transition to rectum are (1) the end of the sigmoid mesentery; (2) the cessation of appendices epiploicae and haustra; (3) the coalescence of the teniae that form a complete longitudinal muscular layer; (4) a constriction at the rectosigmoid junction; and (5) the level of division of the superior rectal artery.

The sigmoid colon is supplied by two to four arteries, the first of which is the largest and arises from the left colic (30% of cases) or the inferior mesenteric artery (IMA). As it enters the pelvis, the IMA becomes the superior rectal (hemorrhoidal) artery, which anastomizes caudally with the middle rectal artery, the terminal branch of the hypogastric artery.

RECTUM

This begins at the end of the sigmoid mesentery in front of the third sacral vertebra and extends to the upper limit of the anal canal, the anorectal junction. It measures 10–15 cm in length and is characterized by a proximal ventral curve (sacral flexure), corresponding to the curvature of the sacrum and then to the levator ani.

The rectum is enveloped by part of the endopelvic fascia, the rectal fascia (fascia propria recti) that is continuous with the endopelvic fascia covering the levator ani. The rectum is divided craniocaudally into two levels, the pelvic rectum (peritoneal and subperitoneal) and the perineal rectum or anal canal.

The proximal third of the rectum is intraperitoneal in its anterolateral surface where the peritoneum is continuous with the pararectal fossae. The anterior peritoneal reflection is located at 5–7 cm from the anal margin.

The middle third is covered by the peritoneum anteriorly only, where it is continuous with the peritoneum of the Douglas pouch, and the distal lower third is totally retroperitoneal.

At the level of the pelvic floor and middle third of the vagina (distal third), the rectum forms a 90° angle in a dorsal direction to form the perineal flexure. Thus, it penetrates the pelvic diaphragm and continues caudally into the anus. The perineal rectum corresponds to the surgical anal canal, extended from the anorectal ring to the anal margin. It is surrounded by the levator ani and the anal sphincters and is fixed dorsally to the coccyx by the ligamentum anococcygeum.

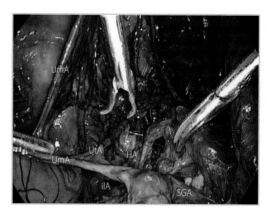

Figure 1.7
Laparoscopic view on a fresh cadaver specimen of the hypogastric vessels' system (right hemipelvis). ilA, Internal iliac artery; SGA, Superior gluteal artery; UmA, Umbilical artery; UtA, Uterine artery; HA, Hypogastric artery.

The mesorectum contains the lymphatics and the division branches of the rectal vessels and nerves; it surrounds the subperitoneal rectum in its dorsal circumference for three fourth and distally, near the levator ani, it becomes thinner at the ends.

The pelvic–subperitoneal space, located among the peritoneum and the pelvic diaphragm, separates the rectum from the lateral pelvic wall and levator ani muscle. This PRS contains the ureters, the hypogastric vessels (**Figure 1.7**) and nervous structures, in relationship with the sacrorectogenitopubic ligaments and the lateral rectal ligaments (the so-called rectal wings).

The middle rectal artery variably originates from the internal iliac artery, umbilical artery, inferior gluteal artery, the lateral sacral artery, or as a branch of the pudendal artery. It has a variable diameter; and extends caudally and medially toward the lateral aspects of the rectum, along the so-called rectal pillars (rectal wings). It ends in two branches; the first (posterior branch) vascularizes the medial portion of the rectum and forms an anastomose with the superior rectal artery; the second (anterior branch with larger diameter) reaches the vagina through the rectovaginal septum.

PELVIC LYMPH NODES

The lymph nodes of the pelvic wall receive lymphatics from the perineum, the lower extremities, the lower abdominal wall, and the pelvic viscera (except the sigmoid). They are covered in a thin layer of endopelvic fascia, which is adherent to the adventitia of the pelvis vessels.

They have been classified into different groups by many authors:

1. External iliac nodes: they are located laterally, superiorly, and medially to the external iliac artery and vein (median number of nodes: 10, range 6–12). They also include the interiliac nodes, located between the artery and the vein. The proximal limit is given by the bifurcation of the common iliac artery, whereas the distal limit is given by the deep iliac circumflex artery at the level of the Cloquet–Rosenmuller's node

2. Obturator nodes: they include all nodes in the obturator fossa. They have been divided into superficial (median number of nodes: 11, range 8–17) or deep obturator nodes (median number of nodes: 4, range 2–8) with respect to the obturator nerve

3. Hypogastric nodes (median number of nodes: 7, range 4–9): they lie around the internal iliac artery and vein, and include the parametrial nodes (along the uterine artery and vein) and the gluteal lymph nodes, lying in the iliolumbar space in the ischiatic region

4. Common iliac nodes: they lie between the pelvic and aortic nodes, around the common iliac vessels. Deep common iliac nodes may be found dorsally to the iliac vessels at the level of the origin of the obturator nerve and lumbosacral trunk. They drain the pelvic wall

lymphatics, although direct channels from the adnexa, uterus, and cervix do exist (median number of nodes: 7, range 5–10)

5. Presacral nodes: they are located on the ventral surface of the sacrum, caudad to the aortic bifurcation and dorsal to the superior mesenteric plexus and to the mesosigmoid (median number of nodes: 3, range 2–5). They may be considered as distal para-aortic nodes or proximal pelvic nodes.

PELVIC VISCERAL NERVES

The superior hypogastric plexus is a triangular-shaped net of sympathetic fibers that lies in the presacral space at the level of the promontorium, covered by a peritoneal sheet and by the anterior layer of the VPF (**Figure 1.8**). It gives origin to the right and left hypogastric nerves, descending for about 8–10 cm along the lateral sides of mesorectum, into the bilayered VPF, following the ureteral course in a dorsal and caudad directions.

To clearly identify the hypogastric nerves' course toward the inferior hypogastric plexus, it is mandatory to access the lower mesorectum, at the level of the rectal wings, bluntly dissecting into the pararectal fossae down along the so-called holy plane of Heald on the midline. Once identified, the posterior and lateral mesorectal fascia are preserved by the division of the filmy areolar tissue in the relatively avascular plane, between the visceral mesorectal fascia and the parietal endopelvic fascia. The middle and distal portions of hypogastric nerves adhere to the mesorectal fascia.

In presacral space, the hypogastric nerves are very variable in thickness (4–7 mm), completely embedded by fatty tissue and sometimes fraying out in multiple thin nervous fibers.

At this level, along their oblique craniocaudad and mediolateral course, the hypogastric nerves are expected to be approximately from 20 to 5 mm below the course of pelvic ureter.

Parasympathetic innervation of the pelvic viscera, rectosigmoid and anal canal, is provided by the pelvic splanchnic nerves (**Figures 1.9** and **1.10**), from the anterior rami of sacral roots S2–S4. At the level of 3–4 and 1–2 cm they are lateral to the pouch of Douglas. Three to five branches of parasympathetic pelvic splanchnic nerves pierce the parietal endopelvic fascial sheet covering the ventral part of piriformis muscle, joining with the ending branches of each sympathetic hypogastric nerve almost 1 cm ventrally, to form the mixed inferior hypogastric plexus, also known as the pelvic plexus. This plexus is bilaterally located in the presacral portion of the visceral endopelvic fascia between the posterior vaginal fornix and the rectum, at the ventral portion of the lateral rectal ligaments.

The DUV is a constant anatomosurgical landmark, commonly used in nerve-sparing radical pelvic surgery to represent the plane dividing the parametrial 'pars vasculosa' (ventrally and cranially) from 'pars nervosa' (dorsally and caudally). Along the course of the DUV, the lateral ligament of the rectum runs close to the pelvic splanchnic nerves in 30% of cases, transverses the pelvic plexus, and then proceeds with the medial efferent bundle of the pelvic plexus up to the lateral or anterolateral surface of the rectum.

Identification of pelvic splanchnic nerves at their origin from the sacral roots may reveal the path of the parasympathetic bundles, leaving their fibers far from the surgical planes of cleavage. In the course of nerve-sparing radical hysterectomy (NSRH) for cervical cancer, following their course, till their joining with the hypogastric nerves, a safer identification of the origin of pelvic plexuses, caudad to the course of DUV, may be rapidly performed, dividing their efferent bundles, sparing the visceral afferent and efferent fibers for the uterus, the vagina and for the bladder.

The distal part of the inferior hypogastric plexus is located in the posterior part of the vesicouterine ligament, lateral and caudad to the lower ureter. To identify and preserve it, during an NSRH, after developing the ureteral tunnel and entering the so-called 'space of Morrow' medially and ventrally to the ureter, the lateral nervous portion and the medial vascular part of the posterior sheath of the vesicouterine ligament must be dissected. Transection of the fascia pubocervicalis, which consists of the cranial and caudad portions of vesicouterine ligament and vesicovaginal ligaments at its parametrial reflection forming ureteral tunnel, is necessarily performed. In such a way, the surgeon gains a safe access to the paravaginal space.

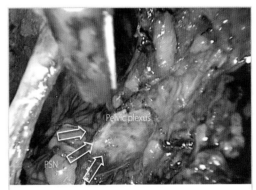
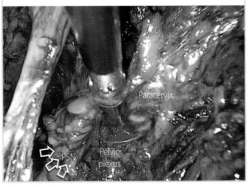

Figure 1.9
Laparoscopic in vivo detail of the pelvic splanchnic nerves (PSN) joining into the pelvic plexus. Preparation obtained in course of laparoscopic nerve-sparing radical hysterectomy for cervical cancer (left hemipelvis).

Figure 1.8 Laparoscopic in vivo isolation of the whole pelvic visceral nerves in course of eradication of deep infiltrating endometriosis with segmental bowel resection. SP, Sacral promontorium; IMP, Inferior mesenteric plexus; SHP, Superior hypogastric plexus; HN, Hypogastric nerves; PSN, Pelvic splanchnic nerves; PP, pelvic plexus; R, Rectum; U, ureter

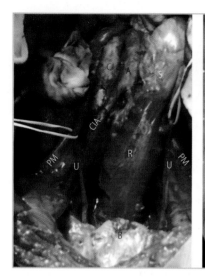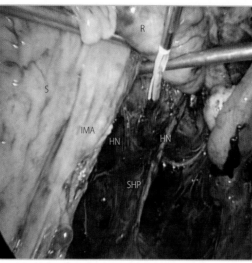

Figure 1.10 Laparotomic (a) and laparoscopic (b) in vivo appearance of the sigmoid and rectum. C, Caval vein; A, Aorta; S, Sigmoid; R, Rectum; PM, Psoas muscle; U, Ureters; B, Bladder; IMA, Inferior mesenteric artery; SHP, superior hypogastric plexus; HN, Hypogastric nerves.

▪ SUGGESTED READING

Ceccaroni M, Clarizia R, Bruni F, et al. Nerve-sparing laparoscopic eradication of deep endometriosis with segmental rectal and parametrial resection: the Negrar method. A single-center, prospective, clinical trial. Surg Endosc 2012; 26:2029–2045.

Ceccaroni M, Clarizia R, Roviglione G, Ruffo G. Neuro-anatomy of the posterior parametrium and surgical considerations for a nerve-sparing approach in radical pelvic surgery. Surg Endosc 2013; 27:4386–4394.

Ceccaroni M, Clarizia R, Roviglione G, et al. Deep rectal and parametrial infiltrating endometriosis with monolateral pudendal nerve involvement: case report and laparoscopic nerve-sparing approach. Eur J Obstet Gynecol Reprod Biol 2010; 153:227–229.

Ceccaroni M, Pontrelli G, Scioscia M, et al. Nerve-sparing laparoscopic radical excision of deep endometriosis with rectal and parametrial resection. J Minim Invasive Gynecol 2010; 17:14–15.

Ceccaroni M, Pontrelli G, Spagnolo E, et al. Parametrial dissection during laparoscopic nerve-sparing radical hysterectomy: a new approach aims to improve patients' postoperative quality of life. Am J Obstet Gynecol 2010; 202:320.

Ceccaroni M, Roviglione G, Spagnolo E, et al. Pelvic dysfunctions and quality of life after nerve-sparing radical hysterectomy: a multicenter comparative study. Anticancer Res 2012; 32:581–588. PubMed PMID: 22287748.

Ercoli A, Delmas V, Fanfani F, et al. Terminologia Anatomica versus unofficial descriptions and nomenclature of the fasciae and ligaments of the female pelvis: a dissection-based comparative study. Am J Obstet Gynecol 2005; 193:1565–1573.

Heald RJ. The 'Holy Plane' of rectal surgery. J R Soc Med 1988; 81:503–508.

Kamina P. Anatomie Clinique. Tome 4°. Paris, Ed Maloine SA, 2008.

Landi S, Ceccaroni M, Perutelli A, et al. Laparoscopic nerve-sparing complete excision of deep endometriosis: is it feasible? Hum Reprod 2006; 21:774–781.

Lang RJ, Davidson ME, Exintaris B. Pyeloureteral motility and ureteral peristalsis: essential role of sensory nerves and endogenous prostaglandins. Exp Physiol 2002; 87:129–146.

Morrow CP, Curtin JP. Gynecologic cancer surgery. London: Churchill-Livingstone Inc., 1996.

Panici PB, Scambia G, Baiocchi G, et al. Anatomical study of para-aortic and pelvic lymph nodes in gynecologic malignancies. Obstet Gynecol 1992;79:498–502.

Querleu D, Morrow CP. Classification of radical hysterectomy. Lancet Oncol 2008; 9:297–303. Review.

Testut L. Traitè d'Anatomie Humaine. Ed Doin, 8th edn, Paris, France, 1931.

Yabuki Y, Asamoto A, Hoshiba T, et al. Dissection of the cardinal ligament in radical hysterectomy for cervical cancer with emphasis on the lateral ligament. Am J Obstet Gynecol 1991; 164:7–14.

Yabuki Y, Asamoto A, Hoshiba T, et al. Radical hysterectomy: an anatomical evaluation of parametrial dissection. Gynecol Oncol 2000; 77:155–163.

Chapter 2 Exposure in laparoscopic surgery

Rodrigo Fernandes, Carolina Meza, Jesús Castellano Moros, Arnaud Wattiez

■ INTRODUCTION

In the past few decades the use of laparoscopic surgery has grown exponentially. During this time, smaller scars with faster and improved recovery time have turned laparoscopy into the gold standard approach for use in both gynecological procedures and other surgical specialties. Today, we know that one of the greatest benefits of laparoscopic surgery is image magnification, which has increased both the knowledge of anatomy and our understanding of different disease processes (Pierre et al. 2009). With the development of high-resolution cameras, the ability to differentiate structures previously unseen during surgery has been realized. Furthermore, with the introduction of 3D technology, depth perception is now possible (Storz, et al. 2012, Tanagho et al. 2012).

As minimally invasive techniques and instruments have evolved so, too, has the surgeon's ability, allowing for more complex procedures to be performed laparoscopically. These types of surgeries are associated with a higher morbidity rate, although this may be related to the surgeon's inexperience. If a specific strategy is adhered to, it can simplify the procedure and potentially minimize complications. The assimilation of these simple gestures into surgical procedure can be called exposure. Exposure in laparoscopy is obtained through a combination of steps that maintain the surgical field while freeing up the assistant. The requirements of these individual steps can vary and should be tailored accordingly. They can be divided into preoperative and intraoperative exposure techniques.

■ PREOPERATIVE EXPOSURE TECHNIQUES

■ Bowel preparation

The debate regarding preoperative bowel preparation and its effect on postoperative morbidity is ongoing. Mechanical bowel preparation prior to colorectal surgical procedures has long been an ingrained practice among surgeons. The rationale for evacuation of fecal content was that it lowered the risk of contamination of the abdominal cavity, thus resulting in fewer infectious complications following surgery (Hughes 1972). This has been challenged in the medical literature, and, in a Cochrane Review with 4599 patients, it was demonstrated that in patients who did not undergo bowel preparation there was no difference in rates of anastomotic leakage, mortality, peritonitis, reoperation, or wound infection (Guenaga et al. 2011). Most of the papers included in the review were related to open surgery; only a few were related to laparoscopy (Bucher et al. 2005, Bretagnol et al. 2010, Moral et al. 2009). These authors suggested that the effect of gravity on fecal matter within the bowel may provide a better surgical overview.

Principles of dissection should be respected, and the surgeon should search for embryological spaces existing between structures so as to maintain an avascular plane. In laparoscopy, the surgeon is often obliged to work with small, delicate instruments, and specific traction and countertraction movements are adopted to facilitate precise dissection. A bowel void of fecal and gaseous content is easier to handle and place above the promontory, free of the pelvis, thereby improving surgical access and exposure. For low-complexity procedures, a low-residue diet between 5 and 7 days preoperatively is sufficient. In deep endometriosis, where bowel surgery may be necessary, we recommend an enema the night before the surgery (Wattiez et al. 2013), whereas colorectal surgeons suggest an additional enema 2–3 hours prior to surgery. When a segmental resection is performed, the proximal segment of the transected bowel usually needs to receive the anvil in order to anastomose the distal segment of the transected bowel using a circular stapler. This can be performed by enlarging one of the port sites or performing a mini laparotomy using a 5 cm Pfannenstiel incision (Wattiez et al. 2013). In the past few years, a novel concept called natural orifice specimen extraction (NOSE) was introduced that enabled colorectal surgeons to reduce the risk of hernias, infection, and pain while improving aesthetic results (Diana et al. 2011, Palanivelu et al. 2008). Using this technique, the specimen is extracted through the anus or vaginally, in cases where a posterior culdotomy is performed due to endometriotic infiltration.

■ INTRAOPERATIVE EXPOSURE TECHNIQUES

■ Exposure strategy

Independent of the complexity of the surgery, the formulation of a surgical strategy remains an important step and should always be observed. Not all exposure techniques need to be adopted during surgery; however, they should be carefully selected because they will influence and will be influenced by the surgical strategy.

Exposure strategy begins with patient positioning, Trendelenburg positioning, and tailored placement of the trocars, all of which can have a significant influence on the surgical procedure. Patient positioning can contribute to an adequate intraoperative exposure. For example, positioning the arms alongside the body will allow the surgeon to move freely and contribute to his or her own ergonomy. Also, positioning the bottom of the pelvis 4 cm away from the table will increase uterine manipulator movements and pelvic structure exposure.

Depending on the case, trocars can be rearranged to give the surgeon better access. Following placement of the 10 mm umbilical trocar and visualization of both the upper and lower abdomen, the patient is placed in Trendelenburg and three additional 5 mm trocars are placed in the lower abdomen, two in the right and left iliac fossas in a range no greater than 2 cm from the anterior iliac spines and a third toward the midline. It is of significant importance for the ergonomy of the surgeon that the middle trocar is at the same level as the lateral trocars or slightly above it, respecting the 8 cm distance from the optical trocar (Wattiez et al. 2013). With this arrangement of trocars the surgeon benefits from an ergonomic positioning with access to the entire pelvis and lower abdomen. Once inside the abdominal cavity, after confirmation that no entry complications have occurred, it is important to gather information and perform a thorough inspection of the abdominal cavity.

Abdominal inspection

The first assessment of the pelvis should include a systematic and detailed anatomical survey. At this point, any kind of surgical act without a correct recognition of the operating field can lead to inadequate dissection, bleeding, and increased rates of complications (Chapron et al. 1998). High-complexity cases like deep endometriosis and patients with numerous previous surgeries usually present with scattered implants, adhesions, and distorted anatomy that requires careful recognition of organs and structures (Chapron et al. 2003).

The inspection should start by ruling out upper abdominal adhesions or endometriotic implants that may explain patient symptoms (Ceccaroni et al. 2013). Looking toward the pelvis, the assessment begins with recognition of the bladder, uterus, adnexa, and bowel, and subsequent structures that allow for identification of important landmarks for dissection. In cases of adhesions, the bowel is often attached to the uterus and left adnexa. The Trendelenburg sequence is used at this time to displace the cecum and small bowel from the pelvis. It is of utmost importance that any kind of dissection in cases where the anatomy is distorted should commence where the tissues and organs are normal and not obscured by disease.

The Trendelenburg sequence

Friedrich Trendelenburg revived a Middle Age habit by placing his patients in lithotomy position. The elevation of the pelvis he described was later assigned his name in 1988 by Mendes de Leon in a publication of pelvic laparotomies and gynecological examination (Cassidy et al. 2014). Trendelenburg defended his eponymous position because it provided better access to intravesical and intraperitoneal procedures mainly by diminishing the local blood supply and also by increasing exposure.

When associated with the Trendelenburg position, the pneumoperitoneum, which makes laparoscopic procedures possible, can lead to cardiorespiratory parameter changes. Findings include decrease in the functional residual capacity and respiratory compliance, increase in respiratory resistance, impairment of arterial oxygenation and increase in dead space (Andersson et al. 2005, Chui et al. 1993, Soro et al. 1997). In a prospective study with 22 patients who underwent laparoscopy for gynecological purposes, the Trendelenburg position was maintained at between 30 and 50° and a pneumoperitoneum pressure of between 12 and 15 mmHg. These changes contributed to a reduction of 44.4% in the compliance of the respiratory system and an increase in expiratory airway resistances of 29.1% (Llorens et al. 2009).

Gasless and low-pressure techniques have been described; however, it has been reported that they can decrease surgical exposure and, as such, should be avoided in high-complexity cases. For ideal exposure during comprehensive laparoscopic surgery of the pelvic floor laparoscopies require the pneumoperitoneum to expand the working area and the Trendelenburg position to free the pelvis from the cecum and small bowel. For cardiorespiratory purposes, a combination of both maneuvers should, at a minimum, always be attempted and a specific sequence should be followed. Attention should be paid

to the patient's position throughout the procedure, because of the risk that the patient may slide upward with increased Trendelenburg angles. Shoulder pieces placed at the beginning of the procedure can prevent this.

With 15 mmHg of pressure and a 30° Trendelenburg, the surgeon manipulates the bowel beginning with the cecum through to the last ileal loop with a well-coordinated sequence of repeated movements. At this point, adhesions that limit the mobility of the colon and small bowel should be removed. Once the bowel is reclined out of the pelvis, the pressure is reduced to 12 mmHg. The last step involves the reduction of the Trendelenburg angle and should be performed with direct vision of the promontory and the pelvic brim; angle reduction should stop just before the bowel starts to descend toward the pelvis.

Uterine manipulation

The pelvis contains numerous structures. Ligaments, vessels, and nerves surround the uterus, bladder, and bowel in a concentric pattern. Unlike the bladder and bowel, the uterus lies in a central position in the pelvis and has a thick wall, making it the perfect pelvic organ for manipulation.

There are numerous types of uterine manipulators on the market, each with differing properties and characteristics. Whether it is for simple procedures or extensive endometriosis cases, there are numerous examples where the uterine manipulator can be useful. The correct exposure of the surfaces and spaces surrounding the uterus during laparoscopic hysterectomy can reduce operating time and minimize complications, especially in cases of an enlarged uterus, adhesions, and deep endometriosis (David-Montefiore et al. 2007). With the uterine manipulator correctly in place, a second assistant standing between the legs of the patient plays a key role during the surgery by moving the uterus in a three-dimensional axis within the pelvis, thus allowing exposure of all important structures (Nakamura et al. 2013).

Moving the uterus posteriorly provides access to the anterior compartment, where both paravesical spaces are found laterally, and the bladder, Retzius space, and anterior uterine wall are found centrally. By placing the uterus anteriorly, the surgeon exposes the posterior compartment, thus making accessible both pararectal fossas laterally, the sigmoid, rectum, and vagina, as well as the rectovaginal space and the posterior wall of the uterus. Lateralization of the uterus allows access to the lateral uterine wall and the adnexa, and to both paravesical and pararectal fossas with all the structures that lie beneath the peritoneum: ureters, vessels, nerves, and nodes.

In addition to the anterior, posterior, and lateral displacement of the uterus, a fourth possibility is craniocaudal movement. Extremely useful, the cranial displacement of the uterus should always be applied in combination with other movements prior to any lateral or anteroposterior movement. Particularly, this maneuver increases the distance between the ureters and the uterine arteries, thus diminishing the risk of ureteral injuries when performing laparoscopic hysterectomies. All these specific movements should be performed in combination and not alone.

The use of uterine manipulation in oncological cases has been extensively discussed (Lee et al. 2013). It is well known that for detailed and precise dissection during nerve-sparing procedures, exposure of the paravesical and pararectal fossas is of particular importance, and, in these instances, the uterine manipulator plays a key role. Some authors warn that the use of the uterine manipulator could increase the risk of introducing malignant cells into the abdominal cavity. In response, some companies have recently developed blunt-tipped manipulators with a backstop security device that diminishes the risk of perforation. Some experts recommend the coagulation of both tubes prior to the placement of this type of uterine manipulator.

The detachment of the sigmoid

The division of the sigmoid from the lateral wall (**Figure 2.1**) allows mobilization of the bowel and access to the left ureter, iliac vessels, infundibulopelvic ligament, and the beginning of the pararectal fossa (**Figure 2.2**). For optimal dissection, the sigmoid at the level of the left pelvic brim must be retracted at a 90° angle away from the pelvic sidewall using an atraumatic forceps. This maneuver reveals a smooth white line that represents the cleavage plane between the peritoneal fold of the sidewall and the sigmoid, the meso-sigmoid peritoneum. The peritoneum should be divided immediately medial to this line using cold scissors, traction, and countertraction while maintaining hemostasis when necessary. These actions will unfold the sigmoid from the pelvic sidewall, revealing the iliac vessels, ureter, and infundibulopelvic ligament on the left pelvic brim. By using the same divergent forces medial to the ureter, an avascular space with a bubbly champagne appearance caused by CO_2 is identified, revealing the entrance to the pararectal fossa.

Ovarian suspension

Ovarian suspension was reportedly first performed by laparotomy in 1970, in a patient receiving radiotherapy for Hodgkin's disease (Ray et al. 1970). The advent of laparoscopic surgery brought about the possibility of ovarian transposition using a minimally invasive approach. Several reports have described laparoscopic oophoropexy as a means of protecting the ovaries from subsequent pelvic irradiation in oncological cases (Tulandi & Al-Took 1998).

Similar techniques have been advocated to reduce postoperative adhesions, as observed by Abuzeid et al. (2002) when they found that temporary suspension of the ovaries for 4–7 days could accomplish this goal. The anatomical position of the adnexa frequently hides access to the pelvic sidewall (Chapman et al. 2007). During deep endometriosis cases, during which the peritoneum of the ovarian fossa is often compromised, a careful retroperitoneal dissection should be performed to identify the path of the ureter and determine whether it is involved by the disease (Cutner et al. 2004). To overcome these difficulties, bilateral suspension of the ovaries permits an optimal exposure of the ovarian fossa (Wattiez et al. 2013).

The technique involves a grasper, which is introduced from the same side on which the ovarian suspension is to be performed. A straight needle on 2-0 polypropylene is inserted perpendicular to the skin and under direct vision lateral to the obliterated umbilical ligament. The inferior epigastric vessels are visualized and avoided. A needle holder is introduced from the port on the contralateral side and grasps the straight needle. The ovary is presented to the straight needle by the grasper on the same side. The needle is the passed through the center of the ovary and is picked up again by the needle holder. Then the needle changes direction, 180° toward the skin, and exits close to the site of insertion. The needle is cut, and the suture is tied to the abdominal wall to enable exposure. Abuzeid et al.'s conclusion was that the technique normally takes less than 5 minutes to be completed on both sides, and, once performed, results in considerable overall time saving during the remainder of the surgery. No injuries were encountered using this method, and anatomy was restored at the end of the procedure. Abuzeid et al. caution that long needle manipulation can be difficult and sometimes dangerous inside the abdomen.

One important advantage of this technique is the possibility of leaving the thread loose on the abdominal wall instead of locking the suspension with a knot. The thread is clamped with forceps over a gauze at the level of the puncture sites thus allowing the surgeon to change the tension on the ovary and thus its position inside the abdomen by simply pulling or releasing the monofilament thread, which allows it to slide smoothly through the tissue.

In 2007, Chapman described a new technique, performed intra-abdominally, with an extracorporeal knot. He used a 75 cm, 2/0 polyglactin suture with a curved needle passing through both ovaries and taking deep bites of the ovarian tissue. Then, with the uterus placed posteriorly, a Roeder knot was performed, positioning both ovaries at the midline over the anterior surface of the uterus. After the procedure, the knot was released and the ovaries returned to their anatomical position. One caveat for this technique is that it can slightly displace the position of the ureters along the pelvic sidewall, so the ureters must be traced before surgery.

Chapman concluded that this maneuver adds only a few minutes to the total operating time, and the view of the pelvic sidewall was judged to be excellent. It was noticed that bleeding at the suture site after removal of the ovarian sutures was minimal. A variation of this technique explores the possibility of attaching the ovaries to the round ligaments, taking care to avoid the vessels of the infundibulopelvic and broad ligament. By performing an intracorporeal single stitch that passes through the ovarian tissue and then through the round ligament bilaterally, both adnexa will remain fixed and will accompany the movement of the uterus. The selection of absorbable suturing materials can also allow the suspension to be left in place at the end of the surgery. This may permit the inflamed dissected area to heal just before the suture is reabsorbed and the adnexus returns to its anatomical position, thus reducing the risk of adhesions. To achieve

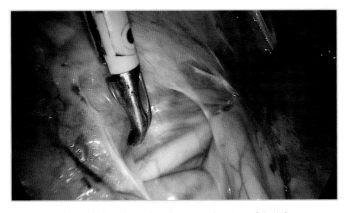

Figure 2.1 Sigmoid physiologic detachment with a view of the left ureter.

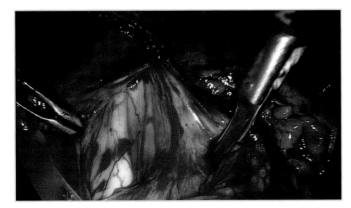

Figure 2.2 View of the ureter at the left pelvic brim and the entrance of the left pararectal fossa medially.

this objective, the use of a monofilament (poliglecaprone 25) 4-0 that will lose 70% of its strength in 2 weeks is recommended to allow time for the ovarian and peritoneal tissues to heal without direct contact between them.

Any laparoscopic surgeon who treats endometriosis appreciates that it is often awkward to operate on the pelvic sidewalls because of the position of the adnexa. The ability to temporarily elevate the adnexa without having to rely on continuous instrumentation offers obvious benefits.

Under the same principle as that described by Cutner et al. (2004), a suspension device was developed to achieve ovarian suspension without having to maneuver straight needles inside the abdomen (**Figure 2.3**). This device consists of a T-shaped insert in a metallic cutting tip sheath and a lock system. The sheath, loaded with a bent T-shape, passes through the abdominal wall and the ovary to be suspended, being careful not to go through the hilum. The plastic device is then pushed inside until its arms open up in a T shape configuration and its body can be grasped. At this point, the inserter is retrieved, the device is adjusted either to a T or J shape, and it is gradually pulled, bringing the adnexa away from the posterior pelvis. Before external locking is performed, variable exposure can be applied according to the needs of the case. At the end of the surgery, the T-shaped device can be cut and removed in two pieces or grasped by the thick arm of the T and pulled out completely (Wattiez et al. 2014). The proposed unpublished advantages of this device are that it is safe, user-friendly, and time-saving with no reported major complications.

Bowel suspension

In certain situations, such as pelvic organ prolapse, deep endometriosis cases, and in obese patients, the position of the bowel may prevent the surgeon from performing an optimal procedure. Suturing techniques or suspension devices can be used to temporarily attach the bowel to the abdominal wall, thus exposing the operating field, giving it a steady position, and keeping the surgeon's assistant free and active for the most important steps. This suspension can be performed by means of straight needle sutures or suspension devices. The place of fixation on the anterior wall should be well-studied and planned in advance by the surgeon. This step is of utmost importance to the surgery because distinct spots of attachment can result in different exposure angles in which centimeters can sometimes make a great difference. The best places of anchorage for suspending the bowel are the epiploical appendices, of which more than one can be used for optimal suspension. The bowel should be displaced by the surgeon or the assistant until the

place of attachment on the anterior wall is selected. Maintaining this position, the optic centers the view on the desired area of dissection to inspect if that point of attachment permits good exposure.

Suspension with straight needles can be challenging. Maneuvering a long straight needle inside the peritoneal cavity can be dangerous and should be performed with care. The needle is introduced through the abdominal wall at the chosen point. The surgeon passes the needle through the epiploical appendices and targets the exit point. At this moment, the assistant moves the bowel along with the suspension to diminish tension and the chance of breaking the attachment.

Fixations with specific suspension devices were introduced a few years ago and spare the surgeon from using straight needles inside the pelvis. The T shape of the plastic device is bent and introduced into the inserter. It is introduced through the epiploical appendices, at which point the surgeon pushes the plastic device forward, making the folded-down T open. For the same reasons explained earlier, the assistant moves the bowel toward the wall while the surgeon pulls the device and fixes it.

Colposacropexy procedures require dissection of the right border of the promontory, continuing medially to the right ureter towards both pararectal fossas. This is one of the most important and delicate steps, where the surgeon deals with the bifurcation of the iliac and the sacral vessels. The combined action of both surgeon and assistant to lift the peritoneum decreases the risk of damaging these vessels and helps to respect the optimal depth of dissection. For a good exposure of this area the sigmoid must be fixed laterally toward the left anterior wall, close to Palmer's point (**Figure 2.4**). Following the same principles, the assistant is also required to help by exposing the right ovarian fossa and the dissection of the puborectalis muscle (Gabriel et al. 2011). At the end of the procedure, peritoneal closure over the dissected area must be performed to cover the mesh. Bimanual coordination of the surgeon facilitated by the exposure of the field and maneuvering of the thread by the assistant are essential to a good hermetic suturing procedure.

Deep endometriosis procedures often require coordinated work between assistant and surgeon. Cases in which bowel attachment to the anterior wall is performed are not common but can be done depending on the judgment of the team. If necessary, the bowel should be attached higher than the optic trocar and closer to the midline, thus permitting both the left and right ovarian and pararectal fossas to be accessed.

The greater abdominal pressure and the higher quantity of fatty tissue in obese patients create a complicated environment. The angle of Trendelenburg positioning is limited due to the risk of cardiovascular problems during anesthesia. Therefore, the small bowel and

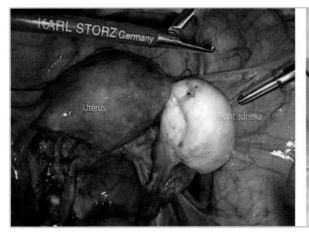
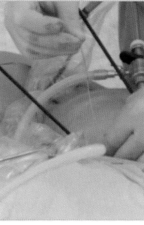

Figure 2.3 Ovarian suspension with exposure of the posterior aspect of the pelvis and ovarian fossa.

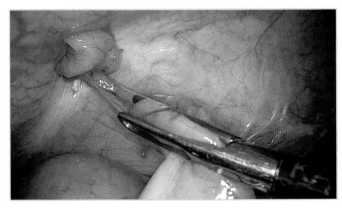

Figure 2.4 Bowel suspension with attachment to the upper left quadrant of the abdominal wall for a colposacropexy procedure.

the sigmoid colon can frequently interfere in the pelvis, impairing the view and the dissection field and sometimes being the reason for conversion (Walker et al. 2009). The use of suspension techniques sigmoid on the sigmoid and maneuvers to pack the small bowel can keep these structures in the upper abdomen.

Cervical suspension

Laparoscopic colposacropexy is the standard technique for pelvic organ prolapse (POP) repair (Gabriel et al. 2011). Vaginal erosion is one of the most frequent complications after POP repair procedures (Deffieux et al. 2012). The literature suggests that to avoid this kind of complication, surgeons should perform supracervical hysterectomy on patients undergoing colposacropexy (Barber et al. 2009). In some cases, access to the rectovaginal space can be challenging to obtain, and the surgeon may need time for careful dissection. At this point, cervical suspension can be performed by a suture exteriorized at the level of the suprapubic region using a thread recovery device, thus exposing the site and facilitating dissection of the posterior compartment while allowing the assistant to be more efficient during the main surgical steps (**Figure 2.5**). In addition, because the cervix has to be closed by a suture placed laparoscopically, this suture can also be used as a temporary cervical suspension with the aim of easing the placement of the posterior mesh.

Uterine suspension

In cases contraindicatory to the use of uterine manipulation, as in virginal patients or when the manipulator is unable to offer optimal anterior displacement, uterine suspension can be helpful to improve exposure of the posterior compartment of the pelvis (**Figure 2.6**). This procedure allows better dissection of the rectovaginal space during deep endometriosis or prolapse surgeries, provides access to posterior wall myomas and facilitates various suturing techniques. The technique consists of introducing a straight needle suture through the pelvic abdominal wall right above the pubis, attaching it at the fundus of the uterus and returning it to the anterior wall. It is suggested that the thread not be knotted, thus allowing for the suspension to be adjusted at any time. A second option uses suspension by the round ligaments by means of straight needles or suspension devices.

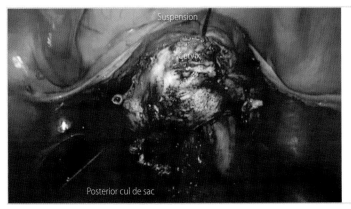
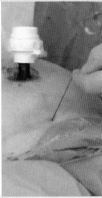

Figure 2.5 Cervix suspension to the anterior abdominal wall exposing the posterior compartment of the pelvis.

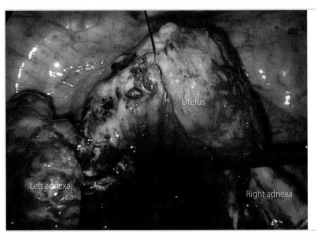
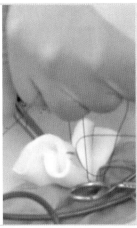

Figure 2.6 Uterine suspension to the anterior abdominal wall by means of a thread.

Peritoneal suspension

Laparoscopic oncologic procedures such as lumboaortic lymphadenectomy often put the surgeon close to delicate structures and vital areas. Depending on the indication, the surgeon needs access to the retroperitoneum from the pelvic brim up to the level of the left renal vein (Medeiros et al. 2013). Both the small bowel and the colon can impair the surgeon's vision; therefore, suspension techniques for exposure are extremely important.

The aim of suspension in this case is to expose the aorta, vena cava, and surrounding retroperitoneal structures that maintain the bowel cranially and laterally. Walker et al. (2009) described lack of exposure as one of the main factors contributing to conversion when performing pelvic or para-aortic lymphadenectomy. The peritoneum is lifted and incised in a longitudinal aspect. By means of suspension devices or sutures with straight needle, the peritoneum is temporarily attached in more than one spot on each side, allowing an adequate view of the retroperitoneal space and producing almost a barrier or natural retractor (**Figure 2.7**). In this way, the surgeon is free to focus on the careful dissection technique required during this procedure, and the assistant is completely active when needed (Kumar et al. 2014).

NOSE procedures

NOSE procedures were first described in 1991, when David Redwine performed a transanal specimen extraction for bowel endometriosis (Redwine & Sharp 1991). In 1993, a fully laparoscopic colectomy with transanal specimen extraction and anvil introduction was performed (Franklin et al. 1993). Following the same principle, similar reports of specimen extractions were also reported via a transvaginal incision (Gill et al. 2002).

The benefits of the NOSE procedure, apart from the lower rate of pain, surgical site infection, and incisional hernia, include the aesthetic aspect because the patient is spared from an enlargement of a lateral port or an abdominal incision. This technique not only requires that both the vagina and rectum remain open to receive the specimen but also that a precise combination of organ manipulation and logistics inside the pelvis be undertaken between the surgeon and the assistant. At this point, a suture or a suspension device can be used to keep organs open, leaving the assistant free to help the surgeon (**Figure 2.8**). This type of exposure is more often applied in transanal NOSE procedures but can also be used when transvaginal specimen extractions are performed.

PERIOPERATIVE INSPECTION

Structures and organ suspension are extremely helpful but should be performed with care. After their removal, all sites where suspension needles or devices were placed should be carefully inspected for bleeding, which can lead to postoperative intra-abdominal hematoma.

CONCLUSION

Laparoscopic surgery contributes not only to better recovery and more aesthetic-looking scars but also allows the surgeon to see better and more clearly, which changes the way we face and deal with

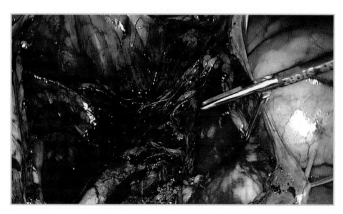

Figure 2.7 Abdominal retroperitoneum and exposure of para-aortic spaces by means of suspender devices.

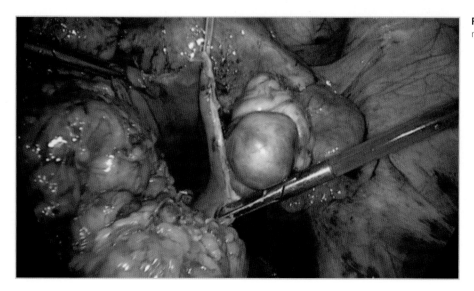

Figure 2.8 Suspender device maintaining the rectum open for specimen extraction.

the human anatomy. The limitation of working in small spaces and dealing with complicated situations obliges the surgeon to use his or her creativity to develop skills and to apply specific strategies for all surgeries. Exposure is a key factor to the success of laparoscopic procedures, whether they are simple or complex. There is no clear evidence published in the literature proving that exposure methods can improve operative time or bring safety and quality to the procedure. Numerous exposure acts can be performed during a single surgery, but not all are necessary. This is why the strategy of exposure should be tailored to the strategy of the surgery in order to to profit most from it.

REFERENCES

Abuzeid MI, Ashraf M, Shamma FN. Temporary ovarian suspension at laparoscopy for prevention of adhesions. J Am Assoc Gynecol Laparosc 2002; 9:98–102.

Andersson LE, Bååth M, Thörne A, Aspelin P, Odeberg-Wernerman S. Effect of carbon dioxide pneumoperitoneum on development of atelectasis during anesthesia, examined by spiral computed tomography. Anesthesiology 2005; 102:293–299.

Barber MD, Brubaker L, Nygaard I, et al. Defining success after surgery for pelvic organ prolapse. Obstet Gynecol 2009; 114:600–609.

Bretagnol F, Panis Y, Rullier E, et al. Rectal cancer surgery with or without bowel preparation: the French GRECCAR III multicenter single-blinded randomized trial. Ann Surg 2010; 252:863–868.

Bucher P, Gervaz P, Soravia C, et al. Randomized clinical trial of mechanical bowel preparation versus no preparation before elective left-sided colorectal surgery. Br J Surg 2005; 92:409–414.

Cassidy L, Bandela S, Wooten C, et al. Friedrich Trendelenburg: historical background and significant medical contributions. Clin Anat 2014; 27:815–820.

Ceccaroni M, Roviglione G, Giampaolino P, et al. Laparoscopic surgical treatment of diaphragmatic endometriosis: a 7-year single-institution retrospective review. Surg Endosc 2013; 27:625–632.

Chapman L, Shama M, Papalampros P, et al. A new technique for temporary ovarian suspension. Am J Obstet Gynecol 2007; 196:494.e1–494.e3.

Chapron C, Fauconnier A, Vieira M, et al. Anatomical distribution of deeply infiltrating endometriosis: surgical implications and proposition for a classification. Hum Reprod 2003; 18:157–161.

Chapron C, Querleu D, Bruhat MA, et al. Surgical complications of diagnostic and operative gynaecological laparoscopy: a series of 29,966 cases. Hum Reprod 1998; 13:867–872.

Chui PT, Gin T, Oh TE. Anaesthesia for laparoscopic general surgery. Anaesth Intensive Care. 1993; 21:163–171.

Cutner A, Lazanakis M, Saridogan E. Laparoscopic ovarian suspension to facilitate surgery for advanced endometriosis. Fertil Steril 2004; 82:702–704.

David-Montefiore E, Rouzier R, Chapron C, Darai E (Collegiale d'Obstetrique et Gynecologie de Paris-Ile de F). Surgical routes and complications of hysterectomy for benign disorders: a prospective observational study in French university hospitals. Hum Reprod 2007; 22:260–265.

Deffieux X, Letouzey V, Savary D, et al. Prevention of complications related to the use of prosthetic meshes in prolapse surgery: guidelines for clinical practice. Eur J Obstet Gynecol Reprod Biol 2012 ;165:170–180.

Diana M, Perretta S, Wall J, et al. Transvaginal specimen extraction in colorectal surgery: current state of the art. Colorectal Dis 2011; 13:e104–111.

Franklin ME Jr, Ramos R, Rosenthal D, Schuessler W. Laparoscopic colonic procedures. World J Surg 1993; 17:51–56.

Gabriel B, Nassif J, Barata S, Wattiez A. Twenty years of laparoscopic sacrocolpopexy: where are we now? Int Urogynecol J 2011 ;22:1165–1169.

Gill IS, Cherullo EE, Meraney AM, et al. Vaginal extraction of the intact specimen following laparoscopic radical nephrectomy. J Urol. 2002; 167:238–241.

Guenaga KF, Matos D, Wille-Jorgensen P. Mechanical bowel preparation for elective colorectal surgery. Cochrane Database Syst Rev 2011:CD001544.

Hughes ESR. Asepsis in large-bowel surgery. Ann R Coll Surg Engl 1972; 51:347–356.

Kumar S, Podratz KC, Bakkum-Gamez JN, et al. Prospective assessment of the prevalence of pelvic, paraaortic and high paraaortic lymph node metastasis in endometrial cancer. Gynecol Oncol 2014 ;132:38–43.

Lee M, Kim YT, Kim SW, et al. Effects of uterine manipulation on surgical outcomes in laparoscopic management of endometrial cancer. Int J Gynecol Cancer 2013 ;23:372–379.

Lloréns J, Ballester M, Tusman G, et al. Adaptive support ventilation for gynaecological laparoscopic surgery in Trendelenburg position: bringing ICU modes of mechanical ventilation to the operating room. Eur J Anaesthesiol 2009 ;26:135–139.

Medeiros L, Rosa DD, Bozzetti MC. Laparoscopy versus laparotomy for FIGO stage I ovarian cancer. Cochrane Database Syst Rev 2008; CD005344.

Moral MA, Aracil XS, Juncá JB, et al. A prospective, randomised, controlled study on the need to mechanically prepare the colon in scheduled colorectal surgery [Estudio prospectivo controlado y aleatorizado sobre la necesidad de la preparación mecánica de colon en la cirugía programada colorrectal]. Cirurgía Española. 2009; 85:20–25.

Nakamura M, Fujii T, Imanishi N, et al. Surgical anatomy imaging associated with cervical cancer treatment: a cadaveric study. Clin Anat 2014; 27:503–510.

Palanivelu C, Rangarajan M, Jategaonkar PA, Anand NV. An innovative technique for colorectal specimen retrieval: a new era of "natural orifice specimen extraction" (N.O.S.E.). Dis Colon Rectum. 2008; 51:1120–1124.

Pierre SA, Ferrandino MN, Simmons WN, et al. High definition laparoscopy: objective assessment of performance characteristics and comparison with standard laparoscopy. J Endourol 2009; 23:523–528.

Ray GR, Trueblood HW, Enright LP, et al. Oophoropexy: a means of preserving ovarian function following pelvic megavoltage radiotherapy for Hodgkin's disease. Radiology 1970; 96:175–180.

Redwine DB, Sharpe DR. Laparoscopic segmental resection of the sigmoid colon for endometriosis. J Laparoendoscop Surg. 1991; 1:217–220. doi: 10.1089/lps.1991.1.217.

Soro M, Cobo R, Paredes I, et al. Changes in lung compliance during laparoscopic surgery using a circular circuit. Rev Esp Anestesiol Reanim. 1997; 44:13.

Storz P, Buess GF, Kunert W, Kirschniak A. 3D HD versus 2D HD: surgical task efficiency in standardised phantom tasks. Surg Endosc 2011; 26:1454–1460.

Tanagho YS, Andriole GL, Paradis AG, et al. 2D versus 3D visualization: impact on laparoscopic proficiency using the fundamentals of laparoscopic surgery skill set. J Laparoendoscop Adv Surg Techn 2012; 22:865–870.

Tulandi T, Al-Took S. Laparoscopic ovarian suspension before irradiation. Fertil Steril 1998; 70:381–383.

Walker, JL, Piedmonte MR, Spirtos NM, et al. Laparoscopy compared with laparotomy for comprehensive surgical staging of uterine cancer: Gynecologic Oncology Group Study LAP2. J Clin Oncol 2009; 27:5331–5336. doi:10.1200/JCO.2009.22.3248.

Wattiez A, Puga M, Albornoz J, Faller E. Surgical strategy in endometriosis. Best Pract Res Clin Obstet Gynaecol 2013; 27:381–392.

Wattiez A, Puga M, Fernandes R, et al. Making the most in exposure: the T-Lift device. Websurg: The e-Surgical Reference. 2014. http://www.websurg.com/MEDIA/?noheader=1&doi=vd01en4118 (Last accessed 02/12/2015).

Chapter 3 Electrosurgery

Craig Sobolewski

HISTORY

The use of electrosurgical instruments is commonplace in most gynecologic abdominal procedures. It is commonly used in many vaginal and operative hysteroscopic procedures. Although it was utilized sparingly by other surgeons in the early part of the twentieth century, it is Dr Harvey Cushing, a Neurosurgeon at Brigham and Women's Hospital in Boston, who is most credited with advancing its eventual widespread acceptance. Dr Cushing was frustrated with the high morbidity associated with hemorrhage during brain tumor resections. Working together with William T. Bovie, a biophysical engineer at Huntington Hospital in Boston, these two men refined the existing electrosurgical system and performed the first successful neurosurgical procedure that utilized electrosurgical technology in 1926. Impressed with its potential, Dr Cushing went on to publish and lecture extensively on the merits of this technology.

Formalized training in the safe and effective use of electrosurgery is lacking in the United States (Feldman et al. 2012). Most hospitals in the United States require documentation of adequate training in order to obtain credentials to permit the use of laser energy, but, in contrast, there is no uniform credentialing process required by hospitals to allow surgeons to operate with devices that apply electrical energy to tissues.

Industry-sponsored events or sales representatives in the hallways outside of the operating rooms provide much of the training around the proper use of new surgical devices. In residency, most education is limited to a trainee mimicking the use of a device after observing a senior resident or attending surgeon utilizing the same instrument. An understanding of the principles of how these electrosurgical instruments interact with tissue is essential to their safe use.

BASIC PRINCIPLES

Radio frequency (RF) electrosurgical instruments are broadly categorized into either monopolar instruments or bipolar instruments. This is an unfortunate historical misnomer since all electrosurgical instruments are 'bipolar' because the electrons have to travel between a positive and a negative pole in order to complete a circuit; hence, there are always two poles (Vilos & Rajakumar 2013). With monopolar instruments, a large portion of the patient becomes part of the circuit. The electrons travel from the electrosurgical generator into a high-power density electrode at the tip of the instrument. A variety of electrical waveforms (both cut and coagulation) can be applied with monopolar instruments. These electrons are discharged in a high concentration into the patient and are distributed throughout the patient until they are ultimately collected at a distant site via a low-power density dispersive electrode (**Figure 3.1**). Another common misnomer in the modern operating room is referring to this second electrode as a 'grounding pad' or 'return electrode.' More appropriately called a 'dispersive electrode,' this large pad is, in fact, another active electrode just like the instrument itself and, if applied incorrectly, can result in tissue damage or burns from the discharge of electrical energy from its surface. Contact quality monitoring was

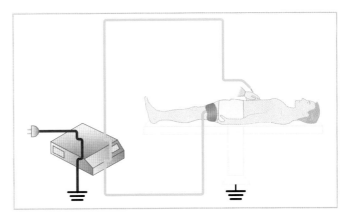

Figure 3.1 A schematic of a circuit created via a monopolar electrosurgical instrument. Note that the current must travel through the patient and return to the generator via a dispersive electrode placed at a location remote from the tip of the instrument.

introduced in the early 1980s in order to minimize this risk. A low-voltage current is passed through the cord attached to specialized dispersive electrode pads that are split down the middle. If a change in voltage or a disruption in this low-voltage current is detected, the primary circuit is shut off rendering the surgical instrument useless until the situation is remedied.

Bipolar instruments consist of two electrodes in close proximity to each other. The only portion of the patient that becomes part of the circuit is the tissue that is held between these two electrodes (**Figure 3.2**). A dispersive electrode is not necessary when using this type of instrument. Bipolar instruments utilize the high-current/low-voltage 'cut' waveform (Vilos & Rajakumar 2013).

These instruments and generators are referred to RF instruments/generators because the electrons that are generated are oscillating between the positive and negative poles at a frequency of >100,000 times per second. Hertz (Hz) is the term utilized to describe cycles per second. The RF portion of the electromagnetic spectrum is between 3 kHz and 300 GHz. Because neuromuscular stimulation does not occur above 100,000 Hz, the patient is not electrocuted and these RF instruments can be used safely during surgical procedures.

Electrosurgical devices create the effect that they have on tissues by generating heat. In fact, all modern surgical energy devices, including ultrasonic energy, laser energy, and plasma energy, work through the creation of heat. With electrosurgery, this heat is generated as the electrons that are flowing through tissue meet up with resistance to that flow. This is referred to as resistive heating (Brill 2011). If high temperatures are generated rapidly, this results in the boiling of the intracellular water. The increased pressure within the cell that subsequently occurs results in the cell wall exploding. As these cells are disrupted, dissection of the tissue occurs. Since the heat dissipates rapidly as steam or plasma, there is very minimal heating of the adjacent tissues.

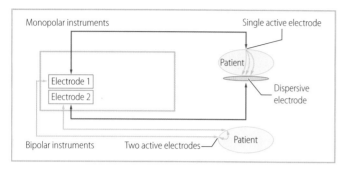

Figure 3.2 A schematic of a circuit created via a bipolar electrosurgical instrument. Note that a dispersive electrode is not necessary since the only portion of the patient that completes the circuit is that tissue between the tines of the instrument itself.

WAVEFORMS

When using monopolar electrosurgical devices, this effect is best achieved with the 'pure cut' waveform. In the pure cut mode, energy is delivered continuously and can be described as a high-current/low-voltage waveform. In contrast, in the 'coagulation mode,' the current is interrupted and, in fact, is only 'on' 6% of the time (Alkatout et al. 2012). This interrupted delivery results in lower tissue temperatures, leading to protein denaturation and the formation of a coagulum. As compared to pure cut current, coagulation current is a low-current/high-voltage form of electrosurgical energy. Voltage is the force that pushes the electrons through the tissue. With higher voltage, the heat that is generated has a greater potential to penetrate the tissue deeply. Therefore, although coagulation current may generate lower tissue temperatures, the higher voltage may result in substantially greater and potentially unrecognized lateral thermal spread (**Figure 3.3**).

It is critically important that the surgeon understands this fundamental difference, especially since the names assigned to these waveforms imply different clinical effects. Although it is true that the word 'cut' sounds potentially more dangerous than the word 'coagulate,' it is quite possible that if the goal is to minimize lateral thermal spread, cut current may be the far safer choice.

The waveform of the current, namely 'cut' or 'coagulation,' is only one of several variables that the surgeon employs in order to achieve the desired clinical effect with electrosurgery (Taheri et al. 2014). Other variables under the control of the surgeon include the shape and size of the electrode, whether the electrode is in direct contact with the tissue or not, and the amount of time the energy is deployed to the tissue. If the electrode has a large surface area, such as a ball shape, the electrons will be distributed over a greater surface area and less heat will be generated than if a needle electrode that highly concentrates electrons at the tip is utilized, for example. Thus, even if the same energy settings were used, such as 25 W of pure cut current, there would be different tissue effects if the surgeon used a ball electrode versus a needle tip. Similarly, in order to most efficiently achieve the cutting or dissection of tissue, the electrode should be held a short distance away from the tissue without direct contact. The cut waveform energy will jump through the short air gap resulting in the delivery of highly concentrated energy bursts. These concentrated bursts of high-current/low-voltage waveform heat the intracellular water rapidly, causing the water to boil, intracellular pressure to increase rapidly, and eventual cell wall disruption resulting in tissue cutting or vaporization. In contrast, placing the electrode in direct contact with the tissue using either the cut or coagulation waveform is described as desiccation. Since the energy does not need to overcome the resistance

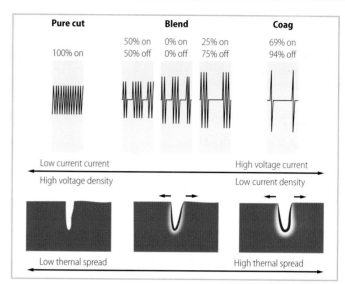

Figure 3.3 Diagram of the variation in waveform between the types of radio frequency current utilized during electrosurgery. As one moves from pure cut, through blend, to pure coagulation current, the amount of time the current is dampened, or 'off', increases. In order to achieve the same power output, the voltage must increase within these dampened currents.

in the air gap between the electrode and the tissue, touching the tissue increases the surface contact area and decreases both the concentration of energy and the rate at which heat is produced. The amount of heat and subsequent thermal effect will differ depending upon the voltage of current used, the shape of electrode, and the amount of time the electrode is in contact with the tissue. Finally, *fulguration* is the technique of using coagulation current in a nontouch fashion to allow this high-voltage current to spark to tissue. Because coagulation current is a dampened current that is 'off' 94% of the time, the sparks are generated intermittently. This allows for brief episodes of cooling in between each burst of energy. This allows for the formation of a coagulum. This technique is useful for achieving hemostasis of large superficial surface areas.

MODERN ADVANCES

As is true with medications, utilizing the lowest 'dose' of electricity over the shortest time that is necessary to achieve one's goal may be the safest way to operate with energized devices. Modern electrosurgical units (ESUs) have evolved into what has been referred to as 'adaptive' generators (Brill 2011). These ESUs are capable of determining the tissue resistance that is encountered by the tip of the electrode and then relaying that information back to the generator. The ESU, in turn, adjusts its internal algorithms in real time to ensure that there are no spikes in voltage and that the power output remains constant over time. This may allow the surgeon to achieve the same clinical effect at the tissue at lower wattage settings or apply the energy for shorter times than required with an older generator that did not have this technology.

In addition to the standard, 'cut,' 'coagulate,' and 'blend' waveforms that surgeons are accustomed to, one ESU manufacturer has utilized this adaptive technology to develop a new waveform. The Valleylab waveform (Covidien, Boulder, Colorado) is created by modulating a coagulation waveform in a way that minimizes the very large voltage spikes that occur with that waveform using the adaptive properties of the ESU. As a result, there is less tissue drag than with pure coagulation current, but improved hemostasis as compared to pure cut current. As a result, surgeons who are accustomed to electrosurgical pencils with only two buttons (yellow for cut and blue for coagulation) now may be exposed to a handheld device with a third button for the application of this new Valleylab waveform.

ELECTROSURGICAL COMPLICATIONS

Surveys have shown that up to 18% of surgeons have experienced a thermal injury complication during laparoscopic surgery (Abu-Rafea et al. 2011, Odell 2013). The fact that a significant portion of the shaft of the typical laparoscopic electrosurgical instrument is not visible on the video monitor creates a potential for unrecognized injury that is unique to laparoscopic procedures. Instrument insulation failure, direct, and capacitive coupling may potentially cause stray energy burns. All of these are more likely to occur with the use of a high-voltage waveform (coagulation current) (Abu-Rafea et al. 2011). A capacitor is created when an insulator (e.g. the coating of the shaft of an instrument) separates two conductors (e.g. the metal conductor inside the shaft and a metal laparoscope). If enough energy is stored within this capacitor, it can discharge spontaneously. In addition to using a high-voltage waveform, excessive 'open-air-activation' can also contribute to this. Open-air-activation refers to activating the button or pedal before the electrode tip is brought near the target tissue, resulting in the accumulation of electrons along the surface of the electrode. This may potentially build up enough energy within the capacitor that it could be spontaneously discharged to surrounding structures, resulting in an injury.

Insulation failure is a more difficult situation to predict and is the most common cause of electrosurgical energy-related thermal injury (Montero et al. 2010). Montero et al. found evidence of an insulation failure in 19% of reusable and 3% of disposable instruments used in cholecystectomy instrument sets at four area hospitals (Montero et al. 2010). A technology referred to as active electrode monitoring (AEM) (Encision Inc., Boulder, Colorado) is designed to detect the occurrence of both insulation failure and capacitive coupling and prevent the consequences of these situations. By integrating a coaxial conductive shield into the shaft of the instrument and running this through the AEM monitor, the system can detect an insulation failure and deactivate the ESU before energy can be delivered (**Figure 3.4**). Although the adaptive properties of modern ESUs have minimized but not eliminated the risk of capacitive coupling by reducing potential high voltage peaks, this is only true in instruments with intact insulation.

In summary, strategies that can help reduce the potential for stray monopolar energy injuries include using low-voltage waveforms (cut current), lower wattage settings, avoiding open-air-activation, and utilizing AEM instrumentation.

In general, bipolar electrosurgical instruments are associated with less risk for unrecognized thermal injuries, but are not completely immune to this possibility. The traditional Kleppinger-style bipolar instrument creates a great deal of lateral thermal spread (Tucker et al. 1992). In fact, that is what the surgeon requires in order to achieve effective tubal desiccation during a laparoscopic sterilization procedure. However, this may be quite undesirable when using such an instrument to control the uterine vasculature when the ureter may be nearby, for example.

MODERN BIPOLAR LAPAROSCOPIC INSTRUMENTS

Dr James Greenwood developed the first bipolar surgical device in 1940. He divided a pair of surgical forceps and attached one side to a monopolar generator and the other side to a ground connector (Vellimarra et al. 2009). The modern generation of bipolar vessel sealer/cutting devices uses the adaptive technology present in today's ESUs to deliver controlled, low-voltage energy with very minimal lateral thermal spread as a result. Currently available advanced bipolar devices on the market in the United States include the PlamaKinetics System (Olympus America, Inc., Center Valley, Pennsylvania), LigaSure (Covidien, Boulder, Colorado), EnSeal (Ethicon Endo-Surgery, Cincinnati, Ohio), and Caiman (Aesculap, Inc., Center Valley, Pennsylvania). Each are approved to seal and cut tissue pedicles up to 7 mm in diameter. All have unique characteristics and many come with different end-effector configurations. All of today's modern bipolar devices offer significant safety advantages over the traditional bipolar instruments of old via more robust tissue seals and substantially less lateral thermal spread.

There have been multiple comparative studies comparing the qualities of several of these advanced electrosurgical instruments against one another. There have been some statistically significant differences seen in blood loss, pain, and operative times, but it is unclear if any of these small differences are clinically relevant. Some animal model ex vivo studies have also shown statistically significant differences in seal time, thermal spread, and particulate smoke creation, but, once again, it is unclear if these differences translate to clinical relevance (Law & Lyons 2013).

ELECTROSURGERY DURING HYSTEROSCOPY

It is possible to use both monopolar and bipolar instrumentations within a fluid environment (Vellimarra et al. 2009). In order for a monopolar instrument to work, a low-viscosity fluid that is electrolyte-free must be utilized. Examples of such fluids include sorbitol, glycine, and mannitol. If the patient absorbs excessive amounts of these high viscosity solutions, serious, even life-threatening complications can occur. Bipolar devices, on the other hand, can be utilized in electrolyte containing solution such as normal saline (Munro 2010). In gynecologic surgery, hysteroscopic resectoscopes that employ either monopolar or bipolar waveform are available. As with open or laparoscopic instruments, capacitive coupling can occur when utilizing a monopolar resectoscope and this can result in injury to the cervix, vagina, or vulva. Munro demonstrated possible mechanisms for this type of injury in an experimental model (Munro 2006). As with abdominal procedures, it is possible that

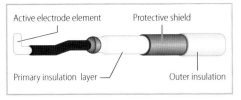

Figure 3.4 A schematic of an active electrode monitored (AEM) device. The shield is dynamically monitored for insulation failure and excessive capacitive coupled current. When a defect is detected, the AEM monitor will shut off the delivery of electrosurgical current protecting the patient from stray energy due to either insulation failure or excessive capacitive coupling. By courtesy of Encision Inc., Boulder, Colorado.

avoiding the use of the high-voltage coagulation waveform may help to lessen the potential risk for capacitance-related injuries during hysteroscopic procedures.

PLASMA ENERGY

The PlasmaJet system (PlasmaSurgical, Roswell, Georgia) is not strictly an electrosurgical device either, but the use of direct current electrical energy is necessary to eventually create the heat needed to treat the tissue. In the case of this system, a beam of argon gas is energized when it passes through a low direct current voltage that is applied between internal bipolar electrodes. This separates the argon gas atoms into positive and negative ions and creates the fourth state of matter known as plasma. The plasma that is created by the PlasmaJet system releases its energy in three ways: light, heat, and kinetic energy. The effect at the tissue level is influenced by how close the jet of ionized gas is held near the tissue, which handpiece is chosen, and which button is pushed on the handpiece. The maximum depth of tissue penetration effect is only 2.0 mm and this is reached after 5 seconds of continuous application.

Ultimately, the safe application of energy-based surgical devices lies in the hand of the surgeon. A sound understanding of the fundamentals of good surgical practice is still of prime importance. Adhering to the standards of careful surgical dissection, appropriate exposure of the surgical field, and a thorough knowledge of anatomy are still necessary regardless of all of the advances in modern technology. A wise surgeon will never ask a surgical instrument to compensate for inadequacies within these basic principles.

REFERENCES

Abu-Rafea B, Vilos G, Al-Obeed O, et al. Monopolar electrosurgery through single-port laparoscopy: a potential hidden hazard for bowel burns. J Minim Invasive Gynecol 2011; 18:734–740.

Alkatout I, Schollmeyer T, Hawaldar N, Sharma N, Mettlker L. Principles and safety measures of electrosurgery in laparoscopy. JSLS 2012; 16:130–139.

Brill A. Electrosurgery: principles and practice to reduce risk and maximize efficiency. Obstet Gynecol Clin North Am 2011; 38(4):687–702.

Feldman L, Fuchshuber P, Jones D, Mischna J, Schwaitzberg S. Surgeons don't know what they don't know about the safe use of energy in surgery. Surg Endosc 2012; 26:2735–2739.

Law K, Lyons S. Comparative studies of energy sources in gynecologic laparoscopy. J Minim Invasive Gynecol 2013; 20:308–318.

Montero PN, Robinson TN, Weaver JS, Stiegmann GV. Insulation failure in laparoscopic instruments. Surg Endosc 2010; 24:462–465.

Munro MG. Complications of hysteroscopic and uterine resectoscopic surgery. Obstet Gynecol Clin North Am 2010; 37:399–425.

Munro MG. Mechanisms of thermal injury to the lower genital tract with radiofrequency resectoscopic surgery. J Minim Invasive Gynecol 2006; 13(1):36–42.

Odell R. Surgical complications specific to monopolar electrosurgical energy: engineering changes that have made electrosurgery safer. J Minim Invasive Gynecol 2013; 20(3):288–298.

Taheri A, Mansoori P, Sandoval L, et al. Electrosurgery Part I. Basics and principles. J Am Acad Dermatol 2014; 70(4):591.e1–591.e14.

Tucker RD, Benda JA, Sievert CE, Engel T. The effect of bipolar electrosurgical coagulation waveform on a rat uterine model of Fallopian tube sterilization. J Gynecol Surg 1992; 8(4)235–241.

Vellimarra A, Sciubba D, Nogle J, Jallo G. Current technological advances if bipolar coagulation. Neurosurgery 2009; 64(ONS Suppl 1):ons11–ons19.

Vilos G, Rajakumar C. Electrosurgical generators and monopolar and bipolar electrosurgery. J Minim Invasive Gynecol 2013; 20(3):279–287.

Chapter 4

Choice of suture materials in minimally invasive gynecologic surgery

James Greenberg

■ INTRODUCTION

Choosing the proper suture material in a minimally invasive surgical procedure is only slightly different than with traditional open operations and relies mostly on answering three basic questions:

1. For how long do the sutured tissues need exogenous support?
2. How much of an inflammatory response within the sutured tissues is acceptable?
3. What are the characteristics and biochemical properties of the available suture materials and how will they affect the two questions above?

Once these questions have been answered, the choice of suture material should be relatively straightforward. Habit, training, and tradition should have less bearing on this decision than evidence-based reasoning. The process of asking and answering these questions to oneself with each portion of each procedure is an important mental exercise that can only lead a surgeon to better outcomes.

■ WOUND HEALING AND INFLAMMATORY RESPONSES

Whether a wound is closed primarily with sutures, staples, or glue or allowed to close by secondary intention, a rudimentary understanding of wound healing is needed before any reasoned decisions can be finalized regarding that choice. For the purposes of this exercise, wound healing can be thought of as occurring in three overlapping phases – inflammation, proliferation and maturation, and remodeling – though in reality, it is one continuous process that starts with the injury and ends months or even years later (**Figure 4.1**) (Li et al. 2007).

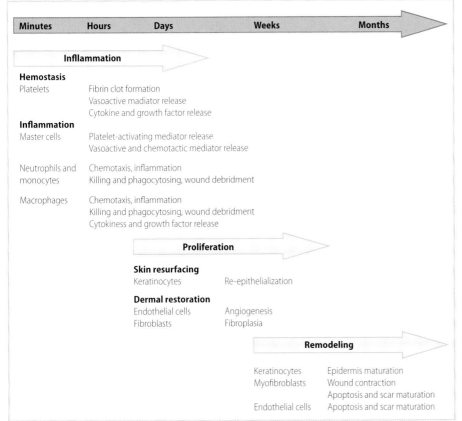

Figure 4.1 Major cells and their effects on normal wound healing.

■ Phase I: inflammation (onset of injury to days 4–6)

The earliest stage of wound healing is marked by vascular responses characterized by blood coagulation and hemostasis in addition to cellular events, including infiltration of leukocytes with varied functions in antimicrobial and cytokine release, which initiates the proliferative response for wound repair. This early hypoxic, ischemic environment is typically populated by macrophages, neutrophils, and platelets. The body's innate response to tissue injury is to limit further injury and repair damage that has already been done. As bleeding from disrupted blood vessels is frequently the earliest consequence of tissue injury, hemostasis is often the first step of wound healing. Insult to cell membranes results in the immediate release of thromboxane A_2 and prostaglandin 2-α (Broughton et al. 2006). These potent vasoconstrictors cause blood vessels to clamp shut thereby minimizing blood loss. Further, damage to the vascular endothelium is a potent initiator of both the intrinsic and extrinsic coagulation cascade inducing platelets to immediately migrate to the area and, secured by von Willebrand's factor, plug the defects in the vasculature (Townsend 2007). Collagen, platelets, thrombin, fibronectin, fibrin, and complement form a fibrin clot that, in turn, serves three major functions:

1. Expresses chemotactic factors (cytokines, prostaglandins, serotonin, etc.) to recruit neutrophils and monocytes to the wound.
2. Serves as a reservoir to concentrate and amplify this cellular signaling milieu (Martin 1997).
3. Provides a support and communication matrix for the arriving inflammatory cells (Gurtner 2008).

Simultaneously, the exposure of platelets to collagen triggers the release of essential growth factors and cytokines, such as platelet-derived growth factor, that will serve to promote deoxyribonucleic acid synthesis in the next phase of wound healing. Activated monocytes in the area become macrophages that will be critical in cellular signaling, angiogenesis, and keratinocyte and fibroblast development, while neutrophils descend upon the wound to kill and phagocytize bacteria and remove necrotic tissue debris (Witte 2006). As the inflammatory process comes to an end, apoptosis of immune cells may be the major key to ending inflammation to allow for the initiation of the proliferation and healing (Wu & Chen 2014).

■ Phase II: proliferation (days 4–14)

The second stage of wound healing is characterized by the rapid formation of new tissue associated with angiogenesis, fibroplasia, and wound contraction. As previously noted, activated monocytes, attracted to the site in the inflammation stage, now transition into macrophages that emit nitrous oxide causing previously constricted blood vessels to dilate and promote the influx of new cells (Witte 2006). Fueled by an expanding variety growth factors, skin edge epithelial cells proliferate to form an eschar and then migrate across the wound to re-establish an intact protective layer. As this is progressing, endothelial cells start to build new capillaries and expand previously established vascular networks (Broughton et al. 2006). Angiogenesis at this stage is essential; while the earliest stages of wound healing can proceed anaerobically, continued proliferation requires large amounts of ATP and cannot occur without an adequate supply of oxygen and nutrients (Kivisaari et al. 1975). Granulation tissue begins to form and fibroblasts are recruited from surrounding intact tissues to initiate the synthesis and deposition of collagen. The entire process is amplified, by both paracrine and autocrine cascades, as a temporary matrix of (weaker) type III collagen, fibronectin, and glycosaminoglycans is laid down in the wound.

■ Phase III: maturation and remodeling (week 1–year 1)

Ideally, the third and final stage of wound healing is characterized by the evolution of the temporary type III collagen, fibronectin, and glycosaminoglycan matrix into an intricately refined and ordered collagen complex. However, not all wound achieve this ideal endpoint. Incomplete tissue regeneration of refining can result in a weak and ineffective scar, while excessive refining yields keloid formation. In this phase, myofibroblasts cause the wound to shrink and contract thereby minimizing the amount of collagen that needs to be deposited. In addition, the wound further contracts as collagen fibers crosslink to increase their strength. The process of collagen deposition will continue to occur over the next 4–6 weeks (Broughton et al. 2006, Townsend 2007). Initially, the collagen is laid down in thin fibrils that run parallel to the wound's surface. As the wound matures, the thin collagen fibers become progressively thicker and reorient themselves in such a fashion as to minimize stress. This yields increasing tensile strength of the wound over the postoperative period. In approximate terms, at 1 week the wound has 3% of its final strength, at 3 weeks 30%, and at 3 months and beyond about 80% (Townsend 2007). It is important to recognize that wounds will never regain the strength of uninjured tissues.

■ EFFECTS OF FOREIGN BODIES AND EXCESS INFLAMMATION ON WOUND HEALING

In a healing wound, the presence of any foreign body – including suture material – induces inflammatory tissue responses that reduce cellular mechanism against infection, interfere with the proliferative phase of wound healing, and ultimately lead to lessened wound strength due to the formation of excessive scar tissue. In this regard, Elek and Conen demonstrated in 1957 that whereas 7.5×10 (Witte 2002) viable staphylococci were typically required to induce an infection when injected intradermally, only as few as 300 bacteria were needed to elicit a similar infection when silk suture was present (Elek & Conen 1957). As briefly described above, some inflammatory response is physiologically necessary after surgical trauma. In optimal circumstances without the presence of foreign bodies or infection, these reactions typically subside within about a week as phase I transitions into phase II. However, some degree of an inflammatory reaction will persist as long as the foreign body – suture material – remains within the tissue. Thus, the degree of the overall inflammatory response and the subsequent integrity of the scar can depend in large part to the chemical nature and physical characteristics of the various suture materials employed in the closure.

■ EFFECTS OF TENSION ON WOUND HEALING

The applied tension to a reapproximated incision can significantly influence wound healing. While an overly loose reapproximation may not allow the opposed sides of a wound to appropriately interact to create fibroblast bridging, excessive tension can cause localized hypoxia, edema, and necrosis. These effects both reduce fibroblast proliferation and yield excessive tissue overlap, both of which lead to reduced strength in the healed wound. To this point, Stone et al. demonstrated in their study in 1986 that tighter knots may be worse for wound healing and strength than looser knots (**Figure 4.2**) (Stone et

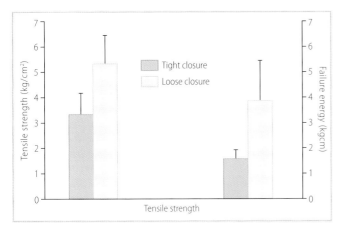

Figure 4.2 Tensile strengths and energy-to-failure of tightly and loosely approximated fascial incisions. Adapted from Stone et al 1986.

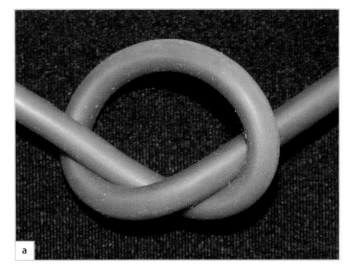

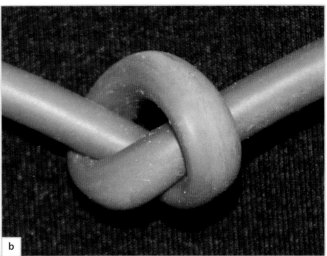

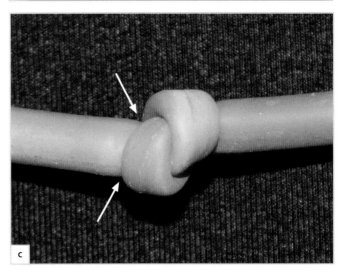

Figure 4.3 (a) Piece of latex tubing early in the knot formation. (b) Piece of latex tubing as the knot begins to tighten. Notice the thinning of the diameter of the tubing. (c) Piece of latex tubing after the knot is tightened. Notice the thinning of the diameter of the tubing and the pinching of the area immediately before the knot (arrows).

al. 1986). Complicating matter is the observation that wound tension within a loop of suture loop will be affected by several factors including the volume (bite) and type of tissue included, the size and diameter of the suture, and the force applied during knotting. Tissues with lower collagen content appear more susceptible to injury due to suture tension than collagenized tissues (Klink et al. 2011). Finally, with a goal of creating appropriate uniform tension across the wound, researchers have investigated the effects of both single suture versus continuous running sutures and as the suture length to wound length (SLWL) ratio. While these data have not been validated in humans, animal models have suggested that, on the fascia, a continuous running suture line produces stronger scars and a SLWL ratio of 4:1 seems to be optimal for wound healing (Höer et al. 2001).

EFFECTS OF SURGICAL KNOTS ON WOUND HEALING

To most surgeons, knots are so integral to the use of suture that their presence in the suture line and their effect on wound healing are often not considered as separate components. Yet surgical knots are simply a necessary evil needed to anchor smooth suture to allow it to function in its role in tissue reapproximation. Other than its anchoring function, the surgical knot offers no benefits whatsoever and introduces a variety of untoward features.

First, the knot is the weakest portion of any suture line and the second weakest point is the portion immediately adjacent to the knot. Surgical knots reduce the tensile strength of all sutures by stretching the material's molecular bonds. A modeled representation of this effect can be appreciated by tying a knot in a piece of rubber tubing (**Figure 4.3a** to **c**) (Greenberg & Goldman 2013). Reductions in suture tensile strength have been reported from 35% to 95%, depending on the studies and suture material used (Chu et al. 1997) and, in a study of suture breakage, failures occurred immediately adjacent to the knot 74% of the time (Marturello et al. 2014). Empirical reasoning would suggest that knot-secured sutures must create an uneven distribution of tension across the wound with the higher tension burdens placed at the knots, where the suture line is its weakest. Moreover, the process of surgical knot tying introduces the potential of human error with observations of significant intra- and interuser variability with regard to perception and measured values for 'appropriate' wound tension (Fischer et al. 2010).

Second, the knot presents the highest density of foreign body material in a suture line and the volume of a knot directly relates to the degree of surrounding inflammatory reaction (van Rijssel et al. 1989). If minimizing the inflammatory reaction in a wound is a component for optimizing wound healing, then minimizing knot sizes or eliminating knots altogether should be beneficial as long as the wound holding strength of the suture line is not compromised.

Finally, with minimally invasive laparoscopic procedures, the ability to quickly and properly tie surgical knots has presented a new challenge. Laparoscopic knot tying is more mentally and physically stressful on surgeons than open knot tying (Berguer et al. 2001, Berguer et al. 2003) and, more importantly, laparoscopically tied knots are often weaker than those tied by hand or robotically (Kadirkamanathan et al. 1996, Lopez et al. 2006). Although the skills necessary to properly perform intra- or extracorporeal knot tying for laparoscopic surgery can be achieved with practice and patience, it is a challenging skill that most surgeons need to master in order to properly perform closed procedures.

CLASSIFICATION AND CHARACTERISTICS OF SUTURE MATERIALS

Choosing the proper suture for a procedure necessitates understanding both the variety of available material characteristic choices and the implications of those properties. Regardless of the material chosen, the ideal suture properties remain the same:

- Adequate strength for the time and forces needed for the wounded tissue to heal
- Minimal tissue reactivity
- Comfortable handling characteristics
- Unfavorable for bacterial growth and easily sterilized
- Nonelectrolytic, noncapillary, nonallergenic, and noncarcinogenic

For suture materials, the full list characteristics can be quite long. For the purposes of this review, this discussion will be limited to suture size, tensile strength, absorbability, filament configuration, stiffness and flexibility, and smooth versus barbed.

Suture size

All sutures materials are available in a variety of sizes (strand diameters). Worldwide, there are currently two standards by which the size of suture material is categorized: the United States Pharmacopoeia (USP) and the European Pharmacopoeia (EP). The USP standard uses a combination of two numerals – a 0 and any other number other than 0 (such as 2-0 or 2/0). The higher the first digit, the smaller the suture diameter. Sizes >0 are denoted by 1, 2, 3, etc. The USP is the more commonly used system in the United States. **Table 4.1** summarizes both the USP and the EP standards and their corresponding knot-tensile strength for synthetic suture. The USP standard code also varies between collagen sutures and synthetic sutures with regard to diameter, while the EP standard corresponds directly to minimum diameter regardless of material. With all suture materials, increasing the size of the suture increases the tensile strength. However, with both standards, there is a marked reduction in the limits of the average minimum of knot-pull tensile strengths between collagen sutures and synthetic sutures for any given size code. For example, 0 USP or (4 EP) chromic gut suture has a minimum diameter of 0.40 mm and is rated to have an average minimum of knot-pull tensile strength of 2.77 kgf, while 0 USP or (3.5 EP) polydioxanone suture has a minimum diameter of 0.35 mm and is rated to have an average minimum of knot-pull tensile strength of 3.90 kgf.

Tensile strength

Each suture material has a standardized tensile strength that is most easily understood as its failure or break load for a given suture size. This tensile strength is the amount of weight in pounds (lb) or kilogram (kg) that is necessary to cause the suture to rupture. As a standard, this measurement is presented in two forms – straight pull and knot pull – to reflect the reduction in any given suture's strength when it is knotted. In practical terms, the knot pull tensile strength most accurately reflects a given smooth suture's in vivo tissue holding capacity since most applications for smooth suture require knotting of the suture. In a straight pull tensile test, tension to rupture is applied at either end of a suture. A knot pull tensile test is the same except that a single knot has been tied in the middle of the strand. As an exception, barbed suture strengths are reported only as straight pull since there is no knot.

Table 4.1 United States Pharmacopoeia and European Pharmacopoeia size codes and corresponding diameters and knot-pull tensile strengths for synthetic sutures

Collagen suture	Synthetic suture		Limits on average diameter (mm)		Knot-pull tensile strength (in kgf) limit on average minimum	
USP size codes	USP size codes	EP size codes	Minimum	Maximum	Collagen	Synthetic
	8-0	0.4	0.04	0.049		0.07
8-0	7-0	0.5	0.05	0.069	0.045	0.14
7-0	6-0	0.7	0.07	0.099	0.07	0.25
6-0	5-0	1	0.10	0.149	0.18	0.68
5-0	4-0	1.5	0.15	0.199	0.38	0.95
4-0	3-0	2	0.20	0.249	0.77	1.77
3-0	2-0	3	0.30	0.339	1.25	2.68
2-0	0	3.5	0.35	0.399	2.00	3.90
0	1	4	0.40	0.499	2.77	5.08
1	2	5	0.50	0.599	3.80	6.35

EP, European Pharmacopoeia; Kgf, kilogram force; USP, United States Pharmacopoeia

All these measurements are reported as in vitro values and reflect only the sutures immediate out-of-the-package strength without regard for the tissue milieu in which they will be placed (**Table 4.2**).

◼ Absorbable versus nonabsorbable (permanent)

All sutures induce a foreign body reaction in all wounds and impede wound at some level. Further, most, if not all sutures, can predispose a wound to infection. In this regard, the 'perfect' suture material retains adequate strength through the healing process and disappears as soon as possible thereafter with minimal associated inflammatory reaction. An essential part of choosing the proper suture is defining the balance between the added strength the suture provides to tissues during wound healing versus the negative effects of that suture material with regard to inflammation. Obviously nonabsorbable suture is permanent. A list of currently available absorbable sutures and their published degradation rates can be found in **Table 4.3** (Tajirian & Goldberg 2010).

Prior to the introduction of the synthetic fibers, nylon, polyester, and polypropylene, in the late 1930s/early 1940s, surgical gut (collagen sutures made from sheep or cow intestines) and silk dominated modern surgery as sutures of choice. While these newer synthetic options expanded the choices of nonabsorbable sutures, surgical gut was still the only absorbable suture option.

Surgical gut is manufactured into one of two preparations: plain or chromic. Processing of both variations is initially the same. The submucosa of sheep intestines or serosa of cow intestines are split into longitudinal ribbons and treated with formaldehyde. Several ribbons are then twisted into strands, dried, ground down, and polished into the correct suture size. The resulting untreated product is called plain gut. If the plain gut is then further tanned in a bath of chromium trioxide, it is called chromic gut. The chromium treatment delays the absorption of the chromic gut and thereby extends its tensile strength for longer periods than plain gut.

Unfortunately with regard to wound healing, the processing and composition of surgical gut make this suture material somewhat of an anachronism in surgery today. First, the grinding and polishing process of the twisted gut multifilaments produces an unpredictable number of weak points and fibril tears. These flaws become readily appreciated with the observation of the sutures' characteristic fraying when tied. Also, these same manufacturing methods make reproducible strength difficult to achieve (Chu et al. 1997). Second, and perhaps more importantly, surgical gut is a foreign protein. As such, it is degraded and absorbed mainly by proteolysis via enzymes from phagocytes and other inflammatory cells. This biologic process tends to yield a less predictable absorption rate and elicit a more intense tissue reaction than hydrolysis by which newer synthetic absorbable sutures are typically broken down. Given these concerns, there is currently little scientific data to support the use of either plain or chromic gut when newer, synthetic absorbable sutures are available.

In the early 1970s, synthetic absorbable sutures were introduced. Because these materials can be produced with uniform chemical compositions under precisely controlled manufacturing conditions, they demonstrate more consistent in vitro and in vivo strength and degradability than their natural collagen analogs. Synthetic materials, such as these, are mostly degraded in vivo via hydrolysis and typically provoke a less-intense inflammatory reaction than their natural protein analogs that, in turn, promote faster wound healing and strength (Barham et al. 1978).

Table 4.2 Mean tensile strengths of 2-0 size smooth sutures and 0 size barbed sutures

Suture	Straight pull strength (kgf)*	Knot pull strength (kgf)*
Chromic surgical gut	4.11	2.05
Polydioxanone (PDS II)	4.89	3.34
Coated polyglactin 910 (Vicryl)	6.93	3.63
Poliglecaprone 25 (Monocryl)	7.26	3.67
Barbed polydioxanone (PDO)	3.89†	N/A
Polyglyconate (Maxon)	7.09	4.41
Barbed poliglecaprone 25 Monoderm	4.64†	N/A

Kgf, kilogram force

*Straight pull strength reflects practical in vivo strength with barbed suture, whereas knot pull strength reflects practical in vivo strength with smooth suture

†0 size barbed suture is rated as 2-0 size smooth suture

Table 4.3 Absorption rates of absorbable sutures

Suture	Time to 50% loss of tensile strength (days)	Time to complete loss of tensile strength (days)	Maximum time to complete absorption (days)
Plain surgical gut*	4–5	14	70
Fast-absorbing coated polyglactin 910 (Vicryl Rapide)	5	14	42
Polyglytone 6211 (Caprosyn)	5–7	21	56
Poliglecaprone 25 (Monocryl)	7	21	119
Chromic surgical gut*	7–10	14–21	120
Coated polyglycolide (Dexon II)	14–21	28	90
Glycomer 631 (Biosyn)	14–21	28	110
Coated polyglactin 910 (Vicryl)	21	28	70
Polyglyconate (Maxon)	28	56	180
Polydioxanone (PDS II)	28–42	90	232

*Extreme variability based on tissue type, infection, and other biological conditions

The first absorbable sutures to be synthesized and commercialized were based on polyglycolic acid. These materials were polyglycolide (Dexon) and glycolide-L-lactide random copolymer or polyglactin 910 (Vicryl). Both are synthesized using a process of melt spinning of chips. The fibers are stretched to several hundred percent of their original length and heat-set to improve their dimensional stability and inhibit shrinkage. Due to their high density of ester functional groups, both of these materials are too rigid in larger diameters to be of practical use as suture. Therefore, individual smaller fibers are braided into multifilament strands of various sizes to allow for a product that has both predictable absorption and strength profiles and acceptable handling characteristics (Chu et al. 1997).

The next major evolution in suture materials came in the 1980s with the introduction of absorbable, synthetic monofilaments. Both poly-*p*-dioxanone or polydioxanone (PDS, PDSII, PDO) and poly (glycolide-trimethylene carbonate) copolymer or polyglyconate (Maxon) are absorbable monofilament sutures that have strength and absorption profiles with the reproducibility of their earlier polymer cousins but with more acceptable stiffness and flexibility characteristics that allow them to be used in a monofilament configuration.

Most recently, advances in biomaterial technology have led to the introduction of segmented block copolymers consisting hard and soft segments that allow for synthetic monofilament sutures with even shorter absorption rates and better handling characteristics. The soft segments translate into improved handling properties (such as pliability), while the hard segments provide strength (Chu et al. 1997). These materials include glycolide and ε-caprolactone or poliglecaprone (http://www.quilldevice.com/general-product-information) (Monocryl, Monoderm), the triblock copolymer glycolide, dioxanone, and trimethylene carbonate or polyglycomer 631 (Biosyn) and the quadblock copolymer glycolide, ε-caprolactone, trimethylene carbonate and lactide or polyglytone 6211 (Caprosyn). These newer monofilament sutures consistently demonstrate better handling profiles, while lowering the complete absorption rates to 119 days, 110 days, and 56 days, respectively. On the multifilament side, the exposure of polyglactin 910 to a gamma radiation sterilization process created a fast-absorbing variety of standard polyglactin 910 (Vicryl Rapide) by weakening the material's molecular bonds to facilitate the hydrolytic process of the suture in vivo. As a result of its pretreatment, this newer suture material has an average absorption of 42 days (Ratner et al. 2012).

Multifilament versus monofilament

As noted above, certain natural and synthetic materials have properties that do not lend themselves to a monofilament design and are better suited being manufactured into multifilament sutures. Multifilament refers to the combining of more than one fiber of suture material into a single strand of finished suture. From the perspective of wound healing alone, there are no advantages of a multifilament over a monofilament. As compared with monofilament sutures, multifilament sutures inflict more microtrauma on tissues as they pass through (Kowalsky et al. 2008). Multifilament sutures also elicit a more intense inflammatory response and produce larger knot volumes than monofilaments of equal sizes (Trimbos et al. 1989, Molokova et al. 2007). Finally, multifilament sutures demonstrate more capillarity with a resultant increase in the transport and spread of micro-organisms (Bucknall 1983) as well as an observed presence of bacteria in the interstices of the braids in the suture strands (Parirokh et al. 2004). However, there are other characteristics of the sutures that can outweigh the beneficial wound healing properties of monofilament as compared with multifilament

sutures. Specifically, currently available multifilament sutures tend to exhibit more favorable handling properties and material flexibility than comparably strong monofilament materials.

Stiffness and flexibility

Stiffness and flexibility are the qualities of suture that describe the strands handling or 'feel.' The suture material's molecular structure determines these qualities of stiffness and flexibility and, in turn, gives strands their memory or recoil and determine the ease with which knots can be tied. Further, it is stiffness and flexibility that tend to be associated with the presence or absence of mechanical irritation from suture due to its ability or inability to comply with the topology of the surrounding tissues (Chu et al. 1997).

As a general rule, at any given diameter, monofilaments tend to have more stiffness and less flexibility than multifilament braided configuration. Natural, twisted multifilament sutures, such as chromic catgut, tend to act more like monofilaments than braided multifilaments in this regard.

Smooth, braided, or barbed

In addition to the other characteristics described previously, suture can be further classified as smooth, braided (and twisted), or barbed based on the strand's surface texture. Not surprisingly, smooth sutures are monofilament strands with a surface that is directionally and topographically uniform. Braided (and twisted) sutures combine thinner suture filaments together to create a multifilament strand that is directionally uniform but topographically varied in a weaved configuration. Barbed sutures by contrast are smooth monofilament suture strands into or onto which angled cuts or protrusions have been made to reconfigure the suture into strands with both directional and topographic variation. From a production perspective, there are essentially two methods of barbed suture manufacturing. The first method involves cutting into the shaft of a strand of smooth suture with a blade of some fashion (**Figure 4.4a** to **c**) (Genova et al. 2011, Maiorino et al. 2012). The second method involves press-forming or compound profile punching in which suture elements protrude from an intact core and serve as the barbs by which tissue holding is achieved (**Figure 4.4d** and **e**) (Lindh et al. 2010). Regardless of the difference in design or production however, barbed sutures are designed to easily pass through tissues in one direction and provide resistance to backward migration. As such, barbed sutures do not require knots for tissue anchors. While on its surface, the elimination of knots has many potential advantages, ensuring adequate wound closure strength and, at least, equivalent inflammation and wound healing are all needed before definitive decisions can be made.

Wound closure strength: knotted suture versus barbed suture

In the assessment of wound closure strength, several studies have been published seeking to address this concern. In 2011, Vakil et al. tested the hypothesis that wound closure using number 2 barbed polydioxanone suture would have equivalent closure integrity to number 1 polyglactin 910 interrupted sutures in arthrotomy closures on cadaveric knees (Vakil et al. 2011). Supporting their hypothesis, they observed that after 2,000 flexion cycles, neither the closures using the smooth interrupted suture nor continuous barbed suture had a single failure. In this same trial, they also sought to determine if cutting the barbed suture line in the closure of the wound would be more likely

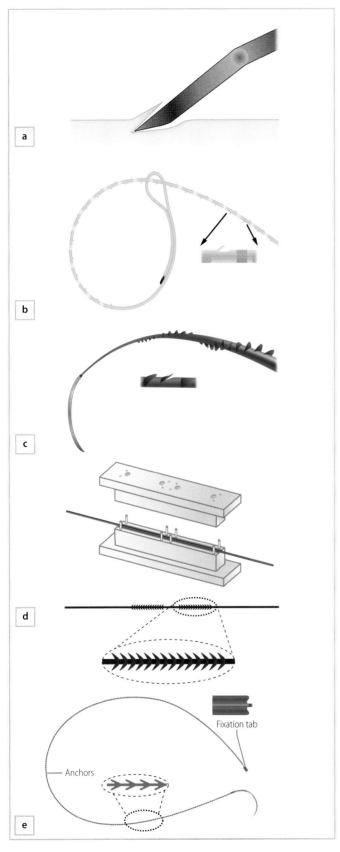

Figure 4.4 (a) Cutting 'barb' into strand of suture. Method for cutting a suture to create tissue retainers of a desired shape and size. (b) V-Loc wound closure device. By courtesy of Covidien, Mansfield, Massachusetts. (c) Quill knotless tissue-closure device. (d) Press forming 'barbs' onto strand of suture. (e) STRATAFIX Symmetric.

to fail than interrupted suture closures. To test this, the integrity of the wounds was further observed after cutting sequential throws/stitches and continuing cyclical testing. Interestingly, they observed that while both smooth and barbed suture closures survived first-throw cutting, the barbed suture fared much better when multiple cuts were made. Once wound closed with interrupted suture sustained three cuts, they all failed, while the barbed suture closures endured up to seven cuts. The authors concluded that wounds closed with barbed suture are at least as strong as those closed with interrupted sutures and are likely better suited to maintaining tissue tension even when portions of the suture line fail.

In another test of wound closure strength, Arbough et al. used a cadaveric canine gastropexy model to compare tensile strength between 2-0 and 3-0 standard glycomer 631 with 2-0 and 3-0 knotless glycomer 631 (Arbaugh et al. 2013). The authors performed 4 cm incisional gastropexies on four groups and then sutured the incisions in a simple continuous fashion using one of the sutures above. Strength of the suture was measured using load to failure, defined as the force (in Newton) required for causing suture breakage or tissue tearing. To measure load to failure, a distraction device was used to stress the sample at a rate of 0.4 mm/s. Authors found that the knotless barbed sutures had a greater load to failure than the smooth standard suture. They found that failure occurred due to tissue tearing, not suture breakage. They concluded that the barbs themselves enabled the higher load to failure in those samples and hypothesized that this is likely due to the barb's ability to distribute the force over a larger contact area and thereby reduce the pressure on localized areas of the wound.

While neither of these studies conclusively established that in vivo wounds closed with barbed sutures are superior in immediate strength to wounds closed with knotted smooth suture, these data and others are suggestive that this technology is at least as good in this realm.

■ Inflammation and wound healing: knotted suture versus barbed suture

While barbed suture may prove to be a superior technology with regard to immediate wound strength, equally important is the consideration of the interaction of barbed suture with tissues over time and how that translates to inflammation and subsequent long-term wound healing. Given the topographic variation in the surface that is created by the barbs, there is a theoretical concern for increased adhesion formation induced by the adherence of nontarget tissues to the exposed barbs as well as an increase in inflammation similar to that seen with braided sutures as compared with smooth sutures.

Studying adhesion formation, Einarsson et al. investigated the impact of barbed suture versus smooth suture on adhesion formation following closure of ovine myometrium (Einarsson et al. 2011). In this animal study, 5 cm myometrial defects were created in each horn of a sheep's bicornuate uterus. One horn was then closed with 2-0 polyglactin 910, and the other with barbed 0 polydioxanone with each sheep acting as her own control. Three months later, the animals were sacrificed, and necropsy was performed to grossly assess adhesion formation. The authors found that adhesion formation was not different between the two groups. The majority of the animals that formed adhesions did so at both horns.

As a follow-up to this study to assess inflammation and wound healing, Einarsson et al. observed at a microscopic level that barbed suture and standard smooth suture had similar histologic effects on cellular composition following myometrial closure in the sheep model (Einarsson et al. 2011). The uterine tissue of the sacrificed animals was fixed and immunohistochemistry was performed to determine the ratio between smooth muscle cells and connective tissue elements, which are generally increased during wound healing. The authors again found no difference between groups: connective tissue cells typical of a proliferating wound were found in equal amounts in myometrium sutured with barbed and smooth suture, suggesting that both sutures confer similar healing characteristics. Sutured myometrium in both groups had more connective tissue cells and fewer smooth muscle cells than myometrium that was not sutured at all. While this early animal clinical data is encouraging, more studies are clearly needed before any final conclusions regarding inflammation and wound healing can be made.

Efficiency: knotted suture versus barbed suture

Efficiency in the operating room is an important factor in minimizing procedural times, affecting cost, infections, and blood loss. Given the difficulty many surgeons experience tying surgical knots using only minimally invasive techniques, knotless barbed sutures offer a potential solution to this challenge. Several researchers have investigated this niche to determine whether or not this newer technology can reduce suturing times.

In an animal model study using porcine bladders, Gözen et al. measured the time to complete the closure of a bladder defect laparoscopically by single expert surgeon with extensive laparoscopic experience performing all the closures (Gözen et al. 2012). The expert surgeon was able to complete the closure in significantly less time using barbed suture (7.13 minutes) as compared with both continuous and interrupted sutures with knots (9.14 minutes with continuous suture and 15.2 minutes with the interrupted group).

Significantly faster closure times with barbed suture were also observed in several in vivo studies. A randomized controlled study by Ting et al. demonstrated 32% faster closure times when using barbed suture (average 9.3 minutes) as compared with closures using knotted suture (average 13.6 minutes) during primary total hip and knee arthroplasties (Ting et al. 2012). Similar findings have been seen in the plastic surgery literature. Grigoryants et al. compared closure time of lipoabdominoplasty wounds using barbed suture in a 2-layer closure to conventional smooth suture in a 3-layer closure (Grigoryants & Baroni 2013). Each surgeon closed half of the wound with barbed suture and the other half of the same wound with knotted suture. At the conclusion of this study, authors demonstrated an approximate 36% faster average closure time using the barbed suture. Finally, in a bariatric surgery study by De Blasi et al., jejunal anastomosis using glycomer 631 barbed suture was 25% faster than anastomosis using knotted suture (De Blasi et al. 2013).

SPECIAL CONSIDERATIONS FOR MINIMALLY INVASIVE PROCEDURES

Suture length

One notable difference with minimally invasive surgery as opposed to open procedures is the need for surgeons to carefully consider a given strand of suture's length in addition to its other characteristics. Suture length that is too short will leave the surgeon either unable to finish the suture line or unable to secure it with a knot. Suture length that is too long will obscure the field with excess material, create tangles, and introduce an unnecessary burden in pulling the suture through the tissue with each pass. For simple figure-of-eight suture closures, a length of 20 cm usually suffices.

Knot tying

Knot tying is one of the more challenging aspects of minimally invasive surgery. A review of the techniques for accomplishing this task is detailed elsewhere in this book but careful consideration of the suture to be tied is of paramount importance and surgeons must be comfortable with their individual skill sets before entering any given procedure. In situations requiring multiple knots, the use of barbed sutures may be helpful. However, the use of barbed sutures should not be considered a replacement for a need master laparoscopic knot tying.

PRACTICAL TIPS

- Either 2-0 or 0 polyglycolic acid based sutures are practical choices to cover the widest variety of applications
- Reabsorbable barbed suture with degradation rates of either 90 or 180 days markedly facilitate closing of long suture lines and convey favorable wound strength profiles

CONCLUSION

The choice of suture material can strongly influence wound healing. Thoughtful consideration of a given suture's variable characteristics should include at a minimum the suture's material composition, diameter, and length as well as the attached needle's size and shape. The practice of choosing sutures by habit alone should be avoided.

REFERENCES

Arbaugh M, Case JB, Monnet E. Biomechanical comparison of glycomer 631 and glycomer 631 knotless for use in canine incisional gastropexy. Vet Surg 2013; 42(2):205–209.

Barham RE, Butz GW, Ansell JS. Comparison of wound strength in normal, radiated and infected tissues closed with polyglycolic acid and chromic catgut sutures. Surg Gynecol Obstet 1978; 146:90t1–7.

Berguer R, Chen J, Smith WD. A comparison of the physical effort required for laparoscopic and open surgical techniques. Arch Surg. 2003; 138:967–970.

Berguer R, Smith WD, Chung YH. Performing laparoscopic surgery is significantly more stressful for the surgeon than open surgery. Surg Endosc. 2001; 15:1204–1207.

Broughton G, Janis JE, Attinger C, et.al. Wound healing: an overview. Plast Reconstr Surg. 2006;117:1e-S.

Bucknall TE. Factors influencing wound complications: a clinical and experimental study. Ann R Coll Surg Engl. 1983;65:71–77.

Chu CC, von Fraunhofer JA, Greisler HP. Wound closure biomaterials and devices. Boca Raton, FL: CRC Press, 1997: 68-122.

De Blasi V, Facy O, Goergen M, Poulain V, De Magistris L, et al. Barbed versus usual suture for closure of the gastrojejunal anastomosis in laparoscopic gastric bypass: a comparative trial. Obes Surg 2013;23:60–63.

Einarsson JI, Grazul-Bilska AT, Vonnahme KA. Barbed vs standard suture: randomized single-blinded comparison of adhesion formation and ease of use in an animal model. J Minim Invasive Gynecol 2011; 18:716–719.

Einarsson JI, Vonnahme KA, Sandberg EM, Grazul-Bilska AT. Barbed compared with standard suture: effects on cellular composition and proliferation of the healing wound in the ovine uterus. Acta Obstet Gynecol Scand 2012; 91:613–619.

Elek SD, Conen PE. The virulence of S. pyogenes for man. A study of the problems of wound infection. Br J Exp Pathol 1957; 38:573–586

Fischer L, Bruckner T, Muller-Stich BP, et al. Variability of surgical knot tying techniques: do we need to standardize? Langenbecks Arch Surg 2010; 395:445–450.

Genova P, Williams RC, Jewett W. Method for cutting a suture to create tissue retainers of a desired shape and size. U.S. Patent 8,015,678, Sep 13, 2011.

Gözen AS, Arslan M, Schulze M, Rassweiler J. Comparison of laparoscopic closure of the bladder with barbed polyglyconate versus polyglactin suture material in the pig bladder model: an experimental in vitro study. J Endourol 2012; 26:732–736.

Greenberg JA, Goldman R. Barbed suture: review of the technology and clinical uses in obstetrics and gynecology. Rev Obstet Gynecol 2013;6:107-115.

Grigoryants V, Baroni A. Effectiveness of wound closure with V-Loc 90 sutures in lipoabdominoplasty patients. Aesthet Surg J 2013; 33:97–101.

Gurtner G. Wound repair and regeneration. Nature 2008; 453:314–321.

Höer J, Klinge U, Schachtrupp A, et al. Influence of suture technique on laparotomy wound healing: an experimental study in the rat. Langenbeck's Arch Surg 2001; 386:218–223.

Kadirkamanathan SS, Shelton JC, Hepworth CC, Laufer JG, Swain CP. A comparison of the strength of knots tied by hand and at laparoscopy. J Am Coll Surg 1996; 182:46–54.

Kivisaari J, Vihersaari T, Renvall S, et.al. Energy metabolism of experimental wounds at various oxygen environments. Ann Surg. 1975; 181:823.

Klink CD, Binnebösel M, Alizai HP, et al. Tension of knotted surgical sutures shows tissue specific rapid loss in a rodent model. BMC Surgery 2011; 11:36.

Kowalsky MS, Dellenbaugh SG, Erlichman DB, et al. Evaluation of suture abrasion against rotator cuff tendon and proximal humerus bone. Arthroscopy 2008; 24:329–334.

Li J, Chen J, Kirsner R. Pathophysiology of acute wound healing. Clin Derm. 2007; 25:9–18.

Lindh D, Nawrocki JG, Collier JP. Tissue holding devices and methods for making the same. U.S. Patent 7,850,894, Dec 14, 2010.

Lopez PJ, Veness J, Wojcik A, Curry J. How reliable is intracorporeal laparoscopic knot tying? J Laparoendosc Adv Surg Tech A 2006; 16:428–432.

Maiorino N, Buchter MS, Primavera M, Kosa TD. Method of forming barbs on a suture. U.S. Patent 8,161,618, Apr 24, 2012.

Martin P. Wound healing: aiming for perfect skin regeneration. Science. 1997; 276:75.

Marturello DM, McFadden MS, Bennett RA, Ragetly GR, Horn G. Knot security and tensile strength of suture materials. Vet Surg 2014; 43:73–79.

Molokova OA, Kecherukov AI, Aliev FSh, et al. Tissue reactions to modern suturing material in colorectal surgery. Bull Exp Biol Med 2007; 143:767–770.

Parirokh M, Asgary S, Eghbal MJ, Stowe S, Kakoei S. A scanning electron microscope study of plaque accumulation on silk and PVDF suture materials in oral mucosa. Int Endod J 2004; 37:776e781.

Ratner BD, HoffmanAS, Schoen FJ, Jack E. Lemons JE. Biomaterials science: an introduction to materials in medicine , 3rd edn. Oxford: Academic Press, 2012:1017.

Stone IK, von Fraunhofer JA, Masterson BJ. The biomechanical effects of tight suture closure upon fascia. Surg Gynecol Obstet 1986; 163:448–452.

Tajirian AL, Goldberg DJ. A review of sutures and other skin closure materials. J Cosmet Laser Ther 2010; 12:296–302.

Ting NT, Moric MM, Della Valle CJ, Levine BR. Use of knotless suture for closure of total hip and knee arthroplasties: a prospective, randomized clinical trial. J Arthroplasty. 2012; 27:1783–1788.

Townsend C. Sabiston Textbook of Surgery, 18th edn. Philadelphia: Saunders, 2007.

Trimbos JB, Brohim R, van Rijssel EJ. Factors relating to the volume of surgical knots. Int J Gynaecol Obstet 1989; 30:355–359.

Vakil JJ, O'Reilly MP, Sutter EG, et al. Knee arthrotomy repair with a continuous barbed suture: a biomechanical study. J Arthroplasty. 2011; 26:710–713.

van Rijssel EJ, Brand R, Admiraal C, Smit I, Trimbos JB. Tissue reaction and surgical knots: the effect of suture size, knot configuration, and knot volume. Obstet Gynecol 1989; 74:64–68.

Witte M. Role of nitric oxide in wound repair. Am J Surg. 2002; 183:406.

Wu YS, Chen SN. Apoptotic cell: linkage of inflammation and wound healing. Frontier Pharm 2014; 5:1–6.

Chapter 5 Hysteroscopy – instrumentation, office and operating room set-up

Morris Wortman

INTRODUCTION

Instrumentation for diagnostic and operative hysteroscopy has made significant improvements in the past quarter century. Prior to late 1980s, the hysteroscope was generally considered a surgical tool in pursuit of an indication. With the advent of endometrial ablation techniques employing both laser (Goldrath 1981) and electrosurgery (DeCherney & Polan 1983, Vancaillie et al. 1989), the hysteroscope had become an indispensable part of the minimally invasive surgical armamentarium for gynecologists. The modern hysteroscope is an essential component in numerous techniques including endometrial ablation (Vancaillie et al. 1989) and resection (Magos et al. 1991), myomectomy and polypectomy (Gimpelson 2000), as well as tubal sterilization (Kerin et al. 2003) and adhesiolysis (March et al. 1978). Recent refinements – including smaller diameter hysteroscopes, resectoscopes, and morcellators – have even allowed the migration of some hospital-based procedures into an office setting (Wortman 2010, Wortman et al. 2013). This chapter will describe the range of instrumentation available for diagnostic hysteroscopy in an office-based setting as well as the equipment for operative hysteroscopy in a hospital or outpatient setting. The author will also suggest an approach to instrument organization or 'set-up' that he has developed over the past 30 years.

INSTRUMENTATION FOR OFFICE-BASED DIAGNOSTIC HYSTEROSCOPY

Although diagnostic hysteroscopy can be performed in an office or ambulatory surgical unit (ASU), we will focus on the instrumentation and set-up for office-based procedures. There are many instances when diagnostic hysteroscopy is more appropriately performed in a hospital or ambulatory surgery center – this is particularly true for the medically compromised patient or when a hysteroscopy serves as a part of a more complex surgical procedure that warrants the ASU environment. The information contained herein is easily transferable to the ASU setting.

The author will address the separate components of a diagnostic hysteroscopy system and how they can be assembled in a manner that allows for efficient use of personnel and equipment. Additionally, several newer and important products will be reviewed that effectively combine many individual components in order to simplify office-based hysteroscopy.

There are three types of hysteroscopic optical devices available.

Rod-lens hysteroscope

The first, the 'rod-lens' hysteroscope (RLH), shown in **Figure 5.1**, has been used for many decades and consists of a series of solid lenses, an angle of view prism, and an illumination fiber placed within a 30 cm tube. The RLH varies from 1.9 to 4.0 mm in outside diameter and its angle of view prism varies from 12 to 30. The RLH is sturdy, inexpensive, and reusable while providing optical clarity unmatched by any other category of hysteroscopic optical device.

The RLH's angle of view prism allows the operator easy visualization of the anterior, posterior, and lateral walls by simply rotating the hysteroscope on its own axis, thereby minimizing the need for aggressive movements within the uterine cavity. The classic RLH is generally assembled with an inflow (internal) and outflow (external) sheath in order to facilitate the continuous flow of irrigation fluid.

Flexible fiberoptic hysteroscope

The second type of hysteroscopic optical device (the flexible fiberoptic hysteroscope (FFH), shown in **Figure 5.2**) has a working length varying from 24 to 29 cm, an outside diameter of 3.1–4.9 mm,

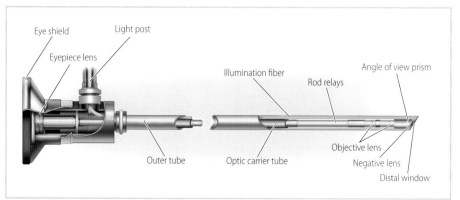

Figure 5.1 Anatomy of a rigid lens hysteroscope.

Eye shield

Light post

Eyepiece lens

Illumination fiber

Rod relays

Angle of view prism

Objective lens

Negative lens

Distal window

Outer tube

Optic carrier tube

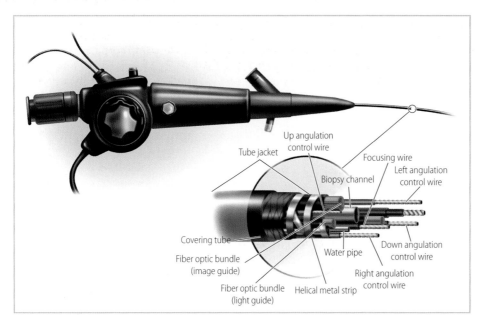

Figure 5.2 Anatomy of a flexible fiberoptic hysteroscope.

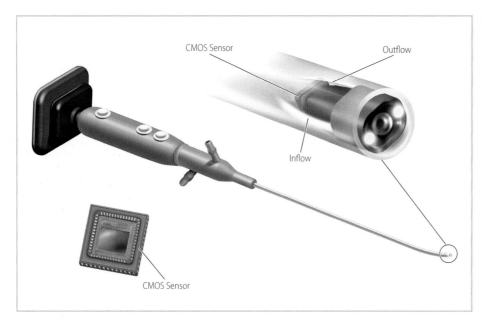

Figure 5.3 Anatomy of EndoSee hysteroscope.

and a 0° viewing angle. Unlike the RLH, the outside diameter of the FFH represents the entire diameter of the scope, the working channel, and the sheath. Although both RLHs and FFHs can be introduced vaginoscopically (Major et al. 1995) – without the use of a speculum or tenaculum – the ability to angulate the FFH's tip allows for easier introduction into and through the endocervical canal. The disadvantages of the FFH include its greater cost, diminished optical clarity, and the vigilant care required during sterilization cycles. The FFH is not equipped with a continuous flow sheath limiting its utility in the presence of blood and debris.

Chip-in-the-tip hysteroscope

The third hysteroscopic optical device (known as a 'chip-in-the tip' (CIT) hysteroscope) is a recent innovation that mounts a complementary metal-oxide-semiconductor (CMOS) chip onto a semirigid cannula. The IDH-4 Invisio Digital Hysteroscope (Olympus, Center Valley, Pennsylvania), is a small diameter (4.0 mm) hysteroscope with a 5 Fr working channel and an inflow port. Additionally, a 5.5 mm outer sheath may be attached to allow continuous flow of distention medium. The digital hysteroscope contains two light-emitting diodes (LEDs) at the tip eliminating the need for an external light source and camera. The flexible tip attached to the rigid insertion portion of the hysteroscope can be deflected 30 to the right and left to optimize the visual field in a variety of clinical settings.

Another example of the CIT hysteroscope (specifically designed for office use) is the EndoSee (EndoSee Corp, Palo Alto, California) shown in **Figure 5.3**. The EndoSee consists of two parts – a reusable handle or 'mini-Tower' and a single-use semirigid sterilely packaged cannula. The reusable handle contains an integrated video display and power supply along with video capture capability. The single-use cannulas are semirigid and contain a CMOS chip, two LEDs for illumination as well as inflow and outflow ports.

In general, the CIT hysteroscope produces an image that is less optically crisp compared to the RLH. Because the CIT hysteroscope has a fixed focal length, it provides adequate but not superb panoramic views. The advantage of the EndoSee hysteroscope is its low acquisition fee and the ability to use it in almost any examination room. Its disposable cannula obviates the need for specialized instrument preparation and sterilization. Finally, the EndoSee even boasts a self-contained image and video capture system.

Hysteroscopic inflow or 'inner' sheath

All hysteroscopes contain a portal that allows for the delivery of distention fluid (usually saline) into the uterine cavity. Some hysteroscopes employ a dedicated inflow sheath (a hollow cylinder) through which the hysteroscope is passed allowing saline to flow between the hysteroscope and the walls of the inner sheath.

In newer hysteroscopes, such as the Campo Compact Hysteroscopy System (Karl Storz Endoscopy, Culver City, California), the inner sheath consists of two parallel channels – one contains the components of an RLH and a second one accommodates the inflow of irrigation fluid. The Campo hysteroscope is based on a 2 mm RLH with an integrated inflow channel – allowing for a combined outside diameter of only 2.9 mm.

Most inner sheaths come in two varieties – those with a dedicated inflow port and those that, in addition, contain an auxiliary working channel. The working channel allows for the introduction of 5 Fr instruments and devices that enable a variety of procedures including tubal occlusion, IUD retrieval, polypectomy, and adhesiolysis.

Hysteroscopic outer sheath

One of the key requirements for high-quality panoramic hysteroscopy is the continuous flow of low-viscosity distention media, generally saline. Saline is carried into the uterine cavity under pressure but is allowed to egress (along with blood, mucus, and debris) through a dedicated outer sheath. The outer sheath generally contains numerous small perforations that facilitate egress (**Figure 5.4**).

For diagnostic hysteroscopy, the outer sheath is passively attached to a dedicated flexible tube that carries effluent to a fluid collection container. Active suction should never be used for diagnostic hysteroscopy as it detracts from the development of adequate intrauterine pressure. Finally, not all diagnostic hysteroscopes are equipped with outer sheaths. The FFH is not equipped with an outer sheath while others (in order to reduce the outside diameter) provide it only as an option.

Light source

Both RLH and FFH require an external light source generally supplied by a 300 W xenon lamp and subsequently transmitted through a flexible fiberoptic cable to the hysteroscope. There are also small self-contained LED systems (**Figure 5.5**) that attach directly to the light post and obviate the need for a fiberoptic light cord and an expensive external light source. The CIT hysteroscope is equipped with an LED at the tip obviating the need for an external light source.

'Combination' systems – light source, video camera, and monitor

There are two different types of 'combination' systems available today. The first combines a light source, video camera, and monitor into a single unit. An example of this system (the Telepak Hysteroscopy System – Karl Storz Endoscopy, Culver City, California) can accommodate either an RLH or FFH (**Figure 5.6**). The second system is the EndoSee Hand Tower (EndoSee Corp Palo Alto, California) featuring a 'mini-tower' that combines a power source and video monitor with a disposable catheter that contains a light source and CIT hysteroscope (**Figure 5.3**).

Image capturing system

It is extremely helpful to have the ability to capture both still images and video as part of hysteroscopic documentation. There are three types of systems available. The first is stand-alone system such as the MediCap (MediCapture Inc Plymouth Meeting, Pennsylvania) that can be used with nearly any commercial medical video system. The second type of image capturing system is one which is already incorporated into some of the costlier video systems and allows images and videos to be downloaded onto a storage device. Finally, both the EndoSee Hand Tower system and the Telepak Hysteroscopy System (Karl Storz

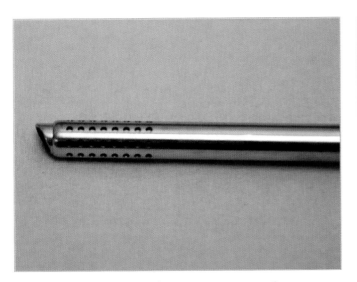

Figure 5.4 Example of outer sheath containing numerous outflow ports.

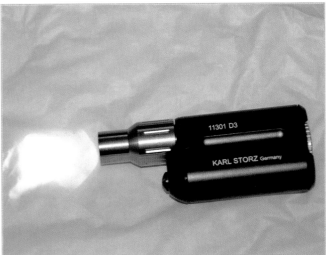

Figure 5.5 Self-contained light-emitting diode source.

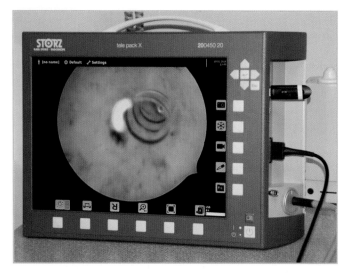

Figure 5.6 Telepak Hysteroscopy System (Karl Storz Endoscopy).

Endoscopy) have incorporated a video and image capturing system into their design.

Uterine distention system

Modern hysteroscopes rely exclusively on the use of normal saline for distention. Physiologic saline is well-tolerated, has excellent optical qualities, and offers few problems in the cleaning and maintenance of equipment. There are at least three methods of administering saline for uterine infusion. The first requires the use of a 50 mL syringe and intravenous (IV) tubing. The second is a gravity-fed system utilizing a 500 mL or 1 L bag of saline with IV tubing attached to the hysteroscope's inflow port. Finally, one can place a 1 L bag of saline into a C-Fusor Pressure Infusor (Smiths Medical, Dublin Ohio) and connect urologic tubing between the fluid containment bag and the hysteroscope's inflow port. The latter arrangement is especially useful when the operator is confronted with active uterine bleeding, a patulous cervix, or an enlarged cavity.

Fluid collection system

A simple office fluid collection system is easily assembled employing a reusable plastic basin and disposable blue pads placed underneath the patient's buttocks. Fluid is allowed to drain into the bucket, which can be kept on the floor in front of the patient or in a designated examination table drawer.

Examination table

Simple office-based diagnostic hysteroscopy can be performed using an ordinary examination table. Special stirrups or electrically operated tables are not necessary for the safe and efficient performance of diagnostic hysteroscopy.

Ancillary equipment

Other useful equipment include an assortment of cervical dilators, flexible plastic cervical os finders, tenaculae, and a variety of vaginal speculums. Although many hysteroscopies can be performed without a speculum, vaginoscopy is not always possible. If paracervical block is to be used, the author recommends the use of Xylocaine 0.5% along with a 24 gauge spinal needle.

Ultrasound

The author prefers to have an ultrasound equipped with both transvaginal and abdominal transducers available at the time of hysteroscopy. The reasons are twofold: first, difficult cervical dilations are not uncommon and the ability to perform sonographic guidance at the time of cervical dilation has virtually eliminated uterine perforation in our practice. Second, ultrasound allows for simultaneous sonohysterography to be performed during selected hysteroscopic examinations. This is especially helpful when assessing submucous leiomyomas that have a large intramural component. Moreover, sonohysterography provides superior information regarding the size of a myoma and its attachment point along with the nature of its relationship to the endometrial cavity.

Monitoring equipment

Our procedure room is equipped with a pulse oximeter as well as an automated blood pressure recording device.

Emergency equipment

Table 5.1 contains a list of recommended equipment that should be kept either on an emergency cart or in the procedure room itself.

SET-UP FOR OFFICE-BASED DIAGNOSTIC HYSTEROSCOPY

Diagnostic hysteroscopy can be performed in almost any standard examination room. Some practitioners prefer to perform them in a designated procedure room, while others prefer to utilize equipment that can be easily moved from room-to-room. The author's diagnostic hysteroscopy setting is a high-volume office-based surgical practice (Wortman 2010) that provides nearly 500 diagnostic hysteroscopies per year. After years of performing diagnostic hysteroscopy in a fixed procedure room, we now use a portable system that allows us to perform our diagnostic procedures in any of our examination rooms. However, we still employ a designated procedure room for our more challenging diagnostic procedures and all of our surgical ones.

Designated procedure room

Our procedure room design is based on (**Figure 5.7**) several important principles:
- *Adequate ingress and egress* are imperative in the event of an emergency that requires patient transfer to a hospital. One must

Table 5.1 Emergency equipment list for office hysteroscopy

• Oxygen administration equipment
• Oxygen canister, nasal cannulas, bag-valve mask, oral airways
• Defibrillator
• Lactated Ringer's or normal saline solution with intravenous tubing
• Medications
– Atropine 0.4 mg/mL
– Epinephrine ampoules (1 mg/mL) with syringes (for SC or IM)
– Diphenhydramine l 50 mg/mL
– Intravenous catheters, lines, and crystalloids
– Albuterol sulfate 0.083%
– Romazicon (flumazenil) 0.1 mg/mL 10 mL vial
– Narcan (naloxone hydrochloride) 0.4 mg/mL
• Ammonia caps

SC, subcutaneous; IM, intramuscular.

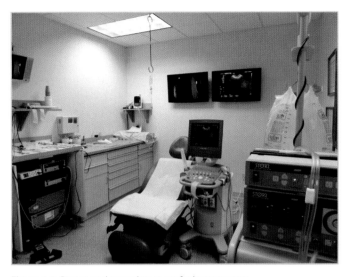

Figure 5.7 Designated procedure room for hysteroscopy.

ascertain that emergency personnel can have adequate access to and from the procedure room.

- *Sufficient room* on all sides of the examination table is important so that staff can move freely about the patient.
- *Floor space should be maximized* by eliminating (wherever possible) free-standing instrumentation. In our procedure room, the video camera, image capturing device, and light source are all built into a cabinet. When the instrumentation is not in use, the cabinet doors are secured and the instrumentation is protected and kept dust-free. Distention fluid is generally hung from ceiling-mounted fixtures. The author also prefers to have wall-mounted monitors so that images can be viewed by the surgeon, the patient, and the staff. Clutter can be further reduced by providing wall mounts for oxygen canisters, a pulse oximeter, and automated blood pressure monitoring equipment.
- *Counter tops should be used in place of instrument tables or Mayo stands.* This represents yet another strategy to maximize floor space allowing staff to move about the patient and providing ingress and egress for emergency personnel.

PERSONNEL

Nearly all of the author's procedures are performed with moderate sedation that requires at least two assistants during diagnostic hysteroscopy. Procedures performed with minimal sedation can often be performed with only a single designated assistant.

INSTRUMENTATION FOR OPERATIVE HYSTEROSCOPY

Experienced physicians have learned that optimum surgical outcomes are achieved when a skilled and practice operating room (OR) team is melded with well-maintained equipment in an atmosphere that fosters unimpeded communication between team members.

The author will review both the instrumentation and OR set-up for operative hysteroscopy primarily focusing on the gynecologic resectoscope. The use of more recent additions to the surgical armamentarium such as hysteroscopic morcellators will also be addressed.

Hysteroscopic surgery involves the use of a complex array of equipment (**Table 5.3**). Prior to any procedure, the author recommends the

Table 5.2 Commercially available uterine distention media

Medium	Osmolarity (mOsmol/L)
Glycine 1.5%	200
Sorbitol 3.3%	185
Mannitol 5%	275
Saline 0.9%	308
Normal serum	285–295

Table 5.3 Suggested instrumentation for ultrasound-guided hysteroscopic surgery

Instrument	Specifics
Continuous flow resectoscopes (CFR)	28 Fr CFR with 27 Fr Loops (Monopolar)
	26 Fr CFR with 24 Fr Loops (Monopolar)
	22 Fr CFR with 19 Fr Loops (Monopolar)
	26 Fr CFR with 24 Fr Loops (Bipolar)
	Operating bridge for vasopressin injection needle
Vasopressin injection needle	40 cm x 21 gauge (Vita Needle Company, Needham, MA)
	N-Tralig Intraligamental Syringe (Integra Miltex, Rietheim-Weiltheim, GE)
Cervical dilators	Hegar
	Pratt
	Denniston
	Os-finders (Cooper Surgical, Trumbull, CT)
Forceps	Ovum forceps (7, 10 and 12 mm)
	Sopher forceps (10, 12 and 14 mm)
Multiple single-toothed tenaculae	
Electrosurgical equipment	Electrosurgical generator (bipolar and unipolar)
	Grounding pads with return electrode monitoring
	Various cutting loops (0, 165, 90 degree)
	Ball-end electrode
Fluid management system	–
Ultrasound scanner	–
Video-cart	–

use of standardized checklists to ascertain that all equipment function properly prior to induction of anesthesia. Additionally, it is of paramount importance that every piece of equipment from hysteroscopes to fluid management systems (FMS) has a useable and functioning duplicate permitting redundancy should any instrument fail during a procedure.

The gynecologic or continuous flow resectoscope

The continuous flow resectoscope (CFR) was first introduced by Karl Storz Endoscopy in 1989. The modern resectoscope (**Figure 5.8**) has changed little in the past 25 years featuring an RLH, inner and outer external sheaths as well as a working element to which one of several types of electrodes can be attached. Typically, the CFR is attached to

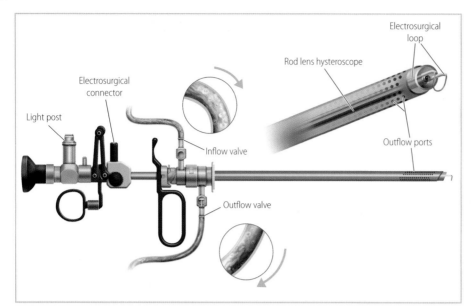

Figure 5.8 Anatomy of a gynecologic resectoscope.

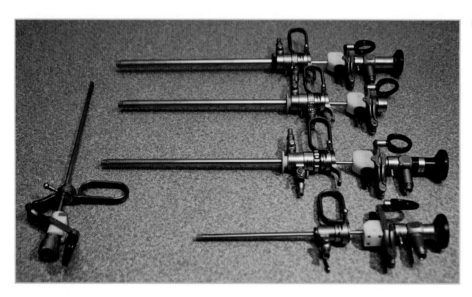

Figure 5.9 Array of gynecologic resectoscopes.

four different components, which include a video camera, a FMS, a light source, and an electrosurgical generator. When first introduced, the CFR operated only as a monopolar instrument utilizing low-viscosity anionic fluids (LVAFs). Today's resectoscope is also available as a bipolar system that permits the use of normal saline for uterine distention.

When Karl Storz Endoscopy first introduced the unipolar resectoscope, it had an overall length of 30 cm along with an outside diameter of 26 Fr permitting a 24 Fr electrosurgical cutting loop or a similar size loop equipped with a 3 mm ball-end electrode. Unipolar CFRs are also available in 30 cm lengths with diameters of 22 and 28 Fr with matching electrodes. The author also employs a much shorter 13 Fr pediatric resectoscope equipped with a unipolar electrosurgical loop. Finally, at least one manufacturer produces a 35 cm long 26 Fr resectoscope that is very useful when working in an enlarged uterine cavity or one that is well suspended.

In addition to a variety of unipolar resectoscopes, the author also utilizes a 26 Fr bipolar resectoscope. The main advantage of a bipolar electrosurgery is that it is compatible with normal saline for distention. However, bipolar electrodes are both expensive and fragile compared to their unipolar counterparts. Although they offer excellent perfor-

mance, when used in a cutting mode they work quite well, their ability to coagulate tissue is quite limited (Ko et al. 2010). **Figure 5.9** shows the array of resectoscopes that we frequently utilize.

Continuous flow bridge

Oftentimes it is helpful to have the ability to inject vasopressin directly into a myoma or its base. It is our practice to utilize a continuous flow bridge that is inserted in place of the resectoscope working element alongside the lens, within the array of inner and outer sheaths. This allows the passage of a 40 cm × 22 gauge needle allowing direct injection of vasopressin into the myoma or its attachment point (Wortman 2013).

Hysteroscopic morcellators

There are presently three commercially available hysteroscopic morcellation systems offered today: the MyoSure (Hologic Inc, Bedford, Massachusetts) and the Truclear System (Smith and Nephew Inc, Andover Massachusetts) are both approved in the United States, while the third, the Intrauterine Bigatti Shaver (IBS) (Karl Storz Endoscopy Tuttlingen, Germany) is approved for use in Europe.

Morcellation systems have three advantages: they utilize normal saline for distention, eliminate floating chips, and cut without electrosurgical energy. Each of the systems feature a cutting blade powered by an electromechanical drive system that enables a combination of reciprocating cutting and rotation to efficiently remove tissue – fibroids or polyps. Additionally, all morcellation systems utilize suction to draw the specimen in contact with the side-facing cutting window of the morcellator. These systems works well with grade 0, 1, and some grade 2 leiomyomas (Emanuel & Wamsteker 2005) with few reports of their efficacy and utility for fibroids >3 cm. One of the disadvantages of these mechanical cutting blades is that their function with very dense leiomyomas may be suboptimal.

The Truclear system is available in two sizes: a 5.6 mm outer diameter and 9.0 mm outer diameter equipped with a 2.9 and 4.0 mm cutting blade, respectively. The MyoSure system is available in a 6.3 and 7.3 mm outside diameter hysteroscope featuring 3 and 4 mm outer diameter cutting devices, respectively. The smaller diameter systems may be used in an office setting.

Light source, video camera, and image capturing system

The free-standing light source, video camera, and image capturing systems that are used for diagnostic procedures also meet the requirements for operative hysteroscopy. They are summarized earlier in this chapter.

Fluid management system

There are many commercially available FMS, and they are commonly composed of two parts:
1. *An infusion pump* that delivers low-viscosity fluids at an increased pressure (a maximum of 140–200 mmHg. There are two types of infusion pumps: inflatable bladder and peristaltic pumps.
   The Dolphin II (Olympus Corp, Center Valley, Pennsylvania) relies on a rigid enclosure that houses an inflatable bladder. A single 3 L bag is placed into the compartment whereupon the bladder is filled with air compressing a 3 L bag of low-viscosity fluid to a pressure up to 140 mmHg. The other type of infusion pump is a peristaltic roller rotation pump available on several systems including the Aquilex (Hologic Inc, Bedford, Massachusetts), the Hamou Endomat (Karl Storz Endoscopy, Culver City California), and Fluid Safe Management System (Stryker Medical, Portage, Michigan).
2. *A fluid collection system* consists of disposable containers generally attached to a scale that weighs the effluent. Some collection systems also include a self-contained suction pump, while others rely on the OR wall suction. The fluid collection system includes tubing that is able collect all the effluent coming from the outflow port of the resectoscope as well as that contained in the fluid collection bag.
   Most FMS are capable of handling several 3 L bags or bottles and allow switching from one to the next in a rapid sequence. The FMS is often equipped with digital readout of the net fluid absorption along with alarms that alert the OR team when a specified fluid deficit has been reached. It is worthwhile noting that FMS vary considerably in the amount of flow they deliver—from 500 mL/min to 800 mL/min. High flow rates are especially important when employing hysteroscopic morcellators, though the author finds them advantageous, especially in cases where significant debris and blood loss can be anticipated.

Fluid collection drapes

There are many excellent commercially available collection drapes available on the market. The author has enjoyed a great deal of success with the Uro Catcher Drape (Allen Medical Systems, Acton, Massachusetts).

Distention media

There are numerous choices commercially available for distention fluid (**Table 5.2**). The author's preference is to use glycine 1.5% for cases involving unipolar electrosurgery and normal saline for cases requiring bipolar electrosurgery. Although some authors (Indman 2000) advocated the use of mannitol 5% because of its iso-osmolarity with serum, it is expensive and available only in 1 L bottles.

Operating room table and stirrups

There are many choices available for OR tables. They all work well and have many more functions than are necessary for operative hysteroscopy. It is worth mentioning that patients undergoing operative hysteroscopy should never be placed in Trendelenburg position as it increases the risk of air emboli during operative hysteroscopy (Wortman 2006). We have found that Allen stirrups (Allen Medical Systems, Acton, Massachusetts) offer a wide variety of positioning options, which is important for providing patient comfort and access for both operative hysteroscopy and simultaneous sonographic guidance.

Electrosurgical generator

The author's preference is to utilize a single generator that can function with both a unipolar and bipolar resectoscope. We employ the Autocon II 400 (Karl Storz Endoscopy, Culver City, California) that can deliver up to 300 W of unmodulated (cutting) current and 120 W of modulated (coagulation) current in a unipolar mode along with a variety of cutting and coagulation bioeffects in a bipolar mode.

Instrument table

The instrument table should contain certain standardized items including:
- One or more resectoscopes as needed for a particular case. It is our practice to have a unipolar and bipolar resectoscope available with appropriate electrodes
- Vasopressin solution containing 5 units in 40 mL saline; 4" needle extender, 20 mL syringe, and four 21 gauge × 1½ needles
- N-Tralig Intraligamental Syringe (Integra Miltex, Rietheim-Weiltheim, Germany)
- Hegar dilators (3-12 mm)
- Four single–toothed tenaculum.

It is worth mentioning that the instrument table contents are reviewed and modified for every patient based on her individualized needs. These modifications are added at the preoperative visit and become part of that patient's preoperative checklist. We have a range of resectoscope options noted above. Sonographically guided myomectomies often call for a variety of additional instrumentation including a Sopher or Blier forceps as well as a myoma injection needle (Vita Needle Company, Needham, Massachusetts) for vasopressin administration. These are reserved only for cases in which their use is anticipated (**Table 5.3**).

■ Ultrasound machine

The ability to perform simultaneous sonographic guidance is an invaluable aid for operative hysteroscopy. The author has found sonography as important adjuvant for hysteroscopic myomectomy, adhesiolysis, reoperative hysteroscopy surgery, and endomyometrial resection (Wortman 2012, Wortman 2013, Wortman et al. 2014). We utilize a Siemens Acuson digital ultrasound machine (Siemens USA, Washington DC) equipped with a variable frequency (2–5 MHz) abdominal transducer and find it an indispensable part of our OR set-up.

■ Operating room set-up for operative hysteroscopy

Physicians frequently underestimate the thought, planning, and coordination that are an essential part of successful operative hysteroscopy. Although much of the set-up for operative hysteroscopy is 'fixed', there are also many occasions that call for individualization of the 'set-up'. Among the items that should be considered for each case are the following:

Ultrasound machine and technician: simple and straightforward cases such as hysteroscopic polypectomy or the resection of a small grade 0 leiomyoma do not require sonographic guidance. However, the excision of a uterine septum or the removal of grade 2 leiomyomas or fibroids >3 cm in diameter can be performed with greater confidence and safety utilizing sonographic guidance.

Hysteroscope or resectoscope diameter: There are many different instruments available today for hysteroscopic resection or ablation.

Unipolar resectoscopes: They vary from 13 to 28 Fr. Smaller diameter loops are well suited for the resection of polyps in the small postmenopausal uterus or for performing reoperative hysteroscopic surgery. Larger loops improve surgical efficiency whenever the anticipated tissue volume is high – an endomyometrial resection performed on a large surface area uterus or one with numerous or larger leiomyomas.

Bipolar resectoscopes: They are preferred when one is concerned about excessive fluid absorption of an LVAF. These resectoscopes are generally limited to 22 and 26 Fr. Morcellators are the tool of choice for many physicians and come in several sizes as well.

Myoma forceps: They are particularly valuable for debulking large myomas. The advantages of these debulking forceps (12 mm ovum forceps, Blier and Sopher forceps) is that they are inexpensive, reusable, and efficient. Importantly, they can be used without exposing the patient to distention fluid. They are best used under sonographic guidance (Wortman 2013).

■ CONCLUSION

The last few decades have seen constant technological advances in both diagnostic and operative hysteroscopy. Diagnostic hysteroscopes have become smaller and better suited to an office-based setting. Recently some hysteroscope manufacturers are even incorporating CMOS chips and producing self-contained mini-Towers that make them affordable for almost any practice. There are also several high-quality combination systems that allow the video system, monitor, light source, and image capturing system to be incorporated into a small portable device that can be utilized in any standard examination room. Operative hysteroscopy has seen many advances including the concomitant use of sonographic guidance as well as the development of a wide array of monopolar and bipolar resectoscopes. In addition, we are beginning to see a variety of electromechanical morcellation devices that are gaining significant acceptance in the gynecologic community. An understanding of these devices and how to integrate them into an office- or hospital-based operating room is essential to providing excellent results and safe outcomes.

■ REFERENCES

DeCherney A, Polan ML. Hysteroscopic management of intrauterine lesions and intractable uterine bleeding. Obstet Gynecol 1983; 61:392–397.

Emanuel MH, Wamsteker K. The intrauterine morcellator: a new hysteroscopic operating technique to remove intrauterine polyps and myomas. J Minim Invasive Gynecol 2005; 12:62–66.

Gimpelson RJ. Hysteroscopic treatment of the patient with intracavity pathology (myomectomy/polypectomy). Obstet Gynecol Clin North Am 2000; 27:327-337.

Goldrath MH. Laser photovaporization of endometrium for the treatment of menorrhagia. Am J Obstet Gynecol 1981; 140:14–19.

Indman PD. Instrumentation and distention media for the hysteroscopic treatment of abnormal uterine bleeding. Obstet Gynecol Clin North Am 2000; 27:305-15.

Kerin JF, Cooper JM, Price T, et al. Hysteroscopic sterilisation using a micro-insert device: results of a multicenter Phase II study. Hum Reprod 2003; 18:1223–1230.

Ko R, Tan AH, Chew BH, et al. Comparison of the thermal and histopathological effects of bipolar and monopolar electrosurgical resection of the prostate in a canine model. BJU Int 2010; 105:1314–1317.

Magos AL, Baumann R, Lockwood GM, Turnbull AC. Experience with the first 250 endometrial resections for menorrhagia. Lancet 1991; 337:1074–1078.

Major T, Bacsko G, Lampe L, Borsos A. Hysteroscopic vaginoscopy in the diagnosis of vaginal bleeding. Surg Technol Int 1995; IV:220–222.

March CM, Israel R, March AD. Hysteroscopic management of intrauterine adhesions. Am J Obstet Gynecol 1978; 130:653–657.

Vancaillie TG. Electrocoagulation of the endometrium with the ball-end resectoscope. Obstet Gynecol 1989; 74:425-427.

Wortman M, Daggett A, Ball C. Operative hysteroscopy in an office-based surgical setting: review of patient safety and satisfaction in 414 cases. J Minim Invasive Gynecol 2013; 20: 56–63.

Wortman M, Daggett A, Deckman A. Ultrasound-guided reoperative hysteroscopy for managing global endometrial ablation failures. J Minim Invasive Gynecol 2014; 21:238–244.

Wortman M. Sonographically guided hysteroscopic myomectomy (SGHM): minimizing the risks and maximizing efficiency. Surg Technol Int 2013; 23:181–189.

Wortman M. Complications of hysteroscopic surgery. In: Issacson K (ed), Complications of gynecologic endoscopy surgery. Philadelphia: Saunders Elsevier, 2006:185–200.

Wortman M. Instituting an office-based surgery program in the gynecologist's office. J Minim Invasive Gynecol 2010; 17:673–683.

Wortman M. Sonographically guided hysteroscopic myomectomy (SGHM): minimizing the risks and maximizing efficiency. Surg Technol Int 2013; 23:181–189.

Wortman M. Sonographically-guided hysteroscopic endomyometrial resection. Surg Technol Int 2012; 21:163–169.

Chapter 6 Laparoscopy – instrumentation and operating room set-up

Giuseppe Di Pierro, Maria Laura Pisaturo, Sergio Schettini

In recent years, manufacturers have made significant improvements in surgical instruments, adapting them to the specific needs of the operator and specific technique to be performed, and improving them as technology has changed and progressed. An appropriate knowledge of laparoscopic surgical instruments is fundamental for the operator, allowing him or her to overcome any unexpected events or setbacks that may occur.

VERESS NEEDLE

The Veress needle was the first instrument used to access the peritoneal cavity in order to create the pneumoperitoneum, and it is still the most widely used access method in laparoscopy. The Veress needle may be either disposable or reusable. It consists of a metal cannula with a sharp chamfer tip. A fenestrated stylet with blunt ends runs within the cannula; the stylet is equipped with a spring mechanism that has a stop positioned over the tip of the outer cannula (**Figure 6.1**).

This system ensures that the tip cuts tissue but, when the tissue does not offer any resistance (i.e. when penetration into the abdominal cavity has occurred), the stylet protrudes beyond the cannula to protect the viscera from iatrogenic lesions. Veress needles come in different lengths from 70 to 150 mm, and their selection depends on the thickness of the patient's abdominal wall. The modern disposable needles are equipped with visual and audio indicators that guide the surgeon during 'blind' insertion.

ELECTRONIC CO_2 INSUFFLATOR

The electronic CO_2 insufflator pumps carbon dioxide into the peritoneal cavity, allowing the creation of the working chamber and maintaining a constant intraperitoneal pressure. Patient safety is guaranteed by built in safety circuits with both audio and visual alarms that signal if overpressure is being reached. The latest-generation electronic insufflators heat the CO_2; preheating the gas to body temperature prevents

cooling of the peritoneum and the consequent risk of hypothermia for the patient (**Figure 6.2**).

In setting the Endoflator, four parameters must be considered:
- Insufflation pressure. This is set by the surgeon before beginning insufflation and kept constant. Pressure should be between 12 and 15 mmHg and should not exceed 18–20 mmHg.
- Intra-abdominal pressure. This should not exceed 25 mmHg in order to avoid the following: compression of the inferior vena cava, with consequent reduction of both venous return and cardiac output and increased risk of deep vein thrombosis; decompression sickness due to venous intravasation; and surgical emphysema.
- Gas flow. Flow can be established by the operator in a variable range between 0 and 30 L/min.
- Total volume of insufflated gas. This can vary from 4 to 5 L, up to a maximum of 7–8 L of CO_2 in wider abdominal cavities.

SUSPENSION SYSTEM OF THE ABDOMINAL WALL

Problems related to the induction and maintenance of a pneumoperitoneum led to the development of alternative techniques to create a intraperitoneal operative space (gasless laparoscopy). The various proposed systems are based on the common principle of mechanically lifting the abdominal wall, implemented through mechanical arms set into the operating table and introduced into the peritoneal cavity subcutaneously. However, none of these systems avoids the so-called

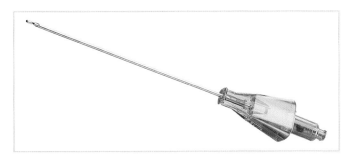

Figure 6.1 Veress needle. With permission from Johnson and Johnson Medical SpA, Italy.

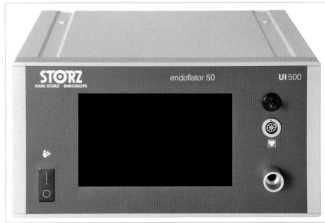

Figure 6.2 Electronic CO_2 endoflator. With permission from Karl Storz Italia.

'tent effect', which does not allow the creation of a homogeneous operative space comparable to that obtained with the insufflation of gas.

TROCAR

Trocars are cannulas used for the introduction of instruments or laparoscopic endoscopes. They allow the surgeon to access the peritoneal cavity and can be introduced either without pneumoperitoneum (direct insertion, open laparoscopy, or optical trocar) or after the pneumoperitoneum has been created (with the Veress needle technique, optical trocar, or expandable trocar). Trocars are equipped with a valve and sealing system that allows the operator to create, maintain, or reduce the pneumoperitoneum. Trocars are either disposable or reusable.

For correct introduction, the trocar should be held in the surgeon's dominant hand so that the proximal part rests on the thenar, with the middle finger resting on the inlet gas control, and the index finger pointed in the direction of the sharp tip of the trocar. Applying constant and controlled force, the trocar is advanced through the abdominal wall using a gentle twirling motion. The angle of inclination at which the trocar is inserted with respect to the abdominal wall should be between 30° and 45°.

Trocars are generally composed of an outer jacket and a stylet. The dimensions of the outer jacket reflect the size of the most commonly used laparoscopic tools (2, 3, 5, 10, or 12 mm), but most trocars are equipped with valved adaptors that allow the use of instruments of lesser gauge while preventing the release of CO_2 during their insertion. The outer jacket is knurled to prevent slippage or dislocation of the trocar during surgical maneuvers or exchange of instruments.

The tip of the stylet makes the entry into the abdominal wall. The stylet may be bladeless (conical), a sharp knife blade, or a sharp pyramidal section (**Figure 6.3**); if there is a blade, it draws back or is covered once the resistance of the muscle wall is breached. The bladeless stylet (**Figure 6.4**) makes a space by spreading out the tissue radially. The most recently developed trocars are transparent and allow the surgeon to observe through a lens the trocar's progression through the tissues into the interior.

There are some specific types of trocars that differ from the traditional design:

- The Hasson trocar is a tool used primarily in patients who have been already subjected to abdominal surgery and are therefore at high risk of adhesions (**Figure 6.5**). It consists of three elements: a cannula-tap to blow the gas, a device for anchoring sutures, and a lid-valve. It is inserted by open technique and fixed to the abdominal wall with sutures; a spacer also allows the surgeon to determine the length of the intra-abdominal portion of the trocar.
- The expandable trocar consists of a stretchable nylon sheath disposed above a disposable Veress needle; once inserted, the sheath expands as it follows the introduction of the trocar (which has a dilatation system inside). This trocar is not equipped with a sharp blade; instead, through progressive expansion, it follows defects in the abdominal wall zone for entry.
- The optical trocar is bladeless; it allows the surgeon to follow the progress of introduction under direct vision through the lens of an endoscope (the optimal is 0° for a better vision) on the tip (**Figures 6.6** and **6.7**). It is used in patients with previous abdominal scars.

ENDOSCOPES

The majority of endoscopes are based on a rod-lens system designed by Harold H. Hopkins. This system consists of a combination of

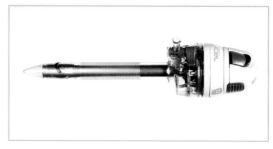

Figure 6.4 Trocar with bladeless stylet. With permission from Johnson and Johnson Medical SpA, Italy.

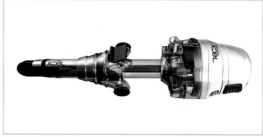

Figure 6.5 Hasson trocar. With permission from Johnson and Johnson Medical SpA, Italy.

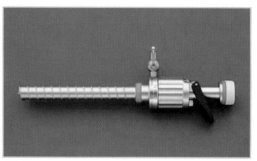

Figure 6.6 Ternamian endotip optical trocar. With permission from Karl Storz Italia.

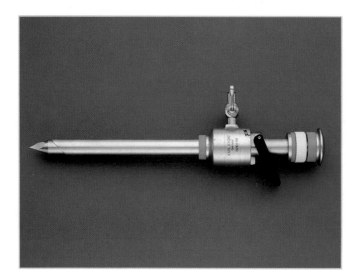

Figure 6.3 Trocar with pyramidal tip. With permission from Karl Storz, Germany.

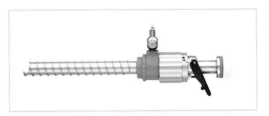

Figure 6.7 Ternamian endotip optical trocar. With permission from Karl Storz Italia.

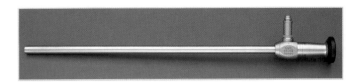

Figure 6.8 Endoscope 0° degree 10 mm. With permission from Karl Storz Italia.

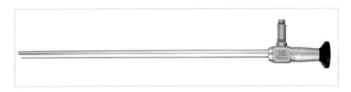

Figure 6.9 Endoscope 30° degree 10 mm. With permission from Karl Storz Italia.

rod-shaped biconvex lenses separated by air, in which light is refracted. The aerial means acts as a negative lens that allows the operator to decrease brightness and image distortion, thus maintaining the focus and the width of the field of view.

Endoscopic diameter varies from 2 to 12 mm; those of the latest generation are equipped with optical fiber viewing systems. Endoscopes can be a rectilinear vision of 0° (**Figure 6.8**), that is the most used in gynecology, or oblique of 30° angle (**Figure 6.9**); for optimal viewing and more panoramic during surgery it has been designed an optical system for adjusting the visual desired between 0° and 120°. Traditional endoscopes allow viewing only in white light mode; in special cases, however (e.g. to detect outbreaks of endometriosis or to assess the perfusion of tissue as a result of anastomosis), newer endoscopes are available that, through stimulation of light at certain wavelengths, exploit the principle of autofluorescence.

VIDEO CAMERA

The video camera is the eye of the operative and is fundamental to successful laparoscopic surgical technique.

Video cameras for endoscopic use are autoclavable. They are based on a system of image capture and processing that uses a charge-coupled device (CCD) or 'chip.' The CCD consists of a microintegrated circuit that has on its surface thousands of photosensitive cells, each of which generates an image point called a pixel. There are two important camera evaluation parameters: (1) chip size as measured in inches (typically 1/2 or 1/4), and (2) the number of pixels it produces (i.e. the number of photosensitive particles present on the chip; at least 800,000). The greater the number of pixels expressed by the CCD, the higher the image quality. A good camera for endoscopic use should also be lightweight and easy to handle, two characteristics generally linked to the weight and ergonomics of the head.

Most cameras used in laparoscopic sugary have a triple CCD in which the light is decomposed by a prism into the three color channels (RGB: red, green, and blue), each of which is analyzed by a specific chip. This produces a clearer picture and provides a feeling of field depth and a greater range of colors. Most cameras are also equipped with automatic zoom and focus. The captured images, after being digitized, are transferred to the monitor (**Figure 6.10**).

More recently, the triple-CCD camera system has been complemented by Full HD (high definition) technology. This allows the operator to obtain images using a color rendering index, which results in significantly better brilliance and detail; in addition, these cameras allow the operator to enlarge the observed image without loss of sharpness (**Figure 6.11**).

The first three-dimensional (3D) view cameras are being developed that, in combination with the latest-generation 3D monitors, generate stereoscopic images that are incredibly close to reality.

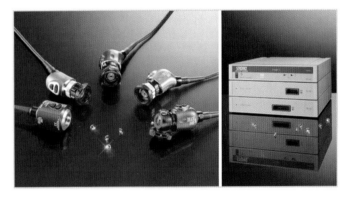

Figure 6.10 Autoclavable high-definition (HD) camera heads. With permission from Karl Storz Italia.

MONITOR

The monitors used for endoscopic surgery are mostly based on a horizontal scanning system. Measured in kHz, the horizontal scanning represents the number of lines drawn horizontally across the screen during 1 second. The image is generated point by point during scanning; the higher the frequency, the more stable and sharper the image. The image resolution also depends on the number of pixels generated (i.e. the number of digital elements that make up the image).

Full HD monitors are available, with some special features (**Figure 6.12**):
- Simultaneous visualization of two full HD images (picture-in-picture)
- High resolution (1920 x 1200 pixels) and 16:9 size
- LED technology that provides excellent color rendering and reduces energy consumption
- High contrast ratio, which allows the surgeon to see even the smallest details
- 3D technology, which offers the surgeon excellent depth perception and subsequent hand–eye coordination.

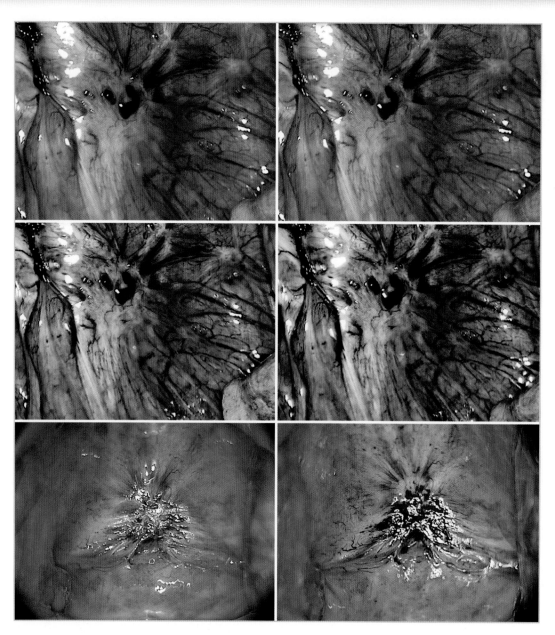

Figure 6.11 Images of full HD video camera. With permission from Karl Storz Italia.

COLD LIGHT SOURCE AND COLD LIGHT CABLE

The light source generates and conveys light into the peritoneal cavity via fiber optic cables. The most important parameter for the choice of a light source is the 'color temperature' of the lamp, which is measured in Kelvin degrees. Given that the best natural light source is the sun (>7000°K), the closer a light's color temperature is to that of the sun, the more realistic the lighting. Another parameter to consider is the wattage of the lamp; the bigger the cavity to illuminate, the greater the power required. Generally 175–250 watts are sufficient for routine endoscopic procedures; light sources currently used can reach a power of 300 watts.

There are three types of light sources, each differing in color spectrum and efficiency. The halogen bulb produces a yellow light and a decrease in performance over time. Metal vapor lamps emit a whiter light but still suffer a decline in performance over time. Xenon lamps (6500°K) are currently the best for color 'reality' and also maintain more consistent performance (in fact, they maintain the same intensity for about 500 hours).

Most light sources are equipped with a system for manually or automatically adjusting brightness; this allows for a constant color temperature and optimal lighting conditions during surgery (**Figure 6.13**).

Fiber optic cables allow the lossless transmission of light from the source to the endoscope. Each cable is formed by a bundle of optical fibers enclosed within a sheath; those most frequently used in laparoscopy have a diameter of between 3.5 and 6 mm and a length of between 180 and 350 cm. The amount of light transmitted is proportional to the number of fibers contained within the cable (**Figure 6.14**).

Optical fibers are subject to wear and breakage; when the percentage of broken fibers reaches 30–35% of the total number in the cable, the cable must be replaced to obtain a sufficient quality of vision.

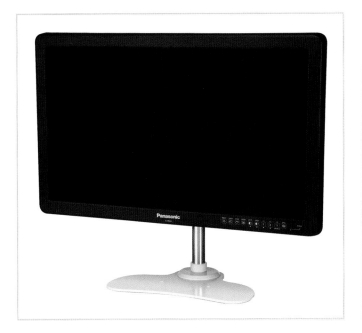

Figure 6.12 3D-2D monitor for endoscopic surgery. With permission from Karl Storz Italia.

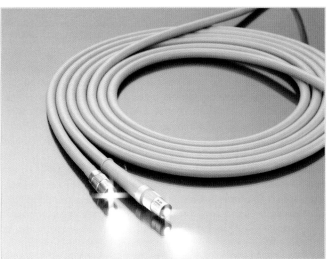

Figure 6.14 Fiber optic light cable. With permission from Karl Storz Italia.

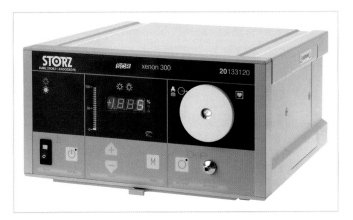

Figure 6.13 Cold light source Xenon 300. With permission from Karl Storz Italia.

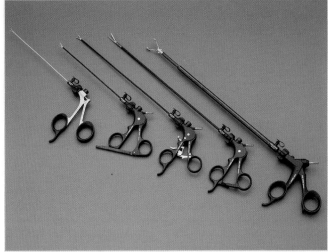

Figure 6.15 Forceps with different diameter and length. With permission from Karl Storz Italia.

Particular care should be taken not to bend or wrap the cord too tightly and not to crush or strike it.

■ FORCEPS AND SCISSORS

Forceps and scissors may be either disposable or reusable. Disposable instruments have the advantage of ensuring high quality standards in terms of sterility and operation. Reusable instruments, although presenting some limitations, help to reduce the cost of endoscopic surgery. In general, ease of use, biocompatibility, radio transparency, reduced light reflection, reliability, and low maintenance costs are the characteristics that must be taken into account in the choice of instruments for laparoscopic surgery.

Laparoscopic instruments have a diameter that ranges from 1.8 to 12 mm, but most are made to be used with 5 and 10 mm trocars.

Tool length varies from 30 to 37 cm, depending on the manufacturer. Smaller instruments (18–25 cm) are usually used in the pediatric field or for cervical interventions. Several manufacturers have marketed longer instruments (about 45 cm) in response to the difficulties of intervention in obese and very tall patients (**Figure 6.15**).

Regarding movement, the traditional laparoscopic instrument is characterized by the basic function of opening and closing; more recently, 360° rotational movement has been introduced, thus allowing a significant increase in freedom of movement.

Three parts make up a tool:
1. The handle: Several kinds of handle are made available for the surgical instruments. Some tools have handles arranged at 90° to the axis of the work, whereas others have a straight handle. For instruments used in electrosurgery, the handle may contain a connector to which the unipolar high-frequency cord is connected.

Some handles feature a locking system that maintains constant grip pressure; this is a very useful feature when the surgeon needs to maintain prolonged traction on a structure because it avoids unnecessary fatigue in the hands.

2. The outer tube: Of variable length and diameter, the tube is generally completely covered by an electrically insulating material.

3. The tip or working insert: In addition to the type of tip (forceps, grasper, pair of scissors), the choice of model to be used depends on the action of the jaws: either single, with one movable jaw and the other fixed, or double, in which both jaws are mobile. In single-action tools, the opening of the instrument is very limited, but the force imposed during closing is much higher; in tools with dual action, the opening is greater, but the grip strength is lower.

Dissecting and grasping forceps used for laparoscopic surgery come in numerous variants (**Figures 6.16–6.18**). A first distinction is made depending on the shape of the distal tip: this is either (1) sharp, (2) with multiple teeth for an atraumatic and accurate grip, (3) tapering, (4) straight, (5) curved, or (6) fenestrated (which allow

a safe and atraumatic grip of tissues). In addition to tip characteristics, forceps jaw surface characteristics are also distinct. Depending on the use for which they are designed, the jaws can be either (1) pronged, for an atraumatic grip of the viscera, or (2) flat, for a very strong grip.

Scissors can be either (1) straight, (2) curved Metzenbaum type (**Figure 6.19**), (3) hooked, or (4) with a sharp or rounded tip.

HIGH-FREQUENCY ELECTROSURGICAL TECHNIQUES

In laparoscopic surgery, high-frequency electrical current can be applied in two ways: monopolar or bipolar. The electrodes used to deliver the current can be disposable or reusable. Electrodes come in different lengths (between 20 and 43 cm) and have a diameter of between 3 and 5 mm.

Monopolar electrosurgery electrodes

There are several forms of monopolar electrodes; selection depends on the indications and the preferences of the surgeon. The most commonly used are those in the form of a spatula (generally blunt) and the hook-shaped (L-, J-. or U-shaped).

Traditionally, one of the major problems with these tools is the limitation of operating angle. To address this issue, new angled or tilted monopolar electrodes were developed to allow the operator to obtain different operating angles. Electrodes can also be equipped with a channel for suction/irrigation.

Bipolar electrosurgery instruments

Tool manufacturers continue to focus on producing single tools that can combine several functions (grasping, dissection, cutting and hemostasis) because the greater the functionality of a single instrument, the less the need to exchange tools during surgery; this consequently reduces operation time and makes surgery simpler. Additionally, instruments have been produced with stems that are adjustable to 360° and with operative inserts that can be quickly replaced.

The most commonly used bipolar instruments are scissors and forceps (**Figure 6.20**). The jaws of the forceps (double or single joint) have different shapes and sizes (**Figures 6.21** and **6.22**); they can be large, thin, flat, multiple toothed, fenestrated, or Maryland type.

Scissors (**Figure 6.23**) can be straight or curved (Metzenbaum), with smooth or toothed surfaces (in the case of difficult to grip tissue structures).

A particular type of bipolar forceps is one that uses a 'Bi-clamp mode'; these automatically stop the power supply once it reaches the optimum level of synthesis or tissue or blood vessels, limiting lateral thermal diffusion.

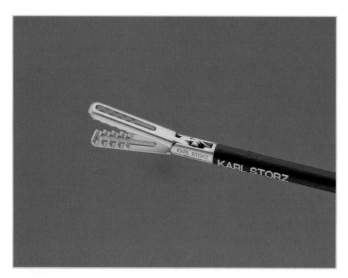

Figure 6.16 Atraumatic double-action jaw grasping forceps. With permission from Karl Storz Italia.

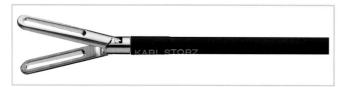

Figure 6.17 Fine atraumatic fenestrated single-action jaw forceps. With permission from Karl Storz Italia.

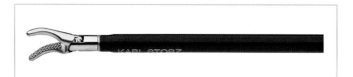

Figure 6.18 Kelly dissecting and grasping forceps with double-action jaws. With permission from Karl Storz Italia.

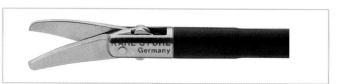

Figure 6.19 Curved double-action jaw scissors (Metzenbaum). With permission from Karl Storz Italia.

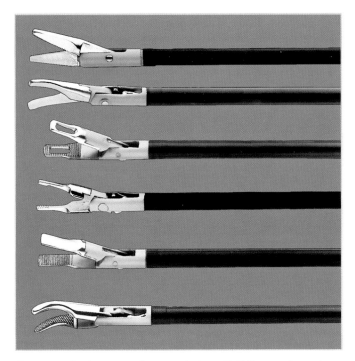

Figure 6.20 Bipolar grasping forceps and scissors (RoBi Clermont-Ferrand type). With permission from Karl Storz Italia.

VESSEL-SEALING TECHNOLOGY

Tools for vessel coagulation use a combination of pressure and either bipolar electric current or electromagnetic high-frequency waves. Hemostasis is achieved through the fusion of collagen and elastin in the vessel wall, which creates a permanent and complete synthesis comparable to that obtained with stitches or clips and superior to that achieved with the standard techniques of bipolar coagulation; the effect is confined to the target tissue or vessel, without charring and with minimal thermal spread to adjacent tissues (**Figure 6.24**). These systems can perform hemostasis on vessels up to 7.5 mm in diameter; the latest devices come with a blade to cut out precoagulated tissue.

In addition, these tools are able to identify the characteristic impedance of the tissue located within the jaws and then distribute the appropriate amount of radiofrequency necessary to carry out vessel synthesis. They are equipped with a safety system that stops the tool when synthesis is obtained and alerts the operator with an audible signal.

ULTRASONIC DISSECTION AND COAGULATION SYSTEMS

Dissection and hemostasis devices based on ultrasonic energy have become an integral part of the standard equipment for laparoscopic

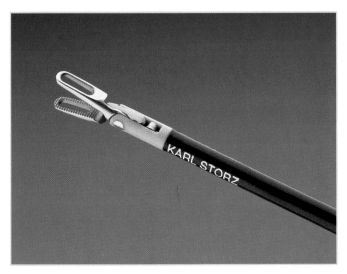

Figure 6.21 Bipolar atraumatic fenestrated double-action jaw grasping forceps. With permission from Karl Storz Italia.

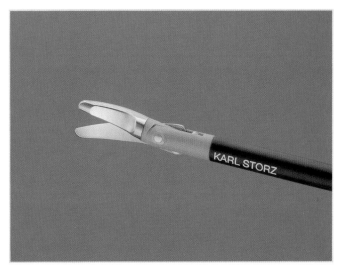

Figure 6.23 Bipolar Metzenbaum scissors. With permission from Karl Storz Italia.

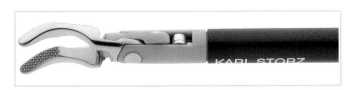

Figure 6.22 Bipolar Kelly forceps. With permission from Karl Storz Italia.

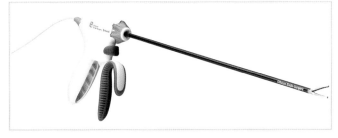

Figure 6.24 Enseal vessel-sealing system. With permission from Johnson and Johnson Medical SpA.

surgery, and they are considered an evolution in electrosurgery. They do not produce smoke, and they combine good cutting capacity with excellent hemostatic characteristics (**Figure 6.25**).

Their operation is based on sending an electrical pulse to the handpiece (which generally is clamp- or hook-shaped), at whose end there is a piezoelectric ceramic element that vibrates at a frequency of 55 kHz; this element transmits the movement to the tissue contained between the tool's jaws. The vibration of the tissue causes heating, which causes collagen denaturation. This process does not produce smoke, only water vapor through the 'cavitation' phenomenon; lateral thermal diffusion is minor compared to traditional electrosurgical systems. The tip temperature reaches and can maintain high temperatures for a few seconds (up to 150 °C); it is appropriate, therefore, to use these devices with extreme caution, using low frequencies and always keeping the tip of the instrument in plain view.

Ultrasonic instruments exert their greatest coagulant power on the vascular structures with a diameter of up to 5 mm. The main drawback of ultrasonic devices is their slowness; this has been improved in the latest models.

Some commercially available systems combine the benefits of both bipolar and ultrasonic energy in a single device, thereby integrating the safe hemostasis of bipolar energy with the speed and precision of ultrasonic dissection. These dual devices may be used on vessels of up to 7 mm in diameter (**Figure 6.26**).

SUCTION/IRRIGATION SYSTEMS

Suction/irrigation systems allow the surgeon a clear view of the surgical field during laparoscopic surgery. In addition to washing the abdominal cavity and suctioning out clots, these tools can provide other functions: (1) hydrodissection, to facilitate anatomical planes of cleavage (using high pressures of up to 1200 mmHg); (2) tissue protection; and (3) adhesion prevention.

These devices have a handle, either straight (**Figure 6.27**) or pistol-grip (**Figure 6.28**), that activates the suction/irrigation system. The suction/irrigation cannulas can be of variable length (from 20 to 43 cm) and diameter, depending on the laparoscopic trocars used. They also can be fitted onto the tip of a needle to puncture and aspirate ovarian cysts or fluid collections.

Suction/irrigation can be obtained through a dedicated system composed of a pump that controls the pressure of the suction/irrigation tool or simply by connecting the device to a vacuum system already present in the operating room and to sacks installed in the upper area of the patient or inserted into a pressure infusion cuff.

SUTURE AND LIGATURE SYSTEMS
Needle holders

These devices come in variable diameters (from 2 to 5 mm) and lengths (from 20 to 43 cm). The handle, usually equipped with a stop function, can be straight (**Figure 6.29**) or ring- or gun-shaped (**Figure 6.30**). The

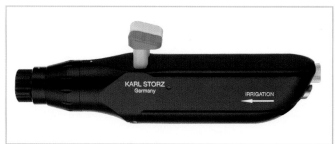

Figure 6.27 Suction irrigation handle (straight). With permission from Karl Storz Italia.

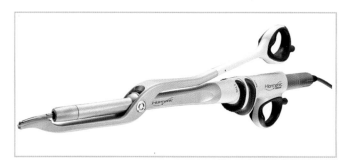

Figure 6.25 Harmonic focus sealing system. With permission from Johnson and Johnson Medical SpA.

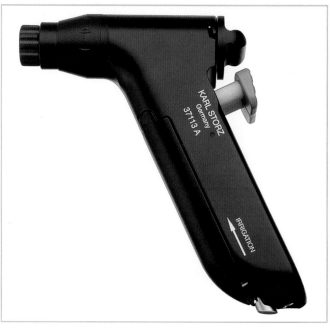

Figure 6.28 Suction irrigation handle (pistol). With permission from Karl Storz Italia.

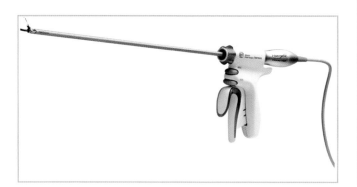

Figure 6.26 Harmonic ACE+ shears. With permission from Johnson and Johnson Medical SpA.

tip is formed by curved or straight (**Figure 6.31**) single-action jaws with microserrated surfaces for a better grip of both the needle and suture thread. To compensate for the reduced freedom of movement inherent in these instruments, needle holders with a tip angled up to 30° are available.

Knot pushers

These tools come in variable diameters and lengths and are used for extracorporeal knotting. They consist of a handle, a stem, and a tip that can be open or closed. The tips are available in different configurations, depending on the surgeon's needs and the characteristics of the suture thread; the tip acts as a guide for the thread (**Figure 6.32**). The extracorporeal knot is positioned and fixed on the desired surgical site. Knot pushers can be equipped with a scalpel to cut the thread directly at knot level.

Clips applicators and surgical staplers

These tools are used to close small blood and lymphatic vessels (**Figure 6.33**). They can be equipped with an interchangeable charging system that contains a dozen clips, or they can require manually inserting individual clips after each application. Applicators are equipped with a stopping device on the handle for better positioning and tightening of clips. Applicators are usually made of titanium, and they can be either disposable or reusable.

In laparoscopic surgery, due to the high difficulty of performing manual endoscopic suturing, surgical staplers have significant applications. Because maximum reliability must be their most important property, they are mostly single-use instruments with various specifications and dimensions according to the tissues on which they are used.

Extraction bags

The use of disposable endoscopic bags in laparoscopy is necessary to prevent the introduction of benign disease (endometriotic debris, dermoid cyst contents, ectopic pregnancies, liquid from ovarian cysts into the peritoneal during extraction, the infection (in case of pyosalpinx), and the dissemination of malignant disease. Bags have a diameter of between 10 and 15 mm and are made of very tough material to withstand the traction exerted by the surgeon during extraction through laparoscopic access (**Figure 6.34**).

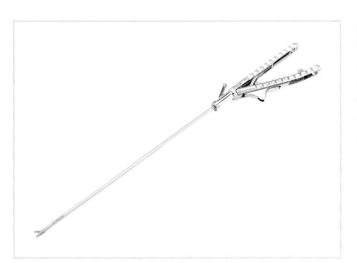

Figure 6.29 Needle holder with straight handle. With permission from Johnson and Johnson Medical SpA.

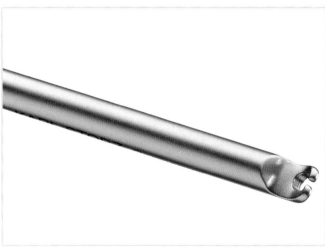

Figure 6.32 Extracorporeal knot tying device. With permission from Karl Storz Italia.

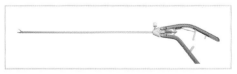

Figure 6.30 Needle holder with gun-shaped handle. Courtesy from Karl Storz GmbH & Co.

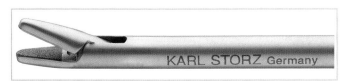

Figure 6.31 Needle holder with straight jaws. With permission from Karl Storz Italia.

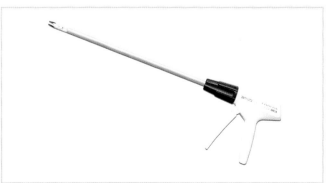

Figure 6.33 Clip applicator. With permission from Johnson and Johnson Medical SpA.

Morcellators

With a diameter of between 12 and 15 mm, manual or electronic morcellators are necessary for some laparoscopic operations such as total or supracervical hysterectomy and myomectomy. The quick removal of anatomical sections depends on the power of the cutting scalpel blades that dissect the sample. The latest-generation electronic morcellators are equipped with powerful engines that produce a blade rotation speed of up to 1200 revolutions per minute, thus greatly reducing surgical time (**Figures 6.35** and **6.36**). Laparoscopic power morcellators have recently come under scrutiny due to the potential risk of disseminating undetected malignancy, and their use has been significantly limited in some countries.

Uterine manipulators

These tools are used to mobilize the uterus during diagnostic or operative laparoscopic procedures. They are available in different shapes and have different characteristics depending on the type of surgery to be performed. Some, such as the Tintara uterine manipulator (**Figure 6.37**), are used to inject into the uterine cavity methylene blue or other contrast media. The Clermont-Ferrand uterine manipulator (**Figure 6.38**) allow the surgeon to perform a total laparoscopic hysterectomy by mobilizing the uterus (anteversion, retroversion,

and lateral displacement are possible) for optimal exposure of the operative field and stretching the vaginal fornices. Manipulators can be either disposable or reusable.

Operating room set-up

Laparoscopic surgery is increasingly a video surgery that requires a whole new series of specific technologies that require space, power (electric or gas), connections, cables, and electrodes. Thus, the traditional layout of the operating room is no longer appropriate to these new needs.

Progress has led to a new generation of 'smart' or 'integrated' operating rooms (**Figure 6.39**). The important features of these operating rooms are as follows:

- Efficiency. The ability to preset configurations for all the connected units for different interventions and/or operators and to recall these settings with a single command drastically reduces the set-up time between various interventions. This increases productivity by allowing a significant increase in treated cases.

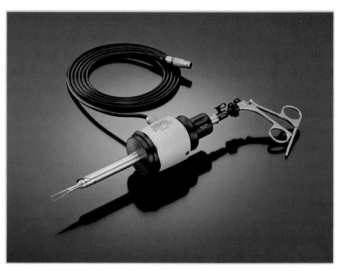

Figure 6.36 The Rotocut G2 morcellator. With permission from Karl Storz Italia.

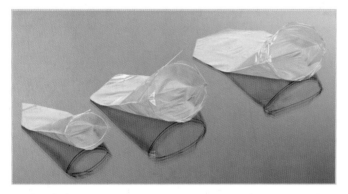

Figure 6.34 Disposable extraction bags. With permission from Karl Storz Italia.

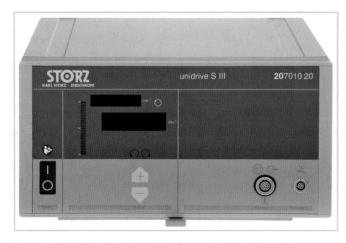

Figure 6.35 Unidrive SIII motor system for use with Rotocut G2. With permission from Karl Storz Italia.

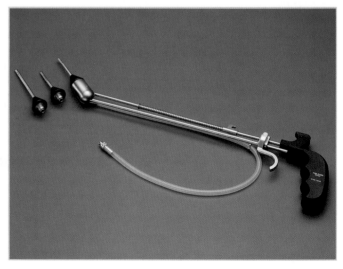

Figure 6.37 The Tintara uterine manipulator. With permission from Karl Storz Italia.

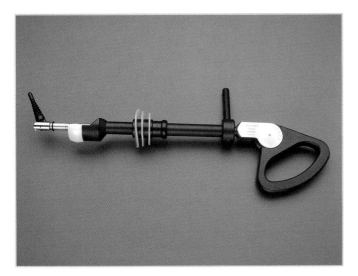

Figure 6.38 The Clermont-Ferrand uterine manipulator. With permission from Karl Storz Italia.

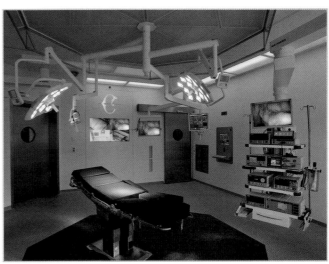

Figure 6.39 The Karl Storz integrated operating room OR1. With permission from Karl Storz Italia.

- Order. The surgeon is able to manage the entire integrated system from a single point on and off the sterile field through voice commands. It is no longer necessary for the operator to have physical access to each unit or subsystem by moving from unit to unit or moving equipment.
- Convenience. All functions of the integrated system, including many environmental functions such as lights, surgical lights, operating table, and phone, can be controlled via a touch screen with a user-friendly graphical interface and also through voice commands. It is also possible to directly view from the sterile field on monitors all archived images related to a diagnostic survey or medical history, as well as to access the internet.
- Economy. The direct control of all equipment involved in the surgical act is returned to operator and to his team, thus reducing the margin of error and especially the time intervals between the operator's request and the concrete result; therefore, operating time can be significantly reduced by eliminating downtime.

The latest-generation operating rooms have the ability to place all electromedical equipment on hanging arms that enable a stable housing of all units and their connections without the need for power and audio/video cables to lay on the floor of the operating room.

The room layout is ideal when each operator can perform his or her task in a comfortable position with a monitor placed at an ideal distance and height for any type of intervention. The latest-generation digital monitors are lightweight, easy to handle, and can be easily installed on mechanical arms anchored to the ceiling so that they can be placed in any position.

The integrated OR allows for an immediate and continuous implementation of additional equipment. Integrated ORs also feature a continuous functionality surveillance of all connected elements, promptly reporting with audible alarms and detailed guidance on the type of encountered problems and the involved equipment. In the integrated system, the failure of one piece of equipment does not interfere with the functionality of the whole system.

A computerized system to capture and store images in digital format allows the surgeon to enter into a single database all images captured from a patient and his or her medical history. From the touch screen in the operating room, it is possible to acquire photos, videos, and audio files and save them to a server for review or have them always available and easily found through computer stations outside the OR. The audio/video signals can be routed to meeting/conference rooms or to other ORs for telemedicine and teaching.

It is possible to interface the hospital information system (which contains all the information related to a patient's clinical history) to the RIS or PACS systems that preserve all a patient's diagnostic imaging (CT, MRI, PET, etc.) as well as to other hospital systems dedicated to, e.g. the storage of anesthesia data, the creation of an electronic medical record, and the management of materials or medications.

Acknowledgments

We would like to thank Karl Storz Italia and Johnson and Johnson SpA for technical support and for permission to reproduce the images.

◼ FURTHER READING

Fanfani F, Gagliardi ML, Fagotti A, Ercoli A, Scambia G. Isterectomia laparoscopica. Rome: CIC Edizioni Internazionali, 2012.

Mage G, Wattiez A, et al. Chirurgia laparoscopica en ginecologia. Rome: Verduci Editore, 2010.

Mencaglia L, Minelli J, Wattiez A. Manual of gynecological laparoscopic surgery, IIth edition. Tuttlingen: Endo-Press, 2008.

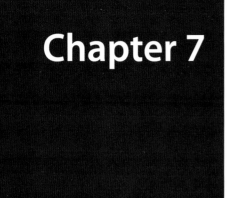

Chapter 7 | Avoiding and managing complications of laparoscopic surgery

Errico Zupi, Gabriele Centini, Jesús Castellano Moros

INTRODUCTION

Laparoscopy brought numerous advantages to gynecological surgery, such as smaller incisions, less postoperative pain, and shorter hospitalizations. However, it presents specific complications that can be related to the technique itself and some general ones that can occur in any surgical procedure. Both types of complications must be recognized and acknowledged before approaching this technique.

The main technique-related complications are those related to first trocar insertion or induction of the pneumoperitoneum. In addition, in laparoscopy, the use of different energy devices is even more essential than in laparotomy, and there are some specific complications related to them. Entry techniques and energy devices have their specific field of application and their own safety rules that, when applied, may reduce the complication rate (Chapron et al. 1997).

One of the main advantages of laparoscopy is image magnification, which can allow more precise and aimed movements but, at the same time, obstructs a general overview. The surgeon has to take into account that injuries can occur outside his field of vision.

Since the rate of laparoscopic complication is strictly related to the difficulty of the procedure and to the surgeon's skills, it is challenging to find homogenous data on it. Taking into account that, compared with laparotomy, laparoscopy is a recently developed approach, not all the techniques are well-standardized. As, on one hand, the rates of complication decrease on basic procedures, on the other hand, surgeons try immediately to do more with the technique. Nevertheless, for benign gynecological surgery, laparoscopy has a lower risk of minor complications (approximately 40% less than in laparotomy), although the major complications rate does not differ.

Chapron et al. (1998) published a study of one of the biggest series of complications in gynecological laparoscopy showing an overall rate of complication of 4.64 per 1000 (Chapron et al. 1998). Incidence seems to increase according to the complexity of the procedure and to the number of organs involved and to decrease with surgeon experience.

The most challenging diseases that the gynecological surgeon may face is deep endometriosis and frozen pelvis, where the rate of complication is reported to be close to 2%, rising to 24% if the bowel is involved (Minelli et al. 2010). In these types of diseases, a complication is more likely to occur because of distorted anatomy that changes the normal relationship between organs and obscures the usual landmarks. Unfortunately, the pelvis is a complex place in which to work, and a gynecological surgeon must have a lot of complementary competencies to be prepared to face all the possibilities that pelvic surgery can offer to him. These competencies are not only related to basic knowledge, such as anatomy or techniques, but also lie on a thin line that separates gynecology from other specialities, such as urology and general surgery.

Although knowing about the risk factors for complications is easily acquired, the surgical skills required to prevent them take much time and energy to learn.

In analyzing a basic gynecological procedure such as hysterectomy, more than one center has reported a drop in the overall complication rate according to the surgeon's experience. Wattiez et al. (2002) reported a reduction of complication from 5.6% to 1.3% in two subsequent 6-year periods in the 1990, and a Finnish group reported a reduction of 11% per year over a period of 20 years (Brummer et al. 2008). In our experience, to reduce complications, the most important thing is to recognize when a procedure is too difficult and remove the scope before beginning the actual surgical procedure.

ENTRY COMPLICATIONS

These are the most common technique-related complications, and they occur during the setup for inserting the first and secondary trocar or inducing the pneumoperitoneum. This inevitable part of the procedure is the most risky because it is blind; even though numerous different techniques have been proposed, none of them has been proved to be totally safe.

Although many tools have been developed and much effort has been made to reduce this type of complication, the rate remains close to 40% of all complications and, unfortunately, may be fatal (Fuller et al. 2005). The most commonly reported major injuries related to entry into the abdominal cavity are related to bowel and major vessels, and the second, in particular, can lead to serious consequences. Fortunately, the overall rate of entry complication is quite rare, between 0.2 and 0.4 per 1000. Regarding minor complications, there are no clear reports and the debate between different techniques is still ongoing (Shirk et al. 2006).

Techniques comparison

Since the first report of laparoscopic complication was published 30 years ago (Levinson 1974), great attention has been paid to developing safer devices such as optical, radially expanding, and retractable shield trocars. Entry techniques can be classified into two main categories: closed (Veress needle, direct entry) and open (Hasson technique). After decades of experience, we believe that, even though each technique has its advantages, none can be considered completely safe. The most commonly used entry technique in gynecological surgery is, classically, the Veress needle, which has been adopted by almost 90% of gynecologists (versus 1% for direct entry techniques and 5% for open techniques).

In considering closed entry, more than one study has demonstrated a higher rate of complications when comparing closed Veress needle entry with direct entry in terms of both major and minor complications and a lower failure rate for open techniques, even if the level of evidence is low (Jiang et al. 2012). A recent comparison of the three different techniques reported a higher overall rate of minor complications associated with the Veress technique when compared with open and direct entry techniques, including omental injury, failed entry, and extraperitoneal insufflation (Angioli et al. 2013). Open and direct entry exhibit no difference in complication rates, but direct entry is faster and is associated with less local infection.

Concerning the type of trocar, a Cochrane review (Ahmad et al. 2012) reported a lower rate of complications using a radially expanding trocar compared with the standard trocar and lower minor complication rates using a blade trocar compared with a blunt one. Optical trocars seem to have some advantages, especially in terms of failure rate (Ahmad et al. 2012).

In our daily practice, we always use the direct entry technique except in cases of median abdominal scar, in which the Veress needle technique on Palmer's point is applied (where the presence of adhesion seems to be lower) (Palmer 1974).

Because there is no evident superiority of one technique over another, an expert surgeon must master all the techniques to be prepared to solve difficult cases; for the beginner, it is more important to become skilled in one technique before moving on to another.

General safety rules

When approaching laparoscopy, the surgeon must take into account that minor entry complications may occur and do all that is possible to reduce this possibility. To do this, few basic rules must be applied. As already stated, the most common complications during this part of the procedure are related to the bowel and vasculature, but the bladder may also be involved.

To reduce the risk of bladder injury, insertion of a Foley catheter before initial abdominal entry is mandatory. Doing so voids the bladder, thus moving it retropubic and making it more difficult to be injured.

Bowel injuries are more frequent in the case of adhesions and thus carefully choosing the entry technique and the placement of the first trocar is very important. The risk of adhesions is related to the type of previous surgeries, and the risk increases with the grade of invasiveness, tissue manipulation, and the occurrence of peritonitis (Robertson et al. 2010).

A prospective study including more than 700 patients demonstrated that, even without previous surgery, the risk of bowel injury due to intestinal attachment under the umbilicus cannot be dismissed. Comparing no previous surgery, laparoscopy, and horizontal and midline incision, the risk was 0.42%, 0.80%, 6.87%, and 31.46%, respectively (Audebert & Gomel 2000). In our experience, a primary umbilical insertion should be avoided in the case of a midline abdominal scar, and the surgeon should opt in favor of a Palmer's point insertion (**Figure 7.1**). To avoid injury to the stomach, a nasogastric tube must be placed before the insertion of the first trocar or the induction of pneumoperitoneum.

Although a bowel injury may not be a grave issue and usually can be easily managed laparoscopically without severe consequences if recognized intraoperatively, a vascular injury, by contrast, may be fatal.

The most commonly injured vessels during the insertion of the first trocar or the Veress needle are the iliac vessels, the aorta, the vena cava, and the aortic bifurcation, all due to their proximity to the umbilicus. The umbilicus lies perpendicularly over the bifurcation, and the distance between these two points is approximately 4 cm. At this level, all the structures of the abdominal wall are fused; this

makes the thickness of the abdominal wall almost constant, even in obese patients (**Figure 7.2**).

To avoid injuries to the midline vessels, it is important to neither place the patient in the Trendelenburg position nor place the legs in a lithotomy position before the insertion of the first trocar. These maneuvers cause a reduction of the distance between the promontorium and the abdominal wall, thus exposing the bifurcation to possible injury. In addition, the entry device must be inserted straight into the pelvis, where the space is wider; on the contrary a lateral deviation may cause iliac vessel injury.

Veress needle safety rules

The Veress needle is the most historically used device for induction of the pneumoperitoneum, and, over decades of experience, a huge number of safety rules have been developed. The needle must be grasped at mid-shaft, as one would a pencil, in order to reduce the length of the active part and avoid a sudden and too deep penetration into the abdominal cavity.

The angle of insertion must be close to 45°, while lifting up the abdominal wall. The valve must be open and the needle inserted using the muscles of the hand (not the arm). By doing so, once the peritoneum has been perforated, the needle's direction will be pointed toward the pelvis, and the flow of air through it will separate the bowel from the abdominal wall.

Once the needle is inserted, there are several techniques available to determine if it is well placed (double click, aspiration-insufflation-aspiration, drop, etc.), but, in our opinion, the most reliable is the assessment of intra-abdominal pressure. To assess abdominal pressure, the insufflator must be connected to the needle with the CO_2

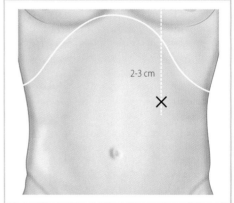

Figure 7.1 Palmer's point. This point is located 2–3 cm under the costal brim at the level of the mid-clavicular line and seems to be associated with fewer adhesions.

2-3 cm

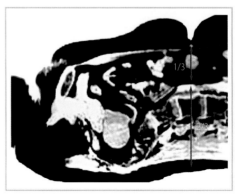

Figure 7.2 The umbilicus. The umbilicus is the thinnest part of the abdomen and is located perpendicularly over the aortic bifurcation. The distance between the abdominal wall and the vessels is one-third of the distance between the skin and the surgical table.

flow turned off. If the needle is properly inserted, the pressure will be lower than 10 mmHg and if the abdominal wall is lifted, the pressure will drop.

First trocar safety rules

Techniques for the insertion of the first trocar do not vary significantly whether a pneumoperitoneum has been already induced (via Veress needle) or not (the direct entry technique). When approaching this step, the surgeon must ensure that the skin incision is large enough to accommodate the trocar's size. Because the skin is not expandable, even few millimeters discrepancy may create a challenge. If the strength necessary to insert the trocar is too great, a too-small incision must be suspected. Applying too much strength to insert the trocar may results in loss of control of the device and in a sudden and deep penetration.

The trocar is inserted with one finger along the main axis of the device. The trocar is gently rotated, and the rate of penetration is kept slow and steady to reduce the risk of uncontrolled entrance. If pneumoperitoneum has been already inducted, a flow of gas through the valve will show that the abdominal cavity has been reached.

With the direct technique, the trocar is placed so that it enters the fascia at a 90° angle and then the abdominal wall is lifted; in this way, the trocar will change its angle in relation to the promontorium without changing its relationship with the fascia. Once the abdominal cavity is reached, the surgeon will feel an easily recognizable loss of resistance.

BOWEL COMPLICATIONS

Bowel complications represent more than 70% of all complications and they may be divided into two main groups: early and delayed. Early bowel complications are mainly related to direct injury due to trocar insertion and tissue manipulation; delayed complications are usually the result of thermal injury, obstruction, and anastomotic leak (**Figure 7.7**).

A review of 28 studies including 329,935 patients reported an incidence of laparoscopy-induced gastrointestinal injury of close to 0.36%. The small intestine was the most frequently injured (55%), and main cause of this injury was the Veress needle (41%), followed by thermal injury (25%), sharp dissection, and tissue manipulation. In 68.9% of bowel injuries, adhesions or a previous laparotomy were noted (van der Voort et al. 2004).

As reported by Chapron et al. (1998), the rate of bowel complication increases exponentially according to the complexity of the procedure. Bowel injuries are not a big issue if recognized immediately and treated intraoperatively, but, unfortunately, 15–50% are misdiagnosed in the first 24 hours, and this is more likely to happen in gynecological surgery. The misdiagnosis may lead to an increase of mortality that is reportedly as high as 3.6% (Bhoyrul et al. 2001).

Safety rules

If injuries caused by trocar insertion are not completely avoidable, a few basic rules may significantly reduce the rate of bowel injury. Electrosurgery, thermal injury, and tissue manipulation are among the main causes of bowel complications, and proper knowledge of instrument function is needed to avoid them.

It is well-known that using a laparoscopic grasper strongly reduces tactile feedback, and this must be taken into account when handling delicate tissues such as bowel. Tissue manipulation usually leads to minor injuries, such as serosa stripping, that are rarely followed by postoperative sequelae. Choose appropriate instruments with atraumatic jaws, such as flat grasper, and take a large bite while handling the bowel may be useful.

The rate of electrosurgical injury is between 2 and 5 per 1000, with bowel perforation occurring in 0.6–3 per 1000 cases. These are mainly due to accidental activation, direct coupling effect, and insulator failure (Wu et al. 2000). When using electrosurgery, lateral thermal spread must be considered while working close to sensitive organs, and this may change from one instrument to another. Because a metal instrument can conduct electrical energy, it can cause damage far from the place where it is applied, and so the coupling effect must be avoided. The coupling effect is more dangerous in laparoscopy than in laparotomy because of the restricted field of vision.

When applying any sort of energy to a device in order to coagulate, the temperature of the instrument's tip rises according to the type of energy and to the application time. On a bipolar instrument, the temperature can rise up to 100°C; on the ultrasonic device, very high temperatures can be reached, and the time needed to cool the device is correspondingly longer. When using ultrasound, the device must not be used to touch the bowel immediately after activation.

Diagnosis and treatment

A diagnosis of bowel injury is done intraoperatively in more than 35% of the cases, and a further 48% are discovered within the first 7 days (Chapron et al. 1999). Bowel injury symptoms may be delayed until 21 days, with mechanical injury presenting earlier than thermal injury (1.7 days versus 4.8 days) (Härkki-Sirén & Kurki 1997).

Any patient with abdominal complaints a few days postsurgery must be evaluated for possible bowel injury. Warning symptoms include nausea, vomiting, ileus, tachycardia, abdominal pain, and fever. In case of high suspicious, surgical exploration is needed; a simple X-ray scan is not sufficient because of the CO_2 remaining in the abdominal cavity after surgery, which may falsify the result.

A CT with oral and/or rectal contrast should be performed, and this can also reveal a hernia or abscess. If examinations are inconclusive and suspicion remains high, a second-look laparoscopy should be considered.

In certain circumstances, such as endometriosis or severe adhesions, the surgeon may be forced to perform a complete exploration of the abdomen at the end of the procedure, to check for signs, such as bowel content leakage or white lesions caused by thermal burns.

The intestinal segments most commonly affected by gynecological surgery are the rectum and the sigmoid. If a lesion is suspected, bowel integrity tests should be performed (blue dye and gas tests). To evaluate for perforation, the pelvis is filled with water and the rectum is filled with at least 60 mL of air injected through a probe or catheter. At the same time, the proximal part of the sigmoid is compressed with blunt forceps to keep the air distal. If a perforation occurs, the surgeon will see rising bubbles.

To assess a thinning or localize a perforation of the rectum of the wall, the rectum should be filled with methylene blue using the same technique as in the previous test. If a full-thickness injury has occurred, antibiotic prophylaxis should be administered (Makai & Isaacson 2009).

Regarding treatment, a small (< 1 cm) partial thickness or thermal injury can be easily repaired with a figure-of-eight stitch made with a 3-0 reabsorbable monofilament suture. To repair a deeper or wider defect, a two-layer interrupted closure may be needed; the involvement of the mucosa during suturing does not make a difference. Large defects that require resection are rare.

If the surgeon is not comfortable dealing with bowel issues, it is always better to ask for a general surgical consultation, even if the injury is diagnosed intraoperatively.

BLADDER COMPLICATIONS

Urinary complications in laparoscopy were, during the early days of the technique, higher than in laparotomy. However, with training and surgeon experience, these complications have decreased while offering the benefits of a minimally invasive procedure (Makinen et al. 2001). The rate of urinary tract injuries during benign gynecological procedures is between 1% and 3%, with approximately two-thirds of these involving the bladder (Nieboer et al. 2009).

Doganay et al. (2011) compared the surgical complications of hysterectomy according to the choice of procedure [abdominal (AH), vaginal (VH), and total laparoscopic hysterectomy (LH)]; he found that 0.7% of bladder injuries occurred in AH, 0.7% in total laparoscopic hysterectomies, and 0.4% in VH. These researchers therefore concluded that there was no significant difference in complications rates among these procedures (Garry et al. 2004). In several reviews that compared LH with AH, the rates of bladder injury were higher in LH, but statistically nonsignificant; although most of the studies included in this analysis were old and showed greater complications with the laparoscopic approach than do recent studies, results are still inconclusive.

Previous cesarean section has been demonstrated to increase the rate of bladder injuries due to the presence of fibrotic tissue at the level of the vesicovaginal septum (Konicxs et al. 2012). Thus, it is important to perform a careful dissection of this anatomical space in cases of previous cesarean section. A bladder injury is more likely to occur during complex procedures, such as deep endometriosis, but it is also the case that sometimes it is the disease itself that requires the bladder to be opened, and, in these cases, this cannot be considered a complication.

Some types of bladder complications may occur postoperatively, caused by the destruction of bladder innervation during procedures that require wide dissection. Deep endometriosis surgery is associated with urinary retention and/or bladder dysfunction (Konicxs et al. 2012). The incidence corresponds to nodule dimension, especially if the lesion requires bilateral dissection of the pararectal space. This is not surprising given the anatomy and the strict relationship of this anatomical space with bladder nerve supply.

The feasibility of a nerve sparing approach while facing deep endometriosis is related to the disease itself, and not to the surgeon, because the nodule may involve nerves that prevent further dissection and in those cases either endometriosis is left in place or part of the nerve is destroyed. Urinary retention generally resolves within a few weeks, occasionally after as long as 9 months. To prevent permanent bladder retention, we prefer to leave some endometriosis unilaterally, when complete excision of the nodule would risk damaging the parasympathetic nerve bilaterally. Another possible complication is vesicovaginal fistula; although this is rare it should be treated immediately by laparoscopy, thus avoiding development of extensive fibrosis (Konicxs et al. 2012).

Safety rules and treatment

A gynecological surgeon may deal with a huge variety of procedures with different levels of complexity, but there are some rules that can reduce the bladder injury rate.

When performing a total hysterectomy, the cleavage between the bladder and anterior vaginal wall has to be developed and the bladder dissected properly and pushed down sufficiently in order to perform the colpotomy (Karaman et al. 2007). To perform this step safely, the surgeon must present the full thickness of the bladder to his assistant. The assistant must be sure to lift the bladder, not only the peritoneum. Once lifted, the bladder will been seen as a weak white line that marks the boundary between the two different layers and shows the correct plane for the dissection (**Figure 7.3**).

Manipulating the uterus upward and downward can help in some cases. This dissection should be performed very carefully in cases of adhesions caused by previous cesarean section. Before performing anterior colpotomy, a vaginal electrically isolated valve is inserted, then pushed toward the site of incision. The bladder is kept at least 1 cm away from this incision. Using this technique, we have not had to perform cystotomy nor have we diagnosed urinary fistulas in our patients so far (Karaman et al. 2007).

Bladder injuries or thickness resection for endometriosis can be easily managed by laparoscopic surgery provided care is taken not to damage the intramural part of the ureter. If the suture is close to the ureter foramen, a stent should be inserted; in cases of wide bladder resection, the bladder should be open as high as possible, permitting the identification of the exact location of the ureters. The bladder wall can be sutured in one or two layers (in our daily practice, we use just one layer) using 3-0 monofilament (Wattiez et al. 2013). A methylene blue test with at least 150 mL must always be carried out to confirm bladder integrity after suturing (Wattiez et al. 2013). A bladder catheter is left in place for 7–10 days; it is unclear whether bladder healing should be checked at the time of catheter removal with a low pressure cystography (Konicxs et al. 2012).

Bladder injury during laparoscopy can be easily recognized by checking the Foley bag at the end of the procedure. If an injury occurred, the bag will be inflated (Nezhat et al. 1993, 1996). An examination of the bladder surface should be performed at the end of the procedure to detect thermal injuries, which appear as white marks on the muscularis.

In the case of thermal injury, a reinforcement stitch (3-0 monofilament, figure-of-eight or single stitch) may be placed to avoid postoperative fistula. This type of lesion may lead to a fistula up to 14 days after surgery. A vesicovaginal fistula can be diagnosed by instilling dye into the bladder via a Foley catheter, followed by direct examination of leakage into the vagina or by placement of a tampon. In patients who develop a vesicovaginal fistula, a urethral catheter should be placed. Some have described early spontaneous closure of surgical fistula (Blaivas et al. 1995, Waaldick 1994).

Cystoscopy should be carried out at the end of the procedure if the suture is close to the ureteral ostium to exclude its involvement during suturing. If the suture is very close to the ureter, and a kinking of the

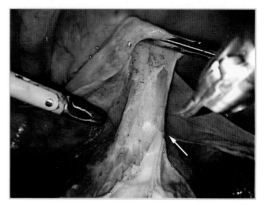

Figure 7.3
Bladder dissection. During vesicovaginal plane dissection, the assistant lifts the bladder, not only the peritoneum, in order to show the correct plane. It is often possible to see a white line on the upper part of the bladder (arrow).

ureter is suspected, a double J stent must be inserted; it must be left in place for 6–8 weeks (Onwudiegwu et al. 1991).

After bladder suturing, an indwelling catheter should be left in place for 10–15 days, according to the size of the lesion and the inflammatory state of the bladder. If there are doubts about the progress of healing, a low-pressure cystography may be performed to assess intra-abdominal leakage (Karaman et al. 2007).

In deep infiltrating endometriosis, the dissection strategy must be clear in order to avoid bladder dysfunction caused by excessive or too lateral pararectal fossa space or bilateral parasympathetic nerve resection; the latter must be considered even if the endometriotic implants are invading both nerves branch because has been demonstrated that conservative resection in at least one side nerve branch decreases bladder dysfunction.

In the case of bilateral dissection of the pararectal fossa, a clamping test of the Foley may be performed to assess the patient's bladder filling sensation. In cases of sensation impairment (filling sensation over 150 mL), the patient may be discharged with a catheter in place. Usually, these symptoms disappear after a few days.

■ URETERAL COMPLICATIONS

The anatomical proximity of the ureteral tract to the uterus and ovaries creates a risk for injury in any gynecological procedure, and ureter injuries are the most dreaded complication in gynecological surgery. Unfortunately, the course of the ureter in the pelvis renders it liable to injury during gynecological operations, particularly during hysterectomies (Wattiez et al. 2002).

The risk of a ureter injury significantly decreases with increasing surgeon experience, with a cutoff level of 30 performed laparoscopic hysterectomies (Wattiez et al. 2002). The reported incidence of ureter injuries during hysterectomies varies between 0% and 2.2% (Härkki-Sirén et al. 1998).

There are high-risk injury zones where most ureteral injuries occur during hysterectomy and other gynecological surgeries (Donnez et al. 2002). Patients with normal anatomy should have minimal risk for all ureteral injures if proper surgical techniques are followed. In women with abnormal anatomy, good surgical technique and anatomical landmarks will greatly reduce the likelihood of these complications (**Figure 7.4**).

Approximately 42% of all ureteral injuries occur in the pelvic brim. The second most common site of ureteral injury during hysterectomy is close to the cervix, where the uterine artery crosses the ureter (Ostrzenski et al. 2003).

Uterine artery bleeding can increase the risk of thermal ureteral injury or even ureteral partial ligation (kinking) when a hemostatic suturing or clipping technique is used.

Ureteral injury risk may be increased depending on the surgical complexity of the procedure, as can happen in deep endometriosis, large uterus hysterectomy, or excessive bleeding (Wattiez et al. 2002).

Ureteral endometriosis is found in about 10% of women with urinary tract endometriosis, and the incidence might be higher in women with rectovaginal nodules (Donnez et al. 2002). If the nodule is bigger than 2 cm, the risk of ureteral involvement increases, as does the rates of complications and injury. Ureteral transection is the most common intraoperative complication. In almost the half of all recognized ureteral injuries, transection often occurs due to dissection of structures close to the course of the ureter without proper ureteral visualization. During deep endometriosis surgery, thermal injury and vascular disruption is also described as possible ureteral complications, with laceration, obstruction, stenosis, and consequent fistula formation (Nezhat & Nezhat 1990).

■ Safety rules and treatment

The safety of advanced laparoscopies is highest in experienced hands; complications are usually related to surgeon inexperience. The ureters should be identified carefully during surgery, and it is essential to follow safety guidelines during the learning phase to decrease serious complications (Chapron et al. 1997).

During hysterectomy, surgeons must observe several safety rules: (1) the full visualization of the ureter avoids the most common injury, which is infundibulum pelvic ligament ligation; (2) recognition of the ureteral trajectory decreases the risk of injury; and (3) opening

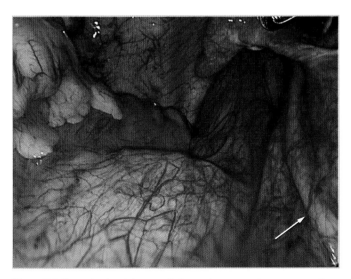

Figure 7.4 Ureter landmark. In case of distorted anatomy, the ureter must be searched for at the level of the pelvic brim where it crosses the external iliac vessels, taking into account that the ureter crosses the external iliac artery on the right side and the common on the left.

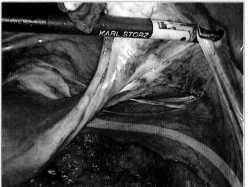

Figure 7.5
Broad ligament fenestration. A window is made on the broad ligament to allow the surgeon to coagulate safely the infundibulopelvic or the utero-ovarian ligament during a hysterectomy. The ureter (highlighted in yellow) remains outside the window.

a window in the broad ligament isolates the vascular ligament, thus permitting proper visualization of the structures beneath this area (**Figure 7.5**).

Manipulating the uterus has been demonstrated to be a safety step that reduces ureteral injury during hysterectomy. After vesicovaginal dissection, pushing the uterus upward separates the ureteral trajectory from the uterine artery ligation site; using an isolated vaginal valve when the colpotomy is performed also decreases the risk of ureteral injury (Garry et al. 2004).

To coagulate the uterine artery, the bipolar device must approach the artery with an angle as close as possible to 90° while the uterine manipulator pushes the uterus cranially to increase the distance between the ureter and the uterine artery. To do so, the bipolar must be placed in the ipsilateral trocar and not in the central one; the position should be changed from left to right according to the uterine artery side passing the bipolar to the assistant, while facing the left side.

In case of distorted anatomy, a careful ureterolysis must be performed, choosing as a starting point the pelvic brim where the ureter is easily recognizable. This is sometimes more difficult on the left side because it is covered by the sigmoid; in these cases, the physiological attachment of the sigmoid has to be freed.

Expectant management may be contemplated in cases of minor ureteral injury. An inadvertently clamped ureter should be released immediately, the ureter trajectory must be inspected, confirmation of normal peristalsis and color should be made, and a ureteral stent should be placed. The Foley catheter and stent should be removed after 10–14 days (Sakellariou et al. 2002). Thermal injury of the ureter or crushing should be managed in the same way. For other more serious injuries, as when the ureter loses its peristaltic mobility or extensive portions of vascularization are removed, resection must be performed.

If the ureteral injury is within 5 cm of the ureteral vesical junction, Utrie (1998) recommended reimplantation. The anastomosis into the bladder should be performed with a psoas hitch to relive tension (Nezhat et al. 2004) (**Figure 7.6**).

For ureteral injuries located >5 cm from the bladder, an end-to-end reanastomosis should be performed over a ureteral stent (Nezhat et al. 1998). After the segment is removed, the ureter is cut diagonally and reanastomozed over an indwelling stent that should be left in place for 10–14 days. Sakellariou et al. (2002) advocated the end-to-end

anastomosis technique closer than 2.5 cm to the bladder if there is no pelvic pathology that would contraindicate the procedure.

To prevent long-term complications such as urinoma or reduced kidney function, ureter injuries should be recognized as soon as possible. A ureteral injury is repaired more easily if discovered intraoperatively, and patients will not need to be subjected to a second major, unplanned, and extensive reoperation.

VASCULAR COMPLICATIONS

In the MAUDE database, vascular injuries were the most common cause of death after laparoscopy. This does not reflect their true incidence because many nonlethal major vascular injuries go unreported, and those that are caused by nontrocar injury are almost never reported. Thus, the true incidence of vascular injuries during laparoscopy is unknown despite being the most devastating complication of this technique.

Laceration injury to the mesentery occurs commonly with trocar insertion, and previous abdominal surgery is the most commonly reported risk factor. Significant omentum adhesions requiring release are a common laparoscopic dilemma. These vessels are encased only in fatty tissue and are retracted and difficult to locate. Mesenteric injuries from trocar insertion are possibly associated with bowel injury or large abdominal vessel injury.

The inferior epigastric vessels are the most common site of vascular trocar injury (Redwine 1997, 2003). The vessels are injured during the placement of the lateral trocars. Large pyramidal or cutting trocars are more likely to cause this injury because their width and triangular cutting path results in lateral laceration of the vessels.

Large-vessel injury is the most catastrophic injury that can occur during laparoscopy. The literature reports an incidence of 0.04–0.5%. Injuries to the large vessels can be the result of trocar insertion, inadvertent perforation by an operating probe, or a perforation during adjacent dissection (Shirk et al. 2006). The large venous structures are more easily damaged than the arterial because of their thinner walls. Their offset anatomic positioning makes it easy to damage the common iliac veins during lymph node dissection and even during sacrocolpopexy.

SAFETY RULES AND MANAGEMENT

Recognition of mesenteric vessel injuries can be difficult, but, when recognized, one should observe for hematoma formation. Mesenteric vessel laceration can be treated by ligation or dissection. However, care should be taken to ensure that achieving hemostasis does not devascularize a segment of bowel; the bowel should be observed for signs of ischemia.

Anatomical landmarks of the abdominal wall must be respected to avoid epigastric injury. Lateral trocars must be placed under visual control and lateral to the rectoabdominal muscles in the so-called safe area (**Figure 7.8**). The superficial vessel may be identified through transillumination and the deep one through direct visualization with the scope. This visual step should be used as safety rule for trocar placement. For lateral ports sites, the use of conical tip or dilating trocars may provide increased safety in this area.

Because of the presence of two bleeding ends, the vessels must be sutured cephalic and caudally of the trocar placement site using a laparoscopic approach and a through-and-through abdominal loop suture. The loop suture can be placed for 8 hours and then removed. Another fast method is to pass a Foley catheter into the abdomen through the trocar and then insufflate the balloon and remove the trocar before pulling it towards the abdominal wall until the bleeding stops, and then blocking it in this position with a laparotomic forceps.

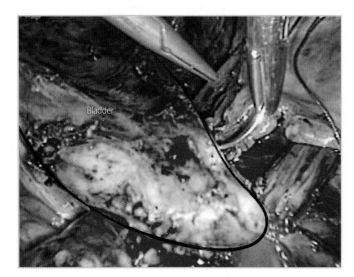

Figure 7.6 Psoas hitch. Releasing the tension on a ureter implantation with a psoas hitch.

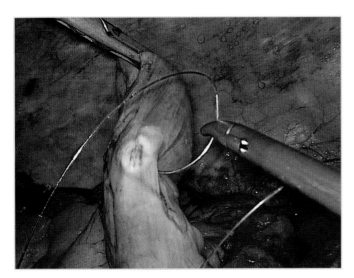

Figure 7.7 Bowel thermal injury. A typical aspect of thermal injury of the bowel.

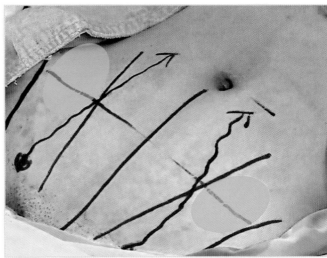

Figure 7.8 Secondary trocar placement. The common landmarks of the abdominal wall (muscles, epigastric vessels, iliac spines) define a safe area to place the lateral trocar (green).

Mayor vascular injury must be avoided. If a large vessel is injured, treatment success depends on rapid recognition and immediate laparotomy using longitudinal incisions to achieve rapid manual tamponade. After hemostasis has been achieved by vascular compression, dissection can proceed with placement of vascular clamps proximal and distal to the injury.

Although large-vessel injury (such as to the iliac vessels) could be laparoscopically managed, when an injury occurs, the surgeon should immediately clamp one end of the vessel with a noncutting instrument and the assistant should clamp the other end of the vessel; the injury is laparoscopically sutured using nonabsorbable 4-0/6-0 thread.

Vascular control below the pelvic brim is basic to all major laparoscopic gynecological procedures. The ability to dissect in the retroperitoneal space is a mandatory skill required for advanced laparoscopic surgery. Anatomic organ vascularization knowledge should be applied in cases of vascular injury, and a vascular branch, such as the hypogastric vessels or the uterine artery, can be sacrificed or even temporarily clamped for hemostatic control.

When the pathologic condition encountered creates a high risk of uncontrolled bleeding, a predissection examination of vital structures such as the ureter and uterine artery is indicated. The uterine artery can be identified and isolated by finding the umbilical ligament. This artery is the first branch of the anterior branch of the hypogastric artery and can be traced safely and ligated distal to this origin point. If there is loss of hemostasis in the broad and/or cardinal ligament, lateral ligation of the uterine artery is the best immediate solution and can be performed by laparoscopic approach.

■ REFERENCES

Ahmad G, O'Flynn H, Duffy JM, et al. Laparoscopic entry techniques. Cochrane Database Syst Rev 2012; 2:CD006583.

Angioli R, Terranova C, De Cicco Nardone C, et al. A comparison of three different entry techniques in gynecological laparoscopic surgery: a randomized prospective trial. Eur J Obstet Gynecol Reprod Biol 2013; 171:339–342.

Audebert AJ, Gomel V. Role of microlaparoscopy in the diagnosis of peritoneal and visceral adhesions and in the prevention of bowel injury associated with blind trocar insertion. Fertil Steril 2000; 73:631–635.

Bhoyrul S, Vierra MA, Nezhat CR, et al. Trocar injuries in laparoscopic surgery. Am Coll Surg 2001; 192:677–683.

Blaivas JG, Heritz DM, Romanzi LJ. Early versus late repair of vesicovaginal fistulas: vaginal and abdominal approaches. J Urol. 1995; 153:1110–1112; discussion 1112–1113.

Brummer TH, Seppälä TT, Härkki PS. National learning curve for laparoscopic hysterectomy and trends in hysterectomy in Finland 2000–2005. Hum Reprod 2008; 23:840–845.

Chapron C, Dubuisson JB, Querleu D, Pierre F. Complications of laparoscopy: a prospective multicentre observational study. Br J Obstet Gynaecol 1997; 104:1419–1420.

Chapron C, Pierre F, Harchaoui Y, et al. Gastrointestinal injuries during gynaecological laparoscopy. Hum Reprod 1999; 14:333–337.

Chapron C, Querleu D, Bruhat MA, et al. Surgical complications of diagnostic and operative gynaecological laparoscopy: a series of 29,966 cases. Hum Reprod 1998; 13:867–872.

Coleman RL, Muller CY. Effects of a laboratory-based skills curriculum on laparoscopic proficiency: a randomized trial. Am J Obstet Gynecol 2002; 186:836–842.

Doğanay M, Yildiz Y, Tonguc E, et al. Abdominal, vaginal and total laparoscopic hysterectomy: perioperative morbidity. Arch Gynecol Obstet 2011;284:385-389.

Donnez J, Nisolle M, Squifflet J. Ureteral endometriosis: a complication of rectovaginal endometriotic (adenomyotic) nodules. Fertil Steril 2002; 77:32–37.

Fuller J, Ashar BS, Carey-Corrado J. Trocar-associated injuries and fatalities: an analysis of 1399 reports to the FDA. J Minim Invasive Gynecol 2005; 12:302–307.

Garry R, Fountain J, Brown J, et al. EVALUATE hysterectomy trial: a multicentre randomised trial comparing abdominal, vaginal and laparoscopic methods of hysterectomy. Health Tech Assess 2004; 8:26.

Härkki-Sirén P, Kurki T. A nationwide analysis of laparoscopic complications. Obstet Gynecol 1997; 89:108–112.

Härkki-Sirén P, Sjoberg J, Tiitinen A. Urinary tract injuries after hysterectomy. Obstet Gynecol 1998; 92:113–118.

Jiang X, Anderson C, Schnatz PF. The safety of direct trocar versus Veress needle for laparoscopic entry: a meta-analysis of randomized clinical trials. J Laparoendosc Adv Surg Tech A 2012; 22:362–370.

Karaman Y, Bingol B, Günenç Z. Prevention of complications in laparoscopic hysterectomy: experience with 1120 cases performed by a single surgeon. J Minim Invasive Gynecol 2007; 14:78–84.

Konicxs P, Ussia A, Adamyan L, et al. Deep endometriosis: definition, diagnosis and treatment. Fertil Steril 2012; 98:564–571.

Levinson CJ. Laparoscopy is easy—except for the complications: a review with suggestions. J Reprod Med 1974; 13:187–194.

Makai G, Isaacson K. Complication in gynecological laparoscopy. Clin Obstet Gynecol 2009; 52:441–411.

Makinen J, Johanson, Tomas C, et al. Morbidity of 10 110 hysterectomies by type approach. Hum Reprod 2001; 16:1473–1478.

Minelli L, Ceccaroni M, Ruffo G, et al. Laparoscopic conservative surgery for stage IV symptomatic endometriosis: short-term surgical complications. Fertil Steril 2010; 94:1218–1222.

Nezhat CH, Malik S, Nezhat F, et al. Laparoscopic ureteroneocystostomy and vesicopsoas hitch for infiltrative endometriosis. JSLS 2004; 8:3–7.

Nezhat C, Nezhat FR. Ureteral injuries at laparoscopy: insight into diagnosis, management, and prevention. Obstet Gynecol 1990; 76:889–890.

Nezhat CR, Nezhat FR. Laparoscopic segmental bladder resection for endometriosis: a report of two cases. Obstet Gynecol 1993; 81:882–884.

Nezhat CH, Nezhat F, Seidman D, Nezhat C. Laparoscopic ureteroureterostomy: a prospective follow-up of 9 patients. Prim Care Update Obstet Gynecol 1998; 5:200.

Nezhat CH, Seidman DS, Nezhat F, et al. Laparoscopic management of intentional and unintentional cystotomy. J Urol 1996; 156:1400–1402.

Nieboer TE, Johnson N. Lethaby A, et al. Surgical approach to hysterectomy for benign gynaecological disease. Cochrane Database Syst Rev 2009; 3:CD003677.

Onwudiegwu U, Makinde OO, Badejo OA, et al. Ureteric injuries associated with gynecologic surgery. Int J Gynaecol Obstet 1991; 34:235–238.

Ostrzenski A, Radolinski B, Ostrzenska KM. A review of laparoscopy ureteral injury in pelvic surgery. Obstet Gynecol Surv. 2003; 58:794–799.

Palmer R. Safety in laparoscopy. J Reprod Med 1974; 13:1–5.

Redwine DB. Complications of sharp and blunt adhesiolysis. In: Corfaman R, Diamond M, DeCherney A (eds), Complications of Endoscopy, 2nd ed. Boston, MA: Blackwell, 1997:78–81.

Redwine DB. Principles of monopolar electrosurgery. In: Redwine DB (ed), Surgical treatment of endometriosis. London: Dunitz, 2003:61–70.

Robertson DL, Lefebvre G, Leyland N, et al. Adhesion prevention in gynaecological surgery. J Obstet Gynaecol Can 2010; 32:598–608.

Sakellariou P, Protopapas AG, Voulgaris Z, et al. Management of ureteric injuries during gynaecological operations: 10 years experience. Eur J Obstet Gynecol Reprod Biol 2002; 101:179–184.

Shirk GJ, Johns A, Redwine DB. Complications of laparoscopic surgery: How to avoid them and how to repair them. J Minim Invasive Gynecol 2006; 13:352–359.

Utrie JW Jr. Bladder and ureteral injury: prevention and management. Clin Obstet Gynecol 1998; 41:755–763.

van der Voort M, Heijnsdijk EA, Gouma DJ. Bowel injury as a complication of laparoscopy. Br J Surg 2004; 91:1253–1258.

Waaldick K. The immediate surgical management of fresh obstetrics fistulas with catheter and/or early closure. Int J Gynaecol Obstet 1994; 45:11–16.

Wattiez A, Puga M, Albornoz J, Faller E. Surgical strategy in endometriosis. Best Pract Res Clin Obstet Gynecol 2013; 27:381–392.

Wattiez A, Soriano D, Cohen SB, et al. The learning curve of total laparoscopic hysterectomy: comparative analysis of 1647 cases. J Am Assoc Gynecol Laparosc 2002; 9:339–345.

Wu MP, Ou CS, Chen SL, et al. Complications and recommended practices for electrosurgery in laparoscopy. Am J Surg 2000; 179:67–73.

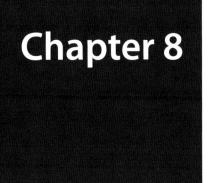

Chapter 8

Complications of hysteroscopic surgery – how to avoid and manage

Jan Bosteels, Bruno van Herendael

INTRODUCTION

Hysteroscopic surgery in general has a low risk of adverse events with an incidence of around 0.28% of 13,600 procedures according to an often cited large Dutch multicenter study (Janssen et al. 2000). A similar incidence of 0.24% was found in a German observational study that included 21,676 procedures (Aydeniz et al. 2002). It is clear that the risk of complications is increased in more complex operative procedures, e.g. in hysteroscopic myomectomy the risk might be as high as 10% (Propst et al. 2000). Complications of hysteroscopic surgery may be due to patient positioning, anesthesia, access problems, the use of distending media, gas emboli, perforation of the uterine wall, bleeding, the use of electrosurgical instruments, infection, or may be caused by the formation of intrauterine adhesions (IUAs), the dissemination of endometrial cancer cells, or unwanted pregnancy (Loffer 1995). The complications discussed in this chapter do not constitute an exhaustive list. We have limited the discussion to the most frequently occurring or potentially life-threatening complications for didactical and practical reasons. Randomized controlled trials (RCTs) on the effectiveness of strategies to prevent complications do exist; nevertheless, since adverse events are rare, an RCT is not an ideal study design to measure surgical complications. A large body of the presented evidence on complications due to hysteroscopic surgery is based on observational studies with an inherent high risk of bias.

METHODS

In preparing this chapter, we searched the Cochrane Database of Systematic Reviews (CDSR), Issue 1 of 12, January 2014 using the simple and broad search strategy 'MeSH descriptor: [Hysteroscopy] explode all trees.' We retrieved 308 records including 6 Cochrane reviews, 23 other reviews, 254 trials, 9 technology assessments, and 16 economic evaluations. We conducted a search in MEDLINE through PubMed using ['complications' (Subheading) OR complications(Text Word) AND (hysteroscopy)]. This search retrieved 1505 records including 232 reviews and 49 systematic reviews (SRs). We decided to include only the reviews retrieved in MEDLINE. Our search in these two electronic databases resulted in 589 records. We used specialized software (EndNote) to remove 34 duplicates. The remaining 555 records were screened for eligibility by screening the titles and abstracts. After removing 394 articles that were clearly irrelevant, we retrieved 161 records of potentially eligible studies. We also searched clinical practice guidelines through National Guideline Clearinghouse or the websites of international societies in obstetrics and gynecology.

We only included SRs of observational studies or RCTs studying interventions for the prevention of complications in hysteroscopic surgery. We excluded studies on patient compliance, pain management, or diagnostic accuracy.

RESULTS

We decided to use a simplified classification between distension medium-related complications and other adverse events for didactical reasons only. Other review authors have used different classifications, e.g. according to the phase of the intervention (Cooper & Brady 2000).

Complications related to the use of distension media

The use of distension media in hysteroscopic surgery enables to convert the virtual cavity of the uterus to a suitable working space by overcoming the resistance of the uterine musculature. Moreover, the preset pressure has to be sufficient to prevent the mixing of blood into the distension medium; otherwise, the blurred vision would increase the likelihood of adverse events. The intravasation of distending media can however contribute to potentially very troublesome complications in operative surgery.

Use of gas as distension medium

Carbon dioxide is a very safe distension medium due to its rapid absorption into the blood and its clearance during pulmonary ventilation (Salat-Baroux et al. 1984). It is not suitable for the use of operative hysteroscopy or when the patient is bleeding. High-quality evidence from RCTs has demonstrated that the use of carbon dioxide is associated with increased patient discomfort, reduced patient satisfaction, and longer intervention times compared to the use of distension fluids (Pellicano et al. 2003, Brusco et al. 2003). Significant adverse events have been reported in the literature including gas emboli (Mahmoud & Fraser 1994, Brink et al. 1994, Groenman et al. 2008). Therefore, carbon dioxide is almost never used in present day hysteroscopic surgery.

Use of fluid as distension medium

Most hysteroscopic procedures are done using fluid distension media. The type of solution is determined by the choice of the electrosurgical modality and the surgeon's practice (Bradley 2002). In general, electrolytic fluids are used with bipolar instruments and nonelectrolytic fluids are used with monopolar instrumentation. There is always one basic rule of thumb for the use of fluid distension media: the surgical team needs to be very vigilant in the monitoring of fluid use. Regardless of their nature, all fluids used in hysteroscopic surgery can be associated with serious life-threatening complications. High-viscosity distending media, e. g. Hyskon (a hyperosmolar solution of 32% dextran in 10% glucose) were often used in the past because they have the advantage of being immiscible with blood (Cooper & Brady 2000). Their use could lead to anaphylactic reactions in 1:1,500–1:300,000 procedures (Borten et al. 1983), pulmonary edema (Lukascko 1985), and disseminated intravascular coagulopathy (Iediekin et al. 1990). High-viscosity distending media are moreover not suitable for use in the continuous flow hysteroscopes, needed to do operative procedures. We therefore have distinguished between electrolytic and nonelectrolytic fluid distension media since this reflects present daily practice. The incidence of fluid overload due to excessive intravasation associated with operative hysteroscopy is estimated in the literature between 0.1% and 0.2% (Aydeniz et al. 2002, Janssen et al. 2000).

Electrolytic fluids

The isotonic electrolytic fluids most often used in operative hysteroscopy are normal saline and Ringer's lactate. In case of excessive intravascular absorption, their physiologic osmolality in general prevents hyponatremia or hypoosmolality. As a general principle, the excessive intravasation of isotonic electrolytic fluids will lead to hypervolemia, which is more amenable to treatment and less dangerous than fluid overload due to nonelectrolytic fluids [American Association of Gynecologic Laparoscopists (AAGL) 2013].

Nonelectrolytic fluids

Electrolytic fluid distending media are not suitable for use with monopolar instrumentation because they disperse the electric current. The electrolyte-free low-viscosity media include 3% sorbitol, 1.5% glycine, 5% mannitol, and combined solutions of sorbitol and mannitol. In general, the excessive intravasation of this type of distending media will cause hypervolemia in combination with hyponatremia and hypo-osmolality. This may lead to the transurethral resection of the prostate) syndrome first described in urological surgery. This potentially life-threatening syndrome is characterized by hyponatremia, hypo-osmolality, nausea, vomiting, and neurologic symptoms including muscular twitching, blurring of the vision, grand-mal seizures, agitation, and if left undiagnosed or inadequately treated, lethargy, coma, convulsions, and even death (Arieff 1987). Premenopausal women are 25 times more likely than men or postmenopausal women to die or have permanent brain damage should hyponatremic encephalopathy occur (Ayus et al. 1992). Moreover, additional complications may develop on top, related to some specific characteristics of the nonelectrolytic fluid distension medium used. Sorbitol is a reduced form of dextrose; when absorbed in the systemic circulation, it is either excreted by the kidney or metabolized by the fructose pathway. Its use is therefore not suited for use in diabetic patients. Glycine is a nonconductive amino-acid with a plasma half-life of 85 minutes; it is uniquely metabolized in the liver to ammonia and free water, further decreasing plasma osmolality. Due to its toxic effect on the central nervous system, the consequences of the excess fluid absorption are aggravated by a hyperammonemic encephalopathy characterized by transient blindness, muscle pain, and memory loss. Mannitol is an isomer of sorbitol; it may act as an osmotic diuretic by increasing both the sodium and extracellular water excretion since it is not absorbed by the renal tubules (AAGL 2013).

◼ Other complications
Complications related to the patient positioning and anesthesia

Nerve trauma, direct trauma, and acute compartment syndrome may be encountered as complications related to patient positioning in the lithotomy position (Munro 2010).

Femoral neuropathy is due to a combination of excessive hip flexion, abduction, and external hip rotation leading to an extreme angulation of the femoral nerve beneath the inguinal ligament and resulting in compression and damage to the femoral nerve. This injury usually resolves spontaneously but may take several months of intensive and painful physiotherapy. The sciatic and peroneal nerves are fixed to the sciatic notch and the neck of the fibula, making them vulnerable to stretch injury. Excessive hip flexion, especially with a straight knee or excessive pressure over the head of the fibula from a stirrup, may lead to neural injury with a drop foot and lateral lower extremity paresthesia.

The acute compartment syndrome occurs when increased pressure in the muscle of an osteofascial compartment compromises local vascular perfusion causing ischemia. The period of ischemia is followed by reperfusion, capillary leakage from the ischemic tissue, and a further increase in tissue edema leading to neuromuscular compromise. This causes rhabdomyolysis and possible serious sequelae including permanent disability (Dua et al. 2002).

Finally, as is the case with any surgical procedure, there is a spectrum of anesthesia-related complications that may be fatal for the patient. These include adverse events related to the use of anxiolytics and systemic analgesics in general anesthesia and allergic reactions, systemic injection of local anesthetics, and overdose associated with the use of local anesthesia (Erickson et al. 2010).

Trauma to the uterus and cervix

Traumatic injuries caused by hysteroscopy are more frequent during operative hysteroscopy than diagnostic procedures because more dilatation is necessary for the introduction of the larger caliber hysteroscopes (Loffer 1995). Cervical lacerations are caused by the tenaculum during dilatation, especially when a single-toothed instrument is used. If the bleeding is brisk, suturing may be required. The cervix or the uterus may be perforated during dilatation or insertion of the hysteroscope. The incidence of perforation varies from 4 to 13 per 1,000 procedures as reported in the literature (Grimes 1982). Perforations caused by Hegar dilators require no treatment. Most full-thickness perforations are near the fundus if proper traction on the tenaculum is applied. In most cases, the procedure cannot be continued due to loss of adequate distension. Perforations due to the hysteroscopic procedure usually occur as a consequence of either poor visualization or lack of adequate uterine distension. When mechanical or thermal energy is used, visceral lesions may occur (Cooper & Brady 2000). Anterior wall perforations may lead to bladder injury. Ureteral damage is associated with posterior or lateral perforations due to difficult endometrial resection or intramural myomectomy. Perforations in the lateral uterine wall may cause vascular lesions in the iliac vessels, mesenteric artery, aorta, and presacral vessels (Valle 1998). These lesions may cause broad ligament hematomas or significant hemorrhage and should be treated without any delay when diagnosed or suspected. Any perforation associated with the concomitant use of electrosurgery or laser carries a high risk of visceral injury. These cases should be explored by laparoscopy for damage to the bladder, ureters, bowel, and vessels. In doubt a laparotomy should be done to discount visceral trauma fully. Patients treated or suspected for visceral injury should be kept under close medical surveillance for several days until full recovery. Penetrating thermal injury to the bowel has been reported to be managed successfully with primary repair (Sullivan et al. 1992).

Air or gas embolism

Air embolism is a very rare but potentially fatal complication of hysteroscopic surgery. It was documented in relation with hysteroscopic surgery for the first time in 1985. An overview of several cases including fatalities has been published in the literature (Brooks 1997). A more recent overview (Groenman et al. 2008) included 13 cases with a mortality rate of nearly 50%. The early detection of gas or air embolism based on altered-electrocardiographic patterns, an acute rise in the pulmonary artery pressure, or aspiration of air from a central venous line should lead to end the procedure, turning the patient to the left side to elevate and keep gas in the right side of the heart and start cardiopulmonary resuscitation. During any hysteroscopic procedure, slight anti-Trendelenburg position can be adopted to minimize the negative aspiration pressure during the cardiac cycle. Cervical trauma should be minimal and the cervical canal should be occluded as long as possible – leaving the Hegar dilator in situ after dilatation to be replaced by the operative hysteroscope. It is likewise important to try to minimize taking in and out the instruments as much as possible.

Bleeding

Intra- or postoperative bleeding is the second most common complication of hysteroscopic surgery: it occurs in 2.5 per 1000 procedures (Hulka et al. 1995). The incidence rates are higher for hysteroscopic resection of fibroids, especially with an intramural component (2–3%), and for endometrial ablation or resection procedures (0.2–2.2%) (Loffer 1994). Problematic bleeding during an operative hysteroscopy is rare because the pressure of the distension medium decreases blood loss from venous vessels. At the base of most fibroids, arterial vessels can deliver enough blood into the distension medium to blur adequate vision. Electrocoagulation with a wire loop or a roller-ball or barrel can stop such bleeding. At the end of the procedure, decreasing the intrauterine pressure while visualizing the entire uterine cavity can reveal any occult bleeding. To stop troublesome bleeding at the end of the procedure, a Foley catheter may be inserted in the uterine cavity and its balloon may be filled with 20–30 mL of saline. Take into account that this maneuver is extremely painful for the patient. The bleeding usually stops due to the tamponade and the balloon catheter may be removed in 2–24 hours (Goldrath 1983). If this fails to stop the bleeding, vasopressin (20 U in 20 mL normal saline) may be injected into the cervix to inhibit bleeding from the lower segment. Misoprostol can be given intrarectally if needed. If these methods fail, uterine artery embolization may be considered by an interventional radiologist. If all other methods fail, hysterectomy may be indicated in case of profuse life-threatening bleeding (Cooper & Brady 2000).

Infection

The incidence of endomyometritis following hysteroscopy is extremely low, ranging from 0.01% to 1.42% (Munro 2010). Routine antibiotic prophylaxis is not recommended for the general population undergoing hysteroscopic surgery according to the ACOG (2009) (level B recommendation according to the method described by the US Preventive Services Task Force) and Society of Obstetricians and Gynecologists of Canada (SOCG) guidelines (Van Eyk et al. 2012) (II-2D using the Canadian Task Force on Preventive Health Care System for the quality of evidence assessment). The risk of infectious complications might be higher following synechiolysis or after resectoscopy in women with a history of pelvic inflammatory disease (PID) ; therefore, the ACOG guideline states that antibiotic prophylaxis may be considered for hysteroscopic interventions in women with a history of PID or tubal damage (2009) (level C recommendation).

Late complications

Intrauterine adhesions

IUA formation is the major long-term complication of operative hysteroscopy in women of reproductive age. According to an RCT on the effectiveness of preoperative treatment before operative hysteroscopy, the incidence of postsurgical IUAs at second-look hysteroscopy was 3.6% after polyp removal, 6.7% after resection of uterine septa, 31.3% after removal of a single fibroid, and 45.5% after resection of multiple fibroids (Taskin et al. 2000). The postoperative formation of IUAs is undesirable in women wishing to conceive or to preserve their fertility.

The removal of several fibroids or fibroids on opposing walls probably increases this risk. Recurrence of intrauterine synechiae is even more challenging. When extensive adhesions are lysed, little normal endometrium may remain to be re-epithelialized and the risk of recurrence is very high. Especially in the lateral and fundal parts, it is very difficult to keep the walls separated (Loffer 1995).

Hematometra

Hematometra following an endometrial resection or ablation occurs very infrequently: about 1–2% of women will develop symptomatic hematometra following these procedures (Hill et al. 1992). Hematometra may develop if scarring or narrowing of the endometrial cavity occurs in women of reproductive age or those using hormone replacement therapy: cyclic or chronic lower pelvic pain is the most dominant symptom. Most cases can be treated by cervical dilatation, although some cases need to be treated by synechiolysis to approach hematometra in the uterine fundus (Hill et al. 1992). When the endometrium in the cornual region is inadequately treated, a postablation tubal sterilization syndrome may develop, characterized by crampy, unilateral or bilateral cyclic pelvic pain accompanied by vaginal spotting. Identifying and avoiding the lower uterine segment and cervix is very important in the prevention of hematometra. For decreasing the risk of a postablation tubal sterilization syndrome, the endometrium in the cornual region should be effectively destroyed (Loffer 1995).

Iatrogenic adenomyosis

At present, there is still controversy whether endometrial resection or ablation may cause iatrogenic adenomyosis. It is clear that adenomyosis may be already present before the hysteroscopic intervention. Others have hypothesized that endometrial resection is more prone to cause iatrogenic adenomyosis than ablation because resection might not uniformly remove all of the deeper lying normal endometrium (McLucas & Perrella 1995).

Unplanned pregnancy

Although a transcervical tubal sterilization is technically very feasible due to the easy approach of both ostia by hysteroscopy, pregnancies do occur after hysteroscopic sterilizations (Loffer 1993); however, they are less common with the newer generation devices. Unplanned pregnancies may be observed in women who were not sterilized previously following endometrial ablation. The incidence in the literature varies from 0.2% to 1.6% (Whitlaw et al. 1992). Pregnancies following operative hysteroscopic procedures must be considered as being at high risk of a variety of medical problems including miscarriage, ectopic pregnancy, uterine rupture, premature birth, intrauterine growth restriction, and higher risk of placenta accreta/percreta (Loffer 1995).

Dissemination of endometrial cancer cells

A recent systematic review and meta-analysis (Polyzos et al. 2010) has demonstrated a significantly higher occurrence of malignant peritoneal cytology following hysteroscopy versus no hysteroscopy in women with proven endometrial carcinoma [the odds ratio (OR) was 1.8, 95% confidence interval (CI) 1.1–2.8, $P = 0.013$, 9 studies, 1015 women]. There was a higher rate of disease upstaging compared with no hysteroscopy (OR 2.6, 95% CI 1.5–4.6, $P = 0.001$, 9 studies, 1015 women). The use of normal saline increased the rate of malignant peritoneal cytology compared to no hysteroscopy (OR 2.9, 95% CI 1.5–5.6, $P = 0.002$, 9 studies, 1015 women); there was no evidence for an increased occurrence of malignant endometrial cells in the peritoneal cytology in the intervention group when inflated media pressure reached or exceeded 100 mmHg (OR 3.2, 95% CI 0.94–11, $P = 0.06$). The authors concluded that additional randomized studies are needed to investigate if the increased risk of disseminating malignant endometrial cells affects the prognosis.

DISCUSSION

The most appropriate way to manage complications is by timely prevention of adverse events. This should ideally start long before the actual intervention itself. We will discuss several strategies according to the phase of the intervention.

Preoperative phase

In recent literature, several SRs with meta-analysis have reported on the effectiveness of misoprostol before hysteroscopy to prime the cervix (Crane & Healy 2006, Selk & Kroft 2011, Gkrozou et al. 2011). One SR including 10 studies demonstrated a reduced need for further cervical dilatation [risk ratio (RR) was 0.61, 95% CI 0.51–0.73], a lower rate of cervical laceration (RR 0.22, 95% CI 0.09–0.56), and increased cervical dilatation (weighted mean difference was 2.64, 95% CI 1.73–3.54) in premenopausal women treated by misoprostol prior to hysteroscopy (Crane & Healy 2006). There was an increased incidence of side effects following the administration of misoprostol for cervical priming before operative hysteroscopy, including vaginal bleeding (RR 11.09, 95% CI 3.08–40.00), cramping (RR 7.98, 95% CI 3.38–18.84), and elevated temperature (RR 5.24, 95% CI 1.37–20.09). The authors concluded that the use of misoprostol for cervical priming before hysteroscopy might be beneficial but additional studies are needed to identify the dosage, route of administration, and the timing of the administration of misoprostol to the intended intervention. Moreover, additional research is needed on the effectiveness of misoprostol in postmenopausal women or those treated with gonadotropin-releasing hormone (GnRH) agonists. The second SR with meta-analysis included 17 RCTs comparing misoprostol versus placebo prior to hysteroscopy (Gkrozou et al. 2011). Following the use of misoprostol, there was a decrease in the need for cervical dilatation in a combined population of pre- and postmenopausal women (RR 0.75, 95% CI 0.59–0.96, $P = 0.02$, 7 studies, 707 women); there was evidence for substantial statistical heterogeneity [Chi^2 = 17.19, df = 6 ($P = 0.009$); I^2 = 65%]. There was no evidence favoring the use of misoprostol for decreasing the incidence of cervical tears (RR 0.47, 95% CI 0.22–1.01, $P = 0.05$, 8 studies, 828 women). The authors concluded that there is insufficient evidence to recommend the routine use of misoprostol before every hysteroscopy. A third SR and meta-analysis (Selk & Kroft 2011) included seven RCTs. There was no evidence for an effect favoring the use of misoprostol for increasing cervical dilatation [the mean difference was 0.85 mm, 95% CI 0.58–2.27 mm, $P = 0.24$, 6 studies, 506 women); there was evidence for substantial statistical heterogeneity (Chi^2 = 411.01, df = 7 (P <0.001); I^2 = 98%]. There was no evidence for an effect favoring the use of misoprostol on surgical complications (cervical lacerations, uterine perforation, and false passage): the RR was 0.65, 95% CI 0.19–2.26, $P = 0.50$, 7 studies, 545 women. There was an increase in side effects (cramps, vaginal bleeding, nausea, and diarrhea) in the intervention group (RR 4.28, 95% CI 1.43–12.85, $P = 0.01$, 4 studies, 374 women). The authors concluded that their findings did not rule out a possible benefit of misoprostol on cervical dilatation or surgical complications. There was evidence for an increase in side effects associated with the routine use of misoprostol before hysteroscopy. The present evidence does not support the routine use of preoperative misoprostol in all women before hysteroscopy (Selk & Kroft 2011). It is clear that there is, at present, no definitive evidence for recommending the routine use of misoprostol in all women before hysteroscopy. This evidence is based on clinically diverse populations of pre- and postmenopausal women before diagnostic and/or operative hysteroscopies. Moreover, there are large differences between the dosage used and the route and the timing of the administration. Women should be counseled that there is an increase in side effects and that definitive evidence of a benefit is lacking; a reappraisal of the present evidence using, e.g. the systematic approach proposed by the Cochrane collaboration is needed to study the effectiveness of the use of misoprostol in a properly defined high-risk subgroup and if this evidence is not definitive, pragmatic RCTs are needed before recommending the use of misoprostol as a cervical priming agent.

There is consistent evidence from five observational studies that the use of GnRH agonists might reduce the degree of fluid overload associated with the use of distending media and the impact of hyponatremic hypotonic encephalopathy (AAGL 2013). One RCT (Mavrelos et al. 2010) demonstrated a trend for a decreased fluid overload in the group treated with GnRH as compared to the control groups but the differences were not statistically significant. The use of GnRH analogs might be considered in women with large submucous fibroids (>4 cm) before hysteroscopic myomectomy to shrink the diameters of the fibroids and to decrease the incidence of serous fluid overload.

The risks of fluid overload related to the use of fluid distending media may be reduced by limiting the degree of preoperative hydration with oral or intravenous fluids (AAGL 2013). It is advisable to obtain baseline levels of the serum electrolytes in women taking diuretics or with medical conditions predisposing to electrolyte imbalance during surgery (AAGL 2013).

The risk of the fluid overload increases when the myometrial integrity is breached, e.g. during hysteroscopic removal of fibroids. Women should have been counseled that more than one procedure might be required (Evidence level B).

Operative phase

Three RCTs have demonstrated the effectiveness of injecting dilute vasopressin into the cervix immediately prior to hysteroscopy in decreasing the incidence of serous fluid intravasation (Corson et al. 1994, Phillips et al. 1996, Goldenberg et al. 1996) (Evidence level A). All three studies have demonstrated the greatest impact on women undergoing hysteroscopic myomectomy. Large systemic doses of vasopressin have resulted in cardiovascular collapse, myocardial infarction, and death. Therefore, the AAGL guidelines do not recommend using vasopressin in concentrations that exceed 0.4 U/mL (2013).

During surgery, the uterine cavity distension pressure should be the lowest pressure that sufficiently distends the cavity: it should be below the mean arterial pressure according to the AAGL guidelines (2013) (Evidence level A). It is always important to purge the air bells out of the automated pump system and tubing: the liquid-containing bag should be changed during the procedure before it gets empty (Evidence level C).

The statements on the limits of fluid intravasation are based on expert opinion. In healthy women, a fluid deficit of 1000 mL has been suggested as the upper limit when using hypotonic distension media and 2500 mL when using isotonic solutions. For the elderly and women with comorbidity, e.g. compromised cardiovascular health, the AAGL guidelines recommend a maximum fluid deficit of 750 mL. The use of normal saline is recommended, whenever possible, given the additional risks of hyponatremia and hypo-osmolality associated with the use of the nonelectrolytic fluid distension media with monopolar surgery. When the limits of fluid intravasation have been reached, the measurement of serum electrolytes and osmolality is recommended.

The use of an automated fluid management is highly recommended in operative hysteroscopy. Although necessary, its use is not by itself sufficient to prevent all cases of fluid overload. The surgical team needs to monitor accurately the fluid input and output. The anesthesiologist should closely monitor the vital parameters.

The addition of 2% ethanol to a mannitol/sorbitol distension medium has proved to be useful for screening for rapid fluid intravasation in women treated for resection of uterine fibroids, endometrium ablation, or septum resection (Evidence level A) (Aydeniz et al. 1995). The use of oxytocin infusion was associated with lower levels of ethanol in the blood, smaller decreases in serum sodium, and decreased glycine deficit compared to a control group in women undergoing transcervical resection of the endometrium for abnormal uterine bleeding (Evidence level A)

(Shokeir et al. 2011). There was a trend for a decrease in operative blood loss measured by hematocrit but the differences were not statistically significant.

Postoperative phase

When serious complications occur such as fluid overload or gas embolism, monitoring the patient on the intensive care unit under close surveillance of a dedicated team with adequate knowledge of the pathophysiology and treatment of the condition is mandatory. Before leaving the hospital or the day care unit, all women treated by hysteroscopy should be informed to seek assistance of the treating physician without any delay in case of severe bleeding, abdominal pain, fever of unknown origin, or malaise.

REFERENCES

AAGL. AAGL Practice Report: Practice guidelines for the management of hysteroscopic distending media. JMIG 2013; 20:137–148.

American College of Obstetricians and Gynecologists (ACOG). Antibiotic prophylaxis for gynaecologic procedures.Washington (DC) 2009 ACOG Practice Bulletin no. 104.

Arieff AI. Hyponatremia associated with permanent brain damage. Adv Intern Med 1987; 32:325–344.

Aydeniz B, Wallwiener D, Rimbach S, et al. Is co-administration of ethanol to the distension medium in surgical hysteroscopy a screening method to prevent fluid overload? A prospective randomized comparative study of ablative versus non-ablative hysteroscopy and various ethanol concentrations. Gynakol Geburtshilfliche Rundsch 1995; 35:108–112

Aydeniz B, Gruber IV, Schauf B, et al. A multicenter survey of complications associated with 21,676 operative hysteroscopies. Eur J Obstet Gynecol Reprod Biol 2002; 104:160–164.

Ayus JC, Wheeler JM, Arieff AI. Postoperative hyponatremic encephalopathy in menstruant women. Ann Intern Med 1992; 117:891–897.

Borten M, Siebert CP, Taymor ML. Recurrent anaphylactic reaction to intraperitoneal dextran 75 used for prevention of postsurgical adhesions. Obstet Gynecol 1983; 61:755.

Bradley LD. Complications in hysteroscopy: prevention, treatment and legal risk. Curr Opin Obstet Gynecol 2002; 14:409–415.

Brink DM, DeJong P, Fawcus S, et al. Carbon dioxide embolism following diagnostic hysteroscopy. Br J Obstet Gynaecol 1994; 101:717–718.

Brooks PG. Venous air embolism during operative hysteroscopy. J Am Assoc Gynecol Laparosc 1997; 4:309–422.

Brusco GF, Arena S, Angelini A. Use of carbon dioxide versus normal saline for diagnostic hysteroscopy. Fertil Steril 2003; 79:993–997.

Cooper JM, Brady RM. Intraoperative and early postoperative complications of operative hysteroscopy. Obstet Gynecol Clin North Am 2000; 27:347–366.

Corson SL, Brooks PG, Serden SP, Batzer FR, Gocial B. Effects of vasopressin administration during hysteroscopic surgery. J Reprod Med 1994; 39:419–423.

Crane JMG, Healy S. Use of misoprostol before hysteroscopy: a systematic review. J Obstet Gynaecol Can 2006; 28:373–379.

Dua RS, Bankes MJ, Dowd GS, et al. Compartment syndrome following pelvic surgery in the lithotomy position. Ann R Coll Surg Engl 2002; 84:170–171.

Erickson TB, Kirkpatrick DH, DeFrancesco MS, et al. Executive summary of the American College of Obstetricians and Gynecologists Presidential Task Force on patient safety in the office setting: reinvigorating safety in office-based gynecologic surgery. Obstet Gynecol 2010; 115:147–151.

Gkrozou F, Koliopoulos G, Vrekoussis T, et al. A systematic review and meta-analysis of randomized studies comparing misoprostol versus placebo for cervical ripening prior to hysteroscopy. Eur J Obstet Gynecol Reprod Biol 2011; 158:17–23.

Goldenberg M, Cohen SB, Etchin A, Mashiach S, Seidman S. The effect of intracervical vasopressin on the systemic absorption of glycine during hysteroscopic endometrial ablation. Obstet Gynecol 1996; 87:1025–1029.

Goldrath MJ. Uterine tamponade for the control of acute uterine bleeding. Am J Obstet Gynecol 1983; 147:869–872.

Grimes DA. Diagnostic dilation and curettage: a reappraisal. Am J Obstet Gynecol 1982; 142:1–6.

Groenman FA, Peters LW, Rademaker BPM, Bakkum EA. Embolism of air and gas in hysteroscopic procedures: pathophysiology and implication for daily practice. JMIG 2008; 15:241–247.

Hill D, Maher P, Wood C, et al. Complications of operative hysteroscopy. Gynaecol Endosc 1992; 1:185–189.

Hulka JF, Peterson JA, Philips JM, et al. Operative hysteroscopy: American Association of Gynecologic Laparoscopists 1993 membership survey. J Am Assoc Gynecol Laparosc 1995; 2:131–132.

Iediekin R, Olsfanger D, Kessler I. Disseminated intravascular coagulopathy and adult respiratory distress syndrome: life-threatening complications of hysteroscopy. Am J Obstet Gynecol 1990; 44:162.

Janssen FW, Vredevoogd CB, van Ulzen K, et al. Complications of hysteroscopy: a prospective, multicenter study. Obstet Gynecol 2000; 96:266–270.

Loffer FD. Hysteroscopic tubal occlusion. In: Sutton C, Diamond M (Eds), Endoscopic surgery for gynaecologists. London: WB Saunders, 1993:345–354.

Loffer FD. Removing intrauterine lesions: Myomectomy and polypectomy. In: Bieber EJ, Loffer FD (Eds), The gynecologic resectoscope. Cambridge: Blackwell Scientific, 1994:186–194.

Loffer FD. Complications of hysteroscopy—their cause, prevention, and correction. J AAGL 1995; 3:11–23.

Lukascko P. Noncardiogenic pulmonary edema secondary to intrauterine instillation of 32% dextran 70. Fertil Steril 1985; 44:560–561.

Mahmoud F, Fraser IS. CO2 hysteroscopy and embolism. Gynaecol Endosc 1994; 3:91–95.1995; 4:123–127.

Mavrelos D, Ben-Nagi J, Davies A, et al. The value of pre-operative treatment with GnRH analogues in women with submucous fibroids: a double-blind, placebo-controlled randomized trial. Hum Reprod 2010; 25:2264–2269.

McLucas B, Perrella R. Does endometrial resection cause adenomyosis? Gynaecol Endosc 1995; 4:123–127.

Munro MG. Complications of hysteroscopic and uterine resectoscopic surgery. Obstet Gynecol Clin North Am 2010; 37:399–425.

Pellicano M, Guida M, Zullo F, et al. Carbon dioxide versus normal saline as a uterine distension medium for diagnostic hysteroscopy in infertile patients: a prospective, randomized, multicenter study. Fertil Steril 2003; 79:418–421.

Phillips PR, Nathanson HG, Milim SJ, et al. The effect of dilute vasopressin solution on blood loss during operative hysteroscopy: a randomized controlled trial. Obstet Gynecol 1996; 88:761–766.

Polyzos NP, Mauri D, Tsioras S, et al. Intraperitoneal dissemination of endometrial cancer cells after hysteroscopy. A systematic review and meta-analysis. Int J Gynecol Cancer 2010; 20:261–267.

Propst AM, Liberman RF, Harlow BL, et al. Complications of hysteroscopic surgery: predicting patients at risk. Obstet Gynecol 2000; 96:517–520.

Salat-Baroux J, Hamou JE, Maillard G, et al. Complications from microhysteroscopy. In: Siegler AM, LIndemann HJ (eds), Hysteroscopy: principles in practice. Philadelphia: JB Lippincott, 1984:112–117.

Selk A, Kroft J. Misoprostol in operative hysteroscopy. A systematic review and meta-analysis. Obstet Gynecol 2011; 118:941–949.

Shokeir T, El-Lakkany N, Sadek E, El-Shamy M, Abu Hashim H. An RCT: use of oxytocin drip during hysteroscopic endometrial resection and its effect on operative blood loss and glycine deficit. JMIG 2011; 18:489–493.

Sullivan B, Kenney P, Siebel M. Hysteroscopic resection of fibroid with thermal injury to sigmoid. Obstet Gynecol 1992; 80:546–547.

Taskin O, Sadik S, Onoglu A, et al. Role of endometrial suppression on the frequency of intrauterine adhesions after resectoscopic surgery. J Am Assoc Gynecol Laparosc 2000; 7:351–354.

Valle RF. Urinary tract, gastrointestinal, and vascular injuries with uterine perforation. In: Hysteroscopic complications and solutions. Postgraduate course syllabus. Int Cong Gynaecol Endosc 1998:30–35.

Van Eyk N, van Schalkwyk J, Infectious Diseases Committee. Antibiotic prophylaxis in gynaecologic procedures. SOGC Clinical practice guideline. J Obstet Gynaecol Can 2012; 34:382–391.

Whitlaw NL, Garry R, Sutton CJG. Pregnancy following endometrial ablation: 2 case reports. Gynaecol Endosc 1992; 1:129–132.

Chapter 9 Laparoscopy in pregnancy

Jessica A Shepherd, Shan M Biscette

Nonobstetrical surgery is required in pregnancy in up to 1 in 500 women and the most common surgeries are those related to acute appendicitis, cholecystitis, and some form of intestinal obstruction. Those related to pelvic conditions include ovarian cysts, ovarian torsion, or symptomatic masses. Other indications for surgery include trauma injuries, complications of inflammatory bowel disorders, and rarely adrenal, hepatic, and splenic disorders.

Pregnancy was once considered a relative contraindication to laparoscopy out of concern that lack of blood flow to the fetus and placenta could induce abortion. Over time this has been re-evaluated, and laparoscopy is now recognized as a practical mode of surgical access in pregnancy. In one review, Affleck et al. noted no fetal loss, uterine injury, or birth defects among 67 pregnant women who underwent laparoscopic procedures. Laparoscopy is generally safer than open surgery because it offers the patient a quicker recovery, less incidence of thromboembolic events, and decreased incidence of postoperative ileus. Whenever possible, however, surgery should be delayed until the second trimester to reduce the risk of miscarriage and potential teratogenic effects.

■ NONOBSTETRIC SURGERY IN PREGNANCY

Appendectomy is the most common nonobstetric surgery performed in pregnancy; the laparoscopic approach has become progressively utilized as the mode of access and is considered by many to be the standard of care. Prompt evaluation of the pregnant patient is essential to decrease morbidity, especially if there is a high clinical suspicion of appendicitis. The incidence of acute appendicitis is highest in the second trimester and lowest in the third. Of note, perforation of the appendix occurs twice as often in the third trimester (69%) compared to the first and second trimesters.

The diagnosis of appendicitis can be complex as the presentation can be obscured by the anatomic shift of the appendix with the gravid uterus. When the diagnosis of appendicitis by ultrasound is equivocal, the surgeon may then choose to proceed with admitting the patient for observation and serial examinations, CT scan, or diagnostic laparoscopy for early diagnosis and decreased risk of rupture. When considering diagnosis and imaging, studies show that 25% of all pregnant women with acute appendicitis will progress to perforation, hence the need for careful examination of these patients. Delaying surgery for >24 hours can increase the perforation rate to 66% compared to 0% when these patients are taken for diagnostic laparoscopy within 24 hours.

Gallstones are also common in pregnancy and occur in approximately 12% of all pregnancies (de Bari 2014). Physiologic changes occurring during pregnancy predispose the pregnant woman to biliary disease and gallstone formation. Although gallstones occur in up to 12% of pregnant patients, only 0.05% will become symptomatic, and 40% of those with symptoms will need surgical intervention (Halkic 2006). The incidence of symptomatic cholelithiasis is 30–40% higher in pregnant patients as compared to the general population.

Early surgical management of symptomatic cholelithiasis is favored over conservative management in the pregnant patient as a delay in aggressive management can lead to increased morbidity and fetal loss. There is a 13% increased risk of gallstone pancreatitis with an associated 15% risk of maternal mortality in cases that are managed conservatively (Thomas 1998). The rate of fetal loss also increases from 5% to 60% in cases that are managed nonsurgically as compared to those managed surgically (Thomas). Conservative management of women presenting in the first trimester results in a 92% recurrence rate, a 64% recurrence rate in the second trimester, and 44% recurrence rate in the third trimester (Graham). Additionally, an increased rate of hospitalization, spontaneous abortions, preterm labor, and preterm delivery is observed when symptomatic cases are managed conservatively (Reedy 1997, Shay 2001).

Surgery is indicated in any trimester for cases of failed medical therapy, evidence of obstructive jaundice, gallstone pancreatitis, or peritonitis. Laparoscopic access to the right upper quadrant is feasible even with advancing gestational age; however, the proximity of the gravid uterus in the late third trimester may necessitate modifications in the laparoscopic approach.

■ ADNEXAL MASSES

Adnexal masses are diagnosed in approximately 1 in 600 pregnancies (Fatum 2001). The majorities of these masses are benign and comprise mature cystic teratomas, functional cysts, and benign cystadenomas. Malignancy is encountered in 1–8% of adnexal masses (Whitecar 1999).

Observation of adnexal masses encountered in the first trimester is reasonable in cases of functional cysts, as these tend to resolve spontaneously by the second trimester. Surgical intervention is reserved for masses that persist into the second trimester, are symptomatic, or show malignant characteristics. Careful consideration should be given to potential complications that can occur with observation of large adnexal masses such as adnexal torsion, ovarian cyst rupture, peritonitis, or hemorrhage. Approximately 10–15% of adnexal masses undergo torsion (Webb & Yen 2015). The presenting symptoms of adnexal torsion are often nonspecific and diagnostic imaging may not always yield unequivocal results. Early laparoscopic evaluation provides an opportunity to diagnose adnexal torsion as well as offer treatment in the form of detorsion or cystectomy, often with ovarian preservation. In cases of late diagnosis of adnexal torsion resulting in a nonviable ovary, oophorectomy is indicated and postoperative initiation of progesterone therapy is recommended if the corpus luteum is removed, and the gestation is <12 weeks.

■ PHYSIOLOGIC CHANGES

The physiologic changes in pregnancy are essential to consider when preparing a pregnant patient for surgery. Significant cardiovascular and pulmonary changes occur that include increases in blood volume, cardiac output, oxygen consumption and CO_2 production, and decreases in functional residual capacity. The alterations seen during the establishment and maintenance of pneumoperitoneum as well as position changes will be heightened in pregnancy, as the diaphragm is limited in its expansion. These limitations will increase the peak airway pressure and decrease functional reserve capacity. Therefore, it is prudent to communicate with anesthesia when the patient is in Trendelenburg position as the intrathoracic pressure will be increased and possibly create an atmosphere of hypercapnia and hypoxemia. The fetus is sensitive to increased levels of maternal CO_2 that can lead to fetal acidosis, which predisposes the need for careful intraoperative maternal monitoring and fetal monitoring postoperatively.

Within pregnancy, there is the phenomenon of increased total body water that will become an important feature for anesthesia and fluid replacement. Maternal blood volume increases 40–45% mostly within the second trimester. Fluid replacement preoperatively, intraoperatively, and postoperatively should be carefully managed to prevent excessive cardiac strain as cardiac output is increased from the fifth week of gestation.

PREOPERATIVE ASSESSMENT

Patients should have blood tests sent and have cross-matched blood for all major surgeries. As there are changes in the respiratory system, it is important to establish aspiration prophylaxis and recognize the decreased requirements for anesthesia and postoperative intravenous medications. If there are any concerns of maternal cardiopulmonary issues, an ECG should be done to rule out any complications. ECG changes during pregnancy include left-axis deviation, premature beats, and nonspecific ST and T-wave changes.

Evaluation of the fetus is also required both preoperatively and postoperatively to ensure continued viability.

Due to the changes physiologically in pregnancy, each patient should be specifically triaged preoperatively for:

- Any risks that would be increased with admistration of anesthesia
- Techniques to maintain pneumoperitoneum safely
- Any additional factors that would increase the risk of thromboembolic events (Srivastava 2010)

Anesthesia

During laparoscopy, the use of CO_2 for intraperitoneal insufflation has caused some concern for effects to the fetus. With the potential effects of acidosis once a consideration, there have been no long-term adverse side effects noted with the use of CO_2 for pneumoperitoneum. For the anesthesiologist, maintaining maternal physiological function while optimizing uteroplacental blood flow and oxygen delivery is a principal part of the procedure.

Most laparoscopic surgeons use 12–15 mmHg for the maintenance of the pneumoperitoneum and also position the patient in a left decubitus position away from the inferior vena cava after the first trimester to prevent hypotension. This positioning of the patient will allow left uterine displacement. When insufflating and performing the procedure, it is also important to maintain end-tidal CO_2 between 32–34 mmHg and observe that maternal blood pressures stay within 20% of baseline (Srivastava). Fetal heart tones are taken prior to anesthesia preoperatively as well as postoperatively to ensure fetal well-being and no effects of hypoxemia, and the patient can also be monitored with a tocometer to confirm that there is no stimulation of the myometrium from oxytocic effects.

Imaging

For patients who present with a pelvic mass or abdominal pain, the radiographic study chosen depends on the complexity and urgency of the presentation. Ultrasonographic imaging during pregnancy is safe and useful for the identification of a pelvic mass or to find the etiology of acute abdominal pain in the pregnant patient. The degree of discomfort of the patient should be taken into consideration to allow expeditious and accurate diagnosis and should also take precedence over concerns for ionizing radiation. When consulting with radiology for imaging studies on a pregnant patient, the amount of radiation dosage should be limited to 5–10 rads (Table 9.1).

Concern over substantial exposure to radiation is warranted as it may lead to chromosomal mutations, neurologic abnormalities, mental retardation, and increase the risk of childhood leukemia. The dosage necessary for each type of radiation varies and should be addressed before choosing which one is appropriate. Another important feature of radiation risk is fetal age as mortality is greatest when there is exposure prior to oocyte implantation within the first week of conception. The recommended dosage from this time, the first week of conception, through to 25 weeks of gestational age is <5–10 rads. Between weeks 10 and 17 gestation, one must be aware of the sensitivity to possible CNS teratogenesis and it is advisable to avoid nonurgent X-rays. When patients consent for radiographic studies, it should be explained that exposure of the fetus to 0.5 rad will increase the risk of spontaneous abortion, malformations, and mental retardation to one additional case in 6,000 above baseline risk. Studies show that at ≤5 rads the risk to the fetus is negligible and risk is increased when the dosage is >15 rads. Recommendations include 5–10 rads as a cumulative dose of radiation in pregnancy while a single diagnostic study should not surpass 5 rads.

OPERATIVE TECHNIQUE

These procedures begin with proper consent of the patient that outlines risks, benefits, and alternatives. Each patient must understand the risk of fetal loss with the procedure. Elective surgery should not be done in pregnancy, and for emergent cases, surgery is often delayed until the second trimester to reduce the risk of both teratogenicity and miscarriage. Foley catheters should be placed in all patients as the risk of bladder perforation can be increased with the displacement of the bladder by the gravid uterus. A nasogastric tube should be inserted by anesthesia to decrease the risk of gastric perforation. Once the patient is placed in the left lateral position, careful consideration should be taken to the level of rise of the gravid uterus. For patients in the first trimester, peritoneal access can be obtained via Veress needle or open laparoscopy as both are safe to use. Once the primary trocar has been placed, the remaining accessory trocars can be placed according to the procedure type and the surgical teams' preference. **Figure 9.1**

Table 9.1 Amount of radiation dosage in different imaging studies

Study	Radiation dosage (Rads)
Chest radiograph	<0.001
Abdominal series	0.245
Pelvic radiograph	0.04
Upper gastrointestinal series	0.05–0.1
Barium enema	0.3–4
HIDA scan	0.15
Chest CT scan	0.01–0.2
Abdominal CT scan	0.8–3
Pelvic CT scan	2.2

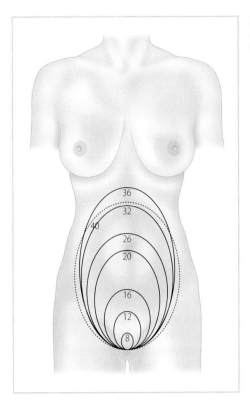

Figure 9.1
Abdominal levels for gravid uterus.

shows the level of height that the gravid uterus occupies and how to adjust the trocar entry.

Once the trocars have been safely inserted and the abdomen and uterus have been surveyed for any injury, the use of CO_2 for insufflation should remain within 10–15 mmHg. Increased pressures of CO_2 are not advised as the diaphragm in a pregnant patient is displaced upward and results in decreased residual lung volume as well as functional residual capacity. These efforts will help reduce any potential pulmonary physiology in addition to adverse outcomes to the fetus.

VENOUS THROMBOEMBOLIC PROPHYLAXIS

Pregnancy is associated with a hypercoagulable state owing to increased venous stasis and changes in the coagulation pathway. The increased plasma levels of fibrinogen and all clotting factors, except XI and XIII, place the patient at an increased risk of thromboembolic complications, which remain a common source of morbidity and mortality associated with pregnancy. The incidence of deep venous thrombosis (DVT) in pregnancy is 0.1–0.2% and the increase in vascular compliance leads to venous stasis (James 2006), which is exacerbated under anesthesia.

There is concern that the utilization of pneumoperitoneum in laparoscopy and the compression of the major abdominal vessels by the gravid uterus may further increase the risk of DVT as a result of decreased venous return. The compression of the gravid uterus impedes venous return and worsens as gestational age increases due to the size of the uterus.

Research pertaining to prophylaxis in the pregnant patient is sparse; therefore, general principles of laparoscopic surgery are often applied to this population. Recommendations for prophylaxis include the use of pneumatic compression devices both intraoperatively and postoperatively, as well as early ambulation. Heparin-based therapy may be utilized in women who require anticoagulation as this does not cross the placenta and therefore does not affect the fetus. Though there is no data for the use of unfractionated or low molecular weight heparin for prophylaxis in this patient population, heparin has been proven safe and is the agent of choice.

CONCLUSION

Laparoscopy in pregnancy provides a form of surgical intervention that can be performed at all gestational ages and offers numerous benefits: shorter recovery times, decreased analgesia, and decreased risk to the fetus as well as shorter hospital stays. Although there was initially concern with laparoscopy regarding the physiologic changes and positioning of the patient, evidence indicates that it does not pose a risk. Each case must be assessed carefully, especially for those patients with cardiovascular and pulmonary diseases. Fetal heart rate should be documented and evaluated pre- and postoperatively and tocolytic agents started for any uterine activity.

With the advances in laparoscopic surgery, it is feasible in pregnancy with stricter guidelines that need to be adhered to. The benefits of laparoscopic surgery are the same as for those patients that are non pregnant and allow a shorter recovery which is especially beneficial in pregnancy. Another aspect to consider is the surgical expertise of the surgeon and which approach is most appropriate for the procedure. Surgeons who are not comfortable with offering a laparoscopic approach to pregnant patients may want to consider referring the patient to an experienced laparoscopic surgeon.

Although there are limited studies of laparoscopic surgery in pregnancy, there appears to be a promising future for using this technique.

REFERENCES

Halkic N, Tempia-Caliera AA, Ksontini R et al. Laparoscopic management of appendicitis and symptomatic cholelithiasis during pregnancy. Langenbecks Arch Surg 2006; 391:467–471.

Fatum M, Rojansky N. Laparoscopic surgery during pregnancy. Obstet Gynecol Surv 2001; 56:50–59.

Thomas SJ, Brisson P. Laparoscopic appendectomy and cholecystectomy during pregnancy: six case reports. JSLS 1998, 2:41–46.

Shay DC, Bhavani-Shankar K, Datta S. Laparoscopic surgery during pregnancy. Anesthesiol Clin N Am 2001; 19:57–67.

Reedy MB, Galan HL, Richards WE, et al. Laparoscopy during pregnancy. A survey of laparoendoscopic surgeons. J Reprod Med 1997; 42:33–38.

Whitecar PM, Turner S, Higby KM. Adnexal masses in pregnancy: a review of 130 cases undergoing surgical management. Am J Obstet Gynecol 1999; 181:19–24.

Webb KE, Sakhel K, Chauhan SP, Abuhamad AZ. Adnexal mass during pregnancy: a review. Am J Perinatol 2015; 32:1010–1016.

Yen C-F, Lin S-L, Murk W, et al. Risk analysis of torsion and malignancy for adnexal masses during pregnancy. Fertil Steril 2009; 91:1895–1902.

de Bari O, Wang TY, Liu M, et al. Cholesterol cholelithiasis in pregnant women: pathogenesis, prevention and treatment. Ann Hepatol 2014; 13:728–745.

Srivastava A, Niranjan A. Secrets of safe laparoscopic surgery: Anaesthetic and surgical considerations. J Minim Access Surg 2010;6:728–745.

James AH, Jamison MG, Brancazio LR, Myers ER. Venous thromboembolism during pregnancy and the postpartum period: incidence, risk factors, and mortality. Am J Obstet Gynecol 2006; 194:1311–1315.

Chapter 10 | Laparoscopic tissue extraction

Sarah L Cohen, Mobolaji O Ajao

INTRODUCTION

The advent of minimally invasive gynecologic surgery has been accompanied by novel procedure-related challenges, including the retrieval of surgical specimens through small abdominal wall incisions. There are limited gynecologic procedures in which the tissue removed is likely to be smaller or at least close to the size of the laparoscopic ports (e.g. peritoneal biopsies or adnexal surgery for small cystic lesions). As more advanced procedures are now being performed laparoscopically, there is an increasing need for methods to extricate larger specimens. Various techniques and devices have been developed to retrieve larger specimens from the abdominal cavity without compromising the minimally invasive approach; this chapter will review the available means of tissue removal during laparoscopic surgery.

EXTENSION OF PORT SITES

Most laparoscopic instruments are designed to be utilized with ports ranging from 5 to 15 mm in size. In addition to up-sizing to a larger trocar, one simple option is to enlarge the skin and fascial incisions under direct vision to accommodate specimen removal. This may be performed with a combination of sharp dissection and blunt stretching in order to achieve desired incision dimensions. This particular technique may be most useful for cases of adnexal or small myoma removal. Additionally, several single incision access ports are available and may be employed with an incision size of 2–3 cm, thereby accommodating specimen removal as well. It is suggested that the fascia is closed when the defect measures >10 mm to prevent port site hernia formation (Kadar et al. 1993, Montz et al. 1994).

SPECIMEN RETRIEVAL BAG

Specimen retrieval bags are particularly useful for removing a structure intact with the goal of avoiding spillage or contamination of the abdominal cavity (see **Figures 10.1** and **10.2**). For example, with a cystic adnexal mass, the specimen is isolated within a specimen retrieval bag and then removed from the abdomen intact or following decompression in an enclosed space. This approach minimizes the risk of chemical peritonitis that may accompany rupture of dermoid cysts, as well as the risk of spread of malignant cells in cases of ovarian cancer.

Choices of specimen retrieval bags include free bags introduced into the abdomen with grasping instruments versus bags introduced via a syringe/plunger introducer tube. The diameter of the introducer shaft is typically 10–15 mm, and the bags are designed with a draw string or pull tab in place at the open end. The capacity of these specimen containment devices varies depending on the manufacturer, ranging anywhere from 175 to 1500 cc when using an introducer, or up to 3000 cc with free-standing bags.

The technique for specimen removal using a retrieval bag begins with insertion of the bag via a ≥10 mm port. The specimen is placed into the bag using gentle maneuvering and with assistance of a laparoscopic grasper. The bag is then cinched down and subsequently withdrawn from the abdominal cavity. If the specimen is unable to be removed intact via the trocar site, the bag may be brought through the skin incision at this site and opened. Next, the specimen can be decompressed or removed via manual morcellation. In some instances, such as ovarian cystectomy for a large cystic adnexal mass, it may be useful to place a specimen retrieval bag underneath the adnexa prior to beginning surgical dissection in an attempt to contain any spillage that could occur during this process (Nezhat et al. 1999).

COLPOTOMY AND CULDOTOMY

When a total laparoscopic hysterectomy or trachelectomy is performed, the circumferential incision about the cervix provides an opening of 5–6 cm in length that communicates with a natural orifice: the vagina. Normal-sized uteri and adnexae can be delivered through the vaginal incision without difficulty. A specimen bag can also be inserted into the abdomen and the specimen placed into the bag prior to removal via colpotomy to allow for contained extraction when decompression/morcellation is necessary. The size of this defect often causes significant loss of pneumoperitoneum; the vagina can be occluded to maintain insufflation using a glove filled with sponges or other occlusive device such as the bulb end from a bulb syringe.

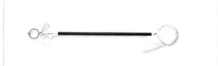

Figure 10.1 EndoCatch Gold 10 mm specimen pouch. By courtesy of Covidien, Mannsfield, Massachusetts.

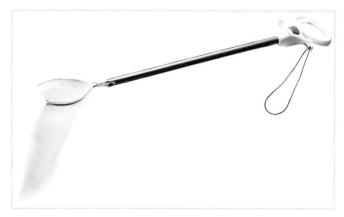

Figure 10.2 Anchor TRS100SB tissue retrieval system. With permission from Anchor Products Company, Addison, Illinois.

Culdotomy is an incision that connects the posterior vaginal fornix with the pouch of Douglas, and hence the peritoneal cavity. Access can be gained via a transvaginal or transabdominal approach, and can be performed with the uterus and cervix in situ. After performing a culdotomy incision, the specimen can be removed either directly or with the aid of a specimen retrieval bag. Due to the lack of a restrictive fascia layer, there is increased pliability in the vaginal wall compared to the abdominal wall. This allows for easier extraction of specimens through vaginal incisions when compared with abdominal incisions of comparable length. Additionally, patients may experience decreased postoperative pain with transvaginal as compared to transumbilical specimen retrieval (Ghezzi et al. 2012).

In order to perform culdotomy under laparoscopic guidance, a sponge stick or vaginal probe can be placed in the posterior fornix of the vagina to create a bulge visible laparoscopically, which can serve as a guide. The posterior vaginal wall is then incised using either sharp dissection or energy device of choice, taking care to remain medial to the uterosacral ligaments. A receiving instrument, such as a ring forceps, is then inserted through the vagina into the peritoneal cavity to accept the specimen or specimen retrieval bag. It is critical to perform this step under direct visualization to avoid entrapping tissue such as bowel along with the specimen during the removal process. After extraction of the specimen, the culdotomy is examined for extensions and closed either with laparoscopic or vaginal approach to suturing. An adjunct to this method is transvaginal trocar placement in the posterior vaginal fornix. Similar to the technique described above, a location in the posterior vaginal wall just inferior to the cervicovaginal junction and medial to uterosacral ligaments is identified. A long trocar is introduced at this location under laparoscopic guidance, with care to avoid injury of the rectosigmoid during this step. One advantage to this approach is ease of maintenance of pneumoperitoneum with the trocar as opposed to open culdotomy incision. An endoscopic bag can be placed through this port for retrieval of the specimen if necessary (see **Figure 10.3**) (Pillai & Yoong. 2010, Watrelot et al. 2010, Wyman et al. 2012).

Of note, patient selection is critical when planning specimen retrieval via culdotomy. If the posterior cul-de-sac is obliterated by endometriosis or adhesive disease, there may be higher risk of visceral or vascular injury. Additionally, prior hysterectomy can result in distortion of anatomy and make culdotomy more difficult. It is prudent to carefully inspect the pelvic anatomy prior to attempting culdotomy, and pursue alternate specimen retrieval technique as indicated (Ghezzi et al. 2002, Ghezzi et al. 2012, Gill et al. 2002, Uccella et al. 2013, Wang et al. 1999, Wang et al. 2006).

MINILAPAROTOMY

Minilaparotomy, in conjunction with laparoscopy, provides a larger intra-abdominal access for operating or tissue extraction when compared to the traditional laparoscopic port sites. A 2-4 cm incision is typically utilized, and may be created in the suprapubic region or as an extension of the umbilical site. Following the laparoscopic portion of the procedure, the minilaparotomy is performed and the specimen can then be removed intact or placed in a specimen retrieval bag and decompressed/morcellated via this site (Fanfani et al. 2005, Glasser 2005, Nezhat et al. 1994, Pelosi & Pelosi 1997).

Hand-assisted laparoscopic surgery is another alternative to this technique that combines the advantages of both laparotomy and laparoscopy. In hand-assisted cases, tactile feedback and manual retraction are possible, while preserving with the benefits of minimally invasive surgery including decreased postoperative pain and shorter convalescence. This technique involves making a minilaparotomy incision through which an airtight hand port can be placed. This enables maintenance of pneumoperitoneum, while providing an enlarged access point into the abdomen. Through this hand port, the surgeon's hand can be inserted into the abdominal cavity to assist with dissection and tissue retraction. (see **Figure 10.4**). When the specimen is ready to be delivered, it can be removed through the minilaparotomy site as described above (Tusheva et al. 2013).

MORCELLATION

Morcellation entails mechanically decreasing the size of the specimen in order to facilitate tissue extraction via smaller incisions. In gynecologic laparoscopy, this technique is commonly employed with myomectomy or hysterectomy specimens, and may be accomplished either manually with a scalpel or via power morcellation. Manual morcellation techniques have been described in

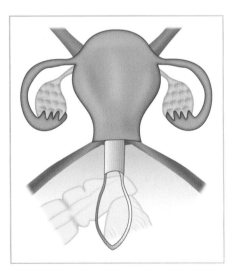

Figure 10.3 Specimen retrieval bag introduced via posterior fornix of vagina. With permission from Ghezzi F, Raio L, Mueller MD, et al. Vaginal extraction of pelvic masses following operative laparoscopy. Surg Endosc 2002;16:1691-1696.

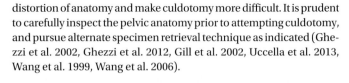

Figure 10.4 Hand-assisted laparoscopy. From Tusheva OA et al. (2013). Figure 10.5 Uterine specimen within insufflated Lahey bag. By courtesy of Dr Karen Wang, Brigham and Women's Hospital, Boston, MA.

prior sections of this chapter as being accomplished through a port site, colpotomy, or minilaparotomy. It is recommended to enclose the specimen within a retrieval bag prior to morcellation via any site in order to decrease potential tissue spread during the mincing process.

In 1993, Steiner first described a hand-held power device for tissue morcellation during laparoscopy. There are currently several electromechanical morcellator devices available, most of which rely on a blade for tissue cutting and some which utilize bipolar energy (Steiner et al. 1993). After the specimen has been completely detached, the morcellator is introduced through a 12–15 mm incision under laparoscopic vision. Manufacturer and device-specific instructions should be followed, but the general principles of operation are similar. A grasping forceps or tenaculum that passes through the cannula of the morcellator grasps the specimen and pulls it toward the morcellator. Prior to activating the morcellator device, the grasper and tissue should be circumferentially visualized to ensure that vital tissue is not included. Morcellation can then be activated, ensuring to keep the specimen and blade in view at all times. Tips for success include ensuring that the specimen is elevated to the morcellator to minimize movement of that device. This can be facilitated by an assistant presenting the tissue to the morcellator with a grasper. In procedures where morcellation is utilized, the abdomen should be systematically surveyed upon at completion of the procedure. Any fragments of devitalized tissue should be removed to decrease the chance of infection, postoperative pain, seeding, or implantation (Cucinella et al. 2011, Hutchins & Reinoehl 1998, Lieng et al. 2006, Paul & Koshy 2006).

Contraindications to electromechanical morcellation include biopsy proven malignancy or high suspicion of malignancy. Open power morcellation has been commonly practiced within the abdominal cavity during gynecologic and general surgery procedures (such as splenectomy and nephrectomy); however, it has come under scrutiny recently due to concerns of disseminating tissue during this process. Spread of benign tissue during morcellation has been documented, with endometriosis, adenomyosis, or myomas being either spread about the peritoneal cavity during morcellation or inadvertently left behind. The typical presentation in these cases is pain that can present weeks to years after the initial surgical procedure (Bogusiewicz et al. 2013, Donnez et al. 2007, Hilger & Magrina 2006, Larrain et al. 2010, Sepilian et al. 2003).

Of particular concern is the issue of disseminating an occult malignancy during the morcellation process, with potential for upstaging the disease and worsening survival outcome. A common indication for morcellation is uterine leiomyomata, a benign condition that may be difficult to distinguish from uterine sarcoma preoperatively. The incidence of occult malignancy of the uterus may be as high as 1 in 350 women undergoing surgery for presumed fibroid disease according to a literature review by the US Food and Drug Administration, although this is a conversational estimate and some authors report a much lower incidence (1 in 8000 cases, or fewer) (Kho & Nezhat 2014, Leibsohn et al. 1990, Parker et al. 1994, Pritts et al. 2015). MRI, in addition to serum markers of lactate dehydrogenase, may be helpful in preoperative detection of leiomyosarcoma, though definitive diagnosis still rests with pathologic confirmation (Goto et al. 2002, Sato et al. 2014, Schwartz et al. 1998).

Due to these concerns, closed laparoscopic morcellation techniques have been proposed that allow for power morcellation within a containment system, thereby minimizing the risk of tissue spread. One such option involves the off-label use of a specimen retrieval bag, such as the Lahey bag, for containment of the specimen (Cohen et al. 2014; Einarsson et al. 2014). Once the specimen is placed within the bag laparoscopically, the opening of the bag is exteriorized via a 1.5–2 cm umbilical incision and then insufflated. The specimen may then be morcellated under direct laparoscopic vision within the insufflated specimen bag (**Figures 10.5** and **10.6**). At this time, the degree to which use of containment bags mitigates risks associated with morcellation is unknown.

◼ CONCLUSION

A variety of specimen retrieval techniques exist for use in minimally invasive gynecologic surgery. In light of concerns regarding potential for spread of tissue during the surgical morcellation process, it is recommended to contain specimens within an enclosed bag prior to decompression of a mass or cutting into tissue, no matter the route of specimen removal. As more challenging procedures with larger pathology are undertaken with minimally invasive techniques, innovations in specimen removal will no doubt follow. It is important that surgeons become familiar with the range of options so that the process of tissue extraction can be individualized and optimized for each unique operation.

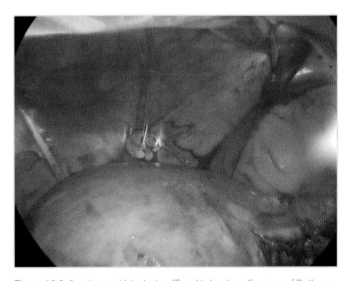

Figure 10.5 Specimen within the insufflated Lahey bag. Courtesy of Dr Karen Wang, Brigham and Women's Hospital, Boston, MA.

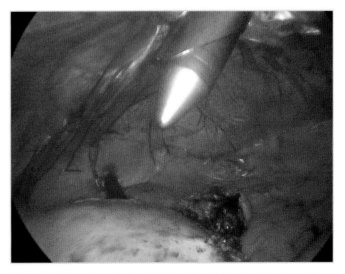

Figure 10.6 Morcellator device within insufflated Lahey bag. Courtesy of Dr Karen Wang, Brigham and Women's Hospital, Boston, MA.

REFERENCES

Bogusiewicz M, Rosinska-Bogusiewicz K, Walczyna B, Drop A, Rechberger T. Leiomyomatosis peritonealis disseminata with formation of endometrial cysts within tumors arising after supracervical laparoscopic hysterectomy. Ginekol Pol 2013; 84:68–71.

Cohen SL, Einarsson JI, Wang KC, et al. Contained power morcellation within an insufflated isolation bag. Obstet Gynecol 2014; 124:491-497.

Cucinella G, Granese R, Calagna G, Somigliana E, Perino A. Parasitic myomas after laparoscopic surgery: an emerging complication in the use of morcellator? Description of four cases. Fertil Steril 2011; 96:e90–96.

Donnez O, Squifflet J, Leconte I, Jadoul P, Donnez J. Posthysterectomy pelvic adenomyotic masses observed in 8 cases out of a series of 1405 laparoscopic subtotal hysterectomies. J Minim Invasive Gynecol 2007; 14:156–160.

Einarsson JI, Cohen SL, Fuchs N, Wang KC. In-bag morcellation. J Minim Invasive Gynecol 2014; 21:951-953.

Fanfani F, Fagotti A, Bifulco G, et al. A prospective study of laparoscopy versus minilaparotomy in the treatment of uterine myomas. J Minim Invasive Gynecol 2005; 12:470–474.

Ghezzi F, Raio L, Mueller MD, et al. Vaginal extraction of pelvic masses following operative laparoscopy. Surg Endosc 2002; 16:1691–1696.

Ghezzi F, Cromi A, Uccella S, et al. Transumbilical versus transvaginal retrieval of surgical specimens at laparoscopy: a randomized trial. Am J Obstet Gynecol 2012; 207:112 e111–116.

Gill IS, Cherullo EE, Meraney AM, et al. Vaginal extraction of the intact specimen following laparoscopic radical nephrectomy. J Urol 2002; 167:238–241.

Glasser MH. Minilaparotomy myomectomy: a minimally invasive alternative for the large fibroid uterus. J Minim Invasive Gynecol 2005; 12:275–283.

Goto A, Takeuchi S, Sugimura K, Maruo T. Usefulness of Gd-DTPA contrast-enhanced dynamic MRI and serum determination of LDH and its isozymes in the differential diagnosis of leiomyosarcoma from degenerated leiomyoma of the uterus. Int J Gynecol Cancer 2002; 12:354–361.

Hilger WS, Magrina JF. Removal of pelvic leiomyomata and endometriosis five years after supracervical hysterectomy. Obstet Gynecol 2006; 108:772–774.

Hutchins FL, Jr., Reinoehl EM. Retained myoma after laparoscopic supracervical hysterectomy with morcellation. J Am Assoc Gynecol Laparosc 1998; 5:293–295.

Kadar N, Reich H, Liu CY, Manko GF, Gimpelson R. Incisional hernias after major laparoscopic gynecologic procedures. Am J Obstet Gynecol 1993; 168:1493–1495.

Kho KA, Nezhat CH. Evaluating the risks of electric uterine morcellation. JAMA 2014; 311:905-906.

Larrain D, Rabischong B, Khoo CK, et al. "Iatrogenic" parasitic myomas: unusual late complication of laparoscopic morcellation procedures. J Minim Invasive Gynecol 2010; 17:719–724.

Leibsohn S, d'Ablaing G, Mishell DR, Jr., Schlaerth JB. Leiomyosarcoma in a series of hysterectomies performed for presumed uterine leiomyomas. Am J Obstet Gynecol 1990; 162:968–974; discussion 974–966.

Lieng M, Istre O, Busund B, Qvigstad E. Severe complications caused by retained tissue in laparoscopic supracervical hysterectomy. J Minim Invasive Gynecol 2006; 13:231–233.

Montz FJ, Holschneider CH, Munro MG. Incisional hernia following laparoscopy: a survey of the American Association of Gynecologic Laparoscopists. Obstet Gynecol 1994; 84:881–884.

Nezhat C, Nezhat F, Bess O, Nezhat CH, Mashiach R. Laparoscopically assisted myomectomy: a report of a new technique in 57 cases. Int J Fertil Menopausal Stud 1994; 39:39–44.

Nezhat CR, Kalyoncu S, Nezhat CH, et al. Laparoscopic management of ovarian dermoid cysts: ten years' experience. JSLS 1999; 3:179–184.

Parker WH, Fu YS, Berek JS. Uterine sarcoma in patients operated on for presumed leiomyoma and rapidly growing leiomyoma. Obstet Gynecol 1994; 83:414–418.

Paul PG, Koshy AK. Multiple peritoneal parasitic myomas after laparoscopic myomectomy and morcellation. Fertil Steril 2006; 85:492–493.

Pelosi MA, 3rd, Pelosi MA. The suprapubic cruciate incision for laparoscopic-assisted microceliotomy. JSLS 1997; 1:269–272.

Pillai R, Yoong W. Posterior colpotomy revisited: a forgotten route for retrieving larger benign ovarian lesions following laparoscopic excision. Arch Gynecol Obstet 2010; 281:609–611.

Pritts EA, Vanness DJ, Berek JS, et al. The prevalence of occult leiomyosarcoma at surgery for presumed uterine fibroids: a meta-analysis. Gynecol Surg 2015; 12:165-177.

Sato K, Yuasa N, Fujita M, Fukushima Y. Clinical application of diffusion-weighted imaging for preoperative differentiation between uterine leiomyoma and leiomyosarcoma. Am J Obstet Gynecol 2014; 210:368(e1-8).

Schwartz LB, Zawin M, Carcangiu ML, Lange R, McCarthy S. Does pelvic magnetic resonance imaging differentiate among the histologic subtypes of uterine leiomyomata? Fertil Steril 1998; 70:580–587.

Sepilian V, Della Badia C. Iatrogenic endometriosis caused by uterine morcellation during a supracervical hysterectomy. Obstet Gynecol 2003; 102:1125–1127.

Steiner RA, Wight E, Tadir Y, Haller U. Electrical cutting device for laparoscopic removal of tissue from the abdominal cavity. Obstet Gynecol 1993; 81:471–474.

Tusheva OA, Cohen SL, Einarsson JI. Hand-assisted approach to laparoscopic myomectomy and hysterectomy. J Minim Invasive Gynecol 2013; 20:234–237.

Uccella S, Cromi A, Bogani G, et al. Transvaginal specimen extraction at laparoscopy without concomitant hysterectomy: our experience and systematic review of the literature. J Minim Invasive Gynecol 2013; 20:583–590.

Wang PH, Lee WL, Yuan CC, Chao HT. A prospective, randomized comparison of port wound and culdotomy for extracting mature teratomas laparoscopically. J Am Assoc Gynecol Laparosc 1999; 6:483–486.

Wang CJ, Yuen LT, Lee CL, Kay N, Soong YK. A prospective comparison of morcellator and culdotomy for extracting of uterine myomas laparoscopically in nullipara. J Minim Invasive Gynecol 2006; 13:463–466.

Watrelot A, Nassif J, Law WS, Marescaux J, Wattiez A. Safe and simplified endoscopic technique in transvaginal NOTES. Surg Laparosc Endosc Percutan Tech 2010; 20:e92–94.

Wyman A, Fuhrig L, Bedaiwy MA, Debernardo R, Coffey G. A novel technique for transvaginal retrieval of enlarged pelvic viscera during minimally invasive surgery. Minim Invasive Surg 2012; 2012:454120.

Chapter 11 · Single-port surgery

Kevin JE Stepp, Patricia J Mattingly

INTRODUCTION

Since the late 1980s and early 1990s, conventional laparoscopy has established its place in the gynecologist's surgical armamentarium. Conventional laparoscopic instrumentation and access devices have vastly improved and robotic-assisted laparoscopic surgery continues to evolve. Although conventional laparoscopic and robotic hysterectomy techniques are still minimally invasive approaches, they require three to five small incisions in the abdominal wall. Each additional port carries a small but not negligible risk for port site complications (Tracy et al. 2008).

In an effort to minimize surgical risks and improve cosmesis, there is a renewed interest in single-port laparoscopy. The first cases of single-port laparoscopy in gynecology were with tubal ligation in the 1972 and then with laparoscopic-assisted vaginal hysterectomy in 1991 (Wheeless 1972, Pelosi & Pelosi 1991). With new instrumentation and better visualization, gynecologists began re-exploring single-port laparoscopy again in 2007. The advent of purpose-built multichannel ports for laparoscopy has enabled surgeons to complete laparoscopic surgeries through a single small incision that can be concealed at the base of the umbilicus, rendering a virtually scar less result.

Since its first description, authors around the world use multiple terms to describe laparoscopy carried out via a single port. However, a recent multispecialty international consortium has recommended the name laparoendoscopic single-site surgery (LESS) (Gill et al. 2010). LESS is meant to recognize and include subtle differences in technique such as using a single port with or without multiple channels or using multiple ports through a single skin incision.

LESS is a feasible alternative to standard laparoscopic technique, with comparable surgical outcomes of blood loss, length of hospital stay, and intraoperative and postoperative complications (Chen et al. 2011, Jung et al. 2011). Most studies currently available comparing LESS hysterectomy to conventional laparoscopy have a median uterine weight <300 g. However, Song et al. demonstrated that LESS hysterectomy is also a safe and feasible option when removing a uterus weighing ≥500 g. Increased uterine weight was associated with longer operative times and blood loss but was not associated with an increased need to convert to traditional laparoscopy (Song et al. 2013). With few exceptions, currently available studies demonstrate comparable operative times between LESS and standard laparoscopic technique. Escobar et al. (2010) examined the learning curve for LESS and found similar results when compared to published conventional laparoscopic learning curves.

LESS may represent a superior alternative to traditional laparoscopy with respect to cosmetic results and postoperative pain. Several retrospective studies suggest the potential for decreased pain with single-port laparoscopy; however, the few, available randomized controlled trials to date have conflicting results (Chen et al. 2011, Fagotti et al. 2011, Jung et al. 2011, Christian et al. 2012, Hoyer-Sorensen et al. 2012). Fagotti et al. and Chen et al. showed lower postoperative pain in patients undergoing single-port procedures, while Christian et al., Jung et al. and Hoyer-Sorensen et al. found no evidence of reduction in postoperative pain. Cosmetic outcomes were found to be better among patients having undergone LESS as compared to conventional laparoscopy (Fagotti et al. 2011, Song et al. 2013, Yoo & Shim 2013).

The objective of this chapter is to illustrate an effective, efficient, and reproducible technique to perform LESS in gynecology. The basic concepts illustrated here are easily understood, replicated, and useful in learning the LESS technique. Although many of these techniques work well for complex surgical cases, we strongly recommend surgeons first become familiar with the technique for simple procedures with benign indications. As with any surgical approach, complicating factors, such as endometriosis, large fibroid uteri, malignancy, and significant adhesions, represent an additional layer of complexity and are not addressed here. We recommend that those cases be reserved for experienced LESS surgeons.

Challenges unique to the LESS surgical approach include an in-line view, instrument crowding, and lack of triangulation. Understanding the principles and techniques described here will help the surgeon proceed efficiently, and avoid external and internal clashing and prevent frustration.

PORTS AND GAINING ACCESS

Various access devices and techniques have been described for peritoneal access. Regardless of the method used, the skin incision should be created to provide the most cosmetically appealing result. The umbilicus itself is a scar with its own unique folds and shape. In some patients, a vertical skin incision is preferable. However, the omega incision first described by pediatric surgeons in 1986 may produce a better cosmetic result and provide additional space for specimen removal while maintaining excellent cosmesis (Hong et al. 2006, Huang et al. 2009) (**Figure 11.1**). It has been postulated by some that an omega umbilical incision may carry an increased risk of infection. However, a retrospective study in gynecology compared

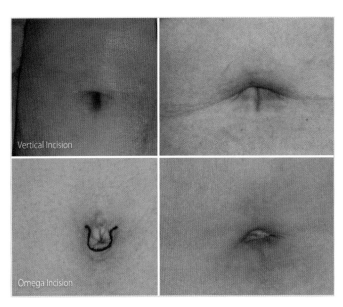

Figure 11.1 Incision options. Top: vertical skin incision before (left) and after (right). Bottom: omega incision before (left) and after (right).

vertical and circumferential umbilical incisions in 120 patients that underwent a LESS procedure and did not find a difference in rates of infection (Kane & Stepp 2011). Limiting the size of the incision may exert unnecessary tension on the skin edges that could lead to pressure necrosis. Although this condition usually heals well, this risk should be considered while making the skin incision and selecting the appropriate port for each patient.

The majority of commercially available LESS ports have two attachments that can be used for insufflation, outflow, smoke evacuation, or an additional insufflation port as necessary (**Figure 11.2**). Surgeons also successfully use noncommercial ports constructed from retractors, gloves, and other materials readily available in any operating room (Lee et al. 2009).

Ports that utilize a single fascial incision maximize space for additional instruments. However, ports that have multiple channels or cannulas minimize instrument friction and unintended crossing at the level of the fascia. These ports typically come at the expense of needing a slightly larger fascial incision. When necessary, conversion to two-port or multiport conventional laparoscopy should not be considered a complication.

SETUP AND INSTRUMENTATION

The majority of gynecologic surgical procedures can be performed using conventional straight instrumentation available in all operating rooms. Specialized articulating and curved instruments, specifically designed for LESS, may help overcome the lack of triangulation and demonstrate some advantages in certain situations. However, there is generally a learning curve associated with these newer devices. We recommend mimizing the number of learning curves. Therefore, we recommend beginning with simple procedures using conventional instrumentation.

An articulating camera has some significant advantages over conventional laparoscopes in LESS and is preferred by most experts. However, bariatric length or longer, 30° or 45° laparoscopes can also be used in LESS with the techniques and principles described here. Conventional laparoscopes have a light cable perpendicular to the scope, making for a burdensome configuration that can exacerbate external crowding and clashing. In contrast, articulating cameras are designed with a light source in the same axis as the scope to help minimize external crowding (**Figure 11.3B**). If a nonarticulating

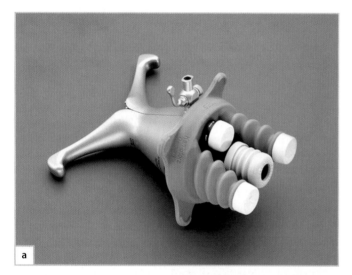

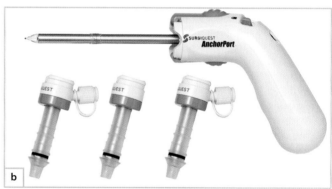

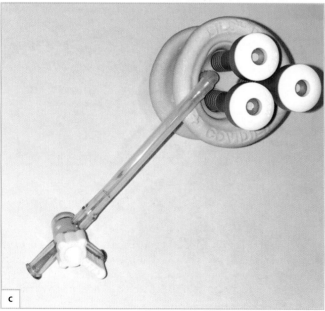

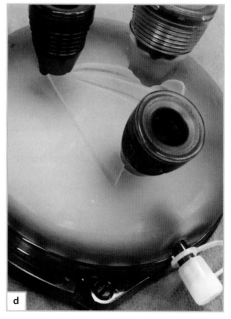

Figure 11.2 *Continue*

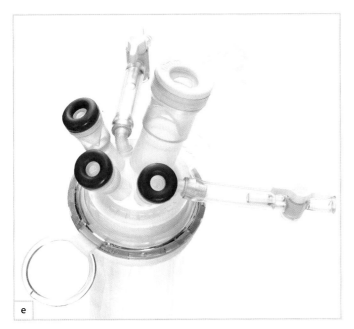

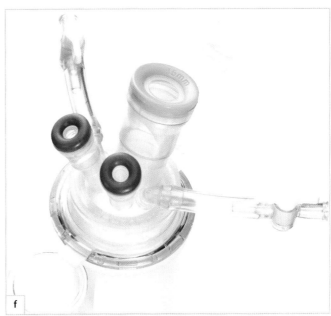

Figure 11.2 LESS ports. (a) The X-CONE (© 2016 Photo courtesy of Karl Storz Endoscopy-America, Inc, El Segundo, CA). (b) The AnchorPort Trocar device (Surgiquest Inc., Orange, Connecticut). (c) SILS Port. (d) GelPoint. (e) TriPort Plus (Advanced Surgical Concepts, Wicklow, Ireland). (f) TriPort 15 (Advanced Surgical Concepts, Wicklow, Ireland).

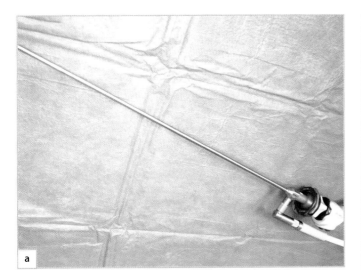

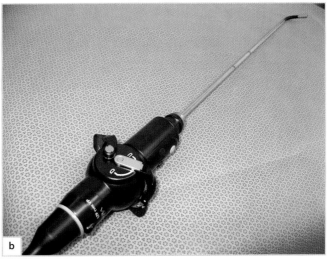

Figure 11.3 Laparoscope options. (a) 30° or 45° laparoscope for laparoendoscopic single-site surgery with 90° light cord adaptor (inset). (b) Articulating laparoscope (Advanced Surgical Concepts, Wicklow, Ireland)

laparoscope is used, we recommend using a 90° adaptor to minimize interference with the light cord (**Figure 11.3A** and inset).

KEY STEPS

There are a few key steps and principles for an efficient LESS procedure. We present a simplified technique that is useful in all gynecologic procedures. This technique when strictly followed will eliminate extraneous or duplicative movements. These steps will maximize space between instruments and avoid extracorporeal and intracorporeal clashing and crossing, also known as 'sword fighting.' In addition

to the steps below, we have developed four core principles for LESS (**Table 11.1**).

Step 1: Orientation of the port and camera placement

The surgeon should choose the port so that the advantages and disadvantages of the specific port are well suited to the complexity of the case. Once securely placed in the peritoneal cavity, the port should be oriented as in **Figure 11.4**. The channels or valves should be oriented so that the laparoscope can be placed through the most cephalad channel. This allows the camera to be placed as close to the chest wall as possible externally while elevating the internal end of the laparoscope toward the anterior abdominal wall. Then, use the

Table 11.1 Core principles for laparoendoscopic single-site surgery

1.   Always retract in such a way that the handle of the instrument moves laterally, away from the camera and central area above the umbilicus. This prevents extracorporeal clashing of instruments.
2.   Plan the procedure and choose instrumentation and techniques that minimize the need for instrument exchanges. Devices that are multifunctional are strongly encouraged.
3.   Use a uterine manipulator. For hysterectomy, we suggest one with a colpotomizer or ring to delineate the vaginal fornix.
4.   If significant difficulty is encountered at any time during the procedure, an additional port can always be considered.

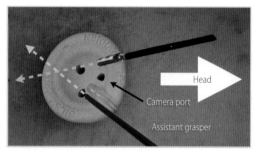

Figure 11.4 Port orientation and camera placement. The laparoscope is placed through the cephalad channel, valve, or cannula.

articulation or angle of the scope to position the camera and light cord low and laterally (**Figure 11.5**). Externally, this positions the assistant's hand and the external aspect of the camera away from the umbilicus to allow space for other instruments and permit the primary surgeon to operate directly above the umbilical port. The greater the angle of the scope (30°, 45°, or flexible), the easier it is to get the laparoscope and camera away from the operative field and avoid clashing.

Step 2: Insert the assistant instrument/grasper

The instructions that follow assume the primary surgeon is on the patient's left side. (This process could be reversed if the surgeon is standing on the opposite side.)

According to the core principles, all retraction by any assistant grasper should be performed by lateral retraction of the handle away from midline. Always retract in such a way that the handle of the instrument moves laterally, away from the camera and central area above the umbilicus. This means that the tissue is actually being retracted across the pelvis toward the contralateral side. This maximizes room for the laparoscope and other instruments externally preventing extracorporeal clashing of instruments. For example, to retract a uterus to the right, an assistant grasper instrument is inserted through the left port channel and controlled with the surgeon's left hand by moving the handle laterally externally to deviate the uterus to the right (**Figure 11.6**). Additionally, a uterine manipulator is a valuable tool to assist with pelvic exposure.

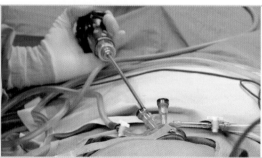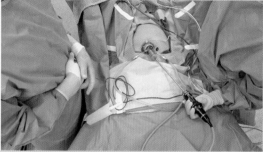

Figure 11.5 Camera placement. The camera should be placed first prior to any additional instruments. Use the articulation or angle of the scope to position the camera and light cord low and lateral.

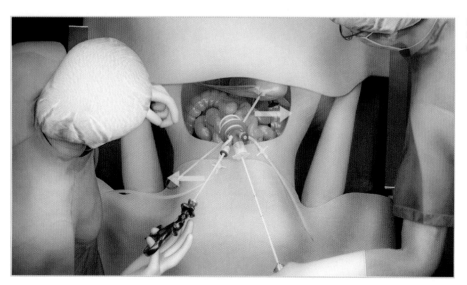

Figure 11.6 Insertion of the assistant grasper. Retraction is always in a way that the handle moves laterally, away from the midline.

Step 3: Insert the operating electrosurgical instrument

The operating instrument will be inserted through the right channel (**Figure 11.7**). It will enter the internal operative field through the center and usually be directed straight toward the surgical target. In the event that the instrument handles interfere with each other or the camera, the handles should be positioned opposite to each other (**Figure 11.7**).

Early in one's learning curve, we believe the simplest option is to set up and expose the surgical target in a systematic way then insert the primary operative instrument (scissors, bipolar vessel sealer, etc.). In this way, the assistant grasper can be applied and good exposure is maintained. Then the surgeon can focus on the dominant/operative hand. Until the surgeon is experienced with LESS, it is easy to get frustrated with retraction across the table or clashing when both hands are moving simultaneously. Therefore, simpler procedures that can be accomplished in a straightforward routine process with little variation are most suited for learning a LESS approach. As the surgeon becomes more experienced, more complex procedures become easily feasible.

SPECIMEN EXTRACTION

One potential advantage of the LESS technique is for specimen extraction. Specimens can be more easily removed through the slightly larger skin incision (15–25 mm versus 12 mm for standard open laparoscopy). Extracorporeal morcellation can be accomplished through the larger incision. Some ports include a wound protector. These ports have a removable portion of the port that reveals a wound protector that facilitates easy extraction of specimens and allows easy replacement of the port [Triport (Advanced Surgical Concepts, Wicklow, Ireland), Gelpoint (Applied Medical, Rancho Santa Margarita, California)]. Because the camera and instruments enter through a single-port site, completely contained intracorporeal morcellation can be performed by inserting a large surgical bag through the port, then creating a pseudopneumoperitoneum directly within the bag. The camera, mechanical morcellator, and an assistant grasper can be inserted through the port and into the bag to perform the morcellation within a contained system. Any small pieces would remain in the bag.

This would minimize or eliminate the risk of potential spread of benign or malignant tissue (**Figure 11.8**).

SUTURING

Laparoscopic suturing requires the most skill. Therefore, we recommend traditional suturing be considered only by those experienced with LESS. If laparoscopic suturing is necessary, we strongly suggest utilizing suturing assist devices such as the Endostitch (Covidien, Norwalk, Connecticut), barbed suture, and Laparo-Ty (Ethicon Endo Surgery, Inc. Cincinnati, Ohio). In the case of a total hysterectomy, the authors suggest closing the vaginal cuff from a vaginal approach until the surgeon is experienced with LESS.

RISKS SPECIFIC TO LESS

As with any laparoscopic technique, it is imperative that surgeons have thorough knowledge of electrosurgery to avoid electrosurgical complications. Surgeons should be aware of the different types of electrosurgical complications. There may be a theoretical increased risk

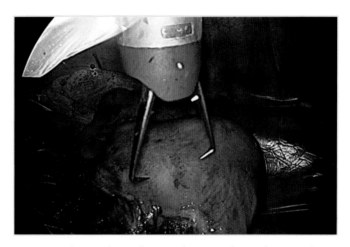

Figure 11.8 Contained morcellation in a bag. Internal view of uterus and morcellator contained within a pseudopneumoperitoneum.

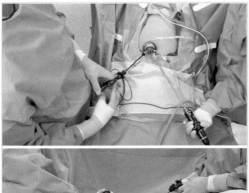
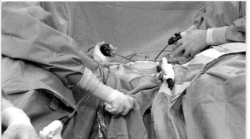
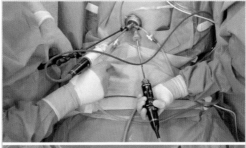
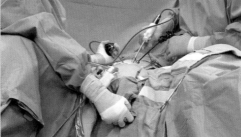

Figure 11.7 External instrument position. External view showing setup and instrument positions without clashing. Note handles of the bipolar device and assistant grasper are facing opposite directions.

of capacitive coupling when performing LESS. Working with instruments in close quarters may predispose them to insulation damage. Therefore, we recommend meticulous inspection of the instruments. Disposable electrosurgical instruments may have decreased risk of insulation damage and thus lower risk of direct coupling. We believe good technique should mitigate these risks.

CONCLUSION

The feasibility of LESS in most laparoscopic procedures is demonstrated in multiple case reports and series in the medical literature.

Several studies have addressed the potential advantages and disadvantages of LESS compared to conventional laparoscopy. There are few randomized trials. A recent meta-analysis of six randomized controlled trials by Song et al. found no significant difference between any of their primary outcome measures including perioperative complications, conversation rates, postoperative pain, and cosmesis (Song et al. 2013). Their conclusions were consistent with other studies with the exception of their assessment of cosmetic preferences. At least three randomized controlled trials to date have shown superior patient satisfaction with LESS cosmetic results (Fagotti et al. 2011, Song et al. 2013, Yoo & Shim 2013).

REFERENCES

Chen YJ, Wang PH, Ocampo EJ, et al. Single-port compared with conventional laparoscopic-assisted vaginal hysterectomy: a randomized controlled trial. Obstet Gynecol 2011; 117:906–912.

Christian HS, Vistad I, Ballard K, et al. Is single-port laparoscopy for benign adnexal disease less painful than conventional laparoscopy? A single-center randomized controlled trial. Fertil Steril 2012; 98:973–979.

Escobar PF, Starks DC, Fader AN, et al. Single-port risk-reducing salpingo-oophorectomy with and without hysterectomy: surgical outcomes and learning curve analysis. Gynecol Oncol 2010; 119:43–47.

Fagotti A, Bottoni C, Vizzielli G, et al. Postoperative pain after conventional laparoscopy and laparoendoscopic single site surgery (LESS) for benign adnexal disease: a randomized trial. Fertil Steril 2011; 96:255–259.

Gill IS, Advincula AP, Aron M. Consensus statement of the consortium for laparoendoscopic single-site surgery. Surg Endosc 2010; 24:762–768.

Hong SH, Seo SI, Kim JC, Hwang TK. Cosmetic circumumbilical incision for extraction of specimen after laparoscopic radical prostatectomy. J Endourol 2006; 20:519–521.

Hoyer-Sorensen C, Vistad I, Ballard K. Is single-port laparoscopy for benign adnexal disease less painful than conventional laparoscopy? A single-center randomized controlled trial. Fertil Steril 2012; 98:973–979.

Huang CK, Houng JY, Chiang CJ, et al. Single incision transumbilical laparoscopic roux-en-y gastric bypass: a first case report. Obes Surg 2009; 19:1711–1715.

Jung YK, Lee M, Yim GW. A randomized prospective study of single-port and four-port approaches for hysterectomy in terms of postoperative pain. Surg Endos 2011; 25:2462–2469.

Kane S, Stepp KJ. Circumumbilical (Omega) incision for laparoendoscopic single-site surgery. Oral Presentation: Society Gynecologic Surgeons Annual Clinical Meeting, San Antonio, Texas, April 2011.

Lee YY, Kim TJ, Kim CJ, et al. Single-port access laparoscopic-assisted vaginal hysterectomy: a novel method with a wound retractor and a glove. J Minim Invasive Gynecol 2009; 16:450–453.

Pelosi MA, Pelosi MA 3rd. Laparoscopic hysterectomy with bilateral salpingo-oophorectomy using a single umbilical puncture. N J Med 1991; 88:721–726.

Song T, Cho J, Kim TJ, Kim IR, et al. Cosmetic outcomes of laparoendoscopic single-site hysterectomy compared with multi-port surgery: Randomized controlled trial. J Minim Invasive Gynecol 2013; 20:460–467.

Song T, Lee Y, Kim ML, et al. Single-port access total laparoscopic hysterectomy for large uterus. Gynecol Obstet Invest 2013; 75:16–20.

Song T, Kim ML, Jung YW, et al. Laparoendoscopic single-site versus conventional laparoscopic gynecologic surgery: a metaanalysis of randomized controlled trials. Am J Obstet Gynecol 2013; 209:317.e1–17.e9

Tracy CR, Raman JD, Cadeddu JA, Rane A. Laparoendoscopic single-site surgery in urology: where have we been and where are we heading? Nat Clin Pract Urol 2008; 5:561–568.

Wheeless CR, Jr. Elimination of second incision in laparoscopic sterilization. Obstet Gynecol 1972; 39:134–136.

Yoo EH, Shim E. Single-port access compared with three-port laparoscopic adnexal surgery in a randomized controlled trial. J Int Med Res 2013; 41:673–680.

Chapter 12 — Surgical management of a uterine septum

Olav Istre

▮ INTRODUCTION

Uterine anomalies result from a defect in the development or fusion of the paired Müllerian ducts during embryogenesis, and are the most common types of malformations of the female reproductive system (**Figure 12.1**). The septate uterus is the most common structural uterine anomaly, and results from failure of the partition between the two fused Müllerian ducts to resorb (Taylor & Gomel 2008). Congenital malformations may be associated with recurrent pregnancy loss, preterm labor, abnormal fetal presentation, and infertility (Heinonen et al. 1982). The overall frequency of uterine malformations was 4.0% (Raga et al. 1997). Infertile patients (6.3%) had a significantly (P<0.05) higher incidence of Müllerian anomalies, in comparison with fertile patients (3.8%). Septate (33.6%) and arcuate (32.8%) uteri were the most common malformations observed (Raga et al. 1997). The septate uterus is associated with the highest incidence of reproductive failure among the Müllerian anomalies (Fedele et al. 1993). Between 38% and 79% of pregnancies in women with septate uteri ended in miscarriage (Homer et al. 2000, Raga et al. 1997). Such outcomes are thought to be a result of poor blood supply, rendering the septum inhospitable to the implanting embryo (Fedele et al. 1996).

▮ DIAGNOSIS OF UTERINE SEPTUM

Diagnosis is established with hysterosalpingography, MRI, and ultrasound. The diagnostic accuracy of hysterosalpingography in patients with septate uteri has been reported to be between 20% and 60% (Braun et al. 2005, Pellerito et al. 1992). Transvaginal ultrasonography is more accurate, with a sensitivity of 100% and a specificity of 80% in the diagnosis of the septate uterus (Pellerito et al. 1992). Three-dimensional sonography (3DULS) is associated with an even higher diagnostic accuracy of 92% (Wu et al. 1997) and hysterosonography, with a 100% diagnostic accuracy in the largest series published to date (Alborzi et al. 2002). The benefit of 3DULS is the view of the uterus in the coronal plane, which allows the operator to distinguish between arcuate, septate, and bicornuate uteri, thereby eliminating the need for simultaneous laparoscopy. 3DULS and 3D saline infusion sonohysterography are proving to be as accurate as MRI and less expensive.

Three-dimensional imaging allows for simultaneous delineation of the external fundal contour and the internal cavity of the uterus (**Figures 12.2** and **12.3**). 3DULS in combination with sonohysterography may ultimately become the gold standard for the diagnosis of Müllerian anomalies as it becomes a more common tool in the office and physicians become more skilled in using it to evaluate Müllerian anomalies.

Recently, the European Society of Human Reproduction and Embryology and the European Society of Gynecological Endoscopy have come to a consensus on a new classification system that allows for a descriptive classification, separating uterine and cervical/vaginal anatomy (Grimbizi et al. 2013).

This chapter describes the diversity of clinical presentations, management strategies, and reports the obstetric outcomes. In the investigated studies, several different methods and instruments for hysteroscopic septoplasty have been described, namely scissors, resectoscope, and argon laser. Data on the impact of the hysteroscopic technique on the reproductive outcome, however, are rare.

Fedele et al. could not find a difference while comparing the reproductive outcome results obtained with microscissors, argon laser, and resectoscope, in their series (Fedele et al. 1993). Thus, it is unclear, whether the use of a specific instrument may improve outcome and further comparative trials should be encouraged. Operative hysteroscopy may be performed using monopolar or bipolar electrosurgery. Bipolar electrosurgery uses isotonic saline as distention medium and may be safer and more effective for hysteroscopic surgery compared to monopolar electrosurgery.

In my own practice, total of 114 women were investigated and their fertility outcome was followed for an average of 2 years. Patients with some degree of Müllerian malformation, as detected at their local gynecologist on transvaginal ultrasound or at our department during admission for any condition, connected to the anomaly.

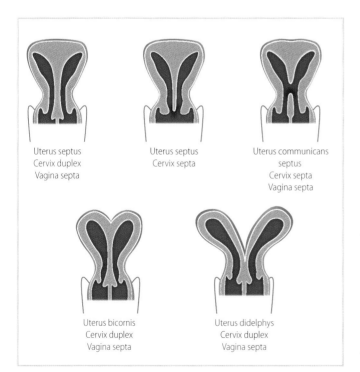

Uterus septus
Cervix duplex
Vagina septa

Uterus septus
Cervix septa

Uterus communicans septus
Cervix septa
Vagina septa

Uterus bicornis
Cervix duplex
Vagina septa

Uterus didelphys
Cervix duplex
Vagina septa

Figure 12.1 Different types of uterine malformations.

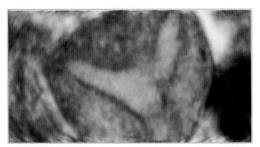

Figure 12 2
Three-dimensional ultrasound scan of the septum.

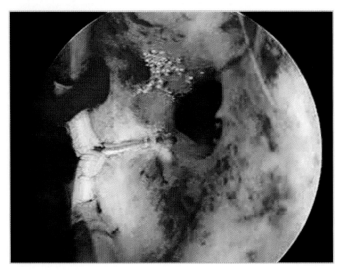

Figure 12.3 Hysteroscopic view of septum uteri.

The patients were assessed using B-mode, 3DULS examinations using a Voluson 730 Expert (General Electric Healthcare, Zipf, Austria) with a vaginal multifrequency probe (5–9 Hz). An initial B-mode examination provided morphologic evaluation of the pelvic organs, including uterine size and endometrium thickness, followed by a saline infusion sonography in most of the patients with findings suggestive of a uterine septum.

SURGICAL TECHNIQUE

The operations are performed under general anesthesia using the following surgical technique. During hysteroscopy, the automatic pressure cuff (Olympus, Center Valley, Pennsylvania) maintains an infusion pressure of 100 mmHg, and suction of 10–15 mmHg is applied to the outflow tube to achieve a sufficient flow. The transcervical resection with a resectoscope (Olympus), Ch. 26 model WA 22061 with 12 optic 22001A (Hamburg, Germany), using sodium chloride 0.9% (Braun, Melsungen, Germany) as irrigant, with a needle of 5 mm is then used to perform the metroplasty. The needle is used with a bipolar cutting current of 280 W to incise the lower segments of the septum from side-to-side until the tubal ostia are visualized. The high power is needed for the ignition of the plasma only. A couple of milliseconds after the ignition, the generator automatically regulates the power down to normal values around 100 W. The septum excision is stopped approximately 10 mm from the line between the two ostia. In six patients from our series, a total uterine septum was identified. In these cases, the incision was made horizontally toward the other obliterated cavity, starting just after the internal os. In cases with a double cervix, the same procedure was performed leaving the cervices intact (**Figure 12.2**).

OPERATIVE RESULTS

One hundred and fourteen women underwent hysteroscopic examination. In cases with a larger septum, a resection was performed, with a mean age of 31 (range 19–42) years. In eight cases, the septum was found to be small and not in need of resection. Uterine septa were found as part of the workup for the following events: infertility workup (33.3%), first trimester miscarriage (22.8%), three or more miscarriages (22.8%), Cesarean section (11.4%), premature delivery (7.9%), and normal delivery (1.8%) (**Table 12.1**). We evaluated the septum size in the 114 women. Ten (8.8%) had a septum consisting one-quarter of their uterus, 18 (15.8%) had a septum one-half of their uterus, and 86 (75.4%) had a septum larger than one-half of their uterus. Six women had a total septum, and were included in the group with a septum larger than one-half of their uterus. The different diagnostic events leading to diagnosis of the uterine septum per septum size are given in **Table 12.2**. The uterine septum was successfully resected in all 106 women. No intra- or postoperative complications were noted.

OBSTETRIC COURSE

There are few studies that have looked at the pregnancy outcome after septum resection and most of the small studies are in line with our findings. Hysteroscopic metroplasty in women with a septate uterus and infertility improves the clinical pregnancy and live birth rates in patients. If such a patient is looking for a spontaneous pregnancy, this is more likely to occur during the first 15 months following the procedure (Bakas 2012).

In my own study, 103 out of 114 women desired a future pregnancy. Seventy-two (69.9%) of these women achieved a successful pregnancy after metroplasty, with 63 (87.5%) subsequent term deliveries, and 9 (12.5%) premature deliveries. Twenty-two (30.6%) of the 72 women had live births delivered by Cesarean section. Twenty-four (23.3%) women who desired future fertility did not become pregnant, and 7 (6.8%) had a spontaneous miscarriage. Eleven women were not interested in future fertility; however, they opted for surgery at time of diagnosis. In examining the outcomes in women divided up by group of septum diagnosis, we found the following rates of live births following metroplasty: infertility workup (56.3%), miscarriage (77.6%), normal/premature delivery (80%), and Cesarean section (66.7%) (**Table 12.1**). We found different pregnancy outcomes after metroplasty of the various septum sizes as is seen in **Table 12.2**. To compare the pregnancy outcome after metroplasty of a different septum size, the material was divided in two groups: one group with a septum size of one-quarter or one-half and one other group with a septum size larger than one-half of their uterus (**Table 12.3**). The pregnancy outcome of a septum size one-quarter or one-half is significantly different from the pregnancy outcome after metroplasty of septum larger than one-half of the uterus (χ^2 test: $P<0.001$). There were only four women in our study with the combination of a septum consisting one-quarter of their uterus and the diagnosis following a first trimester miscarriage. After metroplasty, none of these women became pregnant, although all four had desired fertility. ANOVA linear regression showed no significant difference in age in the different events leading to diagnosis ($P<0.708$) and no significant difference in age and pregnancy outcome ($P<0.160$).

COMPARISON WITH CURRENT LITERATURE

In our study, we performed hysteroscopic metroplasty solely based on ULS findings. No patients underwent laparoscopy. No intra- or

Table 12.1 Pregnancy outcome after metroplasty

Pregnancy outcome	Infertility workup (33.3%)	Miscarriage* (45.6%)	Normal/premature delivery (9.7%)	Cesarean section (11.4%)	Total group
Successful pregnancy	18 (56.3%) (3 premature)	38 (77.6%) (4 premature)	8 (80%) (1 premature)	8 (66.7%) (1 premature)	72 (69.9%)
Miscarriage	3	4	0	0	7 (6.8%)
No pregnancy	11	7	2	4	24 (23.3%)
Desired fertility	32	49	10	12	103 (100%)
Undesired fertility	6	3	1	1	11
Total	38	52	11	13	114

*26 women had a single first trimester miscarriage, 26 had ≥3 miscarriages.

Table 12.2 Event leading to diagnosis and pregnancy outcome after metroplasty for different septum sizes

Diagnostic event	Septum size: ¼ uterus 10 patients (8.8%)	Septum size: ½ uterus 18 patients (15.8%)	Septum size: >½ uterus 86 patients (75.4%)
Infertility workup	4 (40%)	7 (39%)	27 (31%)
First trimester miscarriage	4 (40%)	4 (22%)	18 (21%)
Premature delivery	0	2 (11%)	7 (8%)
Normal delivery	0	1 (6%)	1 (1%)
>3 miscarriages	1 (10%)	3 (17%)	22 (26%)
Cesarean section	1 (10%)	1 (6%)	11 (13%)
Pearson χ^2:	P = 0.754	–	–
Pregnancy outcome after metroplasty			
No pregnancy	7 (70%)	6 (40%)	11 (14.1%)
Successful pregnancy	3 (30%)	5 (33.3%)	64 (82%)
Miscarriage	0	4 (26.7%)	3 (3.8%)
Desired fertility	10	15 (100%)	78 (100%)
Undesired fertility	0	3	8

Table 12.3 Diagnostic event and pregnancy outcome when septum size is divided into two groups

Pregnancy outcome	Septum size ¼ or ½ uterus	Septum size >½ uterus
No pregnancy	13 (46.4%)	11 (12.8%)
Premature delivery	0	9 (10.5%)
Normal delivery	8 (28.6%)	55 (64%)
Miscarriage	4 (14.3%)	3 (3.5%)
Undesired fertility	3 (10.7%)	8 (9.3%)
Total	28	86
Pearson χ^{2}*	19.081†	Df = 1; P = 0.000

*The χ^2 test requires no cells to have a count <5. In order to have a valid χ^2 test, we divided the four groups into two groups. No pregnancy and miscarriage are combined in unwanted outcome, and normal and premature delivery in successful pregnancy.
†0 cells (0%) have expected count <5: the minimum expected count is 10.32.

postoperative complications occurred. Based on our experience in this study, we believe metroplasty of the uterine septum can be safely performed as an office procedure. This corresponds to the study of Ghi et al. (2009), demonstrating ULS and 3DULS to be extremely accurate (positive predictive value 96.3% and negative predictive value 100%) for the diagnosis and classification of congenital uterine anomalies. They suggest women diagnosed with malformations amenable to treatment with a resectoscope may avoid a diagnostic pelviscopy by using operative hysteroscopy with the addition of 3DULS. In the present study, we used this strategy of diagnosis and management as 3DULS was followed by operative hysteroscopy. Our findings indicated an excellent prognosis for successful pregnancy after metroplasty of the uterine septum. Seventy-two women (69.9%) delivered a healthy baby. This was consistent with previous studies. Homer et al. (2000) found in their review a live birth rate of 64% in a total of 658 patients. In our study the live birth rate was different per diagnostic event. We found a lower live birth rate after metroplasty when the septum was diagnosed during infertility workup (56.3%), thus indicating that multiple factors were contributing to the patient's infertility. In approximately 40% of these patients, other factors (e.g. male factor and

tubal factors) were found during infertility workup. The lower live birth rate with unexplained infertility and a uterine septum is seen in other studies as well: Homer et al. (2000) found a crude pregnancy rate of 48%, Pabuccu and Gomel (2004) found a live birth rate of 29.5%, and Mollo et al. (2009) found a live birth rate of 34.1%. All lower than the overall live birth rate of 64% observed by Homer et al. and our live birth rates with other diagnostic events. This suggests again that when the uterine septum is diagnosed during infertility workup, there are coexisting factors such as genetic, infective, endocrine, immune, and thrombophilic factors that play a role in their infertility (Pabuccu & Gomel 2004). Therefore, in the past, removal of the uterine septum in these cases was subject to debate.

The lower live birth rate after metroplasty makes it questionable to perform correction of the uterine septum, as these patients may benefit from concentrating on other infertility treatments. However, in certain cases, prophylactic resection of the uterine septum continues to be recommended: women with longstanding (>6 months) unexplained infertility in whom an extensive workup has ruled out other factors, women >35 years of age, women undergoing laparoscopy and hysteroscopy for other reasons (septal incision at the same time is opportune and appears logical), and women pursuing assisted reproductive technologies (Homer et al. 2000). Mollo et al. (2009) have recently addressed this question. They concluded metroplasty in women with unexplained infertility and a uterine septum improved their live birth rate compared with women with unexplained infertility and no septate uterus (Rai & Regan 2006). The live birth rate was 34.1% after metroplasty in the septate uterus group compared with 18.9% when there was no uterine septum present (χ^2 test: $P<0.05$). We found women with prior miscarriages leading to diagnosis of a uterine septum had the highest live birth rate after metroplasty. Previous studies also reported a significant improvement after metroplasty in this group. Homer et al. (2000) found the overall miscarriage rate dropped from 88% to 5.9% after hysteroscopic metroplasty. In our study, four women had a septum size of one-quarter of their uterus diagnosed after a first trimester miscarriage; despite desired fertility, none of these four women achieved a live birth following metroplasty. Further studies with larger numbers are required to evaluate the need of metroplasty in this group of women. The highest rate of live births after metroplasty in our study was in the group of women with the largest septum (larger than one-half of the uterus). In this group, 82% had a live birth compared with 33.2% and 30% when the septum is one-half or one-quarter of their uterus, respectively (χ^2: $P<0.05$). If a septum extends over more than one-half of the uterine cavity, we strongly recommend metroplasty. There is no reason to wait for these women to prove bad obstetric outcome before surgical management, especially since outpatient hysteroscopic metroplasty of the uterine septum is a minor procedure with rare complications.

CONCLUSION

Hysteroscopic septum resection is a safe and effective method for patients with history of infertility or recurrent miscarriage.

REFERENCES

Alborzi S, Dehbashi S, Parsanezhad ME. Differential diagnosis of septate and bicornuate uterus by sonohysterography eliminates the need for laparoscopy. Fertil Steril 2002; 78:176–178.

Bakas P. Hysteroscopic resection of uterine septum and reproductive outcome in women with unexplained infertility. Gynecol Obstet Invest 2012; 73(4):321–325

Braun P, Grau FV, Pons RM, Enguix DP. Is hysterosalpingography able to diagnose all uterine malformations correctly? A retrospective study. Eur J Radiol 2005; 53:274–279.

Fedele L, Arcaini L, Parazzini F, Vercellini P, Di NG. Reproductive prognosis after hysteroscopic metroplasty in 102 women: life-table analysis. Fertil Steril 1993; 59:768–772.

Fedele L, Bianchi S, Agnoli B, Tozzi L, Vignali M. Urinary tract anomalies associated with unicornuate uterus. J Urol 1996; 155:847–848.

Ghi T, Casadio P, Kuleva M, et al. Accuracy of three-dimensional ultrasound in diagnosis and classification of congenital uterine anomalies. Fertil Steril 2009; 92:808–813.

Grimbizis G, Gordts S, Di Spiezio Sardo A, et al. The ESHRE-ESGE consensus on the classification of the female genital tract congenital anomalies. Gynecol Surg 2013; 10:199–212.

Heinonen PK, Saarikoski S, Pystynen P. Reproductive performance of women with uterine anomalies. An evaluation of 182 cases. Acta Obstet Gynecol Scand 1982; 61:157–162.

Homer HA, Li TC, Cooke ID. The septate uterus: a review of management and reproductive outcome. Fertil Steril 2000; 73:1–14.

Mollo A, De FP, Colacurci N, et al. Hysteroscopic resection of the septum improves the pregnancy rate of women with unexplained infertility: a prospective controlled trial. Fertil Steril 2009; 91:2628–2631.

Pabuccu R, Gomel V. Reproductive outcome after hysteroscopic metroplasty in women with septate uterus and otherwise unexplained infertility. Fertil Steril 2004; 81:1675–1678.

Pellerito JS, McCarthy SM, Doyle MB, Glickman MG, DeCherney AH. Diagnosis of uterine anomalies: relative accuracy of MR imaging, endovaginal sonography, and hysterosalpingography Radiology 1992; 183:795–800.

Raga F, Bauset C, Remohi J, et al. Reproductive impact of congenital Mullerian anomalies. Hum Reprod 1997; 12:2277–2281.

Rai R, Regan L. Recurrent miscarriage. Lancet 2006; 368:601–611.

Taylor E, Gomel V. The uterus and fertility. Fertil Steril 2008; 89:1–16.

Wu MH, Hsu CC, Huang KE. Detection of congenital Mullerian duct anomalies using three-dimensional ultrasound. J Clin Ultrasound 1997; 25:487–492.

Chapter 13 Endometrial ablation

Olivier Garbin, K Wou, Hervé Fernandez, Amélie Gervaise

INTRODUCTION

Endometrial ablation destroys the endometrium by removing the basal layer of endometrial glands. This procedure requires reaching the superficial layer of the myometrium. It should be offered to patients with functional menorrhagia who no longer wish for fertility preservation. The main goal of this minimally invasive treatment is to avoid the need for hysterectomy. Therefore, it should be considered in cases of failure in medical treatments (nonsteroidal anti-inflammatory drugs, antifibrinolytics, levonorgestrel-releasing intrauterine system) (**Figure 13.1**).

Endometrial ablation can be performed with various energies: electricity, heat, cold, microwave, and laser. The first techniques used for endometrial ablation were done by resectoscope during operative hysteroscopy and are very efficacious. Although simple, these techniques require a certain degree of surgical dexterity, and they have an extensive learning curve. Along with the related complications and risks, these have limited endometrial ablation's popularity and use in favor of newer techniques (referred to as second-generation techniques) in the 1990s. The newer techniques are generally performed without the need for concurrent hysteroscopy; instead, a device is introduced into the uterine cavity to deliver energy to destroy the endometrium (so-called nonresectoscopic endometrial ablation). This procedure also requires less surgical skills from the operator and may be safer and faster.

SET-UP

Endometrial ablation is best performed during the earlier phase of the menstrual cycle. For transcervical resection techniques, a thin endometrium may facilitate the surgical procedure and offer better visualization of the entire cavity. Preoperative preparation of the endometrium through the use of gonadotropin-releasing hormone agonists or danazol may be considered to optimize surgical results, although no studies have thus far proved its benefits (Tan & Lethaby 2013).

A pelvic ultrasound must be done preoperatively to measure the uterus and rule out other pathological lesions that may explain the menorrhagia (**Figure 13.1**). An endometrial biopsy should be done before surgery. However, in patients with no risk factors and a normal endometrium on ultrasound, the biopsy can be performed at the beginning of the surgery.

A preoperative course of anti-inflammatory drugs may diminish postoperative uterine cramping and pain (100 mg of ketoprofen in 50 mL of normal saline perfusing over 10 minutes or a suppository of the same dose along with 1000 mg of paracetamol). This treatment can reduce the release of prostaglandins, relax the uterus and the patient, and reduce postoperative cramping. It may sometimes take up to 6 hours before the patient feels the effects of this treatment; it can then be repeated in the immediate postoperative period and every 4–6 hours thereafter.

For the second-generation techniques mentioned earlier, local anesthesia is possible if the conditions are favorable and if it meets the wishes of a motivated, informed, and relaxed patient.

TRANSCERVICAL ENDOMETRIAL RESECTION

Instrumentation

Transcervical endometrial resection (endometrial resection by hysteroscopy) is usually performed using a resectoscope of 26 or 27 Fr under electronic instillation of a distention media that is compatible with the energy source used. The resectoscope includes:
- A loop electrode (mono- or bipolar)
- A rollerball electrode (mono- or bipolar), or
- A vaporizing bar with bipolar current

Some resectoscopes use an operative hysteroscope with laser fiber, most often Nd-YAG.

Key steps of the procedure

The initial step of the intervention is a diagnostic hysteroscopy followed by an endometrial biopsy if not done previously. The endocervical canal is then dilated according to the size of the hysteroscope to be used.

It is easier to initiate the process by coagulation using a rollerball electrode (with a cutting current), starting from the fundus and cornua. In doing so, the surgeon can avoid floating resected tissues from

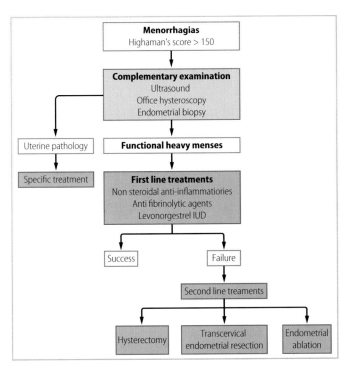

Figure 13.1 Algorithm in treating menorrhagia.

hindering clear visualization of the fundus and ostia toward the end of the surgery. The coagulation electrode is then replaced with a resecting electrode. Some operators may prefer to start the resection with a loop electrode followed by the ball, to destroy the remaining endometrium at the level of the fundus and ostia. If necessary, coagulation is finally used on previously resected areas.

The resection usually starts at the posterior uterine wall, moving from the fundus to the isthmus in a continuous smooth movement using flexion of the forearm toward to the upper arm. The first resected specimen is used to determine the required depth of satisfactory resection, stopping on the muscular wall as defined by the outer circular fibers of the myometrium before the layer of the venous plexus (**Figure 13.2**). In partial endometrial resection, for patients who do not wish for total amenorrhea, a 1 cm endometrial stripe is left below the isthmus (**Figure 13.3**). Endometrial resection is typically done using a counterclockwise technique, including the posterior wall, the left sidewall, the anterior wall, and the right sidewall (**Figures 13.2** and **13.4**). The lateral walls of the uterine isthmus must be carefully resected because of its proximity to the uterine vessels. Also, the endocervical portion should not be resected to avoid endocervical adhesions; it can lead to hematometria and subsequent pelvic pain. Hemostasis of the bleeding vessels is obtained with further coagulation as needed. At the end of the surgery, the resection will be completed by restoring the anatomical landmarks and removing further tissues to reconstruct a regular uterine cavity. To do so, some operators will use only the ball electrode in cutting mode to destroy the endometrium as a whole. This technique causes fewer complications.

Removal of resected tissues is done using the loop electrode or a curette. It is best not to remove these tissues during the operation but instead to place them at the fundus of the cavity. However, in a postmenopausal or smaller uterus, it is often necessary to remove the specimens the procedure progresses. In cases of vaporization using a rollerball or a vaporizing bar, there are no floating specimens to be removed (**Figure 13.5**).

During resection using an Nd-YAG laser, the uterine fundus can be treated by the 'no-touch' technique following a long sweeping motion. The rest of the cavity is treated by the 'in-touch' technique, which consists of creating stripes throughout the uterine walls. This portion of the procedure is usually performed at a power of 100 W.

SECOND-GENERATION TECHNIQUES

Many alternative techniques to hysteroscopic endometrial resection have been developed in the past 15 years. All these techniques have a

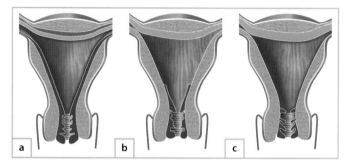

Figure 13.3 Principle of transcervical resection. (a) Uterine cavity with endometrium marked in red. (b) In partial resection of the endometrium, a 1 cm rim of endometrium is left below the isthmus if patient does not want to be amenorrheic. (c) In total endometrial resection, all of the endometrium is resected.

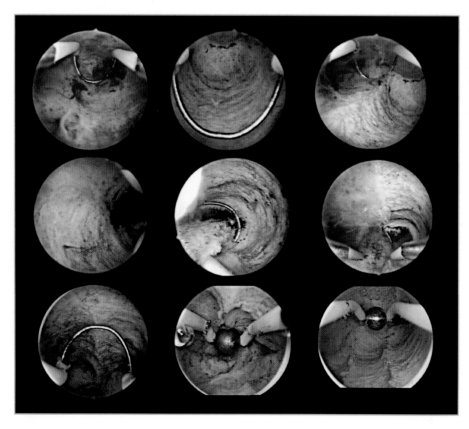

Figure 13.2 Endometrial resection. (a) Start with first specimen. (b) First endometrial specimen from posterior wall removing the base of the glands. (c) The second specimen is aligned lateral to the first. (d and f) Resection of the right and left lateral walls. (f and g) Resection of the anterior surface. (h) Destruction of the endometrium at the fundus and cornua with rollerball electrode. I: Coagulation and final appearance. Reproduced from Fernandez H, Garbin O, Gervaise A. Hystéroscopie et Fertiloscopie. Copyright © 2013, Elsevier Masson SAS: all rights reserved.

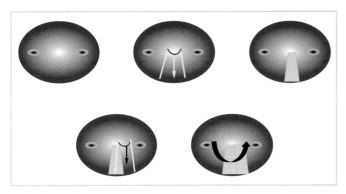

Figure 13.4 Principle of transcervical resection. Achieving the first two endometrial specimens. The first one is taken from the posterior wall, removing with it the base of the glands. To achieve the second specimen, the loop is placed just lateral to the first. The same smooth gestures are pursued in a counter-clockwise fashion to complete the resection.

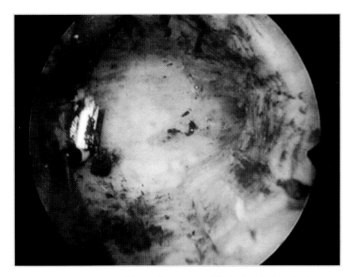

Figure 13.5 Destruction of the endometrium with the bipolar bar. Final aspect. Reproduced from Fernandez H, Garbin O, Gervaise A. Hystéroscopie et Fertiloscopie. Copyright © 2013, Elsevier Masson SAS: all rights reserved.

quick learning curve, requiring the surgeon to perform fewer than five procedures to be proficient. It also eliminates the surgical skills needed in operative hysteroscopy, has a very short operating time, and results in a very low morbidity rate. These techniques include cryotherapy, the direct circulation of hot fluid, interstitial laser, phototherapy,

microwave, radio frequency, and thermocoagulation balloon. Balloon techniques are the most studied. **Table 13.1** shows the main features of these products and techniques. Some of these techniques are still in the developmental stage, others have just appeared on the market, and so-called third-generation techniques are still being studied (e.g. water vaporization).

One-third of interventions can be performed under local anesthesia using lidocaine 1% with 200 milliunits of adrenaline diluted in 20 mL of normal saline for a paracervical block in addition to premedication using anti-inflammatory drugs (see previous section).

Thermal balloons

Several devices are available, under different brands, such as Thermachoice from Ethicon, Thermablate from EAS, and Cavatherm from Endotherapeutics. The device is composed of a flexible plastic catheter: one end has a silicone balloon in which is located a heating electrode; the other end is connected to a central control system that measures pressure in the balloon, regulates the temperature, and monitors the duration of treatment. The central pump circulates dextrose solution within the balloon in order to obtain an even heat distribution on its surface and, therefore, on the endometrium. These three brands of balloons differ essentially in their diameter and the duration of treatment, ranging from 2 minutes for Thermablate to 8 minutes for the other balloon brands. The temperature can reach 173°C for Thermablate and 87°C for the other balloons.

The first step to an operative hysteroscopy is a survey of the uterine cavity if not done previously during a diagnostic hysteroscopy. In our facility, we then perform a curettage for tissue sampling and pathological examination. Then, a hysterometry is used to measure the uterine cavity. Unlike the other two devices, the Thermachoice requires no cervical dilation. The uterine sound is inserted through the endocervical canal to the fundus; the balloon is then inflated and the control generator indicates when the initial pressure stabilizes. At this point, the silicone balloon is perfectly applied to the walls of the uterine cavity. Once the pressure is stable, the central control system is triggered to heat the liquid, which is usually a solution of 5% glucose, to best transmit the temperature. When this is achieved, on average within 30–90 seconds, the therapeutic cycle starts and lasts for a pre-programmed duration (**Figure 13.6**).

Each device is automatically deactivated when the pressure is either too low or too high. At the end of the treatment cycle, it is common to wait 30–60 seconds before deflating the balloon before its removal for safety reasons.

The immediate consequences are typically identified during the first month by the presence of serosanguineous discharge resulting from the resorption phenomenon from intracavitary burns. A hysteroscopy performed 2 months later can reveal major synechia in the uterine cavity.

Table 13.1 Comparison of the different techniques available for endometrial ablation

System	Energy	Temperature (°C)	Dilatation	Duration (min)	Security	Adaptability
Thermachoice	Heat	87	No	8	Good	No
Thermablate	Heat	173	Yes	2	Good	No
Cavatherm	Heat	87	Yes	8	Good	No
HTA	Heat	90	Yes	15	Good	Yes
Microsulis	Microwave	80	Yes	4	Average	Yes
Novasure	Bipolar	Undetermined	Yes	2	Good	No
Her Option	Cold	−100	No	5	Average	Yes

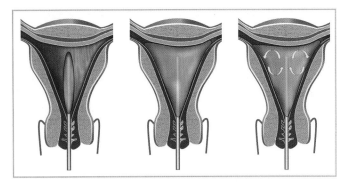

Figure 13.6 Principle of balloon thermocoagulation of the endometrium. The probe is inserted through the cervix to the fundus. The balloon is then inflated. It is closely applied to the walls of the uterine cavity. Once the pressure is stabilized, the heating of the liquid is triggered. When adequate temperature is reached, the treatment cycle can start.

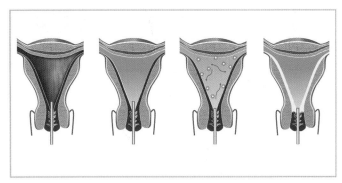

Figure 13.7 Endometrial thermocoagulation with the instillation of hot fluid by hysteroscopy. This requires direct visualization by hysteroscopy. The system consists of instilling hot fluid at low pressure to avoid tubal passage. The heat generated raises the temperature of the serosa to cause destruction of the endometrium.

Instillation of hot serum fluid

The Hydro Therm Ablator (HTA) system from Boston Scientific requires direct visualization by hysteroscopy. This system instills warm saline between 70°C and 85°C over a period of 15 minutes at low pressure (50–55 mm Hg) to avoid tubal passage and intraperitoneal burn (**Figure 13.7**). The heat generated raises the temperature of the serosa to 45°C. The operating time is 8–10 minutes at 90°C. The thickness of endometrial necrosis is 2–4 mm. This system can be used for distorted uterine cavities, as in cases of uterine septum, for example.

Microwave

The Microsulis, from Hologic, has not been commercially available since 2011, for marketing reasons rather than for medical reasons. An 8 mm wand that rotates up and down is inserted into the uterine cavity after dilating the cervix to number 8 Hegar. The distal end of the device delivers heat that must reach a temperature between 70°C and 80°C so that the treatment cycle can start. It is necessary to mobilize the device under computer control by making side-to-side movements in order to sweep across the cavity and deliver a controlled temperature to the contacted tissue. When the device enters an untreated area, it decreases the temperature before increasing it again when it is within a treated area. The computer screen will show a temperature curve and allow the operator to achieve a uniform treatment of the cavity. The device will then gradually exteriorize out of the cavity. Once the isthmus is reached, a marker will reach the external cervical os, and the device can then be removed. The destruction of the endometrium should be to a depth of about 6 mm.

Radio frequency

The Novasure system from Hologic supplies power at 150 W radio frequency to destroy the endometrium. The Novasure consists of a mesh that opens into the shape of the uterus and wherein a bipolar plug is inserted (**Figure 13.8**). The apparatus includes a suction system that keeps the mesh in direct contact with the endometrium throughout the procedure. An initial hysteroscopy is done to measure the distance between the fundus and the internal cervical os (this distance can be determined by ultrasound prior to the procedure). This distance is entered into the generator. Cervical dilatation to Hegar number 8 is required. The device is then introduced into the uterine cavity and the interostial distance (endocervical canal length) is measured on a handle attached to the device and then entered into the generator

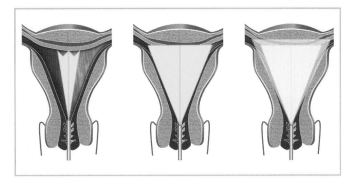

Figure 13.8 Destruction of the endometrium by radio frequency. This device consists of a mesh that expands into the shape of the uterus and wherein a bipolar current is distributed.

system. Once this is achieved, the cervix is sealed by a valve that sits on the introducer. The injection of CO_2 can verify the absence of perforation. Destruction is initiated and lasts between 90 and 120 seconds. The operating time is 90 seconds. The destruction is done to a depth of 4–4.5 mm in the cavity and 2.2–2.9 mm at the level of the uterine horns (**Figure 13.9**).

Cryotherapy

Endometrial cryotherapy is a non-hysteroscopic procedure that uses low temperatures to freeze and destroy the endometrium. The Her Option device by Cryogen is typical. A cryotherapy probe of 5.5 mm in diameter is inserted to the fundus under ultrasound guidance. The probe is then cooled by infusion of liquid nitrogen or a mixture of compressed gas at –100°C. The end of the probe is first placed into one of uterine cornua and then the other to generate an ice ball that destroys the endometrium at that level. Each cycle of freezing is followed by a heating cycle (thawing) to allow the withdrawal of the probe. Additional cycles of freezing/thawing can be done as deemed necessary. This technique leads to destruction to a depth of more than 11 mm.

Which technique to choose?

The second-generation techniques are less complex, faster, easily reproducible, and have fewer complications than transcervical resection. However, they are more expensive and require the purchase of specific generators and disposable devices.

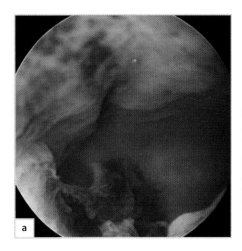
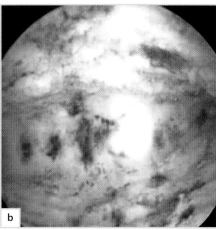

Figure 13.9 Destruction of the endometrium by radio frequency. Hysteroscopic aspect before (a) and after the destruction (b).

When choosing among the second-generation techniques, the operator must take into account the patient's choice to be in amenorrhea or not (most likely with Novasure than with the other balloons; see the 'Complications and postoperative follow-up' section), the shape of the cavity (for anatomically distorted uteri, only Microsulis and HTA devices are possible), and safety (**Table 13.1**).

COMPLICATIONS AND POSTOPERATIVE FOLLOW-UP

Complications

The complication rate for transcervical resection is 4.4% (Overton et al. 1997). Techniques using coagulation ball or laser cause fewer complications than the loop electrode. Uterine perforation may occur either during cervical dilatation or during resection. Hemorrhage is usually mild and disappears within a few hours. More severe bleeding complications have sometimes required the use of hysterectomy to attain satisfactory hemostasis (Overton et al. 1997). Post-hysteroscopic endometritis occurs in 1–5% of cases (Causland et al. 1993).

Second-generation techniques cause less complications than does transcervical resection. The balloons seem safest. Some systems are capable of detecting changes in pressure or leaks, both of which may indicate a perforation (balloons, Novasure, HTA). The Microsulis and Her Option devices do not feature these safety devices (**Table 13.1**). In case of doubt, ultrasound may be necessary to ensure proper positioning of the device. Occasionally, severe complications including deaths and severe burns of adjacent organs have been reported after activation of a device that was wrongly placed intra-abdominally (Brown & Blank 2012).

Late complications have also been reported (Sharp 2012). Subsequent pregnancies are not uncommon (0.7%), and these may be complicated by spontaneous abortions, late mid-trimester pregnancy losses, preterm delivery, and abnormal placentation. Some patients may demonstrate pelvic pain caused by the obstruction of menstrual flow (pain related to obstructed menses). Some cancers have been reported following endometrial ablation; as a result, at-risk women probably do not benefit from these techniques.

Postoperative follow-up

Patients may have pelvic pain for 24–48 hours after the procedure, which justifies the prescription of analgesic treatment with anti-inflammatory medications in the absence of contraindications or allergies. Serosanguineous vaginal discharge may persist for several days or even weeks. Sexual intercourse may resume 7–10 days after surgery.

The introduction of contraception (if necessary) is essential. This can be achieved by implementing an intraoperative levonorgestrel intrauterine device (IUD) or, alternatively, tubal implants.

ALTERNATIVES

Two alternatives to endometrial ablation can be considered: the insertion of a levonorgestrel IUD or hysterectomy.

The insertion of a levonorgestrel IUD is a valid alternative to all techniques of endometrial ablation. In a French multicenter prospective study, 50 patients awaiting hysterectomy or endometrial ablation for the treatment of menorrhagia received a levonorgestrel IUD in the meantime. The study showed that 90% actually waived the planned procedure at 12 months with 86% satisfaction (Yazbeck et al. 2006).

In an earlier meta-analysis, Lethaby et al. concluded that endometrial resection was more effective than levonorgestrel IUD in terms of reducing the amount of bleeding, but overall satisfaction was lower (Lethaby et al. 2005).

In a recent randomized controlled trial (RCT) comparing the levonorgestrel IUD to the thermocoagulation balloon for endometrial ablation in women with menorrhagia, the efficacy of the IUD is greater than thermocoagulation in terms of the need for hysterectomy, amount of bleeding, hemoglobin level, and overall satisfaction (Silva-Filho et al. 2013).

In the latest Cochrane review published in 2013, hysterectomy is found to be superior to endometrial ablation in terms of long-term satisfaction despite a high degree of satisfaction for endometrial ablation. Hysterectomy requires longer operating time, a hospital stay, and a longer recovery period, and it has more perioperative complications than endometrial ablation. Endometrial ablation has an initially lower cost than hysterectomy, but this benefit fades over time because of the need for reoperation (Fergusson et al. 2013).

CONTRAINDICATIONS

The usual contraindications of these treatments are undiagnosed vaginal bleeding, pregnancy, pelvic infection or gynecological malignancies, enlarged uterus (with hysterometry >11 cm), submucosal fibroids, polyps, and women seeking pregnancy. Uterine malformations are a contraindication for second-generation techniques (**Table 13.1**).

SUMMARY OF EVIDENCE

For transcervical resection, the largest series report success rates of 70–97%, amenorrhea rates of 10–60%, and complication rates of 4–7% (O'Connor et al. 1996; Overton et al. 1997). In RCTs, the rates of reoperation (hysterectomy or repeat resection) after transcervical resection vary from 10% to 38% for follow-up periods ranging from 4 months to 5 years (Cooper & Erickson, 2000, Crosignani et al. 1997, Dickersin et al. 2007, Dwyer et al. 1993, Gannon et al. 1991, O'Connor et al. 1997, Parkin et al. 1994, Pinion et al. 1994).

Several studies have compared different first-generation techniques and have been the subject of a Cochrane review (Lethaby et al. 2009). These methods have the same therapeutic efficacy with similar rates of satisfaction. Success rates ranged from 70% to 97%, and the rate of amenorrhea was between 10% and 60%. The rollerball procedure is the fastest and safest technology. Laser surgery requires the longest operating time, with a greater risk of volume overload. Resection by loop electrode exposes the patient to greater risk of complications (7% vs. 4% in laser and rollerball, respectively).

Another RCT compares the use of monopolar loop with glycine solution versus two types of bipolar loop with normal saline for endometrial resection, but also for resection of polyps and myomas (Berg et al. 2009). The absorption of glycine is less than that of normal saline but causes more hyponatremia. As a result, the monopolar technique is the fastest of the two, and the authors attribute this to the larger size of the monopolar loop.

For second-generation techniques, radio frequency and microwave yield higher rates of amenorrhea than does the balloon, with similar rates of satisfaction. Radio frequency and microwave techniques are more effective than HTA from the standpoint of treating bleeding. Radio frequency induces a higher rate of amenorrhea and less dissatisfaction than does HTA. Cryotherapy is less likely to result in amenorrhea when compared to radio frequency or microwave (Daniels et al. 2012).

A meta-analysis on the comparison of transcervical resection and second-generation techniques has been published recently (Lethaby et al. 2013). There is no significant difference between these first- and second-generation techniques in the efficacy of treating bleeding (measured by the improvement in hemoglobin) and patient satisfaction. The second-generation techniques are faster and often performed under local rather than general anesthesia.

The risks of fluid overload, uterine perforation, cervical laceration, and hematometria are increased with transcervical resection as are nausea, vomiting, and uterine cramping in the immediate postoperative period. The risk of hysterectomy also appears higher with transcervical resection.

PRACTICAL TIPS

Whichever technique is being used, a good patient selection is essential. These techniques should be reserved for clinically significant menorrhagia. The patient should be informed of the details of the procedure and its expected benefits, risks of failure, complications, and therapeutic alternatives. Contraceptive methods must be discussed before the procedure.

An endometrial biopsy should be done systematically, at the latest on the day of the procedure.

The anti-inflammatory medications should be given to the patient the night prior to the procedure and, if possible, at least 1 hour before surgery to obtain good postoperative analgesia.

For transcervical resection, the operation should be planned during the follicular phase of the menstrual cycle, and the endometrium should be prepared to reduce its thickness. The rollerball is used in section to destroy the endometrium. One should avoid the subisthmic portion of the endometrium to prevent adhesions and hematometria. Care must be taken so that the thinning does not go too deeply into the lateral walls and subisthmic area and avoids the uterine vessels and its collaterals. One must be wary of large cavities, which result in long and difficult surgery and lower success rates.

For second-generation techniques, the manufacturer's instructions should be carefully followed.

CONCLUSION

New technologies in the field of endometrial ablation play an important role in the management of functional menorrhagia. They can be considered after failure of medical treatments (nonsteroidal anti-inflammatory drugs, anti-fibrinolytic medications, levonorgestrel IUD) and as an alternative to hysterectomy. At present, the second-generation techniques are safer and less operator-dependent than transcervical resection.

REFERENCES

Berg A, Sandvik L, Langebrekke A, Istre O. A randomized trial comparing monopolar electrodes using glycine 1.5% with two different types of bipolar electrodes (TCRis, Versapoint) using saline, in hysteroscopic surgery. Fertil Steril 2009; 91:1273–1278.

Brown J, Blank K. Minimally invasive endometrial ablation device complications and use outside of the manufacturers' instructions. Obstet Gynecol 2012; 120:865–870.

Causland V, Fields A, Townsend E. Tuboovarian abscesses after operative hysteroscopy. J Reprod Med 1993; 38:198–200.

Cooper JM, Erickson ML. Global endometrial ablation technologies. Obstet Gynecol Clin North Am 2000; 27:385–396.

Crosignani PG, Vercellini P, Apolone G, et al. Endometrial resection versus vaginal hysterectomy for menorrhagia: long-term clinical and quality-of-life outcomes. Am J Obstet Gynecol 1997; 177:95–101.

Daniels JP, Middleton LJ, Champaneria R, et al., International Heavy Menstrual Bleeding IPD Meta-analysis Collaborative Group. Second generation endometrial ablation techniques for heavy menstrual bleeding: network meta-analysis. BMJ 2012; 344:e2564.

Dickersin K, Munro MG, Clark M, et al. Hysterectomy compared with endometrial ablation for dysfunctional uterine bleeding: a randomized controlled trial. Obstet Gynecol 2007; 110:1279–1289.

Dwyer N, Hutton J, Stirrat GM. Randomised controlled trial comparing endometrial resection with abdominal hysterectomy for the surgical treatment of menorrhagia. Br J Obstet Gynaecol 1993; 100:237–243.

Fergusson RJ, Lethaby A, Shepperd S, Farquhar C. Endometrial resection and ablation versus hysterectomy for heavy menstrual bleeding. Cochrane Database Syst Rev 2013; 29:CD000329.

Gannon MJ, Holt EM, Fairbank J, et al. A randomised trial comparing endometrial resection and abdominal hysterectomy for the treatment of menorrhagia. BMJ 1991; 30:1362–1364.

Lethaby AE, Cooke I, Rees M. Progesterone or progestogen-releasing intrauterine systems for heavy menstrual bleeding. Cochrane Database Syst Rev 2005; 4:CD002126.

Lethaby A, Hickey M, Garry R, Penninx J. Endometrial resection/ablation techniques for heavy menstrual bleeding. Cochrane Database Syst Rev 2009; 4:CD001501.

Lethaby A, Penninx J, Hickey M, et al. Endometrial resection and ablation techniques for heavy menstrual bleeding. Cochrane Database Syst Rev 2013; 30:CD001501.

O'Connor H, Broadbent JA, Magos AL, McPherson K. Medical Research Council randomised trial of endometrial resection versus hysterectomy in management of menorrhagia. Lancet 1997; 29:897–901.

O'Connor H, Magos A. Endometrial resection for the treatment of menorrhagia. N Engl J Med 1996; 18(335):151–156.

Overton C, Hargreaves J, Maresh M. A national survey of the complications of endometrial destruction for menstrual disorders: the MISTLETOE study. Minimally Invasive Surgical Techniques-Laser, EndoThermal or Endoresection. Br J Obstet Gynaecol 1997; 104:1351–1359.

Parkin DE, Abramovich DR, Naji A, et al. Randomised trial of hysterectomy, endometrial laser ablation, and transcervical endometrial resection for dysfunctional uterine bleeding. BMJ 1994; 15:979–983.

Pinion SB, Parkin DE, Abramovich DR, et al. Randomised trial of hysterectomy, endometrial laser ablation, and transcervical endometrial resection for dysfunctional uterine bleeding. BMJ 1994; 309:979–983.

Sharp HT. Endometrial ablation: post-operative complications. Am J Obstet Gynecol 2012; 207:242–247.

Silva-Filho AL, Pereira Fde A, de Souza SS, et al. Five-year follow-up of levonorgestrel-releasing intrauterine system versus thermal balloon ablation for the treatment of heavy menstrual bleeding: a randomized controlled trial. Contraception 2013; 87:409–415.

Tan YH, Lethaby A. Pre-operative endometrial thinning agents before endometrial destruction for heavy menstrual bleeding. Cochrane Database Syst Rev 2013; 15:CD010241.

Yazbeck C, Omnes S, Vacher-Lavenu MC, Madelenat P. Levonorgestrel-releasing intrauterine system in the treatment of dysfunctional uterine bleeding: a French multicenter study. Gynecol Obstet Fertil 2006; 34:906–913.

Chapter 14 · Hysteroscopic management of uterine fibroids and polyps

Megan Loring, Keith B Isaacson

INTRODUCTION

Uterine fibroids and endometrial polyps are common gynecologic abnormalities among premenopausal and postmenopausal women. The presence of these pathologies often leads to symptoms such as recurrent pregnancy loss, infertility, abnormal uterine bleeding, and postmenopausal bleeding, all of which require treatment. Since the advent of operative hysteroscopy, both submucosal fibroids and endometrial polyps can be easily treated via a hysteroscopic approach – a minimally invasive, nonincisional procedure utilizing the natural orifice of the cervix. Depending on the size of the pathology and the experience of the surgeon, hysteroscopic myomectomy or polypectomy can be performed safely in an office setting as well as in an operating room.

PRESURGICAL EVALUATION

Presence of polyps

Abnormal uterine bleeding such as midcycle spotting or postmenopausal bleeding in women should prompt physicians to pursue an evaluation of the uterine cavity that at the very least includes a vaginal probe pelvic ultrasound and possibly an endometrial biopsy, depending on the woman's age. An endometrial polyp most often appears as a hyper- or hypoechoic lesion within the uterine lumen on transvaginal ultrasound (TVUS). When color Doppler is applied, it is common to find a feeding vessel to an endometrial polyp. In premenopausal women, the ultrasound is best performed before cycle day 10 when the endometrial lining should be thin (<5 mm). Filling the uterine cavity with saline while performing the TVUS [saline infusion sonohysterography (SIS)] will more clearly delineate the size and location of an endometrial polypoid lesion. One must be careful not to mistake an intrauterine blood clot as an endometrial polyp. In addition to TVUS and SIS, office hysteroscopy is also an excellent tool to diagnose uterine polyps. Several studies have compared the sensitivity and specificity of these three modalities, and most suggest that office hysteroscopy and SIS have similar sensitivities near 95%, with slightly higher specificity for the hysteroscopy and lower sensitivity and specificity for the TVUS than both SIS and office hysteroscopy (Salim et al. 2011). With imaging suggestive of an endometrial polyp, patients can then be counseled regarding hysteroscopic removal.

CHARACTERIZATION OF FIBROIDS

Women who are potential candidates for hysteroscopic myomectomy must have fibroid characteristics that are amenable to this surgical approach. Preoperative imaging such as transvaginal ultrasonography has been shown to have good diagnostic accuracy for most

diseases of the uterine cavity. This modality, with the addition of three-dimensional imaging or saline sonohysterography is the best noninvasive option to determine the size of lesion and the depth of myometrial penetration of fibroids (Di Naro et al. 1996, Jorizzo et al. 1999). Diagnostic office hysteroscopy allows the surgeon to confirm of the presence of the submucosal fibroid, as well as to directly assess the intracavity component, size, and exact location of the pathology (Di Speizio Sardo et al. 2008). Additional advantages of office hysteroscopy are that it demonstrates the vascularity of the submucosal myomas; it allows the surgeon to reduce and inflate the intrauterine pressure that can alter the subtype of myoma; and it gives the surgeon the exact view of the uterine cavity that will be seen at the time of hysteroscopy myoma removal.

Submucosal fibroids are most commonly classified by the European Society for Gynecologic Endoscopy (ESGE) according to extent of myometrial involvement; see **Table 14.1** and **Figure 14.1** (Wamsteker et al. 1993). Although the recently published International Federation of Gynecology and Obstetrics (FIGO) classification will likely replace the ESGE classification, we will refer mostly to the ESGE system since most previously published and recent data refer to the ESGE nomenclature. In brief, the new FIGO classification includes the previously

Table 14.1 European Society of Gynecologic Endoscopy classification of submucosal fibroids

Fibroid type	Submucous fibroid location
Type 0	Completely within the endometrial cavity
Type 1	Extends <50% into the myometrium
Type 2	Extends 50% or more within the myometrium

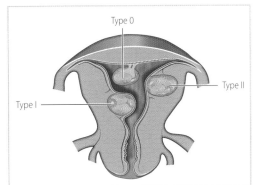

Figure 14.1 Types of submucosal myomas based on the depth of myometrial penetration.

classified submucosal myomas as types 0, 1, and 2, but is extended to include intramural myomas (types 3, 4, 5), subserosal myomas (types 6 and 7), and cervical myomas (type 8; Munro et al. 2011).

The ESGE classification system dictates surgical options and can shape patients' expectations by helping a practitioner to predict the ability to resect the complete fibroid in one procedure (Isaacson 2003). Observational studies showed complete resection rates to vary: type 0 (96–97%), type I (86–90%), and type II (61–83%; Wamsteker et al. 1993, Van Dongen et al. 2006). As a general rule, type 0 and type I fibroids can usually be removed in one procedure whereas type II commonly necessitates two procedures for complete resection. The amount of myometrial penetration in the submucosal fibroid is also related to fluid absorption during hysteroscopy. Specifically, the volume of fluid absorbed during the procedure increases significantly with the degree of myometrial penetration (type 0: 450 mL, type I: 957 mL, type II: 1682 mL; Emanuel et al. 1997). These parameters can be used when counseling patients and setting expectations regarding an upcoming hysteroscopic myomectomy. Until 2006, all hysteroscopic resections were performed with monopolar energy and electrolyte-free media. With the advent of bipolar resection and the use of physiologic distention media, the previously used ESGE classification predictions of one- or two-stage procedures are being rewritten. Women with multiple fibroids or bulk symptoms might be better served by performing laparoscopic myomectomy, either concomitant with or in lieu of hysteroscopy myomectomy.

CONTRAINDICATIONS

Contraindications to hysteroscopic polypectomy or myomectomy parallel general contraindications for hysteroscopy: active pelvic infection, intrauterine pregnancy, known cervical or uterine cancer. Medical comorbidities such as coronary artery disease, chronic obstructive pulmonary disease, or bleeding diatheses must be managed with primary care physicians or anesthesiologists to ensure the patient is safe to undergo a planned procedure.

PROCEDURE LOCATION

Operative hysteroscopy can be safely performed either in an office setting or in an operating room. The choice of location depends on the size of the lesion, the experience of the surgeon, and the motivation of the patient. Office procedures are generally performed without any anesthesia or at most with nonsteroidal anti-inflammatory drugs (NSAIDs) and/or local paracervical blocks. Office operative hysteroscopy is now feasible because of technologic advances – smaller-diameter hysteroscopes with continuous flow system features and a working channel. The 'see-and-treat' approach of office operative hysteroscopy is gaining popularity, as it is convenient for both the patient and the doctor and is a tremendous cost-saving one (Cicinelli 2010). Other advantages include reduced anesthesia risks and faster patient recovery with less time away from work and home (Di Speizio Sardo et al. 2010). Main limitations are patient discomfort, as well as limitations in equipment and office staffing. Keys to a successful operative hysteroscopy in the office setting include operator experience, trained staff, and an examination room with an easy, ergonomic set-up for hysteroscopy (see **Figure 14.2**). In general, office procedures should be completed within 10–15 minutes. Most importantly, the size of polyp or fibroid should not be larger than the diameter of the internal cervical os. Larger pathology will require either cervical dilation or techniques to cut the pathology into small pieces with either a pair of scissors, a bipolar electrode, or a morcellator. Otherwise, removing a tissue fragment larger than the

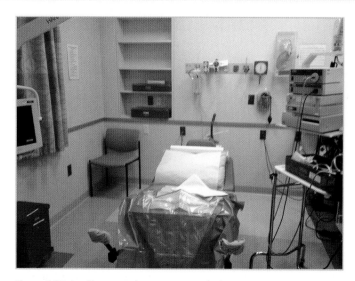

Figure 14.2 In-office procedure room set-up for hysteroscopy.

cervical canal may be too painful for a patient to tolerate. In a recent review of the literature, Cicinelli found that for office polypectomy without anesthesia, the procedure was well tolerated by women as long as the polyp was <2 cm and the procedure was lasted <15 minutes (Cicinelli 2010).

PREOPERATIVE MEDICATIONS

Whether in the office or the operating room, preoperative antibiotics are not indicated for hysteroscopic polypectomy or myomectomy without a history of pelvic inflammatory disease. The role of dilute vasopressin for reducing blood loss, reducing fluid intravasation, and for ease of cervical dilation during operative hysteroscopy in the operating room continues to be debated. A randomized control trial showed that intracervical administration of dilute vasopressin (0.05 U/mL) decreased blood loss, distention media intravasation, and operative time (Phillips et al. 1996). Although statistically significant, the absolute differences were small. Another randomized control trial showed that intracervical dilute vasopressin decreased the amount of force needed to dilate the cervix (Phillips et al. 1997). Again, although statistically significant, the clinical implications of these findings are less clear. In the office, the use of intracervical dilute vasopressin is not indicated due to the small diameter of the hysteroscopic equipment and the low risk of blood loss or fluid intravasation due to the short time of the procedure and the small size of the pathology.

The role of preoperative gonadotropin-releasing hormone agonist (GnRHa), most common leuprolide, is also controversial. Benefits cited in the literature include the ease of surgical scheduling due to hormonally induced thin endometrial lining and improvement in anemia due to GnRH-induced amenorrhea. Most importantly, preoperative leuprolide can reduce uterine and fibroid vascularization. This can limit intraoperative blood loss as well as distention media intravasation (Isaacson 2003, Parazzini et al, 1998). There are no universally accepted guidelines on indication, duration, or dosage for preoperative GnRH agonists. Some experts believe that preoperative GnRH therapy should be reserved for submucosal fibroids of >3 cm or for those suffering from severe anemia (Valle & Baggish 2007). In general, there is only a rare surgical advantage to preoperative treatment, especially in light of potential side effects (hot flushes and vaginal dryness) and high cost of leuprolide (Fedele et al. 1990). Another disadvantage is the shrinkage of myomas, which can make hysteroscopic visualization of type II myomas nearly impossible. More than likely, these are not the cases that will be attempted in an office setting.

OFFICE OPERATIVE HYSTEROSCOPY

Set-up

Keys for successful office hysteroscopy include the presence of proper equipment, an ergonomic set-up, well-trained nurses and medical assistants, and established protocols for managing complications such as medication allergies, vasovagal reactions, and uterine bleeding. Many offices utilize a multipurpose procedure room, but a standard examination room is sufficient, given the limited space required with today's technology. An adjustable bed is essential for the comfort and safety of both the patient and physician. Compact, portable towers are available to keep the camera, light source, video screen, and printer organized (Presthus). Newer technology incorporates the camera and light into the hysteroscope itself, therefore, only requiring a monitor such as a laptop computer to be in the room to perform office hysteroscopic procedures. Office-based procedures are clean and nonsterile. Any instrument used inside the patient should be sterile and the physician should wear sterile gloves; however, a gown and a mask are not required. An under-the-buttocks drape with a pocket to catch fluid is helpful to keep the fluid from soaking the floor and allowing a rough estimate of fluid absorbed by the patient. Large bore 'cysto' tubing with a lure lock adaptor and 1 L normal saline bags for distention media are needed. Office hysteroscopy prepackaged sets that include drapes, tubing, and collection bags are made available by various manufacturers. In addition, it is important to have a hysteroscopic seal through which instruments can be inserted and removed without any leakage on to the operator. During most office operative hysteroscopies, quantitative fluid management is not crucial as procedures should only last 10–15 minutes maximum and it is rare to use >1 L of normal saline; see **Figure 14.2** for an example of an effective procedure room set-up for office hysteroscopy.

Instrumentation

It is advantageous to have a variety of hysteroscopes available for use depending on a patient's indication for office hysteroscopy. For example, a 3.0 mm system with a 2.1 mm 12° or a 30° hysteroscope, or a 3 mm flexible hysteroscope is ideal for diagnostic hysteroscopy. These are noncontinuous flow systems and can only be used when the patient is not actively bleeding. For operative hysteroscopy, a rigid 4.5–5.5 mm continuous flow hysteroscope with 5 Fr working channel is needed. These are available with either a 12° or 30° lenses from various manufacturers. The 5 Fr working channel accommodates mechanical instruments including blunt-tipped scissors, grasping forceps, and a tenaculum, as well as 5 Fr monopolar and bipolar radio frequency (RF) electrodes (Bettocchi et al. 2002, 2004). Current morcellator technologies have been used in the office setting but they are not commonplace due to the expense and the need for high fluid flow and fluid management. A recent pilot study by Dealberti et al. showed promise for a minimonopolar resectoscope (12 Fr) in an office setting without analgesia or local anesthesia. Office polypectomy was successfully performed in 100% (33/33) patients with a mean operating time of 11.5 minutes and a mean visual analog scale tolerability score of 2.5 on a 0–6 scale, indicating mild discomfort only. Drawbacks to this miniresectoscope include its use of monopolar energy, necessitating electrolyte-free distention media (Dealberti et al. 2013).

General technique

The major advantages of office hysteroscopy include the potential to diagnose and treat lesions in a single session that is convenient and efficient for both the patient and the practitioner (Wortman et al. 2013). In the vast majority of cases, no cervical dilation is necessary. Hysteroscopy can be performed completely without anesthesia using a vaginoscopic 'no-touch' technique, or this approach can be supplemented with either oral or intramuscular NSAIDs and with or without a paracervical block if necessary for patient's comfort. A randomized control trial enrolling 130 women compared the vaginoscopic technique with the traditional technique with speculum and tenaculum. The mean pain scores during and after the examinations were significantly lower in the vaginoscopy group compared with the 'traditional' group (Sagiv et al. 2006). In a larger study of 4863 women, 71.9–93.5% of women underwent office operative hysteroscopy using a 'no-touch' technique without discomfort for all pathologies treated except for endometrial polyps larger than the internal cervical os; among them, only 63.6% experienced low or moderate pain (Cicinelli 2010). Perhaps, most important, all office hysteroscopy should be performed during the patients' proliferative phase of the cycle (days 6–11) to avoid endometrial thickness obscuring pathology or menstrual blood obscuring the visual field.

Vaginoscopy

After informed consent is discussed and signed, patients are positioned in low lithotomy in stirrups. The vagina and cervix are then prepped with Betadine using three OB/Gyn applicators. Check inflow/outflow channels and ensure the camera is white-balanced and working properly. Gently spread the labia to allow the placement of the hysteroscope into the vagina. The 1-L normal saline bag is contained within a pressure cuff at 150 mmHg. This is not the pressure within the uterus. The stopcock on the hysteroscope is rotated to the on position until adequate visualization is obtained. If the patient is uncomfortable with the intrauterine pressure, then the stopcock can be rotated to reduce the flow and intrauterine pressure. The hysteroscope, once in the vagina, is directed toward the posterior vaginal fornix; then the operator pulls the scope back to visually locate the cervix and ultimately the cervical os. Once in the external os, it is extremely important to rotate the light cord of the scope while gently advancing toward the uterine cavity. One must remember that when using a 12°–30° hysteroscope, the angle of the scope is opposite to the light cord, so one should be looking at the 12 o'clock position of the cervical canal while advancing the hysteroscope, in order to avoid tunneling into the posterior aspect of the cervix or lower uterine segment.

Polypectomy
Key steps

The majority of endometrial polyps can be removed using mechanical instruments without electrical or mechanical energy. Blunt-tipped or sharp-tipped scissors can be used to cleanly detach the polyp from the endometrium at its base. The polyp is then grasped with either a grasping forceps or a 5 Fr tenaculum to remove the specimen from the uterine cavity. Others have described grasping the base of the polyp with an open forceps and gently detaching it from its implant in the myometrium (Bettocchi et al. 2004). Limitations of these techniques are related to polyp size and the inability of the grasping forceps to completely detach the polyp. Cutting the polyp off at its base eliminates the risk of incomplete removal. If the polyp is larger than the diameter of the internal cervical os, it must be brought out of the cavity in smaller pieces, which can prove to be an arduous process.

To specifically address larger polyps, Bettocchi et al. described a specific polypectomy technique utilizing the 5 Fr Versapoint (Gynecare, Menlo Park, CA) bipolar electrode. The Versapoint Electrosurgical system has a dedicated bipolar generator and three types of electrodes: the Twizzle, used for precise vaporization and cutting; the spring, used for diffusing tissue vaporization, and the ball tip for desiccation. The electrosurgical generator provides various modes of operation: a vapor cut waveform, resembling a cut mode (VC1, VC2, and VC3, where VC3 has the mildest energy flowing into the tissue). There is also a blend waveform (BL1 and BL2) and a desiccation waveform. In his study, Bettocchi preferred using the Twizzle electrode only on the mildest cut mode, VC3, and reduced the default power setting from 100 W to 50 W. He found that these settings maximized patient tolerability and satisfaction with office-based operative hysteroscopic procedures (Bettocchi et al. 2002).

The same authors described removing endometrial polyps intact, using the VersaPoint Twizzle electrode, only if the internal cervical os was wide enough for their extraction. Larger polyps were sliced from the free edge to their base into 2–3 fragments small enough to be pulled through the os using a 5 Fr grasping forceps (see **Figure 14.3**). Care was taken to remove the entire base of the polyp using the Twizzle electrode. Using these techniques, 445 endometrial polyps between 0.5 cm and 4.5 cm were removed in an average of 17 minutes. About 53.7% were removed using the slicing technique while the remaining polyps were able to be removed intact. Patient satisfaction was excellent: 79% of patients reported no discomfort with this office procedure while an additional 15% reported low discomfort.

Office polypectomy can now be done using new hysteroscopic morcellation technology. Both the 5.5 mm Smith and Nephew TruClear system and the 6.5 mm Hologic Myosure device can be used in an ambulatory setting given their small diameter (Emanuel 2013). Limitations for office-based hysteroscopic morcellation include the amount of fluid necessary to complete the procedure and the relatively high cost of the disposable equipment. Potential advantages include rapid resection of an endometrial polyp.

■ Myomectomy
Key steps

Submucosal myomas under 2 cm can also be removed with the VersaPoint Twizzle using the technique described by Bettocchi et al. for larger polyps. Given their higher tissue density, myomas must first be divided into two half spheres, and then each of these slices as described in the office polypectomy section above (see **Figure 14.4**). Likewise, myomas of <1 cm can be removed with blunt-tipped scissors by dissecting the myoma from its myometrial base once the pseudocapsule is identified. The small myoma can then be removed from the cavity with the 5 Fr tenaculum.

Again, patient tolerability of this relates to the size of the fibroid segments being removed through the cervical os.

An additional in-office technique is described by Haimovich et al. that is actually a modification of a method previously described by Bettocchi to address even larger submucous myomas in an office setting. In a pilot study, the first of two planned office procedures consists of preparation of partially intramural myomas. After the classification of the submucous myoma according to the ESGE classification system, the endometrial mucosa and pseudocapsule are incised in an effort to make the fibroid almost entirely intracavitary. This is accomplished using a 4 mm continuous flow hysteroscope with a 2.9 mm rod–lens optical system. Incision is made with a high-power diode laser 1000 mm and diamond probe. During the second office procedure 4 weeks later, the same high-power diode laser is used to excise the myoma or alternatively, mechanical instruments can be used. Myoma is removed if cervical dilation allows, otherwise it is left in the uterine cavity with follow-up ultrasound 2 months postoperatively to ensure expulsion of remnant (Haimovich et al. 2013).

Other operative procedures in the office setting include resection of uterine septa and lysis of adhesions for Asherman's syndrome. Both of these procedures are performed with a 5 Fr scissors and cause no pain unless normal myometrium is encountered. Taking advantage of the difference in innervation, the surgeon can use the sense of pain as a marker for creating a false channel or when to stop cutting an adhesion or septum when the patient is awake with no anesthesia.

■ OPERATIVE HYSTEROSCOPY IN THE OPERATING ROOM

Although there are many benefits of the see-and-treat approach of office hysteroscopy, moving the procedure to an operating room is still often necessary. Factors that necessitate anesthesia and operating room include the following:

1. The presence of a large polyp or fibroid
2. The need for a longer procedure (>20 minutes) to remove all pathology
3. Patient intolerance to office hysteroscopy
4. Patient preference for sedation during procedure

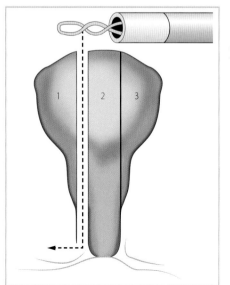

Figure 14.3 Bettocchi's method of larger polyp resection using Gynecare VersaPoint Twizzle tip.

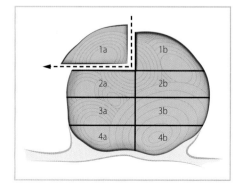

Figure 14.4 Bettocchi's method for myoma resection using Gynecare VersaPoint Twizzle tip.

Set-up

After intravenous anesthesia is given, patients are positioned in dorsal lithotomic position in the operating room with preferably, candy cane stirrups. Of note, operative hysteroscopy can also be accomplished with regional anesthesia on the basis of patient's preference or anesthesiologist's preference, if medical comorbidities are present. It is prudent to ensure the patient is positioned far enough caudad on the operating table – buttocks should be slightly hanging off the edge of the table to allow for full range of motion for the hysteroscope. Draping includes an under-the-buttocks drape with a pocket to collect fluid. Tubing will eventually be attached to the end of this bag to collect all fluid for the fluid management system, explained in detail later. Drapes to cover legs/stirrups, as well as a small drape for the patient's abdomen, are needed to keep instruments sterile if placed atop.

Instrumentation

A key component to successful and safe operative hysteroscopy is an accurate weighted fluid-management system. These systems are available from various manufacturers. It is crucial that operating room staff – nurses, surgical technicians, and physicians – are educated in working with and troubleshooting the fluid-management system. In short, automated fluid-management systems keep track of distention media 'in' and distention media 'out' to determine the net fluid balance. A microprocessor subtracts the collected fluid 'weight out' from the infused fluid 'weight in' to calculate an accurate fluid balance. There are often preset alarms that sound when fluid deficits reach increments of 500 mL to ensure all involved personnel are aware. Errors can occur when a large amount of distention media spills onto the floor and is not accounted for in the 'out' weight calculation (AAGL Advancing Minimally Invasive Gynecology Worldwide et al. 2013); see **Figure 14.5** as an example of a fluid-management system.

Bipolar resectoscopes are quickly becoming the standard of care in hysteroscopy as normal saline can be used as the distention media. Advantages of using isotonic saline include preventing the risk of developing hyponatremia and free water intoxication with excessive absorption as can occur with electrolyte-free media. While fluid overload and rarely pulmonary edema can result from excess absorption of normal saline, these conditions are treatable and not resulted in cerebral edema or cardiac arrhythmias due to electrolyte imbalances (Wamsteker et al. 1993). The second advantage of bipolar resectoscopes is that the proximity of electrodes reduces the risk of electrical burns (Garuti & Luerti 2009). When using physiologic media such as normal saline, once a deficit of 2 L is reached, plans should be made to end the procedure soon. By a 2.5-L deficit, the procedure must be terminated. There are slightly different sizes of resectoscopes available, ranging from a smaller 21 Fr (7 mm) to a standard sized 27 Fr (9 mm) (AAGL 2013).

If bipolar equipment is not available, one must use monopolar resectoscopic technology (or morcellation technology). Similarly, these resectoscopes are available in various sizes, between 7 mm and 9 mm in diameter. Monopolar current requires nonconductive (electrolyte-free) distention media to facilitate the completion of the RF electrical circuit between the active and remotely located dispersive electrode. Examples of electrolyte-free media include 3% sorbitol, 1.5% glycine, 5% mannitol, and a combined solution of sorbitol and mannitol, typically 3% sorbitol and 0.5% mannitol. When using these distention media, the procedure must be absolutely terminated once a deficit of 1 L is reached (AAGL 2013).

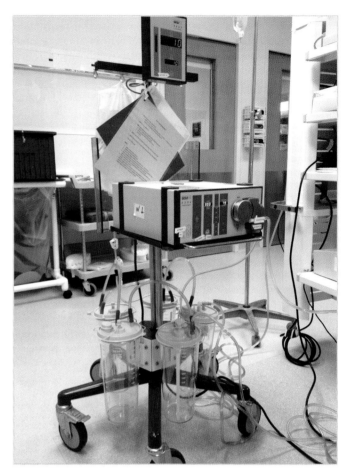

Figure 14.5 A weighted fluid-management system.

Hysteroscopic morcellators have been recently introduced to the global hysteroscopic market: Truclear (Smith and Nephew) and Myosure (Hologic) manufacture disposable systems and Karl Storz endoscopy produces a reusable intrauterine morcellator. The intrauterine morcellator consists of a set of two metal hollow, rigid, disposable tubes that fit into each other. The inner tube rotates within the outer tube, driven by electrically powered control unit activated with a foot pedal. A vacuum source connected to the inner tube causes tissue to be sucked into the cutting window. This tissue is cut or shaved as the inner tube rotates. The hollow tube system is 2.9–4.5 mm, which is introduced into a straight working channel of a 6.5–9 mm rigid hysteroscope. These morcellators can be utilized in cases of polypectomy or myomectomy if the surgeon is aware that the current morcellator technology will not be able to remove the intramural component of a type I or II submucous myoma.

Polypectomy

Hysteroscopic polypectomy in the operating room can be done using the same technique described in the office using mechanical instruments (scissors and grasping forceps or tenaculum). A bipolar electrode such as the VersaPoint or a loop resectoscope can also be used to remove a polyp. With all instruments, the goal is to remove the polyp in its entirety, including the base. With smaller polyps, this can be easily accomplished by simply using the electrode of a resectoscope to detach the polyp at its base. When pathology is larger, one must use the resectoscope loop electrode to cut the polyp in smaller fragments and to allow for easy removal from the uterine cavity. With a resectoscope, one can use the wire-loop electrode to cut the large polyp into small strips, shaving it away until the base is reached. This cutting technique is similar to that described for myomectomy. All polyp fragments should be removed from the cavity, if possible, and sent for pathologic examination. Lastly, a hysteroscopic morcellator can be used for polypectomy. Morcellators are slightly different from each other based on manufacturers; their general mechanism of action is described above in the 'Instrumentation' section. The advantage of morcellators is that tissue fragments are collected in the vacuum system and do not obscure the operative field nor do they have to be removed separately (AlHilli et al. 2013).

Most surgeons develop a preferred method for polypectomy, based on the experience or available equipment. Studies, looking at the optimal tool for polypectomy show virtually equivalent efficacy results. Muzii et al. concluded that operative resectoscopy was the technique of choice for endometrial polyps >2 cm or those with a fundal implant. Smaller, nonfundal polyps were best treated with bipolar electrode excision, based on improved intraoperative speed using this method (Muzii et al. 2007). When polyps have a particularly broad base or are large, >2–2.5 cm, a resectoscope may be preferable based on the data from 240 women by Preutthipan and Herabutya. Lastly, they found polyp recurrence rates to be lowest in the resectoscope group as well; (0% recurrence versus 15% recurrence when grasping forceps used; Preutthipan & Herabutya 2005).

■ Myomectomy
Wire-loop resectoscopic technique (for both bipolar and monopolar resectoscopes)

This resectoscopy is the most common technique for hysteroscopic myomectomy. After anesthesia and proper positioning, the cervix is dilated to accommodate the operative hysteroscope with care being taken not to overdilate. In women with cervical stenosis, preoperative misoprostol can be given to soften the cervix (Choksuchat 2010). Alternatively, dilute vasopressin can be injected intracervically once to facilitate easier cervical dilation in the operating room (Phillips et al. 1997). Fluid-management system is double checked to ensure it be on and working properly. The hysteroscope is placed into the patient's cervix and, once adequate distention is achieved, a thorough survey is taken of the cavity, noting the size/location and type of all present pathologies. It is important to document that both tubal ostia have been visualized insuring the entire cavity has been inspected. If there is >1 fibroid present, care should be taken not to resect both if they are on opposing walls. Otherwise, postoperative adhesions could occur. In addition, if there is a type 0 or I fibroid in addition to a type II, then the former should be done first because more fluid intravasation will occur with the type II myoma. Once the myoma to be resected has been identified, the wire loop is deployed beyond the fibroid and the operator begins to pull the loop back toward himself or herself. Cutting begins when contact is made between loop and tissue. The operator must always take care to keep the loop visible in the surgical field and only apply cut current when pulling the loop back toward the surgeon. Repeated and progressive passages of the cutting loop are made in similar fashion to shave down the fibroid to the myometrium; see **Figures 14.6** and **14.7**.

Type 0

With pedunculated fibroids, the surgeon has the option to simply cut the fibroid stalk or he/she can start from the top to shave down the

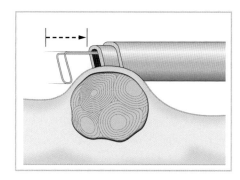

Figure 14.6 Wire-loop fibroid resection. The loop is deployed beyond the fibroid and pulled back toward the surgeon before cutting.

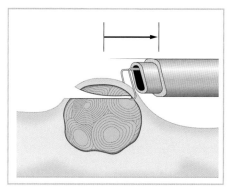

Figure 14.7 Cut current is employed only when tissue contact is made and when the loop is being pulled back toward the surgeon. This happens consecutively until the myometrium is reached.

fibroid in pieces. An advantage of the shaving technique is that the fibroid pieces can be removed from the cervix whereas after a stalk is cut, the fibroid is often difficult to be removed. In this case, the fibroid can be grasped either under direct visualization with an Isaacson optical tenaculum or blindly with Corson forceps. If the tissue is too large to fit through the cervix or cannot be easily grasped, it can remain in the cavity and will be expelled spontaneously. Our preference is to shave the type 0 fibroid from top to stalk.

Types I and II

Technique is similar for fibroids protruding greater or less than 50% in the endometrial cavity. The surgeon starts by shaving the myoma with repetitive sweeps of the loop from the top until the level of the endometrium is reached. Again, care is taken to only activate the foot pedal for cutting current when the loop is moving toward the operator. Once the endometrium is reached, we recommend removing as many fibroid chips as possible by trapping these chips between the loop and resectoscope, and bringing a cluster of chips out through the cervix repeatedly. The operator should always place the distention pressure at the minimum level that will achieve adequate visualization. This allows for minimal fluid intravasation and maximal extension of the myoma from the myometrium into the uterine cavity after the pseudocapsule is reached. A fibroid's pseudocapsule is the junction of the soft myometrial attachment with the dense texture of myoma. The goal is to use blunt dissection with the loop (no RF energy) to tease the myoma within the pseudocapsule from surrounding healthy myometrium and into the uterine cavity. Once in the cavity, the myoma can be shaved to the level of the endometrium once again. Repeat this technique in various areas until the fibroid has been completely removed (see **Figures 14.6** and **14.7**). Remaining tissue fragments should be removed and sent to pathology along with previously collected tissue. If a type I or type II fibroid cannot be completely excised before the fluid deficit is reached, the patient should be counseled about the requirement of a second procedure. Prior to scheduling the second operation, it is prudent to check the patient in about 8–12 weeks postoperatively for follow-up: to verify if bothersome symptoms still present and to conduct office hysteroscopy to ensure the partially resected fibroid does indeed have a resectable intracavitary component. When this is confirmed, the patient undergoes a similar loop resectoscopic procedure as described above.

Fibroid vaporization

Fibroids can also be vaporized using spherical or cylindrical electrodes. These can be either bipolar or monopolar, with a choice of distension media dependent on energy type. The electrode is dragged along the surface of the fibroid until it is a size compatible to extraction with the Isaacson optical tenaculum or blindly using the Corson forceps. Again, current is only applied to the electrode when it is moving toward the operator. Although this technique can be faster than resectoscopic methods, it has several disadvantages. First, no tissue is collected for pathologic examination. Second, vaporization requires high power to be used (200–300 W) and, consequently, numerous gas bubbles are produced and can rapidly enter the bloodstream. Although they dissipate rapidly, complications can develop.

Intrauterine morcellation

For type 0 and type I fibroids (<50% intramural extension), a hysteroscopic morcellator can be used. The exact technique depends on the specific product and the manufacturer used. In brief, the morcellator is used to shave the myoma by placing the side-opening blade of the morcellator up against the myoma tissue to be removed. Unlike the wire-loop technique, the morcellator blade is moved from side to side until the myoma is leveled with the myometrium. These technologies cannot be used for the intramural component of the myoma. The bothersome myoma chips are carried out of the uterine cavity by a vacuum in the morcellator set-up. Preliminary study showed that type 0 myomas were removed more quickly when a morcellator was used compared to traditional resectoscope (mean time: 35.8 minutes versus 14.9 minutes; $P = 0.001$). The authors concluded that this time saving was large because tissue fragments did not have to be removed as a separate procedure as with the resectoscope (Emanuel & Wamsteker 2005). Since the goal of the myomectomy is to remove 100% of the myoma, it is not recommended to use a morcellator for most type I and all type II fibroids as one is unable to identify and dissect out the pseudocapsular plane with this device. Emanuel et al. demonstrated that the rate of symptom recurrence within 3 years was 55% if the entire submucous myoma is not resected.

OUTCOMES

Complete resection of a polyp or fibroid leads to excellent clinical outcomes. In a review to assess endometrial polypectomy in treating abnormal uterine bleeding, 75–100% of patients had improvement in bleeding symptoms with a follow-up period of 2–52 months (Nathani & Clark 2006). As previously stated, the goal during myomectomy is for complete fibroid resection. If this is accomplished, resolution of fibroid-related symptoms occurs in well over 90% of cases. In the case of complete resection, recurrence of menstrual abnormalities is related to growth of new fibroids (Di Speizio Sardo et al. 2008). In patients with an incomplete resection, half pursued repeat surgery for recurrent symptoms within 2 years (Emanuel et al. 1999.) Furthermore, uterine size, fibroid size, and number of fibroids at the time of initial hysteroscopy have independent prognostic value for recurrent abnormal uterine bleeding. In short, the chance for complete resolution of symptoms with hysteroscopic resection decreased when the uterus was enlarged or there were three or more myomas at hysteroscopy

(90% at 5 years vs. 64.8% at 5 years; Emanuel et al. 1999, Hart et al. 1999). In all patients, including complete and incomplete resections, the overall recurrence rate of fibroids or abnormal uterine bleeding is approximately 20% after 3 years of follow-up (Derman et al. 1991, Hart et al. 1999).

ALTERNATIVE TREATMENT APPROACHES

Most endometrial polyps and submucosal fibroids are symptomatic, thus prompting women to seek definitive treatment. In the case of postmenopausal women, endometrial lesions must be removed and sent for pathologic examination to exclude malignancy. Although rare, prevalence of premalignant or malignant endometrial polyps ranges from 0.8% to 8%. In a study of 870 women undergoing endometrial polypectomy, age of >60 and postmenopausal bleeding were independent risk factors for malignancy (Costa-Paiva et al. 2011). Medical management for premenopausal abnormal uterine bleeding can be attempted once endometrial biopsy returns benign; however, the efficacy of this strategy is frequently suboptimal. For example, use of a levonorgestrel (Mirena) intrauterine device for menorrhagia with known intracavitary fibroids can reduce menstrual blood flow, but expulsion rates of around 11% are higher than the general population (Zapata et al. 2010). Endometrial ablation in the setting of submucosal fibroids is also not indicated. Furthermore, uterine artery embolization is contraindicated with known submucosal fibroids as these fibroids will slough off, creating a nidus for intrauterine infection and a chronic foul-smelling discharge. In general, if a fibroid is amenable to hysteroscopic resection, this approach should strongly be recommended. If unresectable, other minimally invasive therapeutics such as MRI-guided focused ultrasound surgery or RF volumetric ablation can be an option for women who have completed childbearing.

PRACTICAL TIPS

1. Be familiar with all the hysteroscopic and fluid monitoring equipment. Be able to assemble and disassemble as well as troubleshoot problems. Do not rely only on the support personnel in the operating room

2. Have a fluid-management protocol that is agreed upon by the gynecology, anesthesia, and nursing departments prior to entering the operating room

3. Cut tissue with the apex of the wire loop and only activate cutting current while drawing the loop toward the surgeon

4. Make it a goal to identify the pseudocapsule and never cut myometrium. This will nearly eliminate the risk of perforation since the fibroids displace but do not invade the myometrium

5. If bleeding vessels encountered during resection, use bipolar desiccation to control bleeding

6. Use the lowest distension media pressure possible to achieve good visualization for reducing fluid intravasation and allowing maximal extension of the myoma into the uterine cavity

7. Know when to stop – do not continue if you are approaching the fluid deficit limit (1 L for electrolyte-free media and 2.5 L for normal saline)

8. Goal is complete resection of myoma and polyp. It may take >1 procedure to accomplish this goal due to fluid intravasation. Set patient expectations at preoperative visit

9. Practice proper preoperative evaluation using either sonohysterography or office hysteroscopy with vaginal probe ultrasound to accurately map submucosal fibroids.

CONCLUSION

Hysteroscopy is one of the most rewarding surgical procedures that the gynecologists can perform. The patients are often severely affected by their preoperative symptoms, and the outcomes for symptom relief are exceptional. All of this is done either in an office setting with little to no anesthesia or in an operating room setting where the patient can be discharged home in a few hours and back to normal activity within 1 day. Hysteroscopy is relatively simple to teach and learn. It should be a standard technique offered to all women being cared for by a general gynecologist.

REFERENCES

AAGL Advancing Minimally Invasive Gynecology Worldwide, Munro MG, Storz K, Abbott JA, et al. AAGL Practice Report: Practice Guidelines for the Management of Hysteroscopic Distending Media. J Minim Invasive Gynecol 2013; 20:137–148.

AlHilli MM, Nixon KE, Hopkins MR, et al. Long-term outcomes after intrauterine morcellation vs hysteroscopic resection of endometrial polyps. J Minim Invasive Gynecol 2013; 20:215–221.

Bettocchi S, Ceci O, Di Venere R, et al. Advanced operative office hysteroscopy without anaesthesia: analysis of 501 cases treated with a 5 Fr. Bipolar electrode. Human Repro 2002; 17:2435.

Bettocchi S, Ceci O, Nappi L, et al. Operative office hysteroscopy without anesthesia: analysis of 4863 cases performed with mechanical instruments. J Am Assoc Gynecol Laparsc 2004; 11:59–61.

Choksuchat C. Clinical use of misoprostol in nonpregnant women: review article. J Minim Invasive Gynecol 2010; 17:449.

Cicinelli E. Hysteroscopy without anesthesia: review of recent literature. J Minim Invasive Gynecol 2010; 17:703.

Costa-Paiva L, Godoy CE, Antunes A, et al. Risk of malignancy in endometrial polyps in premenopausal and postmenopausal women according to clinicopathologic characteristics. Menopause 2011; 18:1278–1282.

Dealberti D, Roboni F, Prigione S, et al. New mini-resectoscope: analysis of preliminary quality results in outpatient hysteroscopic polypectomy. Arch Gynecol Obstet 2013; 288:349–353.

Derman SG, Rehnstrom J, Neuwirth RS. The long-term effectiveness of hysteroscopic treatment of menorrhagia and leiomyomas. Obstet Gynecol 1991; 77: 591–594.

Di Naro E, Bratta FG, Romano F, et al. The diagnosis of benign uterine pathology using transvaginal endohysterosonography. Clin Exp Obstet Gynecol 1996; 23:103–107.

Di Speizio Sardo A, Bettocchi S, Spinelli M, et al. Review of new office-based hysteroscopic procedures 2003-2009. J Minim Invasive Gynecol 2010; 17:436.

Di Spiezio Sardo A, Mazzon I, Bramante S, et al. Hysteroscopic myomectomy: a comprehensive review of surgical techniques. Human Repro Update 2008; 14:101–119.

Emanuel MH. New developments in hysteroscopy. Best Pract Res Clin Obstet Gynaecol 2013; 27:421.

Emanuel MH, Hart A, Wamsteker K, Lammes F. An analysis of fluid loss during transcervical resection of submucous myomas. Fertil Steril 1997; 68:881.

Emanuel MH, Wamsteker K. The Intra Uterine Morcellator: a new hysteroscopic operating technique to remove intrauterine polyps and myomas. J Minim Invasive Gynecol 2005; 12:62–66.

Emanuel MH, Wamsteker K, Hart AAM, Metz G, Lammes FB. Long-term results of hysteroscopic myomectomy for abnormal uterine bleeding. Obstet Gynecol 1999; 93:743–748.

Fedele L, Vercellini P, Bianchi S, Brioschi D, Dorta M. Treatment with GnRH agonists before myomectomy and the risk of short-term fibroid recurrence. Br J Obstet Gynaecol 1990; 97:393–396.

Garuti G, Leurti M. Hysteroscopic bipolar surgery: a valuable progress or a technique under investigation? Curr Opin Obstet Gynecol 2009; 21:329–334.

Hart R, Molnar BG, Magos A. Long term follow up of hysteroscopic myomectomy assessed by survival analysis. Br J Obstet Gynecol 1999; 106:700.

Haimovich S, Mancebo G, Alameda F, et al. Feasibility of a new two-step procedure for office hysteroscopic resection of submucous myomas: results of a pilot study. Eur J Obstet Gynecol Reprod Biol 2013; 168:191–194.

Isaacson K. Hysteroscopic myomectomy:fertility-preserving yet underutilized. OBG Manag. 2003; 15:69-83.

Jorizzo JR, Riccio GJ, Chen MYM, et al. Sonohysterography: the next step in the evaluation of the abnormal endometrium. Radiographics 1999; 19:117–130.

Munro MG, Critchley HO, Fraser IS, FIGO Menstrual Disorder Working Group. The FIGO classification of classes of abnormal uterine bleeding in the reproductive years. Fertil Steril 2011; 75:2004.e3.

Muzii L, Bellati F, Pernice M, et al. Resectoscopic versus bipolar electrode excision of endometrial polyps: a randomized study. Fertil Steril 2007; 87:909.

Nathani F, Clark TJ. Uterine polypectomy in the management of abnormal uterine bleeding: a systematic review. J Minim Invasive Gynecol 2006; 13:260.

Parazzini F, Vercellini P, De Giorgi O, et al. Efficacy of preoperative medical treatment in facilitating hysteroscopic endometrial resection, myomectomy and metroplasty: literature review. Hum Reprod 1998; 13:2592–2597.

Phillips DR, Nathanson HG, Milim SJ, Haselkorn JS. The effect of dilate vasopressin solution on the force needed for cervical dilatation: a randomized control trial. Obstet Gynecol 1997; 89:507. Phillips DR, Nathanson HG, Milim SJ, et al. The effect of dilute vasopressin solution on blood loss during operative hysteroscopy: a randomized control trial. Obstet Gynecol 1996; 88:761.

Preutthipan S, Herabutya Y. Hysteroscopic polypectomy in 240 premenopausal and postmenopausal women. Fertil Steril 2005; 83:705.

Sagiv R, Sadan O, Boaz M, et al. A new approach to office hysteroscopy compared with traditional hysteroscopy: a randomized control trial. Obstet Gynecol 2006; 108:387–392.

Salim S, Won H, Newbitt-Hawes E, Campbell N, Abbott J. Diagnosis and management of endometrial polyps: a critical review of the literature. J Minim Invasive Gynecol 2011; 18:569–581.

Valle RF, Baggish MS. Hysteroscopic myomectomy. In: Baggish MS, Valle RE, Guedj H (eds). Hysteroscopy, visual perspectives of uterine anatomy, physiology and pathology diagnostic and operative hysteroscopy, 3rd edn. Philadephia, PA: Lippincott Williams and wilkins (a Wolters Kluwer business), 2007:385–404.

Van Dongen H, Emanuel MH, Smeets MJ, Trimbos B, Jansen FW. Followup after incomplete hysteroscopic removal of uterine fibroids. Acta Obstet Gynecol Scand 2006; 85:1463.

Wamsteker K, Emanuel MH, de Kriuf JH. Transcervical hysteroscopic resection of submucous fibroids for abnormal uterine bleeding: results regarding the degree of intramural extension. Obstet Gynecol 1993; 82:736.

Wortman M, Daggett A, Ball C. Operative hysteroscopy in an office-based surgical setting: review of patient safety and satisfaction in 414 cases. J Minim Invasive Gynecol 2013; 20: 56–63.

Zapata LB, Whiteman MK, Tepper NK, et al. Intrauterine device use among women with uterine fibroids: a systematic review. Contraception 2010; 82:41–55.

Chapter 15 Hysteroscopic and laparoscopic sterilization

Robert K Zurawin, Jonathan L Zurawin

INTRODUCTION

Female sterilization, first performed in the late 19th century, has become the most widely practiced contraceptive method worldwide and is relied upon by one out of three women of childbearing age (Chan & Westhoff 2010). This chapter will describe interval laparoscopic and hysteroscopic sterilization, comparing the two techniques concentrating on four important areas, conveniently described as the four 'Cs': contraceptive effectiveness, complications, cost, and choice.

HISTORY

Blundell first suggested tubal ligation for sterilization in 1823 before the Medical Society of London, and Lungren was the first to ligate a woman's Fallopian tubes in 1880 in Toledo. Porro performed a Cesarean hysterectomy with the secondary intention of sterilization in 1876 and in 1885. Thomas proposed tubal ligation as a primary sterilization technique. Additional procedural variations were conducted over the following years including the Pomeroy's technique and Uchida's interval/puerperal technique in the 1940s (Zurawin 2015). The first laparoscopic tubal occlusion was performed in 1936 in Switzerland by Bosch. Currently, practiced tubal sterilization techniques include those performed at the time of delivery or shortly thereafter and those performed at a later time, and are referred to as interval sterilization procedures (Bartz & Greenberg 2008, Zurawin 2015). Minilaparotomy with a small infraumbilical incision is the most common procedure in the immediate postpartum period following vaginal delivery, followed by tubal ligation performed at the time of Cesarean section (Guttenmacher 2013).

TUBAL STERILIZATION PROCEDURES IN THE UNITED STATES

The Guttmacher Institute estimates that >2 million women (20–49 years of age) underwent tubal sterilization between 1994 and 1996, half of which were postpartum and half were interval procedures. Of these tubal ligations, postpartum procedures were performed during inpatient hospital stays, whereas only 4% of interval procedures were performed on an inpatient basis (2% of all sterilization procedures). Most interval sterilizations were performed as outpatient procedures in hospital ambulatory surgery centers (ASCs) or in freestanding surgery centers (MacKay et al. 2001).

The percentage of women relying on both female and male sterilization as their primary method of contraception has remained stable since it was studied by the Guttmacher Institute in 1994. The most recent statistics indicate 26.6% of women practicing contraception using tubal sterilization with an additional 10% relying on the vasectomy of their partner (Jones et al. 2012).

Among women aged 20–29, postpartum sterilization rates were higher than interval rates, whereas the reverse was true among women aged 35–49. Women choosing postpartum tubal sterilization tended to be younger than women electing to have an interval procedure (MacKay et al. 2001). The postpartum scenario exposes younger women to higher rates of sterilization regret that is known to be associated with women who undergo sterilization procedures under age 30 (Hollander 1999). In the presence of maternal complications at the time of delivery or any question of viability of the newborn, including prematurity or infection, sterilization should be deferred until after the postpartum period and ideally until the infant is healthy. As neonatal complications may also be associated with higher rates of sudden infant death syndrome (SIDS), it is recommended that sterilization be postponed until after the age when SIDS is less likely to occur.

Around 50 years ago, female sterilization in the United States was generally performed only when pregnancy would be medically contraindicated. During the 1960s, cultural changes of the Baby Boomer generation and books such as *The Feminine Mystique* by Betty Friedan, aided by the development of safe oral hormonal contraception, encouraged women to take greater control over their fertility. However, it should be remembered that at this time the consent of a woman's husband was necessary for her to obtain a prescription for birth control pills. The same decade saw the development of safe, minimally invasive surgical sterilization procedures, but perhaps the most important factor influencing the popularity of surgical sterilization was the adoption by insurance companies of policies that covered these procedures.

Laparoscopy with unipolar electrosurgery was introduced in the 1960s and subsequently abandoned due to safety and efficacy concerns in favor of nonelectrosurgical laparoscopic techniques. Further innovation in 1973 by Hulka resulted in a laparoscopically applied spring clip and in the 1980s Europe embraced the Filshie clip that was adopted by US practitioners in the 1990s. With the development of hysteroscopically guided placement of Essure microinserts for tubal occlusion, the opportunity to offer nonincisional minimally invasive permanent contraception under local anesthesia in the office setting became a reality in 2002. The second hysteroscopic sterilization product Adiana was available for a short period of time but was withdrawn from the market on May 18, 2012. Approximately 700,000 interval tubal occlusions are performed in the United States each year (Chan & Westhoff 2010). Half of those are postpartum and the other half are laparoscopic and hysteroscopic. Hysteroscopic sterilization accounts for approximately 75,000 procedures per year (information on file at Bayer HealthCare Pharmaceuticals).

TECHNIQUES
Laparoscopic sterilization

Since the first laparoscopic tubal sterilization was performed, the technique has undergone several modifications but still fundamentally involves peritoneal entry. Because of the need for pneumoperitoneum with associated discomfort, the vast majority of these procedures are performed under general anesthesia in an operating room.

The technique for laparoscopic sterilization is fundamentally the same for all devices that occlude the tubal lumen. The universally accepted approach to peritoneal access is through the umbilicus, either by direct trocar insertion, Veress needle, or by open Hasson technique. Visualization of the pelvis is accomplished using CO_2 insufflation, although the procedure has been described using gasless technology (Guido et al. 1998) as well as under local anesthesia (Hataska et al. 1997); however, these techniques are rarely used. Occlusion by Falope ring and electrosurgery can be accomplished through a single port using a right-angle scope, while Hulka and Filshie clips require a second midline suprapubic port (Filshie et al. 1981, Hulka et al. 1973). Regardless of the technique, the Fallopian tube is optimally occluded in the isthmic portion.

Electrosurgery

Bipolar electrosurgery electrodes are applied to the isthmic portion of the Fallopian tube and the current is applied until either visual changes indicated coagulation of the tube, or a feedback mechanism on the electrosurgical generator indicates an increase in impedance between the bipolar electrodes consistent with desiccation of the tissue.

Falope ring

A band made of nonreactive silicone is stretched and is slipped over a loop of Fallopian tube using a special applicator. If the tube is edematous, laceration and bleeding can occur. Excessive traction on the tube can also result in laceration and hemorrhage (Yoon & King 1975). Reported failure rate is 1.77%.

Hulka clips

A spring-loaded silastic clip is applied at a right angle to the isthmic portion of the Fallopian tube 2.5–3 cm from the uterotubal junction (UTJ). Although it has the smallest footprint on the Fallopian tube of any occlusive device, it also carries the highest failure rate; reported failure rate is 3.65%.

Filshie clips

The clip (made of titanium with a silicone rubber lining) has the lowest failure rate of all laparoscopic techniques. The clip should be applied at a right angle to the isthmic portion of the Fallopian tube 2–2.5 cm from the UTJ. Silicone rubber expands, possibly preventing residual tubal patency. Potential complications are migration into bladder, vagina, peritoneal cavity, and appendix. The reported failure rate is 0.27%.

Salpingectomy

Recent reports have described the potential benefit of complete salpingectomy in reducing the risk of ovarian cancer (McAlpine et al. 2014). However, these benefits must be weighed against the increased operative risks of salpingectomy and the potential for decreased ovarian reserve leading to premature ovarian failure (Ye et al. 2015). There appears to be no documented evidence of decreased ovarian reserve in very short-term trials of 3 months, but longer study lengths are necessary (Findley et al. 2013, Morelli et al. 2013).

■ HYSTEROSCOPIC STERILIZATION
■ History of hysteroscopic sterilization

The first use of electrosurgery to coagulate the utero-tubal junction was performed in 1878, but these were performed blindly (Kocks 1878). In 1934, Schroeder performed the first direct visualization of the tubal ostia using electrosurgery, by passing an electrode into the intramural portion of the tube under hysteroscopic guidance. The procedure attracted some adherents but was finally abandoned in 1975 because of frequent thermal complications and numerous pregnancies (Greenberg 2008, March & Israel 1975)

Subsequent research focused on nonelectrical nonthermal methods of hysteroscopic sterilization. Several attempts were made using silicone injected through the tubal ostia. Complications were rare but pregnancy rates were high enough to discard this method (Loffer 1984).

In 2002, the Food and Drug Administration (FDA) approved the Essure microinsert system. A polymer matrix implant, Adiana, was approved in 2009. It utilized bipolar, low-level radiofrequency energy delivery, and nonabsorbable silicone matrix inserts, but was withdrawn by the manufacturer in 2012 because of high failure rates.

Essure is indicated for women who desire permanent birth control by bilateral occlusion of the Fallopian tubes. The Essure system includes two radiopaque microinserts each with a dynamically expanding microcoil, composed of a stainless steel inner coil, a nitinol expanding, superelastic outer coil, and polyethylene terephthalate (PET) fibers. The microinsert outer coil contains nitinol, a commonly used component of surgical implants such as orthopedic staples, vena cava filters, dental devices, and intravascular stents. The effectiveness of Essure microinserts is believed to be resulted from the space-filling design of the device coupled with a local, occlusive, benign tissue response to the PET fibers that result in device retention and pregnancy prevention (Cooper 1992). The correct placement of the microinserts is demonstrated in **Figure 15.1**. A hysteroscopic view of the correct placement is demonstrated in **Figure 15.2**.

Following the Essure procedure, patients generally return to normal activities in approximately 24 hours. Essure should not be relied on for contraception until the patient has undergone an Essure confirmation

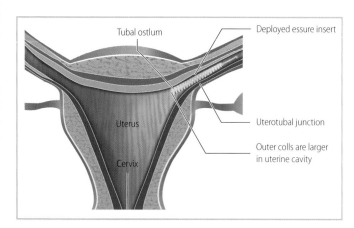

Figure 15.1 Correct placement of the Essure microinserts.

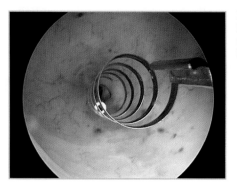

Figure 15.2
Hysteroscopic view of the Essure microinsert in tubal os.

test 3 months after placement, to confirm both bilateral tubal occlusion and satisfactory location of the microinserts, and offers both patients and physicians the opportunity for visual confirmation of proper device placement and occlusion. The protocol for the confirmatory hysterosalpingogram (HSG) differs from the standard HSG required for infertility evaluation. The protocol is notable for requiring lower filling pressure, potentially making the procedure less uncomfortable for the patient. Six specific separate images are required to demonstrate proper placement and occlusion. It is important that radiologists and gynecologists performing confirmatory HSG should follow these protocols, as a misread confirmatory test remains the single most important reason for unintended pregnancy.

A small percentage of patients with correct placement of the microinserts will exhibit patency on HSG at 3 months, but almost all of those will have achieved complete occlusion upon repeat testing at 6 months. The occlusion rates in the phase II trials were 96% at 3 months and 100% at 6 months (Cooper et al. 2003, Kerin et al. 2003). In the phase III trials, 92% of patients were occluded at 3 months but all patients were occluded at 6 months (Cooper et al. 2003). A recent study quotes higher patency rates of 16.1% and 5.8%, respectively, both at 3 and 6 months but did not document subsequent pregnancies, if any (Rodriguez et al. 2013).

Unlike laparoscopic sterilization that is effective immediately postoperatively, patients cannot rely on hysteroscopic sterilization until after at least 3 months and following confirmed occlusion on the confirmation test. The FDA currently requires a HSG at 3 months following the placement of Essure to assess tubal occlusion. The FDA requirement for a confirmation test adds an additional step to the process of hysteroscopic sterilization. The confirmation test does require a procedure involving minor exposure to radiation and patient discomfort. The cost is covered by most insurance plans, with the exception of Medicaid in some parts of the United States.

A number of articles have discussed that the HSG confirmation test required 3 months after the Essure procedure. Guiahi et al did a practice analysis and, as a result of their findings, implemented processes to improve HSG follow-up (Guiahi et al. 2010). Chapa et al. conducted a preprocedure survey of patient preference for hysteroscopic versus laparoscopic sterilization and were able to validate the assumption that such a test provides mental reassurance concerning reliance (Chapa et al. 2012). Outside the United States, a flat plate film of the abdomen is sufficient to determine correct placement of the microinserts. Studies are underway to determine the accuracy of reproducibility of ultrasound to determine correct device placement and occlusion (Veersema et al. 2011). If successful, the procedure could be performed in the gynecologist's office and incur less expense and discomfort for the patient (Simpson & Beitia 2012).

Contraceptive effectiveness
Laparoscopic versus hysteroscopic sterilization

The landmark CREST (US Collabortive Review of Sterilization) study evaluated the effectiveness of the laparoscopic approach and reported a 10-year failure rate of approximately 2% (Jamieson et al. 2000, Peterson et al. 1996). The CREST data further documented a cumulative risk of pregnancy that persists for at least 10 years after tubal sterilization, the etiology of which may be the result of spontaneous tubal reanastomosis.

No pregnancies have been reported in clinical trials and pregnancies reported over 10 years of commercial worldwide. The use of Essure represents 0.15% of total distributed kits (Levy et al. 2007). A 10-year

retrospective review of pregnancy date revealed 748 pregnancies in 497,305 patients or a 99.74% effectiveness rate (Munro et al. 2014).

Most pregnancies appear to have been associated with the patient or physician noncompliance, or misinterpreted confirmation tests. The results of analysis of these commercial data appear similar to those identified in clinical trials, and suggest that the performance of Essure is consistent with the labeled age-adjusted effectiveness of 99.74%. The 10-year commercial experience suggests an estimated rate less than half that reported in CREST.

A 2011 international study of women who had experienced unintended pregnancies after the Essure procedure reported similar findings and concluded that most pregnancies were avoidable and due primarily to patient noncompliance (Veersema et al. 2011).

The US and international medical literature contains numerous hysteroscopic sterilization studies suggesting that female permanent birth control is undergoing another historical shift from traditional tubal ligation to hysteroscopic sterilization. Hysteroscopic sterilization is associated with high rates of effectiveness and patient satisfaction and low rates of complications (Conceptus 2012, Cooper et al. 2003, Kerin et al. 2003). The reliance rate, another proxy for effectiveness, is similarly high at 97% among women with bilateral placement (Conceptus 2012). The reliance rate for tubal ligation modality ranges is outlined in the CREST study.

Cost

A number of worldwide studies have reported the favorable cost-effectiveness of Essure versus laparoscopic tubal ligation. **Table 15.1** compares studies in the United States evaluating in-office Essure versus laparoscopic tubal ligation and operating room (OR) Essure versus laparoscopic tubal ligation report cost savings of up to US$2075 (in-office) to US$180.00 (OR) which includes the cost of the confirmatory HSG.

Two recent papers emphasize the importance of cost-effectiveness in the overall healthcare reform climate. Chapa et al. evaluated physician time effectiveness when performing Essure in the office versus the OR and reported that five in-office Essures were completed within 3 hours versus three in the ASC within 5 hours. The authors suggest that Essure hysteroscopic sterilization performed in physician's office using local anesthesia allows for improved physician time management and productivity compared to performing the procedure in an OR or ASC. Office-based Essure may have substantial cost savings to the healthcare system based on time spent, with maximum patient satisfaction (Chapa et al. 2012). According to a 2010 editorial that evaluated the cost-effectiveness of contraceptive modalities including

Table 15.1 The cost of Essure hysteroscopic sterilization versus laparoscopic tubal ligation

Peer-reviewed publication	Hysteroscopic sterilization (US $)	Laparoscopic sterilization (US $)	Cost savings (US $)
Levie et al. (2005) In-office Essure (Includes HSG)	1374	3449	2075
Kraemer et al. (2009) In-office Essure	2367	3545	1178
Hopkins et al. (2007) OR Essure (includes HSG)	2700	2880	180
HSG, Hysterosalpingogram			

laparoscopic tubal ligation, long-acting reversible contraceptives and hysteroscopic sterilization concluded that 'office hysteroscopic tubal sterilization may be one cost-cutting measure that benefits both the individual patient and greater society' (Barbieri 2010).

Cost comparisons have focused on the differences between the procedures themselves. It is more instructive to look at the long-term cost comparisons between laparoscopic and hysteroscopic sterilizations taking into account the costs related to procedural complications and pregnancy failures with subsequent obstetrical care. Considering the higher rate of operative complications of the laparoscopic approach and lower pregnancy failure rate of hysteroscopic sterilization, the differences are striking and clearly demonstrate both lower short-term and long-term advantages of the hysteroscopic approach (Levie & Chudnoff 2005, Kraemer et al. 2009).

■ COMPLICATIONS

Laparoscopic tubal ligation complications are relatively uncommon, but when they occur they are frequently severe and occasionally life threatening. The estimated mortality rates in the United States are 1–2 deaths per 100,000 procedures. Major complications range from 0.1% to 3.5% for laparoscopic tubal procedures (American College of Obstetricians and Gynecologists 2013). The most common minor complications involve misapplication of the devices. This may take the form of incomplete occlusion, injury to the tube, or placement on the round ligament instead of the Fallopian tube. Many complications are related to the initial insufflation and scope insertion, such as intestinal perforation, abdominal wall vascular injury, and major vascular injury. However, it is the risk of general anesthesia that surpasses all other factors except diabetes in causing complications from laparoscopic sterilization. The risks increase dramatically when the patient is obese or has had prior abdominal surgery (Jamieson et al. 2000). In the largest study of complications of laparoscopic sterilization published in 2000, the incidence of obesity was only 13.6% – far below the current level in the United States (Jamieson et al. 2000). No comparable studies have been conducted since that time, but the obesity rate of reproductive age women in the United States has increased dramatically. More than one-third of women are obese, more than one half of pregnant women are overweight or obese, and 8% of reproductive-aged women are extremely obese (Flegal et al. 2012).

The literature describing these complications does not take into account the epidemic of obesity that greatly increases the risk of injury during laparoscopic entry (Jansen et al. 1997, Scheib et al. 2014).

Obesity is also a national health concern among women in the USA; in 2009–2010, the prevalence of obesity was 35.8% among adult women (Flegal et al. 2012). Essure has been used successfully in obese women, those with chlamydial infection and gonorrhea, and in patients with prior pelvic inflammatory disease (PID) and abdominal surgery (Miner 2004, Warnes et al. 2008).

In addition, the high rate of Cesarean section for delivery adds the dimension of pelvic adhesions to potential complications encountered during a laparoscopic tubal. The current rate of Cesarean section in the United States is 32.8% (Centers for Disease Control and Prevention 2014). Combining the two risk factors of the epidemic of obesity with the high rate of Cesarean section, the opportunity for serious operative complication using a laparoscopic approach is sufficiently high to avoid recommending it as a purely elective procedure.

Finally, the frequency with which the obstetrician gynecologist performs laparoscopic surgery is directly proportional to the rate of complications. More than 50% of American women undergo surgery by low-volume gynecologic surgeons, defined as those who perform fewer than 5.88 laparoscopic hysterectomies per year, or one in every 2 months (Wallenstein et al. 2012).

In contrast, the complications associated with hysteroscopic sterilization are those common to diagnostic hysteroscopy, namely cervical injury from dilation, uterine perforation, and bleeding. The rate of injury from diagnostic hysteroscopy has been estimated to be approximately 0.13% in experienced hands and the addition of tubal cannulation has not been shown to cause significant risk. Uterine perforation has been described following hysteroscopic sterilization but these have been uniformly asymptomatic and discovered at the time of confirmatory HSG. As electrosurgical energy is not used in this procedure, suspected perforations may be managed as 'cold' perforations by observation. Finally, hysteroscopic sterilization is optimally performed in the office setting under local anesthesia, carrying one-third of the odds ratio of risk compared to general anesthesia (Jamieson et al. 2000).

Hatcher et al. compare the safety of laparoscopic tubal sterilization with that of hysteroscopic sterilization. Studies reporting complications associated with laparoscopic sterilization estimate US mortality rates at 1–4 deaths per 100,000 procedures (Hatcher et al. 2012). By comparison, no major life-threatening complications have been reported in the medical literature for hysteroscopic sterilization.

In the clinical trials of Essure, tubal perforations occurred in 1–3% of women, intraperitoneal placement in 0.5–3%, and other improper placements in 0.5% of the cases. Coil expulsion occurred in 0.4–2.2% of subjects (Kerin et al. 2003). A recent study assessed complications associated with Essure in 4306 patients over a 7-year period (Povedano et al. 2012). None of the complications (115/4306; 2.7%) required hospitalization and all patients were discharged <2 hours postprocedures. Around 98.5% of patients had successful microinsert placement. The overall complication rate was 2.7%, with vasovagal syncope being the most common. These include uterine or tubal perforation either by the microinsert or by the hysteroscope itself, coil misplacement, and expulsion of the microinsert devices. No patients had serious complications that required >2 hours of observation in the outpatient unit. The authors concluded that complications associated with the Essure procedure are thought to be uncommon, and are minor when present. Connor's (2009) review draws similar safety conclusions.

In 2015 an increasing number of reports of symptoms, side-effects and complications related to Essure, prompted a review by the Obstetrics and Gynecology Devices Advisory Panel of the Food and Drug Administration (FDA). The report listed over 120 symptoms reported in Essure Medical Device Reports, ranging from pelvic pain and menstrual irregularities, all the way to kidney stones, sleep apnea and degenerative bone disease. The vast majority of these reported symptoms are spurious and deemed to be unrelated to Essure usage (Food and Drug Administration 2015a). Safety and effectiveness data were presented by the FDA and the panel stated that 'hysteroscopic sterilization is an important option for women who are not good candidates for laparoscopic or general surgery (e.g. obese patients, patients who cannot tolerate general anesthesia) and who are well informed of the potential risks of the device (Food and Drug Administration 2015b).

Attribution of a wide variety of symptoms to the hysteroscopic sterilization procedures as well as to the device itself has led to a spate of removal of the devices by various methods – hysteroscopy, salpingectomy, and/or hysterectomy. A recent case series showed that almost 30% of the patients continued to have persistent symptoms after surgery, emphasizing that many of the reported 'symptoms' are unrelated to either the procedure or the device (Brito et al. 2015).

Before considering any sterilization procedure, laparoscopic or hysteroscopic, it is important to take a careful and comprehensive history from the patient of all current symptoms, especially pelvic pain, abnormal bleeding, allergies, and any other chronic condition, and discuss the risks of new symptoms or continuation of current symptoms with the patient.

There are a number of medical conditions such as cardiopulmonary disease, autoimmune disorders, and genetic disorders that render pregnancy life threatening. The same conditions contraindicate an elective procedure such as laparoscopic sterilization under general anesthesia. When counseling patients on their contraceptive options, practitioners should be aware that several papers including the American College of Cardiology/American Heart Association 2008 guidelines for the management of adults with congenital heart disease note that Essure offers an alternative choice for patients with complex congenital heart disease or those with pulmonary artery hypertension (Warnes et al. 2008).

Nickel sensitivity

At its initial release, Essure contained a warning for patients with nickel allergy, based mainly on concerns that patients with contact cutaneous reaction to jewelry-grade nickel alloy, and a positive nickel skin patch test would develop reactions to the nickel–titanium alloy in Essure. This has proved to be untrue. Daily dietary intake of nickel is 1000-fold greater than the amount of nickel released into the bloodstream by the Essure microinsert. The reported incidence of adverse events suspected to be related to nickel hypersensitivity in patients with Essure microinserts is extremely small (0.01%). The incidence of confirmed nickel reactions is even smaller. This very low incidence of clinical reactions is consistent with data from other nickel-containing implantable devices ranging from dental implants to orthopedic prosthesis to cardiac stents, and is reassuring. In 2011, the nickel sensitivity contraindication was removed from the Essure procedure instructions based on research demonstrating a lack of correlation between nickel hypersensitivity and Essure micro-inserts (Conceptus 2012, Zurawin & Zurawin 2011). Patients with nickel sensitivity may utilize Essure and do not require preprocedure skin testing. However, they should be counseled to report any untoward reaction following insertion and be followed appropriately.

CHOICE

Choice is the ultimate determinant in this process. Women who previously rejected the idea of permanent surgical contraception because of their reluctance to undergo anesthesia or even to go to a hospital are now actively seeking hysteroscopic sterilization in their doctor's office. The idea of abdominal scarring, however small, is a turn-off to many people. Patients return to their normal activity within 1 day of hysteroscopic sterilization, compared to several days to a week after laparoscopy for what is, in fact, an elective operative procedure. Out-of-pocket expenses are less. In our patient-driven world of medicine, women will seek physicians who are able to perform hysteroscopic procedures in general, and sterilization in particular. It is clear that this option is not appropriate for all women, as technical and anatomic factors may preclude its universal use. However, for all intents and purposes, laparoscopic tubal occlusion can no longer be regarded as the procedure of choice, and hysteroscopic sterilization should be considered the standard of care.

Choice: patient satisfaction studies

A number of studies report high-level patient satisfaction following the Essure procedure with most women recommending the procedure to a friend (Arjona et al. 2008, Levie et al. 2010). A 2012 patient preference study found that among 100 women who received a preprocedure survey describing tubal ligation versus hysteroscopic sterilization, 93% (93/100) favored hysteroscopic sterilization versus tubal ligation. All 93 viewed the office-based location as an advantage of hysteroscopic sterilization versus laparoscopic sterilization and 94.6% considered the confirmation test (HSG) to be a benefit (Chapa & Venegas 2012).

Patient counseling

As in any medical or surgical intervention, informed consent is of paramount importance (American Congress of Obstetricians and Gynecologists 2009). Even though pregnancy may be achieved following sterilization by the use of advanced reproductive technology or surgical reversal, patients must be counseled about the permanence of the procedure. Surgical reversal or fertility treatments are usually very expensive, hence often are not covered by insurance.

One factor that bears mentioning is the feeling of regret following sterilization. All sterilization procedures have the potential to be accompanied by a degree of regret, which is why it is critical for practitioners to be familiar with the data that report an increased correlation between regret and women under 30 (Wilcox et al. 1991). In addition, sterilization of minors or those with physical or intellectual disabilities either genetic or acquired must comply with legal and ethical guidelines (Paransky & Zurawin 2003). Women should be informed that factors, such as young age, particularly <30, unstable relationship, recent divorce, and low parity, may increase the risk of regret. The highest percentage of women expressing regret underwent postpartum sterilization. Both interval techniques, laparoscopic and hysteroscopic, are associated with the fewest cases of regret (Curtis et al. 2006, Legendre et al. 2013).

By the same token, women should not be denied sterilization due to marital status, age, or even nulliparity, if they have given proper informed consent, but careful documentation is essential before proceeding. The full range of contraceptive options should be discussed, along with their attendant medical or surgical risks, risk of failure, and alternatives. Vasectomy of the male partner should be addressed. A discussion of regret is an important component of the process, and the woman should be given an opportunity to consider her decision and not feel rushed while at the same time respecting her autonomy and right to make decisions about her healthcare.

Other considerations include the assessment of the patient's ability to tolerate an office procedure, her medical and mental health, and her compliance with follow-up care. The safety of each type of sterilization surgery should be assessed keeping in view the patient's medical conditions as discussed above (American College of Obstetricians and Gynecologists 2013).

CONCLUSION

Permanent contraception is a safe and effective option for women who have completed their childbearing years, or for those who either choose not to have children or for whom pregnancy is contraindicated. Tubal occlusion has evolved from large open abdominal operations to periumbilical postpartum procedures to laparoscopic occlusion and hysteroscopic techniques.

The decision as to which procedure should be utilized depends on a thorough discussion with the patient including the following topics:
- Contraceptive effectiveness
- Cost
- Complications
- Choice

Current trends based on all of the above factors suggest that the hysteroscopic route will become the predominant method of interval sterilization as devices continue to evolve and hysteroscopic skills of today's residents and fellows improve.

■ REFERENCES

American Congress of Obstetricians and Gynecologists. ACOG Committee Opinion No. 439: Informed consent. Obstet Gynecol 2009; 114:401–408.

American College of Obstetricians and Gynecologists. ACOG Practice bulletin no. 133: benefits and risks of sterilization. Obstet Gynecol 2013; 121:392–404.

Arjona J E, Mino M, Cordon J, et al. Satisfaction and tolerance with office hysteroscopic tubal sterilization. Fertil Steril 2008; 90:1182–1186.

Barbieri RL. Permanent contraception provides a lesson in cost-effective medicine. OBG Manage 2010; 22:6–10.

Bartz D, Greenberg JA. Sterilization in the United States. Rev Obstet Gynecol 2008; 1:23–32.

Brito LG, Cohen SL, Goggins ER, Wang KC, Einarsson JI. Essure surgical removal and subsequent symptom resolution: case series and follow-up surgery. J Minim Invasive Gynecol 2015; 22:910-913.

Centers for Disease Control and Prevention. Births — Method of Delivery, 2014. http://www.cdc.gov/nchs/fastats/delivery.htm. (Last accessed March 2014.)

Chan LM, Westhoff CL. Tubal sterilization trends in the United States. Fertil Steril 2010; 94:1–6.

Chapa HO, Antonetti AG, Sandate J. Office Versus Hospital Based Essure Procedure: Pareto Principle in Action. J Gynecol Surg 2012; 28:16–19.

Chapa HO, Venegas G. Preprocedure patient preferences and attitudes toward permanent contraceptive options. Patient Prefer Adherence 2012; 6:331–336.

Conceptus. Essure: instructions for use. Mountain View, CA: Conceptus Inc., 2012.

Connor VF. Essure: a review six years later. J Minim Invasive Gynecol 2009; 16:282–290.

Cooper JM. Hysteroscopic sterilization. Clin Obstet Gynecol 1992; 35:282–298.

Cooper JM, Carignan CS, Cher D, et al. Microinsert nonincisional hysteroscopic sterilization. Obstet Gynecol 2003; 102:59–67.

Curtis KM, Mohllajee AP, Peterson HB. Regret following female sterilization at a young age: a systematic review. Contraception 2006; 73:205–210.

Filshie GM, Casey D, Pogmore JR, et al. The titanium/silicone rubber clip for female sterilization. Br J Obstet Gynaecol 1981; 88:655–662.

Findley AD, Siedhoff MT, Hobbs KA, et al. Short-term effects of salpingectomy during laparoscopic hysterectomy on ovarian reserve: a pilot randomized controlled trial. Fertil Steril 2013; 100:1704–1708.

Flegal KM, Carroll MD, Kit BK, Ogden CL. Prevalence of obesity and trends in the distribution of body mass index among US adults, 1999–2010. JAMA 2012; 307:491–497.

Food and Drug Administration. 2015a. www.fda.gov/downloads/AdvisoryCommittees/CommitteesMeetingMaterials/MedicalDevices/MedicalDevicesAdvisoryCommittee/ObstetricsandGynecologyDevices/UCM463486.pdf, page 39.

Food and Drug Administration. 2015b. www.fda.gov/downloads/AdvisoryCommittees/CommitteesMeetingMaterials/MedicalDevices/MedicalDevicesAdvisoryCommittee/ObstetricsandGynecologyDevices/UCM464487.pdf, page 2.

Greenberg JA. Hysteroscopic sterilization: history and current methods. Rev Obstet Gynecol 2008; 1:113–121.

Guiahi M, Goldman KN, McElhinney MM, Olson CG. Improving hysterosalpingogram confirmatory test follow-up after Essure hysteroscopic sterilization. Contraception 2010; 81:520–524.

Guido RS, Brooks K, McKenzie R, et al. A randomized, prospective comparison of pain after gasless laparoscopy and traditional laparoscopy. J Am Assoc Gynecol Laparosc 1998; 5:149–153.

Guttmacher Institute. Contraceptive use in the United States. 2015. http://www.guttmacher.org/pubs/fb_contr_use.html. Last accessed 15 December 2015.

Hataska HH, Sharp HT, Dowling DD, et al. Laparoscopic tubal ligation in a minimally invasive surgical unit under local anesthesia compared to a conventional operating room approach under general anesthesia. J Laparoendosc Adv Surg Tech A 1997; 7:295–299.

Hatcher RA, Trussell J, Nelson AL, et al. Contraceptive technology. New York, NY: Ardent Media, 2012.

Hollander D. Women who are sterilized at age 30 or younger have increased odds of regret. Fam Plann Perspect 1999; 31:308.

Hopkins MR, Creedon DJ, Wagie AE, et al. Retrospective cost analysis comparing Essure hysteroscopic sterilization and laparoscopic bilateral tubal coagulation. J Minim Invasive Gynecol 2007; 14:97–102.

Hulka JF, Fishburne JI, Mercer JP, Omran KF. Laparoscopic sterilization with a spring clip: a report of the first fifty cases. Am J Obstet Gynecol 1973; 116:715–718.

Jamieson DJ, Hillis SD, Duerr A, et al. Complications of interval laparoscopic tubal sterilization: findings from the United States Collaborative Review of Sterilization. Obstet Gynecol 2000; 96:997–1002.

Jansen FW, Kapiteyn K, Trimbos-Kemper T, et al. Complications of laparoscopy: a prospective multicentre observational study. Br J Obstet Gynaecol 1997; 104:595–600.

Jones J, Mosher W, Daniels K. Current contraceptive use in the United States, 2006–2010, and changes in patterns of use since 1995. National Health Statistics Report. Hyattsville, MD: National Center for Health Statistics, 2012.

Kerin JF, Cooper JM, Price T, et al. Hysteroscopic sterilization using a micro-insert device: results of a multicentre Phase II study. Hum Reprod 2003; 18:1223–1230.

Kocks J. A new method of female sterilization. Zentbl Gynäkol 1878; 26:617–618.

Kraemer DF, Yen PY, Nichols M. An economic comparison of female sterilization of hysteroscopic tubal occlusion with laparoscopic bilateral tubal ligation. Contraception 2009; 80:254–260.

Legendre GM, Varoux M, Nazac A, Fernandez H. [Regret following hysteroscopic tubal sterilization.]. J Gynecol Obstet Biol Reprod 2013; 43:387–392.

Levie M, Weiss G, Kaiser B, et al. Analysis of pain and satisfaction with office-based hysteroscopic sterilization. Fertil Steril 2010; 94:1189–1194.

Levie MD, Chudnoff SG. Office hysteroscopic sterilization compared with laparoscopic sterilization: a critical cost analysis. J Minim Invasive Gynecol 2005; 12:318–322.

Levy B, Levie MD, Childers ME. A summary of reported pregnancies after hysteroscopic sterilization. J Minim Invasive Gynecol 2007; 14:271–274.

Loffer FD. Hysteroscopic sterilization with the use of formed-in-place silicone plugs. Am J Obstet Gynecol 1984; 149:261–270.

MacKay AP, Kieke BA Jr, Koonin LM, Beattie K. Tubal sterilization in the United States, 1994-1996. Fam Plann Perspect 2001; 33:161–165.

March CM, Israel R. A critical appraisal of hysteroscopic tubal fulguration for sterilization. Contraception 1975; 11:261–269.

McAlpine JN, Hanley GE, Woo MM, et al. Opportunistic salpingectomy: uptake, risks, and complications of a regional initiative for ovarian cancer prevention. Am J Obstet Gynecol 2014; 210:471.e1–471.e11.

Miner PD. Contraceptive choices for females with congenital heart disease. Prog Pediatr Cardiol 2004; 19:15–24.

Morelli MR, Venturella R, Mocciaro R, et al. Prophylactic salpingectomy in premenopausal low-risk women for ovarian cancer: primum non nocere. Gynecol Oncol 2013; 129:448–451.

Munro MG, Nichols JE, Levy B, et al. Hysteroscopic sterilization: 10-year retrospective analysis of worldwide pregnancy reports. J Minim Invasive Gynecol 2014; 21:245–251.

Paransky OI, Zurawin RK. Management of menstrual problems and contraception in adolescents with mental retardation: a medical, legal, and ethical review with new suggested guidelines. J Pediatr Adolesc Gynecol 2003; 16:223–235.

Peterson HB, Xia Z, Hughes JM, et al. The risk of pregnancy after tubal sterilization: findings from the U.S. Collaborative Review of Sterilization. Am J Obstet Gynecol 1996; 174:1161–1168; discussion 1168–1170.

Povedano B, Arjona JE, Velasco E, et al. Complications of hysteroscopic Essure((R)) sterilisation: report on 4306 procedures performed in a single centre. BJOG 2012; 119:795–799.

Rodriguez AM, Kilic GS, Vu TP, et al. Analysis of tubal patency after essure placement. J Minim Invasive Gynecol 2013; 20:468–472.

Scheib SA, Tanner E 3rd, Green IC, Fader AN. Laparoscopy in the morbidly obese: physiologic considerations and surgical techniques to optimize success. J Minim Invasive Gynecol 2014; 21:182–195.

Simpson WL, Beitia L. Multimodality imaging of the Essure tubal occlusion device. Clin Radiol 2012; 67:e112–e117.

Veersema S, Vleugels M, Koks C, et al. Confirmation of Essure placement using transvaginal ultrasound. J Minim Invasive Gynecol 2011; 18:164–168.

Wallenstein M R, Ananth CV, Kim JH, et al. Effect of surgical volume on outcomes for laparoscopic hysterectomy for benign indications. Obstet Gynecol 2012; 119:709–716.

Warnes CA, Williams RG, Bashore TM, et al. ACC/AHA 2008 guidelines for the management of adults with congenital heart disease: a report of the American College of Cardiology/American Heart Association Task Force on Practice Guidelines (Writing Committee to Develop Guidelines on the Management of Adults With Congenital Heart Disease). Developed in Collaboration With the American Society of Echocardiography, Heart Rhythm Society, International Society for Adult Congenital Heart Disease, Society for Cardiovascular Angiography and Interventions, and Society of Thoracic Surgeons. J Am Coll Cardiol 2008; 52:e143–e263.

Wilcox LS, Chu SY, Eaker ED, et al. Risk factors for regret after tubal sterilization: 5 years of follow-up in a prospective study. Fertil Steril 1991; 55:927–933.

Ye XP, Yang YZ Sun XX. A retrospective analyiss of the effect of salpingectomy on serum antiMullerian hormone level and ovarian reserve. Am J Obstet Gynecol 2015; 212:53.

Yoon IB, King TM. A preliminary and intermediate report on a new laparoscopic tubal ring procedure. J Reprod Med 1975; 15:54–56.

Zurawin RK, Sklar AJ. Tubal sterilization. http://emedicine.medscape.com/article/266799. Last accessed 15 December 2015.

Zurawin RK, Zurawin JL. Adverse events due to suspected nickel hypersensitivity in patients with essure microinserts. J Minim Invasive Gynecol 2011; 18:475–482.

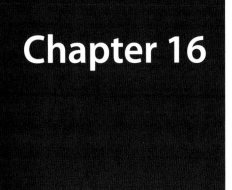

Chapter 16

Laparoscopic management of pelvic organ prolapse

Revaz Botchorishvili

Genital prolapse is a common pathology. With life expectancy set at 80, women run an 11% risk of undergoing surgical treatment for prolapse (Slieker-Ten Hove et al., 2009). The epidemiological data underline that the quality of initial surgical treatment is important because around 30% of patients will be operated several times (DeLancey 2005). Furthermore, although prolapse surgery aims to restore anatomy, the main goal is in fact functional.

Many surgical techniques are used to treat female genital prolapse, and this is in itself proof of how difficult it is to deal with this problem. Treatment of uterine and bladder prolapse by laparotomy using prosthetic mesh was developed by Scali in 1974 (Scali et al. 1974). The principle consists of installing a prosthetic mesh in the intervesi-couterine space and subsequently anchoring it to the promontory. Since 1991, laparoscopy was used for this purpose. Subsequently, the laparoscopic treatment of rectocele by prosthetic reinforcement of the rectovaginal fascia was also developed, as well laparoscopic stress urinary incontinence treatment and paravaginal repair, thus offering a complete range of treatments for all forms of female prolapse (Boughizane et al. 1995, Cheret et al. 2001, Cosson et al. 2000, Cundiff et al. 1997, Dean et al. 2006, Gadonneix et al. 2004, Higgs et al. 2005, Maher et al. 2011, Nezhat et al. 1994, Rivoire et al. 2007, Rozet et al. 2005, Sergent et al. 2011, Wattiez et al. 2001, 2003).

The surgical technique in current use is laparoscopic mesh promontofixation (mesh suspension to the promontory) of the cervix in case of supracervical hysterectomy, of the uterus when this is conserved, or of the vaginal vault in case of posthysterectomy vault prolapse.

LAPAROSCOPIC PROMONTOFIXATION: SURGICAL TECHNIQUE

Setup and instrumentation

The patient is positioned and prepared as for any operative laparoscopy: general anaesthesia; lithotomy position with legs semiflexed at 45°; in-dwelling bladder catheter and uterine cannulation to allow mobilization of the uterus. This cannulation is achieved using a Valtchev-type device (Conkin Surgical Instruments Ltd., North York, Canada) identical to that used for tubal sterility workup (no cervical dilatation) rather than the device used for total hysterectomy (that requires cervical dilatation), with the aim of keeping cervical dilatation and the risks of contamination of the prosthesis to a minimum.

After setting up for laparoscopy, three ancillary ports are required (as for hysterectomy, myomectomy, etc.): one 10 mm umbilical trocar for the optics and two 5 mm trocars, which are inserted in the iliac fossas outside the outer edge of the rectus abdominis muscle, level with or above the anterosuperior iliac spine. The final 5 mm trocar is inserted on the midline at least 8–10 cm from the umbilical trocar (**Figure 16.1**). After dissection is complete, this trocar is replaced by a 10 mm trocar to allow easy insertion of the needles and prosthesis and suturing.

To make it easier to expose the promontory and the pouch of Douglas, temporary suspension of the sigmoid to the abdominal wall is used systematically. This is achieved using a T-Lift device (Vectec, Hauterive, France) introduced through the left sidewall and passed through the epiploic appendices (**Figure 16.2**).

The instruments used are same as for any operative laparoscopy. For prolapse surgery requiring long and precise dissection, the use of RoBi dissecting bipolar forceps (Karl Storz GmbH, Tuttlingen, Germany) is particularly helpful.

The first step is surgical diagnosis with inspection of the peritoneal cavity, especially the ovaries, prior to the following operative phases.

Key steps
Step 1: Exposing the promontory

The first step in approaching the promontory consists of careful anatomical identification of L5–S1, the bifurcation of the aorta, the right ureter, and the lower edge of the left primitive iliac vein and medial sacral vessels. Dissection must go far enough to allow one or two sutures to be placed in the anterior common vertebral ligament

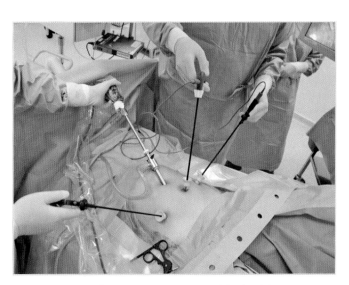

Figure 16.1 Setup of laparoscopy. One 10 mm umbilical and three 5 mm ancillary ports are used. Bipolar forceps are inserted in the left ancillary port and scissors with monopolar connection in the middle.

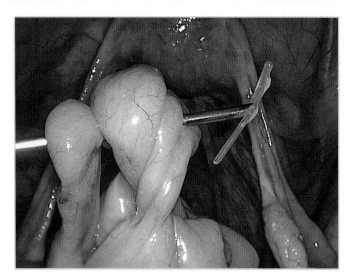

Figure 16.2 Sigmoid colon suspension using T-Lift device. The device is introduced through the left sidewall and passed through the epiploic appendices. This allows perfect exposition of the promontory and of the pouch of Douglas.

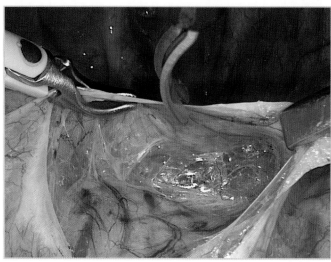

Figure 16.3 Sacral promontory dissection. The assistant pulls on the peritoneum using forceps so that it can be incised vertically downward. Dissection must allow the anterior vertebral ligament to be identified clearly.

without any risk to the surrounding structures. It may be necessary to briefly accentuate the Trendelenburg position so that this procedure can be carried out under good conditions. The assistant pulls on the peritoneum using forceps so that it can be incised vertically downward (**Figure 16.3**). Dissection must allow the anterior vertebral ligament to be identified clearly because any gesture carried out blindly due to inadequate dissection is potentially extremely dangerous in this area. In obese patients and patients with a low aortic bifurcation, particular care must be taken with respect to the left iliac vein, which is often flattened by pneumoperitoneum pressure. The integrity of the right hypogastric nerve should be also respected during dissection (Cosma et al. 2013).

Step 2: Pararectal and rectovaginal dissection

The peritoneal incision started at the promontory is taken forward and caudally toward the pouch of Douglas, running laterally to the rectosigmoid and medially at an adequate distance from the right ureter. This incision will allow the prosthesis to be retroperitonealized at the end of surgery. It is prolonged at the level of the Douglas pouch, medially to the right uterosacral ligament.

Rectovaginal dissection starts after drawing the rectum backward and pushing the uterus forward. The rectum is grasped by the assistant using bowel forceps, then strong traction is applied downward and backward. The peritoneum opposite to the torus uterinus is stretched in an arc; it is coagulated then sectioned 2 cm below its uterine insertion. The cleavage plane is identified as closely as possible to the vaginal wall and is then guided by the relief of the posterior vaginal wall. Dissection of this plane is simple if exposure has been properly achieved. It is made easier by the phenomenon of pneumodissection, the traction applied to the rectum, and the thrust applied to the uterus.

In the rectovaginal plane, the lower limit of dissection lies at the anorectal angle. Dissection continues laterally to the anorectal angle and inward to reveal the levator ani muscles to which the prosthesis will be fixed. At this point, dissection must go far enough to allow easy access for the sutures in this space directly in contact with the pelvic floor. Finally, the space dissected is bordered by the levator ani muscles and pelvic sidewall laterally, the anal–rectal angle medially, the vagina to the front, and the rectum to the back (**Figure 16.4**).

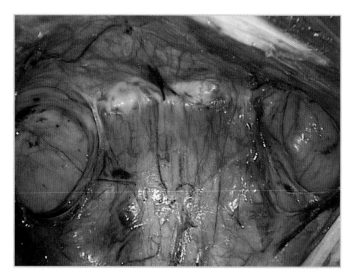

Figure 16.4 Rectovaginal space dissection. The space dissected is bordered by the levator ani muscles and pelvic sidewall laterally, the anal–rectal angle medially, the vagina to the front, and the rectum to the back.

Step 3: Start of supracervical hysterectomy

The standard method was to leave the uterus in place in order to avoid opening the vagina and the consequent risks of infection involving the prosthesis. This technique is possible via laparoscopy without sectioning the round ligaments during dissection of the spaces and taking the prosthesis through the broad ligaments, passing round the uterine pedicles, and avoiding the ureters. It is currently more common to carry out supracervical hysterectomy. There are two advantages with this technique: the cervix is conserved, thus providing a sturdy point to which the prosthesis can be attached firmly, and there is no opening created in the vagina, thus reducing the risk of sepsis due to contact with the prosthesis. In this case, a uterine morcellator is used so that the excised tissues can be extracted without any colpotomy.

The hysterectomy technique is standard and has already been described (Wattiez et al. 2002). Unlike with the simple (total or supracervical) hysterectomy, the anterior dissection is always prolonged beneath the bladder.

Step 4: Vesicovaginal dissection

Dissection of the vesicovaginal space is achieved by pulling up the prevesical peritoneum and bladder, incising the peritoneum, then opening the vesicovaginal space along the midline, and taking the incision downward while pushing the bladder between the internal bladder pillars. Dissection must continue as low as possible, in close proximity to the bladder neck as identified by the outline of the urinary catheter balloon and over a surface wide enough to allow the anterior part of the prosthesis to be spread out completely. The space in which the prosthesis will be installed is triangular and variable in size, with the lower point close to the bladder neck (**Figure 16.5**).

Step 5: End of supracervical hysterectomy

After hemostasis of the uterine pedicles, the cervix is sectioned at the isthmus level after removing the manipulator. Various means can be used for this section. We prefer to use a cold knife in an endoscopic holder (Chardonnens morcellation knife; Karl Storz GmbH, Tuttlingen, Germany) or monopolar cutting device (Supraloop; Karl Storz GmbH, Tuttlingen, Germany). The cervical stump is carefully sutured using two or three stitches of Poliglecaprone 1 (Monocryl, Ethicon, Issy les Moulineaux, France). This phase is important because it protects the prosthesis against any vaginal contamination. Once the hysterectomy has been completed, it is convenient to temporarily suspend the cervical stump to the anterior pelvic sidewall in order to keep the assistant's instrument free to help with suturing.

The uterus is left waiting to be morcellated at the end of the procedure, using a laparoscopic morcellator.

When there has been a previous hysterectomy, the vaginal vault is exposed with the help of a compress held in long-handled forceps inserted into the vagina to make dissection easier. Vesicouterine dissection is, however, more difficult, especially if the vaginal route was used for the hysterectomy. In these cases, there is a greater risk of vaginal or bladder perforation.

If the uterus is conserved, a passage must be prepared through the broad ligament for the two arms of the prosthesis. Dissection is thus continued laterally by opening the two (anterior and posterior) peritoneal layers of the broad ligament, remaining level with the isthmus but at a distance from the uterine pedicle, which is easy to identify. Care must also be taken not to go too deeply into the broad ligament in order to avoid the ureters.

Step 6: Installing the prosthesis

The prosthesis is inserted via the 10 mm trocar. Two polypropylene meshes may be used (Surgymesh, Aspide Medical, La Talaudière, France). The anterior prosthesis consists of a rectangle with a triangular inferior extremity, and the posterior part presenting an inferior inverted V-shape form to avoid compression of the rectum.

The rear part of the tape is fixed first. While this is being done, the cervical stump is lifted upward thanks to a suture taken through the pelvic sidewall using a Reverdin needle. The posterior prosthesis is attached to the levator ani muscles on each side using one stitch (**Figure 16.6**), then to the uterosacral ligaments on each side with one stitch, and one more stitch to the posterior part of the cervix medially. The sutures consist of braided nonresorbable Polyester 0, with a curved 26 mm needle, in 90 cm strands (Ethibond, Ethicon, Issy les Moulineaux, France) or resorbable polydioxanone 2-0 with a curved 26 mm needle, in 70 cm strands (PDS II, Ethicon, Issy les Moulineaux, France). It is easier to take the needle through the levator ani muscles using the right hand, from outside inward. The sutures are closed with extracorporeal knots of the half-hitch type using a knot pusher. Four to six knots are needed to achieve a sturdy anchorage. When the prosthesis is to be fixed to the vaginal vault, particular care must be taken to not transfix the latter.

The anterior prosthesis is placed beneath the bladder and fixed with one nontransfixing stitch to the anterior face of the vagina, then with one stitch level with the extremity of the cervix (**Figure 16.7**). The anterior and posterior prostheses are then attached to each other laterally with one stitch, which also takes up the cervix (**Figure 16.8**). It is essential not to have any stitches that transfix the vagina in order to avoid any risk of contaminating the prosthesis.

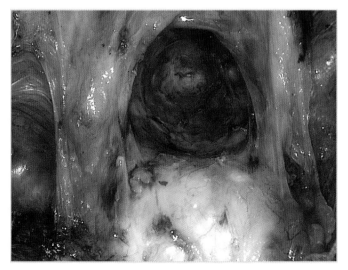

Figure 16.5 Vesicovaginal space dissection. Dissection must continue as low as possible, in close proximity to the bladder neck and over a surface wide enough to allow the anterior part of the prosthesis to be spread out completely.

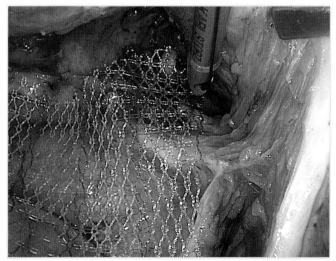

Figure 16.6 Mesh fixation to the levator ani muscles. The posterior prosthesis is attached to the right levator ani muscles with extracorporeal knots of the half-hitch type using knot pusher.

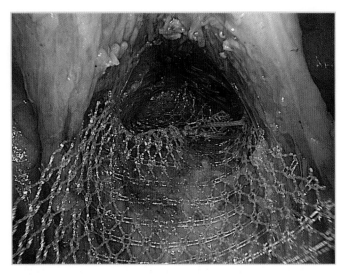

Figure 16.7 Mesh fixation to the anterior vaginal wall. The anterior prosthesis is placed beneath the bladder and fixed with one non-transfixing stitch to the anterior face of the vagina.

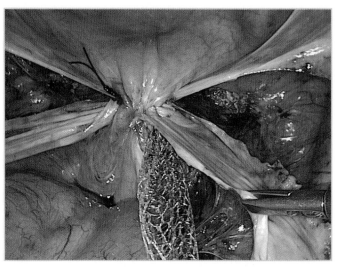

Figure 16.9 Anterior peritonization. This step is achieved by taking up the anterior and posterior peritoneum using a 'back-and-forth' running suture.

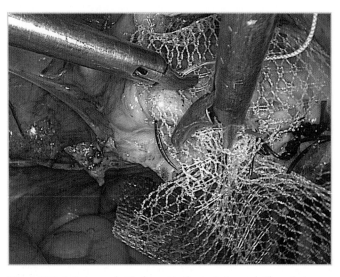

Figure 16.8 Anterior mesh attachment to the posterior mesh. The anterior and posterior prostheses are attached to each other laterally with one stitch that also takes up the cervix.

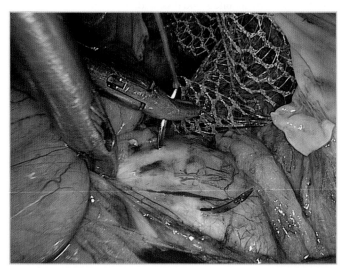

Figure 16.10 Mesh fixation to the promontory. The needle must only take up the fibrous layer of the ligament, meaning it remains visible by transparency, to ensure that the disc is not perforated in any way.

If the uterus is conserved, the two arms of tape are taken through the openings made in the posterior layer of the broad ligament. They are then knotted behind the isthmus using a flat knot in the area deperitonized when the rectovaginal detachment was started.

Step 7: Peritoneal closure

This must be meticulous, aiming at complete retroperitonealization of the prosthesis. It is commenced prior to fixation to the promontory. There are two steps, with an anterior step for vesicouterine and rectovaginal detachment. This step is achieved by taking up the anterior and posterior peritoneum using a 'back-and-forth' running suture (**Figure 16.9**). Then, when the prosthesis is fixed to the promontory, a second running suture closes the line of the incision going from the promontory to the pouch of Douglas. The suture material used is a Poliglecaprone 0 resorbable monofilament type (Monocryl, Ethicon, Issy les Moulineaux, France). Retroperitonealization will prevent

incarceration of a loop of bowel, which otherwise is always possible. The tape is thus routed exclusively behind the peritoneum.

Step 8: Fixing to the promontory

The final step in promontofixation is to fix the prosthesis (single, pre-cut prosthesis or anterior and posterior prostheses together) to the anterior common vertebral ligament. This fixation uses one or two stitches of braided nonresorbable polyester 1, 30 mm curved needle, 75 cm long (Ethibond, Ethicon Issy les Moulineaux, France). The suture is made using the left hand, from the inside toward the outside and from bottom to top (**Figure 16.10**). The needle must only take up the fibrous layer of the ligament to ensure that the disc is not perforated in any way.

We do not recommend the use of staples in this location, for the same reason. In addition, the problem of bleeding in case of injury to the midsacral pedicle arises mainly when the needle is routed too median relative to the promontory and when the promontory has not been sufficiently dissected.

Once the sutures have been taken through the tissues, sustained traction is applied to check that they are firmly attached. The mesh is placed on the promontory in tension-free fashion, then fixed in position. We make a perioperative clinical examination to check that normal anatomical relations are restored by this promontofixation. Note that the traction acts directly on the cervical stump and indirectly on the other tissues, insofar as the prosthesis always remains relatively flexible relative to the vagina on which it is fixed. The final peritoneal closure stitches are made after the mesh has been fixed to the promontory (**Figure 16.11**).

Step 9: Paravaginal repair and Burch colposuspension

The purpose of this phase is to prevent any urinary incontinence revealed by the prolapse repair, on the one hand, and to treat lateral cystocele, on the other hand (Wattiez et al. 2001).

The retropubic space (cave of Retzius) is opened by an incision in the peritoneum above the bladder, running from one umbilical artery to the other, after pulling the peritoneum downward. The urachus is coagulated then sectioned, and dissection must then proceed along a vertical plane toward the pelvic sidewall. The umbilicovesical fascia must be crossed in order to enter the cave of Retzius. Pneumodissection helps to open the space. The right and left Cooper ligaments revealed on each side mark the upper limit of the cave of Retzius. Now the space is opened up completely by simply breaking down the tissues until the internal obturator muscle, lateral cystocele, and arcus tendineus fasciae pelvis are revealed. Dissection continues backward until just below the obturator foramen. The dome formed by the vagina is also exposed by a finger placed in the vaginal fornix.

For the colposuspension, the suture is first taken from top to bottom through the Cooper ligament, then through the vagina, from the inside outward, being careful not to transfix it. Between two and four sutures are made each side. Traction must be moderate (**Figure 16.12**). The surgeon's experience is extremely important in this respect.

The width of tissue taken up in the ligament and in the vagina must be sufficiently broad to ensure a sturdy result. The suture material used is braided polyester 0, with a 26 mm curved needle (Ethibond, Ethicon, Issy les Moulineaux, France). Half-hitches are used for the fixation.

Before carrying out colposuspension, the positive pressure of the pneumoperitoneum allows inspection of the lateral defects that are almost always present in cases of complex prolapse. They show up as hernias running from the arcus tendineus fasciae pelvis to the vagina itself. If there is a paravaginal hernia like this, it must be repaired. This is essential to avoid any risk of recurrence of the cystocele, in particular lateral cystocele.

This paravaginal repair can be made prior to the colposuspension, using separate stitches or a running suture of nonresorbable braided polyester 0 and a 26 mm curved needle (Ethibond, Ethicon, Issy les Moulineaux, France).

The suture runs from the pubourethral ligaments at the front to the sciatic spine to the rear. It may be uni- or bilateral. However, paravaginal repair using sutures requires the needle to be taken through the arcus tendineus fasciae pelvis; however, with lateral defects, this is often thin and/or torn (which is precisely what causes the defect) so cannot be considered as sufficiently sturdy for anchorage and a durable repair. Thus, at present, we prefer to carry out the colposuspension to the Cooper ligament using at least three anchorage points, which thus brings the vagina up level with the arcus tendineus and in effect represents the paravaginal repair. To close the defect completely and encourage fibrosis, a floating prosthetic reinforcement is positioned paravaginally (**Figure 16.13**).

The colposuspension and paravaginal repair phase is completed by peritonization using a running suture of resorbable monofilament material such as Poliglecaprone 0 (Monocryl, Ethicon, Issy les Moulineaux, France).

Uterine morcellation and closure of the aponeurosis at the location of the midline 10 mm trocar are the final steps in the procedure.

▪ AVAILABLE EVIDENCE ON LAPAROSCOPIC TREATMENT FOR GENITAL PROLAPSE

A literature review shows that there is already good available evidence on the laparoscopic approach for genital prolapse, mainly for apical prolapse. A Cochrane review (Maher et al. 2013) compared laparoscopic sacrocolpopexy (LSC) with abdominal sacrocolpopexy (ASC) for vault prolapse treatment: they concluded that LSC presented less blood loss and reduced impatient days, with similar median Patient Global

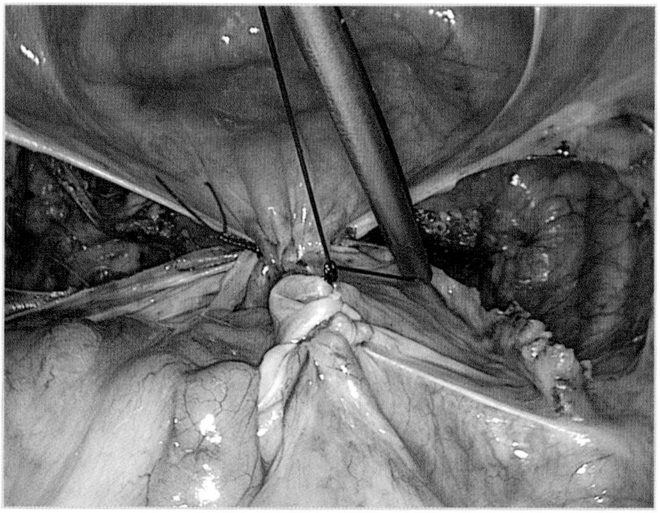

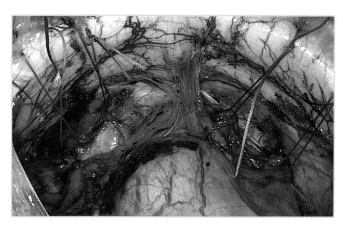

Figure 16.11 Posterior peritonization. The final peritonization stitches are made after the mesh has been fixed to the promontory.

Figure 16.12 Burch colposuspension. For the colposuspension, between two and four sutures are made on each side. Traction must be moderate.

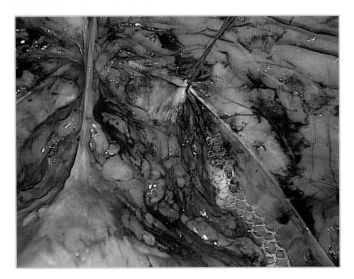

Figure 16.13 Paravaginal repair and floating mesh. To close the defect completely and encourage fibrosis, a floating prosthetic reinforcement is positioned paravaginally before suturing.

Impression of Improvement and similar anatomical results rates, operative time, serious adverse events, and prolapse quality-of-life (QoL) outcome compared to ASC. In the same review, LSC was compared with total vaginal polypropylene mesh kit (vault prolapse), presenting reduced blood loss, reduced impatient days, quicker return to activities of daily living, lower objective recurrence rate (higher point C, higher point Ba, higher point Bp, longer total vaginal length), and higher patient satisfaction despite longer time to perform. Improvement on QoL was similar, as well as mesh exposure risk; however, the reoperation rate related to primary intervention was less likely after LSC. LSC was also compared to robotic sacral colpopexy (RSC) and presented shorter operative time, less use of NSAIDs, lower cost, and similar improvements in objective assessment and functional outcomes.

Specifically regarding the complication rates and management, Khan et al. compared a minimally invasive sacrocolpopexy (LSC and RSC) with ASC, concluding that LSC led to a higher rate of reoperation for anterior wall prolapse, but less medical (primarily cardiopulmonary) complications (Kahn et al. 2013). Antosh et al. also reported similar perioperative complications between LSC and RSC. (Antosh et al. 2013).

Concerning risk of mesh exposure in LSC, Warner et al. concluded, with their cohort study, that 'preserving the integrity of the vaginal cuff led to a lower incidence of mesh exposure and when hysterectomy is indicated, a supracervical technique should be strongly considered as the mesh exposure rate is significantly lower.' Nonetheless, 'if removal of the cervix is indicated, the risk for mesh exposure remains low and should not preclude total hysterectomy, though transvaginal mesh attachment may be preferable' (Warner et al. 2012). According to Tan-Kim et al., concomitant vaginal hysterectomy at the time of LSC results in a high rate of mesh erosion with a sixfold increased risk. Based on these data, the authors proposed supracervical hysterectomy as the procedure of choice in association with LSC unless removal of the cervix is otherwise indicated (Tan-Kim et al. 2011). In regard to obstructive defecatory syndrome, Ramanah et al. reported no improvement and even worsening of obstructive defecatory syndrome after LSC (Ramanah et al. 2012).

About some technical aspects of the surgery, Culligan et al., in their randomized controlled trial, showed that porcine dermis and polypropylene mesh yield comparable short-term (12 months) cure rates (Culligen et al. 2013).

There is a cohort study evaluating the anatomical and functional results of bone anchor fixation of the mesh on LSC. Despite attaching their bone anchors to S2–S4, these researchers concluded that bone anchoring is a 'safe and efficacious treatment (good anatomical outcomes)' (with only 6 months of follow-up), with only case reports of lumbosacral discitis (Withagen et al. 2012).

More prospective randomized clinical trials studies involving more patients, longer follow-up times, appropriate controls, and objective assessment techniques are needed to further evaluate the laparoscopic approach as a minimally invasive method for successful long-term treatment of pelvic organ prolapse and urinary incontinence.

◼ OUR EXPERIENCE

We now have performed >500 laparoscopic promontofixation procedures using a standardized technique without vaginal opening. In our first published series of about 131 patients, we excluded patients who underwent total hysterectomy during the same surgery, patients in whom there was no fixation of the prosthesis to the levator ani muscles, patients operated via the vagina or by laparotomy, and cases where biological meshes were used (Rivoire et al. 2007).

This study only included patients in whom there was no perioperative opening of the vagina. We believe that this technique reduces vaginal erosion complications, and it has gradually become the only technique used in our department except for when there is a specific indication for cervical ablation.

Supracervical hysterectomy was carried out in 101 cases, the uterus was conserved in four cases, and prolapse of the vaginal vault was treated in 26 cases; 109 patients had a Burch colposuspension, 40 paravaginal repair by suturing, and 24 patients had prosthetic paravaginal reinforcement.

The mean operating time was 190 minutes. No conversion to laparotomy was required. The perioperative complication rate and rate of repeat surgery in the immediate postoperative period were 5.8% and 2.9%, respectively. The mean follow-up was 31 months (range 11–79).

No stage 3 or 4 genital prolapse was found 1 month after surgery, and eight patients (8%) presented clinical recurrence at some distance after surgery. Survival analysis showed that after 40 months follow-up, the probability of presenting no recurrence remains stable at 0.8018, with a confidence interval of 95% (0.6689–0.8857).

Patients were asked how satisfied they were overall with respect to the operation and 105 patients (80%) declared they were very satisfied, 23 (18%) that they wer e moderately satisfied, and three patients (2%) were not satisfied.

Complications related to the prosthesis were observed in nine patients (6.9%). Problems with vaginal healing were seen in seven patients (5%), in the form of vaginal mesh erosions. There were no cases of erosion with the polypropylene prostheses; all the erosions occurred when multifilament polyester was used. One prosthesis was removed due to spondylodiscitis, and one other due to a vesicovaginal fistula successfully repaired by laparoscopy.

Concerning bladder function, correction of stress urinary incontinence was inadequate in our series. Fifty-one percent of patients were incontinent preoperatively and 45% postoperatively. It would appear best to treat urinary incontinence preventively in every case since there was a very high frequency of postoperative incontinence when no preventive measures were taken.

CONCLUSION

Many important changes have taken place in the management and treatment of urogenital prolapse over the past few years. The goals are improved QoL for the patients, better surgical management using techniques that are as minimally invasive as possible, and a durable result. Laparoscopy appears to be a feasible approach for surgical correction of urogenital prolapse. It combines the advantages of minimally invasive surgery with a rapid return to normal activities, with the possibility of efficient treatment of prolapse by adapting a reference surgical technique by laparotomy (Ganatra et al. 2009).

Promontofixation by laparoscopy offers the same advantages for treatment of prolapse as does laparotomy (Nygaard et al. 2013, Paraiso et al. 2005). The technique is acceptable in terms of anatomical and functional results concerning the prolapse and also in terms of continuous effectiveness. The complications are minor and similar to, if not better than, the results found with laparotomy. In an environment with an operating room where operative endoscopy has become the technique of reference, the procedure can be used in the great majority of cases. The operating time has become acceptable, lasting <3 hours.

Concurrent treatment of stress urinary incontinence appears to be a weak point in this technique, which might be improved by more frequent use of suburethral tape techniques. In this connection, several technical points need to be stressed.

Importantly, just as with laparotomy, preventive treatment of stress urinary incontinence should be carried out in every case, even in patients who did not have any incontinence preoperatively. The frequency of postoperative incontinence is high when no preventive steps have been taken.

At the same time, it should be said that these cases of postoperative incontinence can be actually easily corrected using suburethral meshes. But this requires a second surgery, which may be disagreeable from the patient's point of view.

Finally, it seems that, in the years to come, we will have two minimally invasive surgical approaches available: laparoscopy and vaginal surgery. A randomized prospective comparison of these two methods is essential (Maher et al. 2011). Moreover, prosthetic devices must be used with caution (De Tayrac & Sentilhes 2013). Only those materials that have been proved to be efficient and innocuous must be used, and the technical recommendations for their installation must be respected.

Further studies are required in order to improve the overall management of patients and our understanding of the prosthetic materials and to make this technique more accessible for everyday surgical practice.

REFERENCES

Antosh DD, Grotzke SA, McDonald MA, et al. Short-term outcomes of robotic versus conventional laparoscopic sacral colpopexy. Female Pelvic Med Reconstr Surg 2012; 18:158–161.

Boughizane S, Alexandre F, Canis M, et al. Laparoscopic procedures for stress incontinence and prolapse. Curr Opin Obstet Gynecol 1995; 7:317–321.

Cheret A, Von Theobald P, Lucas J, et al. Faisabilité de la promontofixation par voie cœlioscopique. J Gynecol Obstet Biol Reprod 2001; 30:139–143.

Cosma S, Menato G, Ceccaroni M, et al. Laparoscopic sacropexy and obstructed defecation syndrome: an anatomoclinical study Int Urogynecol J 2013; 24:1623–1630.

Cosson M, Bogaert E, Narducci F, et al. Promontofixation coelioscopique: résultats à court terme et complications chez 83 patients. J Gynecol Obstet Biol Reprod 2000; 29:746–750.

Culligan PJ, Salamon C, Priestley JL, Shariati A. Porcine dermis compared with polypropylene mesh for laparoscopic sacrocolpopexy: a randomized controlled trial. Obstet Gynecol 2013; 121:143–151.

Cundiff GW, Harris RL, Coates K, et al. Abdominal sacral colpoperineopexy: a new approach for correction of posterior compartment defects and perineal descent associated with vaginal vault prolapse. Am J Obstet Gynecol 1997; 177:1345–1353.

Dean NM, Ellis G, Wilson PD, Herbison GP. Laparoscopic colposuspension for urinary incontinence in women. Cochran Database Syst Rev 2006; 19;3:CD002239.

DeLancey JO. The hidden epidemic of pelvic floor dysfunction: achievable goals for improved prevention and treatment. Am J Obstet Gynecol 2005; 192:1488–1495.

De Tayrac R, Sentilhes L. Complications of pelvic organ prolapse surgery and methods of prevention Int Urogynecol J 2013; 24:1859–1872.

Gadonneix P, Ercoli A, Salet-Lizée D, et al. Laparoscopic sacrocolpopexy with two separate meshes along the anterior and posterior vaginal walls for multicompartment pelvic organ prolapse. J Am Assoc Gynecol Laparosc 2004; 11:29–35.

Ganatra AM, Rozet F, Sanchez-Salas R, et al. The current status of laparoscopic sacrocolpopexy: a review. Eur Urol 2009; 55:1089–1103.

Higgs PJ, Chua HL, Smith A. Long term review of laparoscopic sacrocolpopexy. Br J Obstet Gynaecol 2005; 112:1134–1138.

Khan A, Alperin M, Wu N, et al. Comparative outcomes of open versus laparoscopic sacrocolpopexy among Medicare beneficiaries. Int Urogynecol J 2013; 24:1883–1891.

Maher CF, Feiner B, DeCuyper EM, et al. Laparoscopic sacral colpopexy versus total vaginal mesh for vaginal vault prolapse: a randomised trial. Am J Obstet Gynecol 2011; 204: 360.e1–7.

Maher C, Feiner B, Baessler K, Schmid C. Surgical management of pelvic organ prolapse in women. Cochrane Database Syst Rev 2013; 4:CD004014.

Nezhat CH, Nezhat F, Nezhat C. Laparoscopic sacral colpopexy for vaginal vault prolapse. Obstet Gynecol 1994; 84:885–888.

Nygaard I, Brubaker L, Zyczynski HM, et al. Long-term outcomes following abdominal sacrocolpopexy for pelvic organ prolapse. JAMA 2013; 309:2016–2024.

Paraiso MF, Walters MD, Rackley RR, et al. Laparoscopic and abdominal sacral colpopexies: a comparative cohort study. Am J Obstet Gynecol 2005; 192:1752–1758.

Ramanah R, Ballester M, Chereau E, et al. Anorectal symptoms before and after laparoscopic sacrocolpoperineopexy for pelvic organ prolapse. Int Urogynecol J 2012; 23(6):779–831.

Rivoire C, Botchorishvili R, Canis M, et al. Complete laparoscopic treatment of genital prolapse with meshes including vaginal promontofixation and anterior repair: a series of 138 patients. J Minim Invasive Gynecol 2007; 14(6):712–718.

Rozet F, Mandron E, Arroyo C, et al. Laparoscopic sacral colpopexy approach for genito- urinary prolapse : experience with 363 cases. Eur Urol 2005; 47:230–236.

Scali P, Blondon J, Bethoux A, Gérard M. Operations of support-suspension by upper route in the treatment of vaginal prolapse [Les opérations de soutènement-suspension par voie haute dans le traitement des prolapsus vaginaux]. Journal De Gynecologie, Obstetrique Et Biologie De La Reproduction 1974; 3:365–378.

Sergent F, Resch B, Loisel C, et al. Mid-term outcome of laparoscopic sacrocolpopexy with anterior and posterior polyester mesh for treatment of genitourinary prolapse. Eur J Obstet Gynecol Reprod Biol 2011; 156:217–222.

Slieker-Ten Hove MC, Pool-Goudzwaard AL, Eijkemans MJ, et al. Symptomatic pelvic organ prolapse and possible risk factors in a general population. Am J Obstet Gynecol 2009; 200:184.e1–184.e7.

Tan-Kim J, Menefee S, Luber KM, et al. Prevalence and risk factors for mesh erosion after laparoscopic-assisted sacrocolpopexy. Int Urogynecol J 2011; 22:205–212.

Wattiez A, Canis M, Mage G, Pouly JL, Bruhat MA. Promontofixation for the treatment of prolapse. Urol Clin North Am 2001; 28:151–157.

Wattiez A, Cohen SB, Selvaggi L. Laparoscopic hysterectomy. Curr Opin Obstet Gynecol 2002; 14(4):417–422.

Wattiez A, Mashiach R, Donoso M. Laparoscopic repair of vaginal vault prolapse. Curr Opin Obstet Gynecol 2003; 15:315–319.

Warner WB, Vora S, Hurtado EA, et al. Effect of operative technique on mesh exposure in laparoscopic sacrocolpopexy. Female Pelvic Med Reconstr Surg 2012; 18(2):113–117.

Withagen MI, Vierhout ME, Mannaerts GH, van der Weiden RM. Laparoscopic sacrocolpopexy with bone anchor fixation: short-term anatomic and functional results. Int Urogynecol J 2012; 23(4):481–486.

FURTHER READING

De Tayrac R, Letouzey V. Basic science and clinical aspects of mesh infection in pelvic floor reconstructive surgery. Int Urogynecol J. 2011;22:775–780.

Gigliobianco G, Roman Regueros S, Osman NI, et al. Biomaterials for pelvic floor reconstructive surgery: how can we do better? Biomed Res Int 2015; Article ID 968087.

Moen M. Randomized controlled trials in surgery: are we still missing something important? Int Urogynecol J. 2012;23:1321–1323.

Parkes IL, Shveiky M. Sacrocolpopexy for the treatment of vaginal apical prolapse: evidence based surgery. J Min Inv Gynecol. 2014; 21:546-557.

SET-UP AND INSTRUMENTATION

Operative set-up

Strategic operative set-up is pivotal for a successful case and should not be overlooked. The operative table should be evaluated to ensure adequate positioning capability in regard to table height, Trendelenburg, and removal of the footboard. A right-handed primary surgeon typically stands on the patient's left side. Video screens should be placed at or just below the level of the surgeon's eyes to prevent neck strain. If two video monitors are available, they should be placed just lateral to the patient's legs in line with the opposite-sided surgeon's line of vision (**Figure 17.1**). If a single video monitor is available, it should be placed centrally between the patient's legs. The surgeon should be ergonomically comfortable with shoulders relaxed and elbows slightly bent. Stepstools may be required to achieve this position.

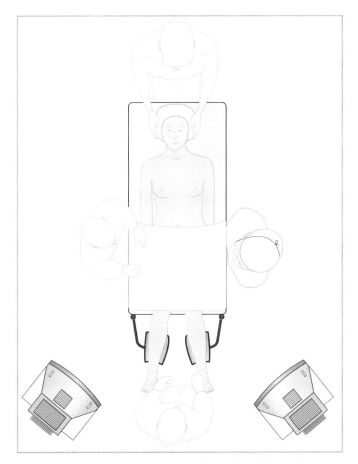

Figure 17.1 Strategic operative set-up should include careful attention to patient, surgeon, and equipment positioning.

Patient positioning and preparation

Meticulous patient preparation and positioning should routinely be performed to both decrease the incidence of postoperative neuropathy and to allow adequate access to the patient and surgical field. The patient should be placed on a foam pad to minimize slippage during steep Trendelenburg positioning. Sequential compression devices should be placed and activated upon initial entry into the operating room. Following induction of general anesthesia and successful intubation, an orogastric tube is inserted to allow for adequate decompression of gastric contents. This step is absolutely essential if a left upper quadrant abdominal entry is planned. The patient is then brought to the bottom of the table so her buttocks are at the table margin. This positioning allows adequate space to place the uterine manipulator.

The patient is then placed in the low dorsal lithotomy position, most commonly utilizing Allen stirrups. The two nerve bundles in the lower extremity at highest risk of injury during gynecologic surgery include the femoral nerve and the common peroneal nerve. Femoral nerve injuries are most commonly associated with incorrect lithotomy positioning. If the hip is placed in excessive flexion or the lower extremity is placed in excessive abduction and external rotation, the femoral nerve can be compressed. When placing the lower extremity in stirrups, it is pivotal to ensure proper hip flexion of no more than 80° as well as appropriate thigh abduction and rotation. Symptoms of femoral nerve injury include limited hip flexion or knee extension.

The common peroneal nerve is also at risk of a compression injury during lower extremity positioning, specifically at the level of the fibular head. This injury can be encountered if the knee and lower leg are positioned with excessive lateral pressure against the stirrup. External pressure can compress the common peroneal nerve between the stirrup and fibular head, causing lateral foot parasthesia and possible foot drop.

Bilateral tucking of the patient's arms in neutral position enhances patient safety in regard to nerve injury and allows the surgeon adequate space for ergonomic positioning. The two nerve bundles, mostly at risk during gynecologic surgery, include the brachial plexus and the ulnar nerve. The brachial plexus is at risk of injury with malpositioned shoulder braces that are placed too medial or lateral, or in extended arms placed on arm boards that are abducted >90° (Bradshaw & Advincula 2010, Dornette 1991, Winfree & Kline 2005). Symptoms of brachial plexus injury vary and can range from upper extremity tingling to paralysis with the characteristic wrist drop.

The ulnar nerve is also at risk of injury if care is not taken during upper extremity positioning. The ulnar nerve runs though the olecranon groove as it passes by the elbow, which places it at increased risk of a compression injury. When arms are tucked, they should be padded and placed in the anatomical to pronated position. This positioning rotates the olecranon process laterally to minimize pressure against the operating room table (Bradshaw & Advincula 2010). If the patient's arms are positioned on the arm board, they should be kept in the supine position to protect the ulnar nerve at the level of the cubital tunnel. Symptoms of an ulnar nerve injury include parasthesia of 4th and 5th digits and the lateral half of the 3rd digit. Motor defects may include the characteristic 'claw hand.'

Once the patient's upper and lower extremities are properly positioned, her abdomen, perineum, and vagina are sterilely prepped and draped. A Foley catheter is inserted into the bladder to deflate the bladder for safe suprapubic port entry and to allow for continuous monitoring of urine output during the case. Prophylactic antibiotics are administered prior to making the first skin incision.

◼ Instrumentation

It is imperative that all necessary equipment is assembled and evaluated prior to patient's transfer to the operating room. A preoperative checklist should include the verification of a functioning camera and light source, power sources for desired electrosurgery equipment, as well as an ample source for CO_2 gas insufflation. Both 5 mm and 10 mm 0° laparoscopes should be available. If a large uterus is present, 30° scopes can also be beneficial for visualization of difficult angles. Warming laparoscopes preoperatively in 120° sterile water can assist with fogging.

Basic laparoscopic equipment may include monopolar or bipolar electrosurgery instruments, atraumatic graspers, suction irrigator, needle graspers, and a uterine manipulator. Simplifying the equipment list can assist with room turnover and staff familiarity with the instruments (Einarsson & Suzuki 2009). Depending on the uterine and adnexal characteristics, ancillary equipment should also be accessible including a uterine morcellator, vaginal or rectal probes, cystoscopy, ureteral stents, and laparoscopic clip appliers.

◼ KEY STEPS OF THE PROCEDURE
◼ Uterine manipulation

Correct placement of the uterine manipulator is pivotal for proper uterine manipulation and appropriate colpotomy location. We use the Pelosi uterine manipulator (Cooper Surgical, Trumbull, CT) as it provides superior uterine manipulation and delineates distinct cervicovaginal margins; however, there are numerous options available. If a colpotomizer cup cannot fit into the vagina, a breisky vaginal retractor or bulb syringe can be used in replacement. In addition, the VCare Uterine Manipulator (ConMed Endosurgery or the RUMI system [Cooper Surgical]) can be used in women with a narrow introitus, as these models provide the option of a small colpotomy cup.

◼ Laparoscopic entry

The majority of laparoscopic complications occur during initial abdominal entry that is arguably the most dangerous step in minimally invasive surgery. It has been shown that 50% of trocar-related injuries to the bowel and vasculature occur with initial entry (Vilos et al. 2009). Opinion continues to be divided regarding the best and safest method of entering the abdomen. A recently updated Cochrane Review revealed a reduction in the incidence of failed entry, extraperitoneal insufflation, and omental injury with the use of an open-entry technique as compared to a closed-entry technique (Ahmed et al. 2012). No difference was found in the incidence of vascular injury or visceral injury between the two techniques. Ultimately, the choice of entry is commonly based on surgeon's preference, dependent on experience and comfort level.

Regardless of the desired method of entry, knowledge of the anterior abdominal wall entry is paramount for safe placement of laparoscopic trocars. The umbilicus is the most common location of entry for both open- and closed-entry techniques, as this is the thinnest portion of the anterior abdominal wall. The umbilicus is devoid of subcutaneous fat and represents the fusion of the three fascial layers including the external oblique, internal oblique, and transversalis. Caution must be exercised in thin patients, as the decreased body fat can bring the great vessels within centimeters of the umbilicus. In addition, the patient should be in supine position during initial entry, as premature Trendelenburg can angle the sacrum and great vessels anteriorly, and increase the risk of vascular injury.

Clinical scenarios that may preclude an umbilical entry include patients with a prior umbilical or ventral hernia repair with mesh, previous surgical procedures causing increased risk of severe adhesions, pregnancy, or a large pelvic mass suspicious of malignancy. In these cases, an alternate site for laparoscopic entry is in the left upper quadrant at Palmer's point. Palmer's point is located approximately 3 cm below the left costal margin in the midclavicular line. An orogastric tube is necessary, when using this technique, to assist in protecting the stomach. Additional underlying structures include the spleen, liver, pancreas, and transverse colon.

Once intraperitoneal access is confirmed, pneumoperitoneum of approximately 15 mmHg is obtained. Initially, the patient is kept in supine position and the area directly below the point of entry is examined in detail to ensure the underlying bowel, bladder, and vessels are intact. The patient is then placed in Trendelenburg position, and accessory ports are inserted under direct visualization. Lateral ports are placed lateral to the inferior epigastric vessels, and medial and superior to the anterior superior iliac spines. Cadaver studies have shown that the inferior epigastric vessels are most commonly 2.6–5.5 cm lateral to midline (Rahn et al. 2010). Skin incisions are made following Langer's lines, which can improve cosmesis. A suprapubic port should be placed above the upper margin of the bladder, located approximately one third of the distance between the pubic symphysis and umbilicus. A Foley should be placed prior to this trocar insertion, and can be backfilled if the bladder margin is difficult to identify.

◼ Round ligament transection

The round ligament is first identified and placed on upward traction, which allows visualization of the avascular portion of the broad ligament. To avoid bleeding, the round ligament should be transected through this clear window, which is most commonly found lateral to the varicose vessels in the broad ligament.

◼ Bladder flap development

Next, focus is placed on creation of the bladder flap. With the assistance of the uterine manipulator, the uterus is placed in the retroverted position and pushed toward the patient's head. The assistant can also apply gentle pressure on the uterine corpus to assist in visualization. An atraumatic grasper is used to skeletonize the anterior leaf of the broad ligament, which is placed on anterior traction to allow CO_2 gas to further dissect this space. The peritoneum is then incised, aiming toward the colpotomy cup, being cognizant to avoid any underlying vasculature. Once the cup is reached, the peritoneal incision is then curved upward, toward the opposite round ligament.

The bladder is then mobilized off of the lower uterine segment. This is accomplished by first placing the bladder on gentle anterior traction using an atraumatic grasper. Utilizing this countertraction, blunt and sharp dissection is performed, staying midline on the cup until endopelvic fascia is visualized. Once the correct vesicouterine plane is identified, it is used as a guide to mobilize the remaining portions of the bladder off of the cervicovaginal junction (**Figure 17.2**). Lateral dissection should be avoided during this step to minimize potential bleeding from the uterine vessels.

Securing the cornual pedicles

The optimal uterine position when securing the upper cornual pedicles is achieved by keeping the uterus in a midline, neutral position with upward traction toward the contralateral side. Whenever possible, a window is created in the avascular portion of the posterior leaf of the broad ligament below the vasculature of the upper pedicles and above the ureter. This technique is utilized whether a salpingo-oophorectomy is being performed or the ovary is conserved. The peritoneal window is then bluntly extended parallel to the cervix, which further skeletonizes the utero-ovarian ligament and infundibulopelvic ligament. This technique will assist in hemostasis when transecting the utero-ovarian ligaments and ensure that the ureter is not included within this pedicle. When transecting the Fallopian tube, the cornual region should be avoided to minimize bleeding. If the adnexa is enlarged, the utero-ovarian ligament can be transected despite an anticipated salpingo-oophorectomy to improve visualization when transecting the uterine vessels. The infundibulopelvic ligament is sealed and divided at the end of the case in these circumstances.

Uterine vessel skeletonization

When transecting the uterine vessels, it is pivotal to first dissect the posterior leaf of the broad ligament and skeletonize the vessels to ensure an adequate seal and minimize the risk of bladder or ureter injury. The uterus should first be placed in a semianteverted position with the round ligaments remaining at the 3 and 9 o'clock positions. This position allows adequate visualization of the posterior cul-de-sac and maintains orientation.

The posterior leaf of the broad ligament is first dissected to the uterosacral ligament, which should be at the level of the colpotomizer cup. This dissection isolates the uterine vessels at the level of the internal os, and further mobilizes the ureter away from the uterine pedicle.

The remaining areolar tissue that surround the uterine vessels should be further divided and retracted in a caudad direction.

Securing the uterine artery

Once the uterine vessels are adequately skeletonized, attention is next placed on uterine artery desiccation and division. Visualization and accessibility is optimized with the uterus maintained in an anatomical, semianteverted position. The assistant should also be instructed to apply firm upward (cephalad) traction to increase the distance between the ureter and uterine pedicle. Using a bipolar instrument or advanced vessel-sealing device, the uterine vessels are coagulated at the level of the internal os, being cognizant to exclude the posterior peritoneum. The instrument should be pressed firmly against the cervix to bounce off of the colpotomizer cup to ensure inclusion of the medial branches.

In patients with a large uterine pedicle, an atraumatic grasper is often used to compress the pedicle inferior to the level of the internal os, which allows the vessel-sealing device to include more of the pedicle (**Figure 17.3**). Coagulation should be limited to tissue superior and medial to the colpotomy cup to decrease the incidence of ureter involvement. Once transected, the uterine pedicle should then be mobilized inferior and lateral to the colpotomizer cup to ensure that the endopelvic fascia is clear of major vasculature.

Colpotomy

In a total laparoscopic hysterectomy, the cervix can be separated from the vagina using a variety of techniques including monopolar energy, bipolar energy, or with a cold knife. The colpotomy is commonly started posteriorly between the two uterosacral ligaments. The uterine position is continuously adjusted with the assistance of the manipulator to ensure adequate visualization of the cervicovaginal junction. Tissue tension provided by proper manipulation can ensure quick separation of the cervix from the vagina and minimize thermal damage to the vaginal cuff. When using monopolar energy, a pure cut current should be utilized to further minimize thermal spread and promote adequate blood supply for healing.

Once the cervix is amputated from the vagina, the specimen can be removed through the vagina. If the specimen is too large, it can be debulked with an electric morcellator, laparoscopically by hand with

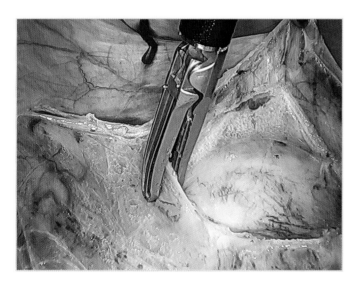

Figure 17.2 The bladder is held on gentle anterior traction allowing adequate mobilization off the lower uterine segment using blunt and sharp dissection.

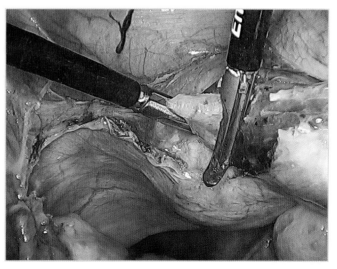

Figure 17.3 The left uterine pedicle is compressed inferiorly with an atraumatic grasper to allow a more complete pedicle at the internal os.

a 10-blade scalpel on a long knife handle, or vaginally until it has an appropriate size to be delivered through the vagina. If the uterus occludes the vagina during removal, it can be left in place to maintain pneumoperitoneum while suturing the vaginal cuff. Alternatively, a glove containing kerlix sponges is placed in the vagina to prohibit the escape of CO_2 gas.

While performing a supracervical hysterectomy, the uterus is amputated from the cervix at the level of the internal os. A reliable anatomic landmark is the uterine attachment of the uterosacral ligament. Uterine amputation can be performed with multiple modalities including a monopolar instrument, monopolar loop, or utilizing a cold knife. Typically, the uterine manipulator is removed once it is reached at the midline, and an instrument is placed in the posterior cul-de-sac to elevate the cervix away from the underlying bowel.

Vaginal cuff closure

Attention is next placed on suturing of the vaginal angles. A modified Richardson technique is employed using a monofilament delayed absorbable suture. This technique incorporates the uterosacral ligament and compresses the small vessels medial to the uterine pedicle to enhance hemostasis. This is secured using an extracorporeal knot tied to maintain elongated suture tails, which are then retracted out of the ipsilateral lower quadrant ports. These 'stay' sutures assist in elevating the vaginal cuff, and place it on tension, which assist in delineating the anatomy. The vaginal cuff is then closed in a transverse fashion, starting at the distal angle, being sure to include vaginal mucosa as well as pubocervical and rectovaginal fascia. Closure can be performed using an interrupted or 'figure-of-eight' sutures, a continuous running suture, or a barbed suture. Regardless of methods, sutures should be placed approximately 1 cm apart (**Figure 17.4**).

ALTERNATIVES: SURGICAL AND NONSURGICAL OPTIONS

In general, hysterectomy is offered to women who have failed or are at high risk of failure for more conservative options. The medical and surgical alternatives to laparoscopic hysterectomy vary on the basis of presenting pathology. The most common benign indications for

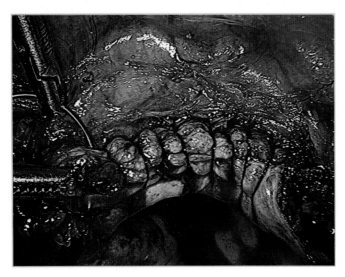

Figure 17.4 The vaginal cuff is closed in a transverse fashion.

laparoscopic hysterectomy include uterine leiomyomas, dysfunctional uterine bleeding, endometriosis, adenomyosis, pelvic organ prolapse, and chronic pelvic pain (Carlson et al. 1993). For an alternative option to be acceptable, it must offer comparable satisfaction rates, have decreased side effects and complication rates, and be cost-effective. The individual treatment goals and priorities of the patient should be included in the decision-making process.

Medical alternatives to hysterectomy

These include both hormonal and nonhormonal medications, and are often used as first-line therapy in women experiencing menorrhagia, dysfunctional uterine bleeding, and dysmenorrhea. The underlying pathology dictates the most effective option. In general, evidence-based reviews suggest that medical therapy typically provides only short-term relief, and subsequent surgical management is high (Marjoribanks et al. 2006).

Nonhormonal agents

In women with dysmenorrhea as the indication for hysterectomy, non-steroidal anti-inflammatory agents are effective at improving symptoms; however, there are no studies documenting improvement in women with dysmenorrhea caused by leiomyomas (American College of Obstetricians and Gynecologists 2008). When menorrhagia is the primary concern, tranexamic acid (TA) is a nonhormonal option that works locally on the endometrium to decrease menstrual blood loss. A systematic review was performed, which showed a menstrual blood loss reduction of 34–54% with the use of TA (Naoulou & Ming 2012). No significant difference was found in regard to the length of menses between TA and placebo. In addition, TA is recommended only during menstruation, which aids in compliance. The recommended dosage of TA varies; however, the US Food and Drug Association have approved TA to be prescribed as 1300 mg every 6 hours for 5 days during each menses (Barbieri 2010). In women with idiopathic or nonfunctional heavy vaginal bleeding, this may be a reasonable first-line therapy.

Hormonal medications

Contraceptive steroids have widely been used in the treatment of dysmenorrhea and menorrhagia, both in women with and without leiomyomas. These methods are often used as first-line therapy; however, these methods have been shown to offer minimal long-term relief, with surgical management ultimately performed (Marjoribanks et al. 2006). Agents including gonadotrophin-releasing hormone (GnRH) agonists, aromatase inhibitors, and progesterone modulators can be effective at reducing heavy vaginal bleeding, but their side effects limit the long-term use (Banu & Manyonda 2005). These agents may also be considered for preoperative use in an attempt to decrease the size of leiomyomas prior to hysterectomy or myomectomy, or to temporarily improve a patient's bleeding profile with the addition of ferrous sulfate.

The intrauterine levonorgestrel intrauterine system (LNG-IUS) is an additional surgical alternative that offers localized endometrial effects shown to be beneficial in the treatment of menorrhagia (Marjoribanks et al. 2006). It offers the advantage of a low-risk office procedure that is cost-effective in comparison to hysterectomies at 1 year (Hurskainen et al. 2001). A few studies have also shown an improvement in bleeding profiles when used in women with leiomyomas; however, these patients have an increased risk of LNG-IUS expulsion and continued vaginal spotting (American College of Obstetricians and Gynecologists 2008, Mercorio et al. 2003).

Ablation

Endometrial ablation may be considered in women who present primarily with abnormal uterine bleeding. This option offers women a shorter operating time, shorter hospital stay, quicker recovery, and fewer postoperative complications than a hysterectomy. However, sexually active women in their reproductive years must continue to use contraception, as pregnancy is contraindicated after this procedure. Women must also be counseled that they will likely experience variable amounts of continued vaginal bleeding after an endometrial ablation. Amenorrhea rates for ablation groups have shown to range between 13–64% as compared to 100% for hysterectomy groups (Dickersin et al. 2007). Despite these uterine bleeding trends, most women have a significant improvement in quality of life after ablation. However, it is important to discuss expectations for postoperative outcomes in detail during preoperative counseling to improve satisfaction.

In addition, women who present with dysmenorrhea and abnormal uterine bleeding are commonly poor candidates for this procedure, as pelvic pain frequently persists or increases after an ablation. Three studies have evaluated postoperative pain at 2–3 years after ablation versus hysterectomy, and have found improved pain in the hysterectomy group (5–19% vs. 24–64%); therefore, this patient population should be counseled with caution (Sculpher et al. 1996, Zupi et al. 2003).

Overall, the evidence has shown to be moderate that vaginal bleeding is better controlled with a hysterectomy versus an ablation (Matteson et al. 2012). Furthermore, women should be counseled that additional surgical intervention is often required. Matteson et al. found that at 1–4 years following ablation, 16–41% of women had undergone additional surgical intervention for vaginal bleeding, with 10–29% eventually being treated with hysterectomy.

Uterine artery embolization (UAE)

This, also known as uterine fibroid embolization, is a nonsurgical option for premenopausal women with bulk symptoms or menorrhagia secondary to leiomyomas. An interventional radiologist typically performs this procedure, in which bilateral uterine arteries are embolized using polyvinyl alcohol particles of trisacryl gelatin microspheres, causing uterine leiomyoma devascularization and involution. Relative contraindications for this procedure include pedunculated or submucosal fibroids, concurrent use of GnRH agonists, significant adenomyosis, and anticipated pregnancy. Once leiomyomas are diagnosed by ultrasound, an MRI should be performed to further characterize the leiomyomas and rule out additional pathology.

A systematic review was performed comparing short- and long-term outcomes of UAE versus surgery, which included hysterectomy or myomectomy (van der Kooij et al. 2010). A total of 4 randomized controlled trials were included with a total of 515 women. In regard to short-term results, a statistical significance was found with shorter length of hospital stay and quicker return to work in the UAE group; however, the majority of hysterectomies were performed by the abdominal approach. If UAE was compared strictly with a laparoscopic approach, the difference would likely be negligible. In the UAE in the treatment of symptomatic fibroid tumors randomized trial, the rates of major complications were similar, with 4.9% in the UAE group and 2.7% in the hysterectomy group (Hehenkamp et al. 2006). Minor complications including postprocedure vaginal discharge, hematoma, and vaginal leiomyoma expulsion have been found to be higher in the UAE group (58% vs. 40%; Hehenkamp et al. 2005).

Long-term outcomes have also been evaluated in multiple studies. At 2-year follow-up, the chance to avoid hysterectomy in patients who underwent UAE was found to be 76.5% (Hehenkamp et al. 2006), while menorrhagia and quality of life were improved in both the hysterectomy and UAE groups (Volkers et al. 2008). Furthermore, at 5-year follow-up, 28% of women in the UAE group required a hysterectomy, all secondary to continued menorrhagia (Hehenkamp et al. 2006). Overall, based on both short-term and long-term data, UAE has shown to be a safe and effective option for appropriate women who desire to avoid a hysterectomy.

Myomectomy

Women who desire uterine preservation and experience menorrhagia, dysmenorrhea, or pelvic bulk symptoms secondary to a leiomyomatous uterus may be a candidate for a myomectomy. Surgical approaches include abdominal, laparoscopic, or hysteroscopic depending on the location and size of the leiomyomas. Women who choose myomectomy risk the possibility of recurrence and possible additional surgical management. In addition, women are at risk of an unexpected hysterectomy secondary to intraoperative complications.

CONTRAINDICATIONS TO A MINIMALLY INVASIVE APPROACH

In the hands of a skilled laparoscopic surgeon, there are a few contraindications to a minimally invasive approach. The experience and skill level of the surgeon remain the primary limiting factor for successful laparoscopic hysterectomy. Medical conditions that preclude laparoscopy include severe cardiopulmonary conditions, which can inhibit adequate Trendelenburg positioning or sufficient pneumoperitoneum. In addition, laparoscopic hysterectomy should be performed with caution in women with suspicious uterine or ovarian masses that cannot be removed intact. When morcellation is contraindicated, specimen retrieval should be well planned with consideration for minilaparotomy versus abdominal approach if the specimen is too large to fit vaginally.

Practical tips

Variations in anatomy secondary to underlying pelvic pathology or previous abdominal surgeries can add an additional dimension of complexity to a laparoscopic hysterectomy. Understanding and mastering additional techniques for more challenging cases can assist in the success of a minimally invasive approach.

Alternative techniques for obtaining visualization

The surgeon should never compromise on exposure and should have a constant knowledge of surrounding structures in case bleeding is encountered. In cases with poor visualization, strategic sutures can be used to retract organs out of the surgical field. A redundant sigmoid colon can be mobilized by placing multiple large stitches using a monofilament suture through the epiploica. The long suture tails are then removed through the lateral port, and the trocar is removed and reinserted. This allows the sutures to lie on the outside of the trocar, avoiding the direct line of entry of instruments for the remainder of the case. The sutures are then clamped with a hemostat against the skin to maintain tension on the sigmoid.

The ovaries can be temporarily retracted in a similar fashion. A monofilament suture on a Keith needle is used to place a single stitch through the ovary. The suture tails can then be extracted in a similar fashion through the lateral port, or through an alternate site with the assistance of a Carter Thomason fascial closure device.

Alternative trocar placement

The umbilical port is routinely used as the optical port whenever feasible. In cases that involve a large fibroid uterus, which extends to the umbilicus or above, the placement of a subxiphoid port can assist with a more 'global' view and maintain midline orientation.

Alternative to uterine artery ligation

Access to the ascending branch of the uterine artery may be limited by underlying pathology including lower uterine segment or cervical fibroids as well as endometriosis. In these situations, it is recommended to enter the retroperitoneal space early and to secure the uterine arteries at their origin off the internal iliac artery. A thorough knowledge of the retroperitoneal space, including the gynecologic pararectal space and the paravesical space, is pivotal for successful execution.

The origin of the uterine artery is routinely located using one of two approaches. The first approach, which is often called the 'anterior approach,' utilizes the identification of the medial umbilical ligament as it courses from the anterior abdominal wall. Once the ligament is identified, it is placed on anterior tension and followed retrogradely to the origin of the uterine artery. The pararectal space is bluntly dissected proximal and medial to the uterine artery to further skeletonize this vessel and allow proper ligation.

The second approach, often called the 'lateral approach,' starts with entry into the retroperitoneum within the pelvic sidewall triangle at the level of the pelvic brim. The sidewall triangle is bordered by the external iliac artery laterally, the infundibulopelvic ligament medially, and the round ligament at its base. Once the peritoneum is incised, the ureter is first identified within the posterior leaf of the broad ligament. The internal iliac artery should be visualized lateral to the ureter, and can often be recognized by its pulsation. Blunt dissection parallel to these structures will develop the pararectal space, with the ureter comprising its medial border. As the surgeon continues to develop the pararectal space anteriorly, the uterine artery will be encountered as it crosses over the ureter. With either of these two approaches, the medial umbilical ligament can be used to mobilize the uterine artery further laterally, which creates additional space for safe ligation of the uterine artery without injury to the ureter (**Figure 17.5**).

Alternative technique for colpotomy

Enlarged, bulky uteri can impair visualization deep in the pelvis, leading to difficulty in creation of the standard colpotomy. In these situations, it is oftentimes helpful to first amputate the uterine corpus at the level of the internal os, similar to the technique in a supracervial hysterectomy. The assistant maximizes the distance between the cervix and underlying structures in the cul-de-sac by placing an instrument posterior to the cervix and elevating it anteriorly. Following

amputation, a standard colpotomy can be performed as described above to remove the cervix.

Alternative techniques for developing the bladder flap

Dense bladder adhesions secondary to prior cesarean sections can make the traditional approach to the development of the bladder flap unfeasible. In situations where bladder anatomy cannot be delineated, backfilling the bladder using irrigation fluid or CO_2 gas can be helpful. In regard to lysis of adhesions, it is helpful to remember that most hysterotomies performed during cesarean section are created at the midline in the lower uterine segment; therefore, adhesions are typically most dense in this area. Typically, decreased adhesions exist laterally and inferiorly to this location. Initiating bladder dissection laterally, between the ascending uterine arteries and bladder, can be helpful in identifying the endopelvic fascia overlying the colpotomizer cup. Once this endopelvic fascia is identified, the bladder is placed on anterior traction, and the uterine artery is skeletonized and ligated. After the uterine blood supply is controlled bilaterally, the plane identified between the endocervical fascia and bladder can be followed medially on the colpotomizer cup, below the level of dense adhesions.

CONCLUSION

Laparoscopic hysterectomy is a safe and effective procedure for women requiring a hysterectomy. Proper and meticulous preoperative set-up is pivotal for a successful case. A strategic and thoughtful approach can increase the efficiency and execution of a minimally invasive technique.

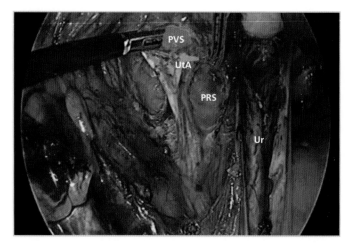

Figure 17.5 Development of the pararectal and paravesical spaces assists in identifying the uterine artery at its origin for ligation. PVS, Paravesical space; PRS, Pararectal space; UtA, Uterine artery; Ur, Ureter.

■ REFERENCES

Ahmed G, O'Flynn H, Duffy JM, Phillips K, Watson A. Laparoscopic entry techniques. Cochrane Database Syst Rev 2012: 15:CD006583.

American Congress of Obstetricians and Gynecologists. ACOG Practice Bulletin: Alternatives to hysterectomy in the management of leiomyomas. Obstet Gynecol 2008; 112:387–400. No 96.

Banu N, Manyonda I. Alternative medical and surgical options to hysterectomy. Best Pract Res Clin Obstet Gynaecol 2005; 19: 431–449.

Barbieri RL. A new (to the US) first-line agent for heavy menstrual bleeding (Editorial). OBG Manage 2010; 22:9–12.

Bradshaw A, Advincula A. Optimizing patient positioning and understanding radiofrequency energy in gynecologic surgery. Clin Obstet Gynecol 2010; 53:511–520.

Carlson K, Nichols D, Schiff I. Indications for Hysterectomy. N Engl J Med 1993; 328:856–860.

Dickersin K, Munro MG, Clark M, (Surgical Treatments Outcomes Project for Dysfunctional Uterine Bleeding (STOP-DUB) Research Group) et al. Hysterectomy compared with endometrial ablation for dysfunctional uterine bleeding: a randomized controlled trial. Obstet Gynecol 2007; 110:1279–1289.

Dornette WHL. Identifying, moving, and positioning the patient. In: Dornette WHL (ed). Legal Issues in anesthesia practice. Philadelphia, PA: FA Davis, 1991:113–124.

Einarsson J, Suzuki Y. Total laparoscopic hysterectomy: 10 steps toward a successful procedure. Rev Obstet Gynecol 2009; 2:57–64.

Hehenkamp WJ, Volkers NA, Birnie E, Reekers JA, Aukum WM. Pain and return to daily activities after uterine artery embolization and hysterectomy in the treatment of symptomatic fibroids: results from the randomized EMMY trial. Cardiovasc Intervent Radiol 2006; 29:179–187. (Level 1).

Hehenkamp WJ, Volkers NA, Donderwinkel PF, et al. Uterine artery embolization versus hysterectomy in the treatment of symptomatic uterine fibroids (EMMY trial): peri- and postprocedural results from a randomized controlled trial. Am J Obstet Gynecol 2005; 93:1618–1629 (Level 1).

Hurskainen R, Teperi J, Rissanen P, et al. Quality of life and cost effectiveness of leveonorgestrel releasing hormone intrauterine system versus hysterectomy for treatment of menorrhagia: a randomized trial. Lancet 2001; 35:273–277.

Marjoribanks J, Lethaby A, Farquhar C. Surgery versus medical therapy for heavy menstrual bleeding. Cochrane Database Syst Rev 2006, 2::CD-003855.

Matteson K, Abed H, Wheeler T, et al. A systematic review comparing hysterectomy with less invasive treatments for abnormal uterine bleeding. J Minim Invasive Gynecol 2012; 19:13–28.

Mercorio F, De Simone R, Di Spiezio Sardo A, et al. The effect of a levonorgestrel-releasing intrauterine device in the treatment of myoma-related menorrhagia. Contraception 2003; 67:277–280.

Naoulou B, Ming TC. Efficacy of tranexamic acid in the treatment of idiopathic and non-functional heavy vaginal bleeding: a systematic review. Acta Obstet Gynecol Scand 2012; 91:529–537.

Rahn DD, Phelan JN, Roshanravan SM, White AB, Corton MM. Anterior abdominal wall nerve and vessel anatomy: clinical implications for gynecologic surgery. Am J Obstet Gynecol 2010; 202:el–e5.

Sculpher MJ, Dwyer N, Byford S, Stirrat GM. Randomised trial comparing hysterectomy and transcervical endometrial resection: effect on health related quality of life and costs two years after surgery. Br J Obstet Gynaecol 1996; 103:142–149.

Van der Kooij S, Hehenkamp WJ, Volkers NA, et al. Uterine artery embolization versus hysterectomy in the treatment of symptomatic uterine fibroids: 5 year outcome in the EMMY trial. Am J Obstet Gynecol 2010; 203:e1–e13.

Vilos GA, Vilos AG, Abu-Rafea B, et al. Three simple steps during closed laparoscopic entry may minimize major injuries. Surg Endosc 2009; 23:758–764.

Volkers NA, Hehenkamp WJ, Birnie E, Aukum WM, Reekers JA. Uterine artery embolization versus hysterectomy in the treatment of symptomatic uterine fibroids: 2 years' outcome from the randomized clinical embolization versus hysterectomy (EMMY trial). Radiology 2008; 246:823–832.

Whiteman M, Hillis S, Jamieson D, et al. Inpatient hysterectomy surveillance in the United States 2000–2004, Am J Obstet Gynecol 2008; 198:34.e1–34.e7.

Winfree CJ, Kline DJ. Intraoperative positioning nerve injuries. Surg Neurol 2005; 63:5–18.

Zupi E, Zullo F, Marconi D, et al. Hysteroscopic endometrial resection versus laparoscopic supracervical hysterectomy for menorrhagia: a prospective randomized trial. Am J Obstet Gynecol 2003; 188:7–12.

Chapter 18 | Laparoscopic myomectomy

Matthew T Siedhoff

INTRODUCTION

As the most common pelvic tumor in women, leiomyomas represent a problem with significant economic and physical toil on reproductive-age women (Munro 2011, Spies et al. 2010, Wechter et al. 2011). Associated symptoms include heavy or, otherwise, abnormal uterine bleeding, resultant anemia, dysmenorrhea, subfertility, abdominal distension or 'bulk' symptoms, adjacent organ pressure, including ureteral or pelvic vessel compression in rare cases (Bonito et al. 2007, Lai et al. 2009, Nishikawa et al. 2000, Phupong et al. 2001). Although not all the cases will have symptoms, 70–80% of women will have sonographically identified fibroids by the age of 50 (Baird et al. 2003). Partly in response to changing patient's preferences regarding hysterectomy (Borah et al. 2013), a number of uterine-preserving procedures have been developed (Bergamini et al. 2005, Hald et al. 2004, Hindley et al. 2004, Liu et al. 2001, Ravina et al. 1995, Woods & Taylor 2013). Myomectomy represents the only one that is recommended in women wishing to become pregnant in the future (American College of Obstetricians and Gynecologists 2008) and the only one that actually extracts the tumor rather than simply shrinks it.

SET-UP AND INSTRUMENTATION

- Laparoscopy operating room
- Table capable of 30°–45° Trendelenburg
- Equipment to accommodate obese patients, e.g. sleds, antiskid pad, chest taping, and shoulder bolsters
- Energy device: monopolar hook electrode or ultrasonic scalpel
- Uterine manipulator
- Four to five trocars
- System for tissue extraction/morcellation, e.g. power morcellator, specimen retrieval bag, and ring self-retaining retractor
- Suture (delayed absorbable, standard, or barbed)
- Vessel ligation, e.g. laparoscopic vessel clip applier, polymer clip applier, and spring-loaded temporary vascular clamps
- Vasopressin
- Laparoscopic injection needle
- Laparoscopic tenaculum
- Laparoscopic corkscrew
- Adhesion barrier

KEY STEPS OF THE PROCEDURE

Set-up: patient positioning and placement of a uterine manipulator

The patient should be positioned in low dorsal lithotomy, as for any advanced pelvic laparoscopy. To prevent lower extremity neuropathy, the legs should be well secured without excess external or internal rotation at the hip, or without overflexion or extension (Irvin et al. 2004). A good rule of thumb is that ipsilateral ankle and hip joints should be aligned with the contralateral shoulder (**Figure 18.1**). The arms should be tucked at the side with the hand in military (thumb-up) position.

Especially in situations where brachial plexus injury is a greater risk, measures such as antiskid pads, shoulder taping, or bolstering should be employed (Shveik et al. 2010).

The bladder is drained with an indwelling Foley catheter and a uterine manipulator is placed (e.g. RUMI, Cooper Surgical, Trumbull, Connecticut; VCare, ConMed, Utica, New York). Besides allowing the movement of the uterus, including anteversion and retroversion for articulating manipulators, having a manipulator makes it very clear when the cavity is entered in removing fibroids with a submucosal component.

A randomized trial demonstrated 400 μg misoprostol placed rectally reduced the need for transfusion during myomectomy (Celik & Sapmaz 2003). Although the numbers were small and the trial involved laparotomies, given the low cost of the medicine and its safety profile, there seems a little downside to adding this measure.

Port placement

Usually, four ports are required for laparoscopic myomectomy. The midline port is typically a 10- or 12-mm one, as this is a common site for specimen retrieval, and the others are of 5 mm. Depending on the preference of the surgeon, a suprapubic 'diamond' configuration (**Figure 18.2a**) or an ipsilateral configuration (**Figure 18.2b** and **c**) can be used. Occasionally, for complex myomectomies, bilateral ipsilateral ports can be useful. This not only allows two-handed ipsilateral operating from both sides but also provides more viewing flexibility via 'port hopping' (**Figure 18.2d** and **e**). Even with large pathology, using an angled telescope (e.g. 30°) will permit the use of the umbilicus for the midline port, although in some cases, a subxiphoid midline port may be helpful to see the top of the uterus (**Figure 18.2f**).

Vessel ligation

If multiple or very large fibroids are to be removed, temporarily clamping the vascular pedicles can help reduce blood loss. From an

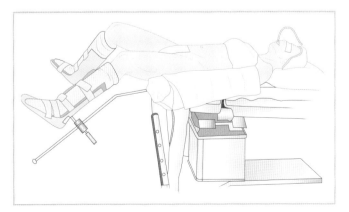

Figure 18.1 Low lithotomy position. The ipsilateral ankle and hip are aligned with the contralateral shoulder.

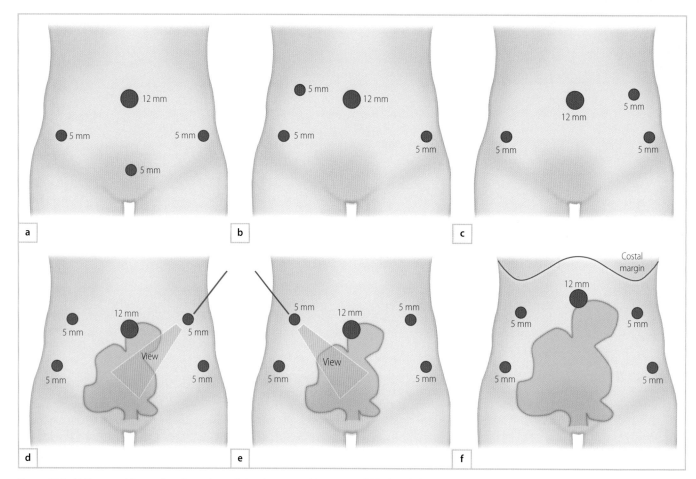

Figure 18.2 (a) Four-port 'diamond' configuration, utilizing the suprapubic position. (b) Right-sided ipsilateral configuration. (c) Left-sided ipsilateral configuration. (d) Bilateral ipsilateral port configuration, viewing from the left upper quadrant. (e) Bilateral ipsilateral port configuration, viewing from the right upper quadrant. (f) Subxiphoid midline port.

anterior or posterior approach, the broad ligament is opened, and the pararectal and paravesical spaces developed (**Figure 18.3a**). If the round ligament is divided to gain better access to the sidewall, it can easily be reapproximated at the end of the procedure with visceral peritoneal closure. The ureter is dissected out; the uterine artery is skeletonized at its origin; and the infundibulopelvic ligament is at the pelvic brim (**Figure 18.3b**). Endoscopic bulldog temporary spring-loaded vascular clamps (e.g. Aesculap, Tuttlingen, Germany) can then be placed across the pedicles Figure 18.3c. Permanent polymer clips are another option for uterine vessel ligation (e.g. Hem-o-lock, Teleflex Medical, Research Triangle Park, North Carolina). Although they can be removed, they are intended to be permanent and thus typically employed only when fertility is not an issue (**Figure 18.3d and e**). The final option for the uterine pedicle is a standard laparoscopic automatic metal hemoclip applier.

Vasopressin injection

This, or synthetic antidiuretic hormone, is a potent vasoconstrictor, and shown to be effective in several trials for reducing blood loss during myomectomy (Kongnyuy & Wiysonge 2011). A laparoscopic needle placed through a lateral port or a spinal needle placed directly through the skin (**Figure 18.4a**) can be used to inject the solution. Another option is to attach an 18-guage needle to sterile infusion tubing (usually standard equipment for the anesthesia team) and bring the needle through

a 10- or 12-mm port (**Figure 18.4b**). The flexible tubing allows the placement of the needle anywhere on the uterus, and the larger gauge (compared with a spinal needle) allows for more rapid injection with less resistance. The goal is to inject over the fibroid, just under the serosa, so that the solution spreads out over a large surface area. Sudden cardiac arrest has occurred with myometrial vasopressin injection (Hobo et al. 2009, Hung et al. 2006, Nezhat et al. 1994), so one must be careful about the concentration and total amount of drug injected (Frishman 2009). Suggested concentrations for laparoscopic myomectomy include 20 units diluted in 100, 200, or 300 mL normal saline. Since the half-life of vasopressin is 10–20 minutes, it is safe to reinject after an hour or so.

Hysterotomy

Some argue that a vertical hysterotomy is the most hemostatic approach since the uterine arteries provide branches from the lateral aspect and thus the center of the uterus should have smaller blood vessels to traverse (**Figure 18.5a**). Others flip this notion by arguing that a vertical incision may traverse multiple vessel branches while a transverse incision may only hit a few (**Figure 18.5b**). In reality, the blood supply over a fibroid is quite variable, and the incision that will allow most ready extraction of the fibroid and reapproximation of the myometrium is probably the best. Most do consider suturing a transverse incision is easier in laparoscopic surgery, however. Other considerations in choosing a hysterotomy include the ability to extract

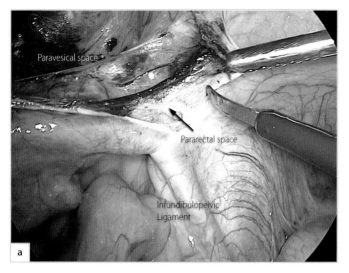

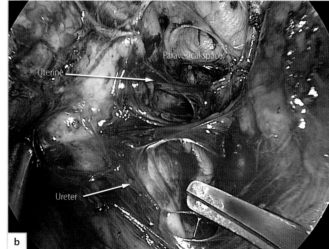

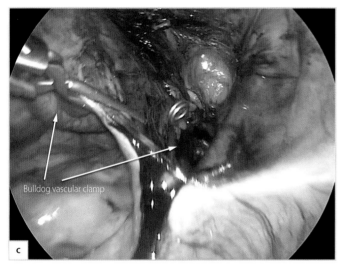

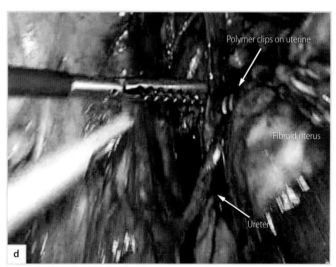

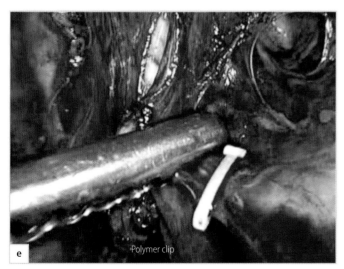

Figure 18.3 (a) Opening the pararectal and paravesical spaces. (b) Skeletonizing the uterine artery to its origin off the internal iliac artery. (c) Bulldog temporary vascular clamps placed on the uterine artery at its origin and the infundibulopelvic ligament at the pelvic brim. (d) Placing polymer clips on the uterine artery at its origin off the internal iliac. (e) Close-up view of the polymer clip.

several fibroids from the same incision and the location of the adnexae – one does not want to, of course, inadvertently injure the ovary or fallopian tube in removing a myoma.

A monopolar hook electrode (**Figure 18.6a**) or ultrasonic instrument (e.g. Harmonic, Ethicon Endo-Surgery, Cincinnati, Ohio; So-

nocision, Covidien, Mansfield, Massachusetts; **Figure 18.6b**) are the most common instruments used to make the incision. The former is readily available in most laparoscopic trays and is reusable; advanced energy devices create less plume and cause less tissue damage to the myometrium.

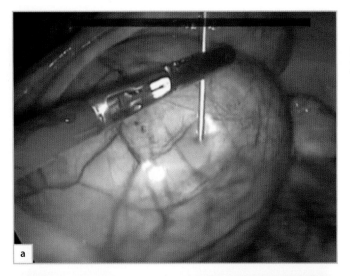

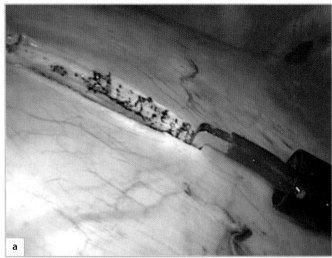

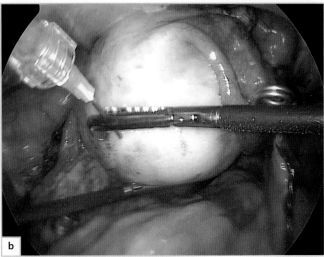

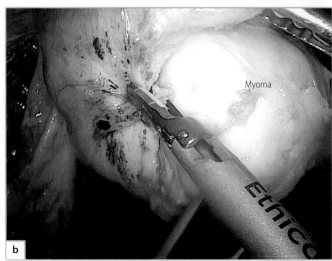

Figure 18.4 (a) Vasopressin injection via a spinal needle inserted directly through the abdomen. (b) Vasopressin injection using sterile infusion tubing connected to an 18-guage needle.

Figure 18.6 (a) Monopolar hook electrode. (b) Ultrasonic energy device.

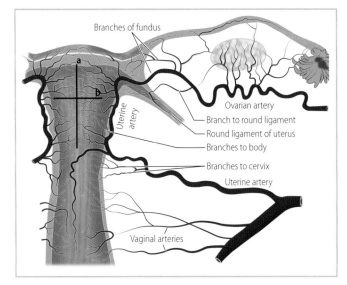

Figure 18.5 (a) Vertical hysterotomy. (b) Transverse hysterotomy.

▇ Tumor extraction

The myoma is grasped with a laparoscopic tenaculum (**Figure 18.7a**) or corkscrew (**Figure 18.7b**) and strong traction is applied. The operator incises myometrial fibers perpendicular to the fibroid and peels away the tissue from the tumor. Repeatedly, rolling the fibroid laterally and vertically allows for separation of the myometrium from all sides, like peeling an orange. For subserosal or pedunculated fibroids, simply incising the tissue below the fibroid is sufficient.

If multiple small fibroids are removed, they can be strung on a suture (known colloquially as creating a 'string of pearls') so that they are not lost in the abdomen during the rest of the procedure (**Figure 18.8a and b**).

▇ Hysterotomy closure

The hysterotomy is closed with delayed-absorbable suture. Traditionally, this was done with interrupted figure-of-eight sutures or using absorbable suture clips (e.g. Lapra-Ty Ethicon Endo-Surgery, Cincinnati, Ohio) throughout a running closure. Most laparoscopists now prefer using barbed suture (Alessandri et al. 2010, Ardovino et

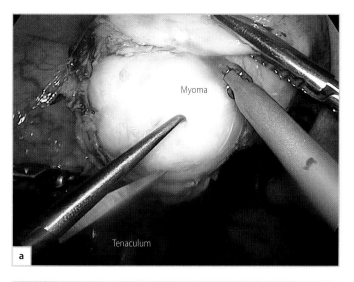

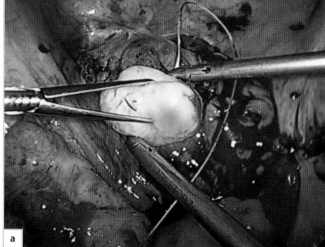

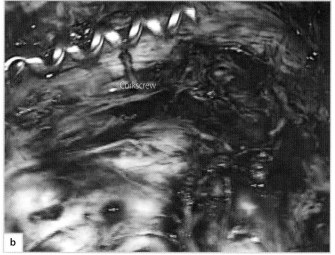

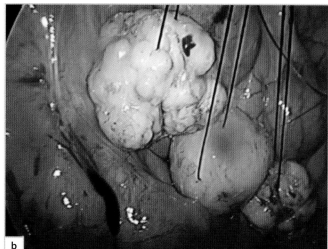

Figure 18.7 (a) Laparoscopic tenaculum. (b) Laparoscopic corkscrew.

Figure 18.8 (a) Placing a suture through a small myoma so it is not lost in the abdomen. (b) Multiple myomas tagged with suture.

al. 2013, Soto et al. 2014, Tulandi & Einarsson 2014; Stratafix, Ethicon, Somerville, NJ; V-Loc, Covidien, Mansfield, Massachusetts). Tiny barbs are cut into the suture so that it holds tightly with each pass; and tying knots are unnecessary, increasing the speed (and thus blood loss) of the closure (**Figure 18.9**). Barbed suture is particularly useful for suturing laparoscopically, where it can be difficult for the assistant to maintain tight countertraction on the suture during closure. The number of layers of suture needed depends on the depth of the defect. The final layer includes the serosa, which can be closed with a 'baseball stich' to present as a smooth surface to the peritoneal cavity as possible. Some place an adhesion barrier (Tinelli et al. 2011; e.g. Interceed, Ethicon, Somerville, New Jersey) over the hysterotomy once complete hemostasis is achieved.

Tissue extraction/morcellation

To remove the myomas in a minimally invasive fashion, morcellation is necessary. This can be done through a colpotomy or minilaparotomy (**Figure 18.10**). The minilaparotomy can be performed by extending the umbilical incision and placing a self-retaining ring retractor

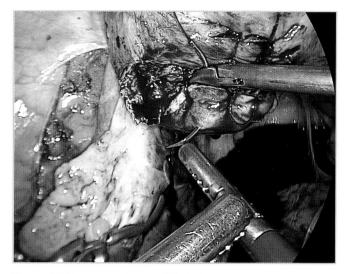

Figure 18.9 Hysterotomy closure with barbed suture.

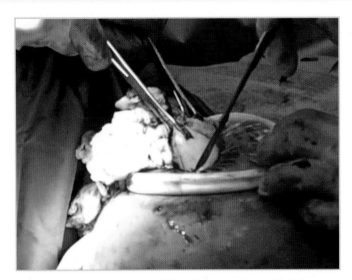

Figure 18.10 Morcellating by hand through a minilaparotomy incision and self-retaining ring retractor.

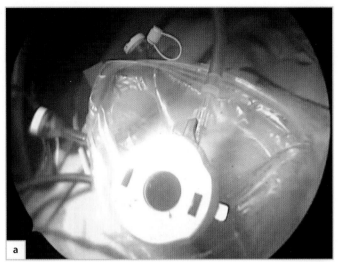

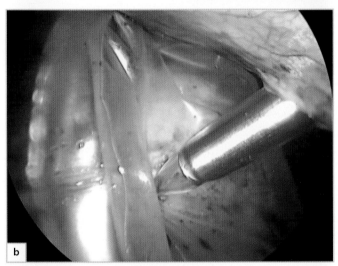

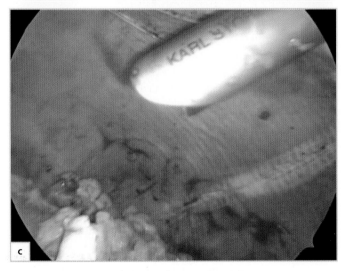

(e.g. Alexis Wound Protector/Retractor, Applied Medical, Rancho Santa Margarita, California). Morcellation is done more commonly using a power or electronic morcellator. These machines use a fast-rotating blade or a bipolar electrode through which tissue is pulled to cut the specimen into strips. Complications such as visceral organ or vessel injury can occur (Milad & Milad 2013), so great care must be taken when using a power morcellator. Because tissue can be spread throughout the peritoneal cavity and inadvertently left behind, causing iatrogenic leiomyomatosis or endometriosis (Kumar et al. 2008, Larrain et al. 2010, Leren et al. 2012, Schuster et al. 2012)or worsening the prognosis if the tumor is actually a sarcoma rather than a leiomyoma (Park et al. 2011), one can perform power morcellation in a specimen retrieval bag. With this technique, the myomas are placed in the bag and the edges of this bag are brought up through the skin of a 12–15-mm trocar site. The trocar is reinserted through the skin incision and into the bag's opening. The bag itself is then insufflated with carbon dioxide via the reinserted trocar (**Figure 18.11a**). A lateral port is then pushed through the side of the bag (penetrating it) and the insufflation tubing connected to this lateral port (**Figure 18.11b**). The larger port is replaced with the morcellator and the laparoscope through the lateral port. Viewing through the lateral port, the specimen is then morcellated, keeping any free tissue fragments contained in the bag (**Figure 18.11c**).

Procedural alternatives
Hysterectomy

For those who are not wishing uterine preservation, hysterectomy is, of course, the most straightforward and definitive treatment for fibroids. Nearly all hysterectomies can now be accomplished with minimally invasive techniques.

Hysteroscopic myomectomy

Submucosal fibroids should be removed hysteroscopically, if feasible. Larger type 1 and type 2 fibroids should be removed by those with extensive experience in operative hysteroscopy. If a submucosal fibroid is particularly large or if there is a very little myometrium surrounding it, a laparoscopic approach may be preferable.

Figure 18.11 (a) The ends of the bag are brought through the skin incision and the 12 mm trocar placed into the bag to insufflate it. (b) A lateral trocar penetrates the side of the bag. (c) The power morcellator is placed into the midline incision and the bag, and the specimen is morcellated within the specimen retrieval bag.

Uterine artery embolization

Uterine artery embolization (UAE) is a procedure performed by an interventional radiologist, where a catheter is threaded up through the femoral artery to the internal iliac artery and to branches of the uterine artery supplying fibroids (Ravina et al. 1995). Embolization material is injected through the catheter, which can reduce bulk, and to a greater extent, bleeding symptoms associated with fibroids.

Magnetic resonance-guided focus ultrasound surgery

This technique uses MRI in three dimensions and high-intensity ultrasound energy to heat and destroy tissue (Hindley et al. 2004). Successful treatment involves reduction of fibroid size and symptoms, but, unlike UAE, it is completely noninvasive.

Laparoscopic volumetric radiofrequency ablation

This involves destruction of myoma tissue via radiofrequency electrodes placed under laparoscopic visualization (Bergamini et al. 2005).

Laparoscopic uterine artery vessel occlusion

With this approach, the treatment principle is similar to UAE. However, the uterine arteries are approached surgically – they are laparoscopically skeletonized and occluded with permanent vessel occlusion clips (Hald et al. 2004, Liu et al. 2001).

Endometrial ablation

Nonresectoscopic global endometrial ablation devices destroy endometrial tissue via radiofrequency, circulating hot water, heated water within a balloon, freezing, or microwave energy (Woods & Taylor 2013) and can be used in the presence of submucosal myomas (Glasser & Zimmerman 2003). This technique is not appropriate for large uteri, will not treat bulk symptoms, and the presence of fibroids represents a risk factor for heavy menstrual bleeding treatment failure (Gemer et al. 2007).

■ CONTRAINDICATIONS TO A MINIMALLY INVASIVE APPROACH

The only absolute contraindications to using laparoscopy to perform myomectomy include those that preclude the use of gynecologic laparoscopy in general, such as baseline disease that prevents sufficient ventilation with insufflation or Trendelenburg position. Beyond that, it is a matter of the surgeon's skill and experience. Laparoscopic myomectomy can be safely performed for myoma weights >1000 g using blood-reduction measures described above. If myomas are to be removed through multiple hysterotomies, the surgeon should consider interval closure before all the tumors are extracted as considerable blood loss can occur if uterine incisions are left open during a long operation. MRI can be very useful for surgery planning and deciding whether a laparoscopic approach is feasible, as it outperforms other imaging modalities in terms of number, size, and location of fibroids (Dueholm et al. 2002). A single large fibroid is usually easier to treat with laparoscopic myomectomy than many small fibroids. In consideration of risks and benefits, the patient should be advised that because laparoscopy precludes direct palpation of the uterus, if many fibroids are present, it may not be possible to identify and remove all of them in laparoscopic myomectomy.

■ CONCLUSION

Laparoscopic myomectomy is a safe and effective alternative to hysterectomy for the treatment of symptomatic leiomyomas. Compared with a laparotomic approach, laparoscopic myomectomy is associated with better cosmesis, less blood loss, fever, postoperative pain, convalescence, wound infection, and adhesions, without reduction in reproductive outcomes (Palomba et al. 2007). Measures such as vessel occlusion, the use of vasopressin, ultrasonic energy devices, and barbed suture can produce a surgery that replicates open myomectomy but with minimally invasive benefits.

■ REFERENCES

Alessandri F, Remorgida V, Venturini PL, Ferrero S. Unidirectional barbed suture versus continuous suture with intracorporeal knots in laparoscopic myomectomy: a randomized study. J Minim Invasive Gynecol 2010; 17:725–729.

American College of Obstetricians and Gynecologists. ACOG practice bulletin. Alternatives to hysterectomy in the management of leiomyomas. Obstet Gynecol 2008; 112:387–400.

Ardovino M, Castaldi MA, Fraternali F, et al. Bidirectional barbed suture in laparoscopic myomectomy: clinical features. J Laparoendosc Adv Surg Tech A. 2013; 23:1006–1010.

Baird DD, Dunson DB, Hill MC, Cousins D, Schectman JM. High cumulative incidence of uterine leiomyoma in black and white women: ultrasound evidence. Am J Obstet Gynecol 2003; 188:100–107.

Bergamini V, Ghezzi F, Cromi A, et al. Laparoscopic radiofrequency thermal ablation: a new approach to symptomatic uterine myomas. Am J Obstet Gynecol 2005; 192:768–773.

Bonito M, Gulemi L, Basili R, Brunetti G, Roselli D. Thrombosis associated with a large uterine myoma: Case report. Clin Exp Obstet Gynecol 2007; 34:188–189.

Borah BJ, Nicholson WK, Bradley L, Stewart EA. The impact of uterine leiomyomas: a national survey of affected women. Am J Obstet Gynecol 2013; 209:319.e1–319.e20.

Celik H, Sapmaz E. Use of a single preoperative dose of misoprostol is efficacious for patients who undergo abdominal myomectomy. Fertil Steril 2003; 79:1207–1210.

Dueholm M, Lundorf E, Sorensen JS, et al. Reproducibility of evaluation of the uterus by transvaginal sonography, hysterosonographic examination, hysteroscopy and magnetic resonance imaging. Hum Reprod 2002; 17:195–200.

Frishman G. Vasopressin: If some is good, is more better? Obstet Gynecol 2009; 113:476–477.

Gemer O, Kruchkovich J, Huerta M, et al. Perioperative predictors of successful hysteroscopic endometrial ablation. Gynecol Obstet Invest 2007; 63:205–208.

Glasser MH, Zimmerman JD. The HydroThermAblator system for management of menorrhagia in women with submucous myomas: 12- to 20-month follow-up. J Am Assoc Gynecol Laparosc 2003; 10:521–527.

Hald K, Langebrekke A, Klow NE, et al. Laparoscopic occlusion of uterine vessels for the treatment of symptomatic fibroids: Initial experience and comparison to uterine artery embolization. Am J Obstet Gynecol 2004; 190:37–43.

Hindley J, Gedroyc WM, Regan L, et al. MRI guidance of focused ultrasound therapy of uterine fibroids: Early results. AJR Am J Roentgenol 2004; 183:1713–1719.

Hobo R, Netsu S, Koyasu Y, Tsutsumi O. Bradycardia and cardiac arrest caused by intramyometrial injection of vasopressin during a laparoscopically assisted myomectomy. Obstet Gynecol 2009; 113:484–486.

Hung MH, Wang YM, Chia YY, Chou YM, Liu K. Intramyometrial injection of vasopressin causes bradycardia and cardiac arrest—report of two cases. Acta Anaesthesiol Taiwan 2006; 44:243–247.

Irvin W, Andersen W, Taylor P, Rice L. Minimizing the risk of neurologic injury in gynecologic surgery. Obstet Gynecol 2004; 103:374–382.

Kongnyuy EJ, Wiysonge CS. Interventions to reduce haemorrhage during myomectomy for fibroids. Cochrane Database Syst Rev 2011; (11):CD005355.

Kumar S, Sharma JB, Verma D, et al. Disseminated peritoneal leiomyomatosis: an unusual complication of laparoscopic myomectomy. Arch Gynecol Obstet. 2008; 278:93–95.

Lai CC, Chang CK, Wang JY. Hypertension secondary to bilateral hydronephrosis caused by a large uterine myoma. Am J Kidney Dis 2009; 54:1187.

Larrain D, Rabischong B, Khoo CK, et al. "Iatrogenic" parasitic myomas: unusual late complication of laparoscopic morcellation procedures. J Minim Invasive Gynecol 2010; 17:719–724.

Leren V, Langebrekke A, Qvigstad E. Parasitic leiomyomas after laparoscopic surgery with morcellation. Acta Obstet Gynecol Scand 2012; 91:1233–1236.

Liu WM, Ng HT, Wu YC, Yen YK, Yuan CC. Laparoscopic bipolar coagulation of uterine vessels: a new method for treating symptomatic fibroids. Fertil Steril 2001; 75:417–422.

Milad MP, Milad EA. Laparoscopic morcellator-related complications. J Minim Invasive Gynecol 2014; 21:486-491.

Munro MG. Uterine leiomyomas, current concepts: pathogenesis, impact on reproductive health, and medical, procedural, and surgical management. Obstet Gynecol Clin North Am 2011; 38:703–731.

Nezhat F, Admon D, Nezhat CH, Dicorpo JE, Nezhat C. Life-threatening hypotension after vasopressin injection during operative laparoscopy, followed by uneventful repeat laparoscopy. J Am Assoc Gynecol Laparosc 1994; 2:83–86.

Nishikawa H, Ideishi M, Nishimura T, et al. Deep venous thrombosis and pulmonary thromboembolism associated with a huge uterine myoma—a case report. Angiology 2000; 51:161–166.

Palomba S, Zupi E, Falbo A, et al. A multicenter randomized, controlled study comparing laparoscopic versus minilaparotomic myomectomy: reproductive outcomes. Fertil Steril 2007; 88:933–941.

Park JY, Park SK, Kim DY, et al. The impact of tumor morcellation during surgery on the prognosis of patients with apparently early uterine leiomyosarcoma. Gynecol Oncol 2011; 122:255–259.

Phupong V, Tresukosol D, Taneepanichskul S, Boonkasemsanti W. Unilateral deep vein thrombosis associated with a large myoma uteri. A case report. J Reprod Med 2001; 46:618–620.

Ravina JH, Herbreteau D, Ciraru-Vigneron N, et al. Arterial embolisation to treat uterine myomata. Lancet 1995; 346:671–672.

Schuster MW, Wheeler TL 2nd, Richter HE. Endometriosis after laparoscopic supracervical hysterectomy with uterine morcellation: a case control study. J Minim Invasive Gynecol 2012; 19:183–187.

Shveiky D, Aseff JN, Iglesia CB. Brachial plexus injury after laparoscopic and robotic surgery. J Minim Invasive Gynecol 2010; 17:414–420.

Soto E, Flyckt R, Falcone T. Minimally invasive myomectomy using unidirectional knotless barbed suture. J Minim Invasive Gynecol 2014; 21:27.

Spies JB, Bradley LD, Guido R, et al. Outcomes from leiomyoma therapies: comparison with normal controls. Obstet Gynecol 2010; 116:641–652.

Tinelli A, Malvasi A, Guido M, et al. Adhesion formation after intracapsular myomectomy with or without adhesion barrier. Fertil Steril 2011; 95:1780–1785.

Tulandi T, Einarsson JI. The use of barbed suture for laparoscopic hysterectomy and myomectomy: a systematic review and meta-analysis. J Minim Invasive Gynecol 2014; 21:210–216.

Wechter ME, Stewart EA, Myers ER, Kho RM, Wu JM. Leiomyoma-related hospitalization and surgery: prevalence and predicted growth based on population trends. Am J Obstet Gynecol 2011; 205:492.e1–492.e5.

Woods S, Taylor B. Global ablation techniques. Obstet Gynecol Clin North Am 2013; 40:687–695.

Chapter 19 | Ectopic pregnancy

Jean Luc Pouly, Benoit Rabischong, Demetrio Larrain, Marianne de Bennetot, Michel Canis, Hubert Manhes

The laparoscopic treatment of ectopic pregnancy (EP) was the first treatment used and defined within this field. It was this technique that demonstrated the feasibility of operative procedures by laparoscopy and opened the door to all other fields of surgery. It should also be noted that this method was devised and used before the era of video, which then led to the rapid expansion of endoscopic surgery.

HISTORY

In 1973, Manhès noted a publication by Shapiro relating to the coagulation of an isthmic pregnancy during laparoscopy. We must remember that, at this time, the suspicion of EP led to a laparoscopy to confirm the diagnosis and then to a laparotomy. In 1975, Manhès had the idea of incising the hematosalpinx, as during laparotomy, and then aspirating the contents of the tube (Bruhat & Manhes 1977). The first surgical interventions were performed using the equipment available at that time: a monopolar electrode for ovarian drilling and a Karman aspiration cannula passed through the abdominal wall.

Between 1975 and 1982, Manhès, Bruhat, and their staff refined the technique until they had treated more than 100 cases (Bruhat et al. 1980). The two major difficulties were gradually resolved: hemostasis was ensured through chemical hemostasis or compression, and non-closure of the tube turned out to be judicious since second-look laparoscopies and control hystero-salpingographies showed spontaneous healing and good tubal permeability. At the same time, other technical aspects were improved, and specifically adapted equipment was designed (Manhes et al. 1983). Although a 16 mm movie demonstrating the laparoscopic procedure was presented in 1979, it was the advent of video in 1983 that allowed this technique to emerge into the limelight and become widespread. In 1986, it became the gold standard procedure to treat tubal pregnancies (Pouly et al. 1986).

During the same period, in 1986, Dubuisson carried out salpingectomy by laparoscopy (Dubuisson et al. 1987). In 1987, the medical treatment of ectopic pregnancy was developed with in situ injection of methotrexate (MTX) by Feichtinger, followed by intramuscular use by Stovall in 1989 (Stovall et al. 1991).

OPERATIVE TECHNIQUES
Conservative treatment

This has not changed much since 1985. In addition to the conventional laparoscopic equipment, a fine monopolar electrode, a 10 mm diameter suction probe, and a set of atraumatic laparoscopic forceps must be available.

The steps of the procedures are detailed in the following sections.

Inspection and aspiration of the hemoperitoneum

The Trendelenburg position and uterine cannulation are used systematically. Evacuation of the hemoperitoneum is achieved by inserting a 10 mm suction device on the midline in the suprapubic position. Washing of the peritoneal cavity is carried out in order to operate under the best possible conditions. Evaluation of the status of the pregnant tube and also the contralateral tube is the first step when deciding whether the treatment can be conservative or not. We will return to this point later.

Salpingotomy

The salpingotomy can be performed with the fine monopolar electrode using the pure cut mode. The electrode must not be pressed on the tube, but just touched gently to improve the current density. This increases the cutting effect and decreases collateral coagulation. Bipolar coagulation should not be used for this step. The incision should be sagittal on the anti-mesenteric side of the tube and on the most internal part of the hematosalpinx, where the trophoblastic tissue is located. The outer part tends to contain clots. The incision should be 15 mm long, which is sufficient to allow introduction of a 10 mm aspiration tube but not too large to cause problems with healing.

Despite some successful reports, 'milking' of the tube must be avoided in all cases where a hematosalpinx is found. In our first publications (Bruhat et al. 1980), we cautioned that 'milking' was complicated by persistent trophoblastic tissue in 25% of the cases versus 5% when a salpingotomy was performed. Thirty years later, this remains true and partially explains the high failure rate in some reports.

Tubal aspiration

Often, a few seconds after the tube is cut, the pregnancy begins to emerge naturally out of the tube. The suction cannula allows the hematosalpinx to be aspirated. Then the cannula is inserted into the Fallopian tube. Successive injection and suction operations are made. If a narrow device is used, there can be a risk of only partial removal of the trophoblastic tissue. This is one of the main causes of failure, and to avoid this risk we developed a special device (Triton).

Verification of tubal emptiness

The edges of the tubal incision are grasped using forceps. The tube must be washed and checked thoroughly to ensure complete removal of the trophoblastic tissue, which appears as a white mass.

Hemostasis

In 1981, the Manhès and Bruhat team came up with the idea of injecting a vasoconstrictor in the mesosalpinx before performing the salpingotomy. They used ornithine vasopressin (Por8). Under these conditions, treatment was achieved without significant bleeding. No secondary hemorrhage was reported (Manhes et al. 1983). Nevertheless Por8 can induce serious cardiac risks in the case of intravascular passage, and the product was banned in France in 1986. It remains in use in other countries, including the United States. Other products that have been tested since then are not very efficient, or present higher risks.

Bleeding in the case of EP comes from the tubal incision or the implantation area of the EP. The first measure is to wait because, in the vast majority of cases, the bleeding will stop by itself after a few minutes. Significant bleeding from the edges of the salpingotomy can be treated by bipolar coagulation using a thin bipolar forceps in order to minimize the number of coagulations and consequent destruction of the tube. Diffuse bleeding in the implantation area can be treated by clamping the mesosalpinx. A long forceps is installed along the tube. It must be left in place for at least 10 minutes to be effective. Ultimately, at the end of the intervention residual seepage should be tolerated, as aggressive coagulations can destroy the Fallopian tube.

Tubal closure

This is unnecessary. At the beginning of our experience, it was not done simply because we were unable to suture during laparoscopy. Later, successive experimental and epidemiological works by Tulandi et al. (1991) demonstrated that the absence of suture leads to minimal obstructions, less damage to tubal folds, and, finally, a faster return of fertility. The rare cases of tubal fistulae are due to excessively extensive coagulations but do not seem to impair fertility.

Peritoneal washing

At the end of the intervention, the peritoneal cavity must be washed and aspirated with the patient placed in an anti-Trendelenburg position to retrieve blood and the washing liquid that has accumulated in the upper part of the abdomen. The use of anti-adhesion products such as icodextrin does not seem necessary in this type of surgery.

Postoperative check-up

The patient can be discharged on the same day if there is little hemoperitoneum; otherwise, the next day. It is mandatory to monitor the relative decrease in human chorionic gonadotropin (hCG) levels according to the diagram shown in **Figure 19.1**. If the fall is insufficient after 48 hours (>40%), complementary treatment with MTX IM is required. In case of a major fall (<10%) subsequent monitoring is not necessary or can be checked at 10 days. For intermediate rates, an hCG assay is required every 2 days (Pouly et al. 1992).

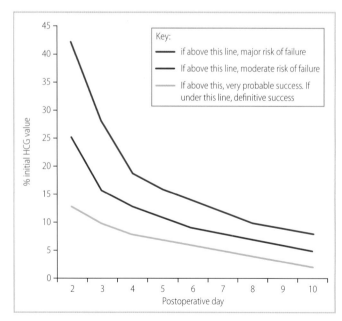

Figure 19.1 Management of the postoperative human chorionic gonadotropin drop. With permission from Pouly et al. (1992).

Salpingectomy

Laparoscopic salpingectomy is performed as a primary procedure or secondarily to a conservative treatment complicated by persistent bleeding. In the initial report, thermocoagulation was used. It has since been replaced by bipolar coagulation.

The salpingectomy can be achieved through the anterograde or retrograde route. The retrograde procedure includes the following steps: the tubal isthmus is coagulated with bipolar cautery and sectioned with scissors. The section is continued in the direction of the infundibulopelvic pedicle, remaining close to the tube and using the same method. Finally, the tubal branch of the infundibulopelvic pedicle is coagulated close to the tube. This technique avoids impairing ovarian vascularization.

The Fallopian tube is then placed in an Endobag and extracted from the abdomen. Peritoneal lavage is carried out in the same way as conservative treatment. The postoperative check-up is limited to an hCG assay 1 week after the intervention. The residual rate must be <2%.

Special situations
Fimbrial pregnancy

For conservative treatment, the 'milking' technique with tubal expression caused by pushing the trophoblastic tissue through the fimbria must be abandoned except in the rare case of fimbrial pregnancy or tuboabdominal abortion and under the absolute condition that there is no hematosalpinx.

Interstitial pregnancies

In the case of ultrasound diagnosis, treatment with MTX IM coupled with ultrasound-guided injection of KCl if there is cardiac activity is one option. If an interstitial pregnancy is found during laparoscopy, surgical treatment can be difficult, with potential bleeding risk during incision of the tube. Coagulation may be ineffective to achieve hemostasis. The only way to solve this problem is to use sutures to take up the entire uterine angle. This requires perfect mastery of the technique of laparoscopic suturing. In cases of rupture and acute bleeding, the situation is the same.

Cervical pregnancies

The basis of treatment is MTX IM. This is preceded by uterine embolization for large-volume cervical pregnancies.

Cesarean section scar pregnancies

These cases can be managed conservatively (i.e. using MTX or embolization). However, successful management has been reported using laparoscopic excision and lower uterine segment reconstruction (Fuchs et al. 2015).

Medical treatment

Medical treatment has become very important in the treatment of EP. It can be used in up to 45% of cases (Rabischong et al. 2011). It involves the intramuscular injection of MTX. The dose is 1 mg/kg limited to 70 mg. Only one injection is made. Repeated injections are used by some authors to improve the effectiveness of the treatment, but this is controversial. In a meta-analysis including 1,327 patients, the overall success rate for MTX treatment was 89%. Success rates for multiple-dose and single-dose protocols were 92.7% and 88.1%, respectively [OR 4.74; 95% CI (1.77,12.62)] (Barnhart et al. 2003). However, single-dose treatment was associated with fewer side effects. Conversely, further studies comparing both regimens found no significant difference (Alleyassin et al. 2006, Mol et al. 2008).

In our opinion, the small difference found in the meta-analysis cannot justify the option of multiple- dose treatment due to the potential severe side effects that can occur with a high dose of MTX. Prior to the injection, a thorough patient history must be taken to rule out hematological, renal, or hepatic disorders.

TREATMENT FAILURES

This is always caused by the persistence of active trophoblastic tissue in the tube after conservative treatment (or in the peritoneum after salpingectomy). But the precise situation depends on the type of initial treatment and to the type of second-line treatment.

For conservative treatment, failure is defined as complete if a second laparoscopy is necessary, and as relative if there is injection of MTX. The same definitions apply for radical treatment by salpingectomy.

For treatment with MTX, the definitions for failures are the same, but it should be noted that second MTX treatment criteria are subjective in view of the very slow fall rates of hCG and frequent pain after the injection (Gabbur et al. 2006).

For conservative laparoscopic treatment, the rate of failure ranges from 5% to 20%, according to one series, which is surprising (Rabischong et al. 2010). This difference is due to four elements, three of which concern the operative procedure:
- 'Milking' should be discouraged.
- The use of an excessively small-diameter suction cannula (5 mm) is a major factor in failures.
- The tubal incision must not be made in the outer part of the hematosalpinx.

The fourth element is the 'activity' of the pregnancy. It has been shown that an active (and/or well- implanted) pregnancy increases the risk of failure. In a recent study, we analyzed the factors predicting failure in 1306 patients with a failure rate of 6.6%. The only data that appeared to have any predictive value were the hCG levels. The OR of failure for this factor was 1.8 [95% CI (1.1,2.8)] for patients with an hCG assay of >1960 UI versus those with less. But, in practice, the difference was low with respective failures of 8.6% and 5.1%, and even in our opinion this cutoff has a poor value (Rabischong et al. 2010).

Many authors consider that the cutoff is much higher and that hCG is not the only criteria. For Hagström, an hCG level >5000 IU/mL associated with a progesterone level higher than 10 ng/mL is an important failure factor (Hagström et al. 1994). The situation is similar in the case of EP with fetal cardiac activity. In these cases, the question arises as to whether salpingectomy should be performed directly or conservative treatment attempted, followed immediately by IM MTX treatment.

The latter solution was proposed in systematic fashion by some authors. Thus, for Grazcykowski (1997), it allows the likelihood of a second laparoscopy to be reduced from 14% to 2%. However, it seems more important to correct the surgical technique to again achieve a 5% rate of relative failures that justify MTX injection rather than to use MTX systematically because this treatment induces serious complications. Treatment with salpingectomy is followed by very rare failures (2%) (Mol et al. 2014). They consist of secondary implantation of trophoblastic tissue in the peritoneal cavity.

For purely medical treatments, the definition of failure is always uncertain, even in cases of secondary laparoscopy. The decision for secondary laparoscopy or a second injection of MTX is often founded on subjective data that make comparison hazardous (Dudley et al. 2004). Elsewhere in our experience, extension of indications was accompanied by a decrease in the failure rate, which is quite illogical (Rabischong et al. 2011). But in any series, the rate of relative failures ranges from 15% to 40%, and the rate of complete failure requiring a laparoscopy from 10% to 30%. Nevertheless, the main factor for failure of MTX is again the activity of the EP as defined by hCG levels. Many publications are interested in this issue and have tried to fix a cutoff level (Rabischong et al. 2011). The most optimistic allow up to 5000 IU/mL (Menon et al. 2007); the most pessimistic reserve this treatment for levels below 1000 (Nazac et al. 2003, Nowak-Markwitz et al. 2009, Potter et al. 2003). For our part, we consider that treatment can be routinely used for rates <1300 IU/mL (Rabischong et al. 2011).

In a large-scale study, we checked the predictive factors of failure of a single-dose MTX treatment in 419 cases with an overall failure rate of 24.5% (a second MTX injection or a laparoscopy required). With more than 20 patterns taken into account, we found only a minor difference for those patients who had previously used contraceptive pills and a major difference according to the hCG level [OR for failures = 3.6 (95% CI (2.1,5.9)] for patients with an hCG level of more than 1300 versus an hCG level of <1300.

Fernandez has even proposed a predictive score for the efficacy of MTX, including other data such as progesterone level, but it is rarely used (Fernandez et al. 1991).

Fertility

EP should be considered as a form of tubal infertility. Overall, only 65–70% of patients wishing to be pregnant after a first EP will subsequently have a child (Graczykowski & Mishell 1997, Hagström et al. 1994, Rabischong et al. 2010). A new EP will occur for 15–20%, and 15–20% will remain infertile. When the number of EP rises, the likelihood of having a child afterward dramatically decreases to 30–40% after two ectopic pregnancies and to less than 15% after three. At the same time, the risk of recurrence increases (Bouyer et al. 2000, 2003, Pouly et al. 1991).

The same applies when there are multiple factors in the history (infertility, salpingitis, tubal plasty, etc.) (Thorburn et al. 1988). We have even recommended in cases of multiple histories to prefer a bilateral salpingectomy rather than to risk a recurrence since the chances of natural procreation are extremely low (Pouly et al. 1991).

In a recent study again based on a large cohort, we demonstrated this strong effect of the history (Dubuisson et al. 1996). In cases of previous infertility, the OR for conception is reduced to 0.51 [95% CI (0.40,0.64)]; in cases of tubal disease, the OR is 0.62 [95% CI (0.50,0.67)]; and after the age of 35, this OR is 0.5 [95% CI (0.37,0.67)].

Therefore, the choice of technique is important in order to optimize the probability of conception and to reduce the risk of recurrence. This topic has led to many cohort studies or comparative studies to clarify this choice. The purpose of this chapter is not to be exhaustive on this subject but simply to outline the main recent issues.

Conservative treatment versus salpingectomy

Conservative treatment results in better fertility than does salpingectomy, of the order of 10%. In a large cohort study, we found that the crude OR for conception was 0.784 [95% CI (0.66,0.931)] in patients treated by salpingectomy versus those treated conservatively. But the adjusted OR was 0.87 [95% CI (0.73,1.04)], thus demonstrating a strong tendency but not a definitively proved difference (that would require 5000 patients to be randomized in order to obtain a clear answer (de Bennetot et al. 2012). Some authors have proposed this treatment as a first-line method (Dubuisson et al. 1996). In the prospective DEMETER study (Fernandez et al. 2013), the cumulative fertility curves were not significantly different between conservative and radical surgery. OR was 1.06 (0.69–1.63) and $P = 0.78$. The 2-year rates of intrauterine pregnancy were 70% after conservative surgery and 64% after radical surgery.

In the prospective ESEP study (Mol et al. 2014), the cumulative ongoing pregnancy rate was 60.7% after salpingotomy and 56.2% after salpingectomy [fecundity rate ratio 1.06, 95% CI (0.81,1.38); $P = 0.678$].

However, in our study (Rabischong et al. 2010), this difference is significant among patients at risk (age >35 years; history of infertility; history of EP; history of salpingitis, adhesions, contralateral fallopian tube deteriorated). For patients without any risk, the difference is low and not significant. In the risk group, the OR for conception was 0.67 [95% CI (0.50,0.91)] in the salpingectomy group versus conservative treatment, but in the no-risk group this OR was 0.99 [95% CI (0.80,1.23)]. But a patient at low risk who is treated by salpingectomy during the first ectopic pregnancy becomes a high-risk patient for the second. It is therefore not really logical to remove the first tube and not the second.

On the other hand, all studies agree that unilateral salpingectomy does not reduce the risk of recurrence (Fernandez et al. 2013, Mol et al. 2014). In our study (de Bennetot et al. 2012), we found that the recurrence rate was 18.5% after either salpingectomy or conservative treatment.

Conservative treatment versus MTX

There is now sufficient data to conclude that the likelihood of having a child is the same after treatment by MTX and salpingotomy. In the same study previously mentioned (de Bennetot et al. 2012), we found that the OR for conception did not differ between MTX and salpingotomy: 1.13 [95% CI (0.88,1.45)]. In the no-risk subgroup this OR was 1.02 [95% CI (0.75,1.23)], and in the risk group it was 1.20 [95% CI (0.77,1.85)].

In the prospective DEMETER study (Fernandez et al. 2013), cumulative fertility curves were not significantly different between medical treatment and conservative surgery. OR was 0.85 (0.59–1.22) $P = 0.37$. The 2-year rates of intrauterine pregnancy were 67% after medical treatment and 71% after conservative surgery. On the other hand, the risk of recurrence seems higher with MTX, but the difference is low: 22.5% versus 18.5% in our experience (de Bennetot et al. 2012).

One of the advantages of laparoscopy over MTX is the ability to check tubal status. On the another hand, a second laparoscopy 3 months after a successful MTX treatment permits a much more efficient check-up than is possible at the time of an EP.

TREATMENT INDICATIONS

Contraindications

The contraindications for laparoscopic treatment are rare. The contraindications for salpingectomy are cases of severe adhesions where the salpingectomy can induce a severe impairment in tubal vascularization.

The contraindications for salpingotomy are relative. They are the cases of very active EP with an hCG level of >10,000 UI. Tubal ruptures and acute bleeding are not contraindications but make the procedure difficult to achieve.

The contraindications for MTX treatment are as follows:
- Signs of rupture or pre-rupture
- Presence of hemoperitoneum
- Hematosalpinx of >4 cm
- Lack of patient compliance for therapeutic monitoring
- Hepatic, renal, hematological disorders

Indications

There are many indications, but the main considerations are:
- The patient's history (ectopic pregnancies, infertility, pelvic inflammatory disease)
- The desire for subsequent pregnancy
- The activity of the pregnancy, mainly determined by the level of hCG
- The contraindication for the MTX treatment
- the local tubal status seen during the laparoscopy

We must also keep in mind that the cost of treatment with MTX is considerably lower than that of surgery even if account is taken of a much greater frequency of failures. This cost is about three times lower for a failure rate of 25% (Vaissade et al. 2003).

Laparoscopic treatment is possible in cases of hemodynamic shock. In most cases, the tube is ruptured, and a salpingectomy is the only available option. The crucial deciding point is the surgeon, who must be trained in laparoscopy and able to achieve hemostasis in a few minutes (Soriano et al. 1997). Blood products should also be readily available.

In cases when there is definitely no desire for childbearing, the choice will be between salpingectomy (because the failure rate is lower) and MTX treatment (because the cost is lower). The arguments of choice will be the clinical context and hCG levels. In cases of hCG of >1500 or in case of doubt concerning the risk of rupture, laparoscopy and salpingectomy are the logical option; if not, MTX is the logical option.

In other cases, it is better to opt for conservative treatment except in the rare case of multiple recurrences, where salpingectomy should be bilateral to avoid any other recurrence.

MTX is logical if there no contraindications. In all other cases, laparoscopic treatment should be used. But in case of infertility, even if there is no contraindication for MTX, laparoscopy could be considered in order to check tubal status.

During laparoscopy, conservative treatment must be attempted. But faced with a catastrophic tubal status or the impossibility of ensuring correct hemostasis, secondary use of salpingectomy may be necessary.

CONCLUSION

Even if laparoscopy remains the gold standard procedure for the treatment of EP, it must be weighed against the possibility of medical MTX treatment that can be applied in 40% of cases.

ACKNOWLEDGMENT

This chapter is presented in memory of Maurice Antoine Bruhat.

REFERENCES

Alleyassin A, Khademi A, Aghahosseini M, et al. Comparison of success rates in the medical management of ectopic pregnancy with single- dose and multiple-dose administration of methotrexate: a prospective, randomized clinical trial. Fertil Steril 2006; 85:1661–1666.

Barnhart KT, Gosman G, Ashby R, Sammel M. The medical management of ectopic pregnancy: a meta-analysis comparing "single dose" and "multidose" regimens. Obstet Gynaecol 2003; 104:778–784.

Bouyer J, Fernandez H, Coste J, et al. Fertility after ectopic pregnancy: 10-year results in the Auvergne Registry. J Gynecol Obstet Biol Reprod (Paris) 2003; 32:431–438.

Bouyer J, Job-Spira N, Pouly JL, et al. Fertility following radical, conservative-surgical or medical treatment for tubal pregnancy: a population-based study. BJOG 2000; 107:714–721.

Bruhat M, Manhes H. Trial treatment of extra-uterine pregnancy during celioscopy. Nouv Presse Med 1977; 6:2606.

Bruhat MA, Manhes H, Mage G, Pouly JL. Treatment of ectopic pregnancy by means of laparoscopy. Fertil Steril 1980; 33:411–414.

de Bennetot M, Rabischong B, Aublet-Cuvelier B, et al. Fertility after tubal ectopic pregnancy: results of a population-based study. Fertil Steril 2012; 98:1271–1276.

Dubuisson JB, Aubriot FX, Cardone V. Laparoscopic salpingectomy for tubal pregnancy. Fertil Steril 1987; 47:225–228.

Dubuisson JB, Morice P, Chapron C, et al. Salpingectomy: the laparoscopic surgical choice for ectopic pregnancy. Hum Reprod 1996; 11:1199–1203.

Dudley PS, Heard MJ, Sangi-Haghpeykar H, et al. Characterizing ectopic pregnancies that rupture despite treatment with methotrexate. Fertil Steril 2004; 82:1374–1378.

Fernandez H, Capmas P, Lucot JP, et al. GROG. Fertility after ectopic pregnancy: the DEMETER randomized trial. Hum Reprod 2013; 28:1247–1253.

Fernandez H, Lelaidier C, Thouvenez V, Frydman R. The use of a pretherapeutic, predictive score to determine inclusion criteria for the non-surgical treatment of ectopic pregnancy. Hum Reprod 1991; 6:995–998.

Fuchs N, Manoucheri E, Verbaan M, Einarsson JI. Laparoscopic management of extrauterine pregnancy in caesarean section scar: description of a surgical technique and review of the literature. BJOG. 2015 Jan; 122(1):137–140.

Gabbur N, Sherer DM, Hellmann M, et al. Do serum beta-human chorionic gonadotropin levels on day 4 following methotrexate treatment of patients with ectopic pregnancy predict successful single-dose therapy? Am J Perinatol. 2006; 23:193–196.

Graczykowski JW, Mishell DR Jr. Methotrexate prophylaxis for persistent ectopic pregnancy after conservative treatment by salpingostomy. Obstet Gynecol 1997; 89:118–122.

Hagström HG, Hahlin M, Bennegarg-Eden B, et al. Prediction of persistent ectopic pregnancy after laparoscopic salpingostomy. Obstet Gynecol 1994; 84:798–802.

Manhès H, Mage G, Pouly JL, et al. Améliorations techniques du traitement coelioscopiques de la grossesse extra-utérine. Nouv Presse Med 1983; 12:1431–1433.

Menon S, Colins J, Barnhart K. Establishing a human chorionic gonadotropin cutoff to guide methotrexate treatment of ectopic pregnancy: a systematic review. Fertil Steril 2007; 87:481–484.

Mol F, Mol BW, Ankun WM, et al. Current evidence on surgery, systemic methotrexate and expectant management in the treatment of tubal ectopic pregnancy: a systematic review and meta-analysis. Hum Reprod Update 2008; 14:309–319.

Mol F, van Mello NM, Strandell A, et al. Salpingotomy versus salpingectomy in women with tubal pregnancy (ESEP study): an open-label, multicentre, randomised controlled trial. Lancet 2014; pii: S0140-6736(14)60123-9.

Nazac A, Gervaise A, Bouyer J, et al. Predictors of success in methotrexate treatment of women with unruptured tubal pregnancy. Ultrasound Obstet Gynecol 2003; 21:181–185.

Nowak-Markwitz E, Michalak M, Olejnik A, Spaczynski M. Cut-off value of human chorionic gonadotropin in relation to the number of methotrexate cycles in the successful treatment of ectopic pregnancy. Fertil Steril 2009; 92:1203–1207.

Potter MB, Lepine LA, Jamieson DJ. Predictors of success with methotrexate treatment for tubal ectopic pregnancy at Grady Memorial Hospital. Am J Obstet Gynaecol 2003; 188:1192–1194.

Pouly JL, Chapron C, Wattiez A, et al. Multifactorial analysis of fertility following conservative laparoscopic treatment of ectopic pregnancies. Fertil Steril 1991; 56:453–460.

Pouly JL, Chapron C, Wattiez A, et al. The drop in the level of hCG after conservative laparoscopic treatment of ectopic pregnancy. J Gynecol Surg 1992; 7:211–217.

Pouly JL, Mahnes H, Mage G, et al. Conservative laparoscopic treatment of 321 ectopic pregnancies. Fertil Steril 1986; 46:1093–1097.

Rabischong B, Larraín D, Pouly JL, et al. Predicting success of laparoscopic salpingostomy for ectopic pregnancy. Obstet Gynecol 2010; 116:701–707.

Rabischong B, Tran X, Sleiman AA, et al. Predictive factors of failure in management of ectopic pregnancy with single-dose methotrexate: a general population-based analysis from the Auvergne Register, France. Fertil Steril 2011; 95:401–404.

Soriano D, Yefet Y, Oelsner G, et al. Operative laparoscopy for management of ectopic pregnancy in patients with hypovolemic shock. J Am Assoc Gynecol Laparosc 1997; 4:363–367.

Stovall TG, Wing FW, Gray LA. Single dose methotrexate for treatment of ectopic pregnancy. Obstet Gynecol 1991; 77:754–757.

Thorburn J, Lundorff P, Lindblom B. Fertility after ectopic pregnancy evaluated in relation to background factors and surgical treatment. Fertil Steril 1988; 49:595–601.

Tulandi T, Guralnick M. Treatment of tubal ectopic pregnancy by salpingotomy with or without tubal suturing and salpingectomy. Fertil Steril 1991; 55:53–55.

Vaissade L, Gerbaud L, Pouly JL, et al. Cost-effectiveness analysis of laparoscopic surgery versus methotrexate: comparison of data recorded in an ectopic pregnancy registry. J Gynecol Obstet Biol Reprod 2003; 32:447–458.

Chapter 20

Cervical incompetence and laparoscopic abdominal cerclage

Valerie To, Togas Tulandi

INTRODUCTION

Cervical incompetence or cervical insufficiency is one of the causes of preterm birth leading to increased perinatal morbidity and mortality. It is found in 0.1–1.0% of all pregnancies and in up to 8% of women with repeated second trimester miscarriages (Ludmir 1988, Drakeley et al. 1998. Cervical insufficiency manifests as painless dilatation of the cervix in the absence of contractions before 37 weeks of gestational age. It leads to premature rupture of membrane and preterm delivery. Treatment involves placement of a cervical cerclage that is most commonly performed through a vaginal approach with MacDonald or Shirodkar techniques (Medical Research Council 1993). However, in some conditions, cervical cerclage cannot be performed vaginally or will not be effective.

INDICATIONS OF ABDOMINAL CERCLAGE

When the intravaginal portion of cervix is either too short or inexistent due to previous conization or loop electrosurgical excision procedure, abdominal cervical cerclage is indicated. Other indications are short cervix related to congenital malformation or severe cervical lacerations. The most common indication of abdominal cervical cerclage is after failed vaginal cerclage. The cerclage is placed transabdominally in the cervicoisthmic portion of the uterus (Delarue 2002). This can be achieved by laparotomy or laparoscopy.

Advantages of the abdominal route include decreased likelihood of slippage of the suture because of high placement, ability to leave the cerclage in situ for future pregnancies, and lack of foreign body in the vagina that could increase the risk of ascending infection and premature labor (Al-Fadhli & Tulandi 2004).

Laparotomy versus laparoscopic approach

The main disadvantage of performing an abdominal cervical cerclage is that the patient will require a second laparotomy for Cesarean delivery. To date, there has not been any randomized trial comparing cervical cerclage to laparotomy or laparoscopic approach. Burger et al. conducted a systematic review of the subject by pooling data from 135 laparoscopic cerclages and 1116 cerclages by laparotomy. Compared to those of laparoscopic abdominal cerclage, the rates of intraoperative and 2 weeks postoperative complications appear to be higher in the laparotomy group but did not reach statistical significance (Burger et al. 2011). The rates of delivery of an infant >34 weeks and of pregnancy complications [preterm premature rupture of membrane (PPROM), chorioamnionitis, premature contractions, and fetal loss] were comparable (Burger et al. 2011, Tulandi et al. 2014). The mean hospitalization time in the laparoscopic group was between 1.8 day and 4 days in the laparotomy group.

Robotic-assisted abdominal cerclage

With the availability of surgical robot, a few authors have reported abdominal cerclage with robotic assistance. The largest case series of robotic-assisted abdominal cerclage performed in a nonpregnant state involved 24 patients (Moore et al. 2012). The surgeries were well tolerated without complications except one conversion to laparotomy due to severe adhesions. This patient developed a port wound infection. In another series of seven patients between 11 and 15 weeks pregnant, there were two conversions and one fetal loss, and a consistent problem with access to the upper cervix due to the soft and enlarged uterus (Foster et al. 2011).

In general, expert laparoscopists could perform laparoscopic abdominal cerclage without robotic assistance. In addition, the use of robot increases the operating time as well as the cost. There has been no study demonstrating the clinical benefit of robotic-assisted abdominal cerclage.

PROCEDURE
Timing

Abdominal cerclage can be done before conception (preconception) or during pregnancy (postconception), ideally in the first trimester. The drawbacks from operating during pregnancy include difficult exposure, increased risk of bleeding, and possible risks to the fetus and the pregnancy (Al-Fadhli & Tulandi 2004). However, there has been a concern in performing the procedure before conception, with respect to eventuality of a subsequent miscarriage. This concern seems unwarranted. During the first trimester, it is still feasible to evacuate the products of conception through the cerclage using an 8 mm suction curette (Delarue 2002, Al-Fadhli & Tulandi 2004). The use of up to a 12 mm suction to evacuate an 18 week miscarriage has also been reported with a subsequent successful delivery at term (Chandiramani et al. 2011). Otherwise, removal of the cerclage can be done laparoscopically. This will be followed by spontaneous expulsion of the fetus within a few days (Agdi &Tulandi 2008). Hysterotomy is not indicated.

In a systematic review by Burger et al., the rates of surgical complications of pre- and postconceptional abdominal cerclage were comparable (Burger et al. 2011). However, the number of patients was small and some of the studies pooled the patients together. Yet, the conversion rate to laparotomy was higher in pregnant patients (4.4% vs. 0.8%)(Burger et al. 2011).

Surgical steps

The procedure is performed under general anesthesia. The patient is positioned in dorsal lithotomy position and an indwelling Foley catheter is placed. In preconceptional abdominal cerclage, we place a uterine manipulator to facilitate exposure. Laparoscopy is started in the usual fashion, with a primary trocar for the camera infraumbilically and two secondary trocars in the lower abdomen, placed higher than the level of the fundus. In pregnant patient, the primary trocar might have to be inserted supraumbilically.

The uterovesical peritoneum is incised and the bladder is separated off the cervix. The uterine vessels are identified but it is not necessary to dissect them. We use a 5 mm Mersilene polyester tape for the cerclage. The needles are removed and the two ends of the tape are tapered. The tape is inserted into the abdominal cavity and placed in the pouch of Douglas.

We use a disposable Endoclose needle (Tyco Healthcare, Mansfield, Massachusetts), which is inserted into the abdominal cavity percutaneously at the level of the cervix. Its tip is directed posteriorly toward the isthmus, between the cervix and the uterine corpus, medial to the uterine vessels and ureter. It pierces the cervical body adjacent to the uterosacral ligament (**Figures 20.1–20.5**). The tapered end of the Mersilene tape is placed into the opening at the tip of the Endoclose and brought anteriorly. The same procedure is repeated on the opposite side. The tape is tied anterior to the cervix using intracorporeal knot tying. In order to have a tight knot, the uterine manipulator is removed before tying the knot. Excess tape is trimmed.

POTENTIAL INTRAOPERATIVE PROBLEMS

- Injury to the uterine vessels: Piercing the cervical body too lateral will cause injury to the uterine vessels. It is imperative to be sure about the location of the vessels before inserting the Endoclose into the cervix. On the other hand, putting it too medial does not provide sufficient strength to the cerclage. The cervical canal could also be entered with placement of the suture too medial.

- The opening at the tip of Endoclose sometimes does not open. This is usually due to a bend on its shaft. In this situation, one can use a needle holder to pull the tip of the Endoclose exposing its opening. Alternatively, other fascial closure devices such as Carter-Thomason device (Cooper Surgical, Trumbull, Connecticut) or Berci fascial closure (Karl Storz Endoskope, Tutlingen, Germany) can be used.

- The suture is closing the upper vagina. The cerclage should be located adjacent to the uterosacral ligament.

- The knot is not tight enough. Intracorporeal knot tying and removal of intrauterine manipulator before tying ensure tight knots.

- The gravid uterus is too large. If the uterus is too large for postconceptional laparoscopic abdominal cerclage, a laparotomy is required. The same technique using fascial closure device is performed.

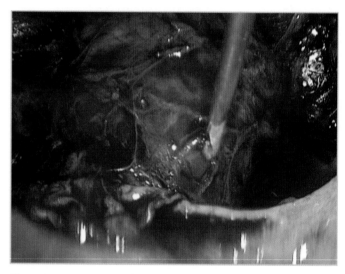

Figure 20.2 Anterior view of the cerclage. The opening at the tip of the Endoclose is demonstrated.

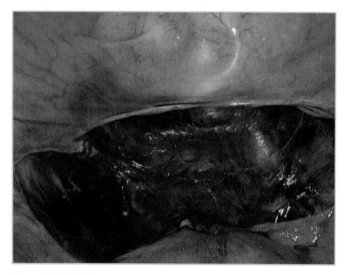

Figure 20.1 Endoclose entry point. The peritoneum between the uterus and the bladder has been incised and the bladder separated off the cervix.

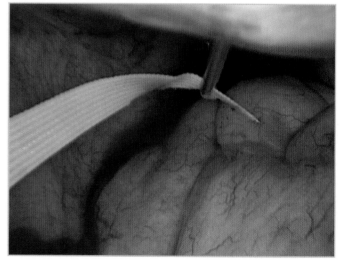

Figure 20.3 Posterior view of the cerclage with the tapered end of the tape inside the Endoclose.

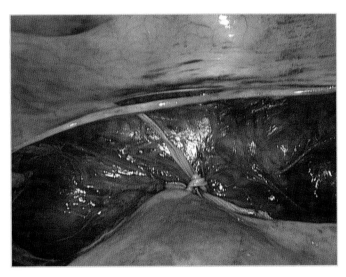

Figure 20.4 End result. The cerclage has been tied using intracorporeal knot tying.

COMPLICATIONS

The most common complication of abdominal cerclage is bleeding from the uterine vessels (Foster et al. 2011). This occurs more often in open abdominal cerclage during the dissection of the uterine vessels. It rarely occurs during abdominal cerclage by laparoscopy (Burger et al. 2011). Other complications including bowel or bladder injury, urinary tract infection, and fever are rarely encountered (0.7%).

Conversion of laparoscopy to laparotomy has been reported in as high as 5.2% of cases, usually with postconceptional abdominal cerclage. Associated fetal loss is uncommon (1.5%). Other complications such as wound infection, wound hematoma, and uterine artery ligation have been reported but not with the laparoscopic technique (Foster et al. 2011).

PREGNANCY OUTCOME

Cervical cerclage reduces premature delivery in high-risk women. However, abdominal cerclage is not a replacement of vaginal cerclage. The results of studies comparing abdominal versus vaginal cervical cerclage have been conflicting. Some studies reported that the results were comparable, while others showed that compared to cervical cerclage by vaginal approach, transabdominal cerclage was associated with fewer preterm births and improved neonatal survival (Foster et al. 2011).

In our institution, most of the abdominal cerclage is performed for those who have failed cervical cerclage by vaginal approach. When comparing laparoscopic and open abdominal placement of a cervical cerclage, successful outcomes (delivery of a viable infant >34 weeks of gestational age) were comparable, ranging from 79% to 90% versus 81–85% (Burger et al. 2011). Fetal survival rate was >84% and the mean gestational age at Cesarean section was over 36 weeks in both groups. Pregnancy complications were <10% with both approaches including PPROM, chorioamnionitis, premature contractions, and uterine rupture and dehiscence. Fetal losses including first trimester miscarriages were <12% in both groups (Burger et al. 2011).

CONTRAINDICATIONS

Contraindications of abdominal cerclage are similar to those of a vaginal cerclage; e.g., when the procedure will be unlikely to prevent preterm birth or improve neonatal outcome. These include fetal anomaly incompatible with life, PPROM, intrauterine infection, active bleeding, and active preterm labor (Norwitz 2013). For a laparoscopic approach, the procedure should ideally be performed around 12 weeks of gestation as a larger uterus may lead to a conversion to laparotomy (Abenhaim & Tulandi 2009).

PATIENT SATISFACTION

In a Dutch cohort of preconceptional laparoscopic abdominal cerclage, all patients reported to be very satisfied with the surgery, regardless of the outcome (70% pregnancy rate and 83% fetal survival rate) (Burger et al. 2012). They felt their recovery was fast without any adverse effects.

CONCLUSION

For women with cervical insufficiency, especially if they have failed a previous vaginal cerclage, laparoscopic cerclage placement provides a viable option in preventing preterm birth without a laparotomy. The procedure is well tolerated by patients and recovery is faster. It is an effective technique with at least comparable outcomes and complications to an open abdominal cerclage (Tulandi et al. 2014). Bleeding can be minimized by not dissecting the uterine vessels. Some studies even suggest that compared to the conventional cervical cerclage vaginally, abdominal cerclage provides better results.

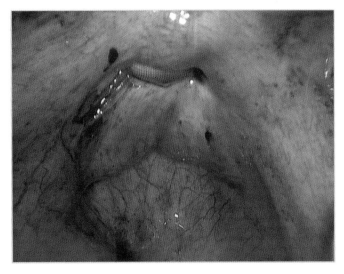

Figure 20.5 Posterior view of the cerclage. The cerclage is located adjacent to the uterosacral ligament.

■ REFERENCES

Abenhaim HA, Tulandi T. Cervical insufficiency: re-evaluating the prophylactic cervical cerclage. J Matern Fetal Neonatal Med 2009; 22:510–516.

Agdi M, Tulandi T. Placement and removal of abdominal cerclage by laparoscopy. Reprod Biomed Online 2008; 16:308–310.

Al-Fadhli R, Tulandi T. Laparoscopic abdominal cerclage. Obstet Gynecol Clin North Am 2004; 31:497–504, viii.

Burger NB, Brolmann HA, Einarsson JI, Langebrekke A, Huirne JA. Effectiveness of abdominal cerclage placed via laparotomy or laparoscopy: systematic review. J Minim Invasive Gynecol 2011; 18:696–704.

Burger NB, Einarsson JI, Brolmann HA, et al. Preconceptional laparoscopic abdominal cerclage: a multicenter cohort study. Am J Obstet Gynecol 2012; 207:273 e1–12.

Chandiramani M, Chappell L, Radford S, Shennan A. Successful pregnancy following mid-trimester evacuation through a transabdominal cervical cerclage. BMJ Case Rep 2011; 2011.

Delarue T. An article about 'Isthmic cerclage by laparoscopy' by P. von Theobald. J Gynecol Obstet Biol Reprod (Paris) 2002; 31(6):604.

Drakeley AJ, Quenby S, Farquharson RG. Mid-trimester loss – appraisal of a screening protocol. Hum Reprod 1998; 13:1975–1980.

Final report of the Medical Research Council/Royal College of Obstetricians and Gynaecologists multicentre randomised trial of cervical cerclage. MRC/RCOG Working Party on Cervical Cerclage. Br J Obstet Gynaecol 1993; 100:516–523.

Foster TL, Moore ES, Sumners JE. Operative complications and fetal morbidity encountered in 300 prophylactic transabdominal cervical cerclage procedures by one obstetric surgeon. J Obstet Gynaecol 2011; 31:713–717.

Ludmir J. Sonographic detection of cervical incompetence. Clin Obstet Gynecol 1988; 31:101–109.

Moore ES, Foster TL, McHugh K, Addleman RN, Sumners JE. Robotic-assisted transabdominal cerclage (RoboTAC) in the non-pregnant patient. J Obstet Gynaecol 2012; 32:643–647.

Norwitz ER. Transvaginal cervical cerclage. In: Basow DS, (ed). UpToDate. Waltham, MA: UpToDate; 2015. last accessed 18 Nov 2015.

Tulandi T, Alghanaim N, Hakeem G, Tan X. Pre and postconceptional abdominal cerclage by laparoscopy or laparotomy. J Minim Invasive Gynecol 2014; 21:987–993.

Chapter 21 Laparoscopic treatment of endometriosis

Arnaud Wattiez, Karolina Afors, Gabriele Centini, Rouba Murtada

INTRODUCTION

Endometriosis is a gynecological condition arising from ectopic deposits of endometrium outside the uterine cavity. Although the prevalence of endometriosis is difficult to determine, it is estimated to affect 5–15% of women mainly of reproductive age, with an increasing prevalence in the last 15–20 years (Redwine 1999).

Endometriosis symptomatology is mainly characterized by pelvic pain (dyspareunia, dysmenorrhea, dysuria, and dyschezia) and infertility (Carneiro et al. 2010). It is a chronic condition, which may result in intermittent or chronic pelvic pain, and can impact significantly on organ function impairing women's quality of life Endometriosis can occur in various locations within the pelvis and the two main forms are endometriomas and deep infiltrating endometriosis (DIE).

An endometrioma is a cystic ovarian mass arising from the implantation of ectopic endometrium on the ovarian surface, commonly at the level of the posterior leaf of the broad ligament. This cyst contains a brown fluid that is typical, if not pathognomonic, of the disease.

Deep endometriosis, on the other hand, is defined as invasion of >5 mm of the peritoneal surface by an endometriotic lesion with the most common location at the rectovaginal septum, uterosacral ligaments, pararectal fossa, and vesicouterine pouch.

Laparoscopy remains the gold standard for the diagnosis of endometriosis with direct visualization of endometriotic implants. Developments in transvaginal sonography (TVS) and magnetic resonance imaging (MRI) have made these tools increasingly useful to aid diagnosis, and evaluate the specific location and extent of infiltrating lesions (Eriksen et al. 2008).

Over the past decade, endoscopic surgery has continued to evolve and has revolutionized the surgical approach to the treatment of endometriosis (Catenacci et al. 2009). A minimally invasive approach has specific advantages that can assist the surgeon facing this complex and multivariable disease. The endoscope allows image magnification and enables the surgeon to select and frame the required picture. This is particularly useful in cases of DIE where laparoscopic image magnification allows the recognition of subtle lesions that were perhaps previously overlooked at laparotomy. In addition, laparoscopy improves precision and fine movement facilitating more complex dissection, making surgeries previously considered too difficult more easily attainable.

STRATEGY IN ENDOMETRIOSIS

Endometriosis is a complex disease. It can lead to anatomical distortion making surgical treatment technically challenging with a resultant higher risk of complications. Endometriosis is multicentric and can affect the entire pelvis including the urinary tract, bowel, and rectovaginal septum. Involvement of these additional organ systems requires a specific expertise and knowledge of what we call 'transversal competencies' to facilitate safe and effective treatment.

A systematic approach is used for the management of endometriosis, making surgery reproducible, less time consuming, with a view to minimizing complications. This type of systematic approach can be further subdivided into general and organ-specific steps (**Figure 21.1**).

General strategy

The aim of the strategy is threefold: achieve exposure, identify important landmarks to preserve during dissection, and separate the diseased tissue from in sano.

A vaginal examination under general anesthesia is performed at the beginning of the procedure. This enables the surgeon to localize any rectovaginal disease that serves as a benchmark in cases where sequential examination may be indicated to adequately identify the limits of the nodule.

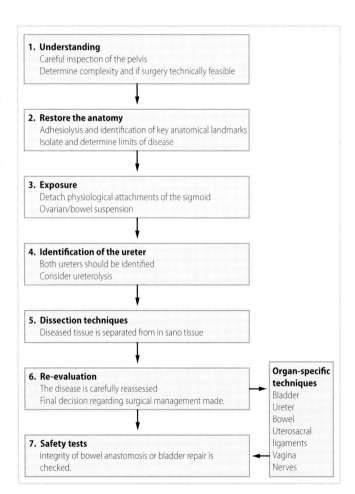

Figure 21.1 Strategic approach for surgical management of endometriosis.

Following insertion of trocars and positioning of the uterine manipulator, the patient is placed in Trendelenburg position. The surgery begins with a thorough inspection of the intra-abdominal cavity. In cases of DIE, exposure of the operative field is essential. Adhesiolysis is performed to restore normal anatomy. Both ovaries are freed from their fossae and any endometriotic cysts are drained to facilitate access to the pouch of Douglas. If necessary, the ovaries are suspended from the anterior abdominal wall using either a T-lift device or suture on a straight needle, which improves exposure and frees the assistant.

The normal physiological attachments of the sigmoid colon are also detached from the left parietal wall by dividing the peritoneum while avoiding entering the retroperitoneal space. There are four advantages to achieving this step:

1. It allows the colon to be mobilized, displaced cranially, and suspended, if needed, giving access to the left adnexa.
2. It allows access to the left infundibulopelvic ligament and identification and subsequent preservation of the adnexae is achieved.
3. The course of the left ureter can be visualized. The ureter is most easily identified at the left of the pelvic brim as it is the first structure medial to the infundibulopelvic ligament. This is a key step in deep endometriosis, as it is often medialized as a result of retraction and fibrosis of the disease process. Once identified, it can then be lateralized and preserved during central dissection.
4. It provides adequate exposure to access to the left pararectal fossa, an avascular space, which can be developed either at the level of the pelvic brim or caudally close to the rectovaginal space in the absence of any anatomical distortion. The sigmoid is pulled cranially and laterally to the right in order to identify the limits of the left pararectal fossa.

At the end of this technical sequence, a new vaginal exam is performed and all the lesions re-evaluated. It is following this second examination that the specific treatment is decided.

Thus, the surgery is tailored according to the location of the endometriotic lesions and severity of the disease, with emphasis on preserving organ function.

■ Specific strategy
Endometrioma

Surgical treatment of endometriomas is not a technically challenging procedure; nevertheless, it is the subject of much debate regarding the impact of cystectomy on ovarian reserve and subsequent fertility. The main objective of surgical treatment is not only to treat the cyst in order to provide pain relief but also preserve the follicle count (ovarian reserve) while avoiding recurrence and minimizing adhesions. Repetitive surgery on the same ovary should be avoided. The chosen technique should aim to eradicate the disease either by means of excision or destruction of the pathological tissue so as to decrease the risk of recurrence, while preserving healthy ovarian tissue. The current available techniques are excision, ablation, or a combined approach. Based on current evidence, excision of endometriomas seems to be the preferred method of treatment due to the reduced risk of recurrence (Hart et al. 2008).

Preoperative workup

Endometriomas are easily diagnosed by TVS, and are typically described as having a 'ground glass echogenicity of the cyst fluid' (Van Holsbeke et al. 2010). Endometriomas serve as a good indicator of deep endometriosis and are associated with more extensive disease in up to 98% of cases (Redwine 1999).

Surgical technique

Excision or endometrioma stripping: Surgery begins with mobilizing the ovary, which causes the endometriotic cyst to rupture and spill its chocolate content. The rupture point is found and enlarged, and the cyst is everted. The bed of the cyst is incised using scissors, preferably avoiding the use of energy. This is to prevent the cyst from fusing with the adjacent stroma, and consequently losing the cleavage plane (**Figure 21.2**). The cyst is stripped using two graspers with opposing divergent forces. The operator and the assistant work in unison, each holding one half of the cyst or ovary in order to strip the cyst capsule free from the ovarian parenchyma. This is particularly important in the case of large endometriomas where during stripping of the cyst identification of normal ovarian tissue and endometrioma may be difficult for the surgeon to distinguish. The stripping technique is for the most part bloodless and hemostasis is usually required only close to the ovarian hilum. Hemostasis can be achieved using bipolar coagulation that should be used sparingly in short bursts to avoid devascularization. An alternative option is suturing the ovary, which closes the dead space thereby minimizing blood loss, in addition to restoring its normal anatomical shape (Ferrero et al. 2012).

Ablation: Ablative treatment consists of aspiration, irrigation, and biopsy of the cyst to exclude malignancy. The thermal effect of either bipolar coagulation, CO_2 laser, or plasma energy is then utilized to destroy the cyst wall.

Combined technique: A combined approach using both excisional and ablative techniques has also been described. It consists of performing a classical excision of the endometrioma utilizing the stripping technique along the cleavage plane to treat 90% of the cyst. The remaining 10% of the cyst wall adjacent to the ovarian hilum is often more vascular due to fusion of the cleavage plane. To avoid excessive bleeding, a partial cystectomy is performed with subsequent ablation of the remaining endometrial foci using either CO_2 laser or bipolar diathermy.

The three-step procedure: For large endometriomas >5–6 cm, a three-step procedure may be considered. The cyst is opened, emptied, irrigated, and biopsied. Following this initial drainage, a 12–week medical treatment with a gonadotropin releasing hormone

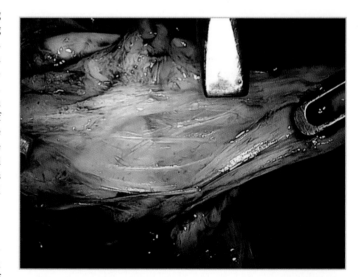

Figure 21.2 Laparoscopic ovarian cystectomy: cleavage plane between cyst wall and ovarian parenchyma is identified and stripping of endometrioma performed.

(GnRH) agonist is prescribed in order to reduce the size of the cyst. A reduction in size of up to 50% has been described in the literature. A second-look laparoscopy may then be performed with ablation of the remaining cyst wall.

Postoperative care and outcomes

Medical treatment can be effective in the secondary prevention of endometriomas by halting the growth and activity of endometriotic lesions. Medical therapies such as progestogens, oral contraceptive pills, and GnRH agonists can be used to achieve this goal. Patients who have undergone surgical treatment of endometriomas who do not wish to conceive immediately but require long-term management may benefit most from oral contraceptives as they can be given indefinitely. Postoperative oral contraceptives have been shown to be effective in decreasing the rate of recurrence of endometriomas (Vercellini et al. 2013).

In a Cochrane review, Hart et al. concluded that compared to ablation, excision yielded better results in terms of dyspareunia (OR = 0,08) and dysmenorrhea (OR = 0,15) relief, reduced recurrence (OR = 0,41), and increased spontaneous pregnancy rates in women with previous subfertility (OR = 5,21) (Hart et al. 2008). With regard to outcomes of assisted reproductive treatments, no conclusion could be reached due to contradictory data (Hart et al. 2008, Benschop et al. 2010). Despite these results being clearly in favor of excision for symptomatic relief, the debate regarding the preferred treatment option in terms of minimizing loss of ovarian reserve is yet to be solved. The effect of cystectomy on ovarian stroma has been demonstrated with histological analyses, showing the removal of healthy ovarian follicles in cystectomy specimens (Muzii et al. 2005, Roman et al. 2010). Measuring serum anti-Müllerian hormone (AMH) and resting follicle count, in addition to observing ovarian response to stimulation, is a useful means of indirectly studying the effect of cystectomy on ovarian reserve. Serum AMH levels remain stable throughout the menstrual cycle, decline with age, and correlate well with resting follicle count, thereby serving as a useful marker. Significant reductions in serum AMH levels in excess of 30% have been documented following endometrioma stripping (Raffi et al. 2012). In cases of bilateral endometrioma surgery, ovarian failure has also been documented in 2.5% of cases (Busacca et al. 2006). The rationale for endometrioma ablation is that it avoids inadvertent excision of normal ovarian tissue and the thermal effect is limited and therefore considered harmless. Data regarding the thermal effect of ablation is lacking and a deleterious effect may still occur, resulting in follicle loss and damage to normal ovarian tissue. Further comparative studies between ablative and excisional techniques are needed to determine their true effect on ovarian reserve.

Regardless of the surgical technique used, a meticulous surgical approach to excision of endometriomas should be adopted. The surgery should be as atraumatic as possible with careful dissection, respect for hemostasis, and sparing use of bipolar coagulation. Surgeons should be mindful of the potential deleterious effect on ovarian reserve and patients should be carefully assessed (preoperative serum AMH levels may be of benefit) and counseled accordingly.

DIE of the posterior compartment

Rectovaginal endometriosis typically refers to infiltrative disease or adenomyosis externa of >5 mm involving the cervix, vagina rectovaginal septum, and rectum. The disease can occur in isolation or extend to cause distortion of pelvic anatomy and in some cases complete obliteration of the pouch of Douglas (**Figure 21.3**). Extent of rectovaginal endometriosis does not often correlate with pain severity, and as a result may remain undiagnosed for many years.

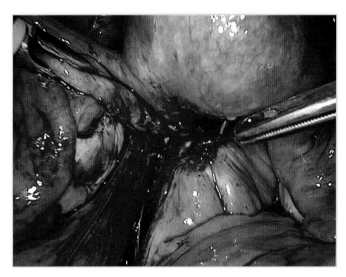

Figure 21.3 Laparoscopic view of a rectovaginal endometriotic nodule.

Correlation between symptoms and various locations of DIE do exist; however, physical examination has limited value for assessing the true extent of the disease (Chapron et al. 2003). Unfortunately, distinguishing between infiltrative and noninfiltrative rectovaginal disease is challenging and no single imaging modality can predict infiltrative disease with certainty. Several techniques such as transrectal/TVS and MRI have been recommended for diagnosing and locating DIE. Regarding the use of transrectal sonography, excluding intestinal endometriosis, it is often poor at detecting DIE at the uterosacral ligaments (Bazot et al. 2009). TVS has been reported as having a slightly lower sensitivity when compared to MRI (78.3% versus 84.4%); however, this may be operator-dependent (Bazot et al. 2009). Rectovaginal endometriosis is often associated with infiltrative disease at various locations and in cases where TVS is equivocal MRI may provide more reliable mapping as to the true extent of the disease.

DIE is more commonly located in the posterior compartment, with a predisposition for the left hemi pelvis, predominantly affecting the uterosacral ligaments. Isolated uterosacral lesions occur in 83% of cases; however, in 16.8% of cases lesions of the vagina, bowel, and bladder may coexist (Chapron et al. 2003).

Laparoscopic surgical excision of isolated uterosacral endometriosis has been demonstrated as an effective method of treatment. Surgical dissection commences with identification of key anatomical landmarks, specifically the ureter, which may be medialized due to the fibrotic effect of the disease process. If the ureter is not clearly seen, ureterolysis may be indicated and the course of the ureter should be followed caudally until it enters the ureteric channel. Any endometriotic nodules involving the uterosacral ligaments can then be dissected and removed safely with minimal risk of ureteric injury.

In cases of bilateral involvement of the uterosacral ligaments or where a coexisting vaginal nodule is present, the ureter should be identified bilaterally and ureterolysis performed if necessary. The pararectal fossa can then be identified and dissected, moving cranially to caudally. Once the pararectal spaces are opened, the vaginal nodule can be approached laterally from both sides. Periodic vaginal examinations may be required to help delineate the limits of the nodule. If attached to the bowel wall, it should be freed by carefully shaving the nodule off. Following its removal from the bowel wall, it will then remain attached to the posterior uterine wall/cervix and vagina. The nodule is then re-evaluated and the disease excised using, e.g. a monopolar hook. All glands and endometriotic disease should be removed even if this results in entering the vagina, which can subsequently be sutured using a 2/0 monofilament.

In cases of bilateral uterosacral disease, care should be taken to preserve nerve supply and function as much as possible. Dissection beyond the level of the uterine vein can result in inadvertent damage to the autonomic splanchnic nerves, which serve an important role in maintaining urinary and bowel function. When dissecting the uterosacral ligaments, the hypogastric inferior plexus may be compromised, putting women at risk of sexual dysfunction and urinary retention requiring intermittent self-catheterization. In patients who underwent radical surgery for DIE of the uterosacral ligaments, postoperative urinary retention was reported in up to 29% of patients (Volpi et al. 2004). In the majority of cases, this was transient; however, symptoms can persist for up to 18 months. As endometriosis is a benign disease affecting young women, care should be taken to dissect and preserve the pelvic autonomic nerves and patients should be informed of these potential adverse effects (Dubernard et al. 2007).

Bowel endometriosis

Bowel endometriosis occurs in 3–37% of cases and in 90% of cases the rectum, sigmoid colon, or both are most commonly involved (Campagnacci et al. 2005). Different laparoscopic techniques have been developed for the management of bowel endometriosis; however, the debate on the preferred approach is far from resolved. Historically, resection of deep endometriotic lesions of the bowel was avoided due to the significant associated morbidity for what is essentially a benign disease affecting women wishing to safeguard their fertility. With improved understanding of the disease process and development of innovative techniques, in the hands of an experienced surgeon, the morbidity associated with bowel resection is more acceptable.

Preoperative workup

Preoperative diagnosis of bowel endometriosis is difficult and no consensus exists on the most appropriate tool for diagnosing intestinal involvement. Several techniques such as transrectal/TVS, MRI, computed tomography, colonoscopy, and barium enema have been proposed. However, the practicality of their use is dependent on availability and also expertise in interpreting radiological findings. Endorectal ultrasonography has been demonstrated as having a high sensitivity for detecting and assessing degree of infiltration of the rectal wall. However, endorectal ultrasound may be limited in detecting multifocal lesions or nodules located further away from the probe. Regarding TVS, a sensitivity and specificity of 98% and 100% has been reported. Similarly MRI has demonstrated a sensitivity of 83% and specificity of 98% (Abrao et al. 2007, Piketty et al. 2009). Double contrast barium enema has also been shown to be effective, specifically in detecting stenotic bowel lesions with a sensitivity of 93.7% and specificity of 94.2% (Faccioli et al. 2010). Despite these results reported in the literature, relying solely on imaging may nevertheless lead to under and over treatment of some women. In cases where bowel resection was performed based on imaging findings alone, no rectal involvement was found in up to 29% of cases based on histological findings.

Surgical technique

Several laparoscopic surgical options exist for the management of bowel endometriosis, including 'shaving' for more superficial disease,

discoid excision, and segmental resections [mini-Pfannenstiel or NOSE (natural orifice specimen extraction) specimen extraction]. There is no clear evidence that these surgical techniques are the most effective form of treatment with regard to outcomes and complications. A meta-analysis comparing these different techniques was attempted; however, the data was insufficiently detailed and varied greatly with regard to extent of disease and outcomes making any meaningful comparison impossible.

Selection of a specific surgical strategy is often dependent on the surgeon's expertise and experience following careful evaluation of the lesion.

Shaving: Laparoscopic 'shaving' or 'skinning' involves dissecting largely superficial disease from the bowel wall (whether this be the serosa or muscularis layer) without entering the bowel lumen. Exposed areas of bowel mucosa are identified and sutured using interrupted 3/0 Monocryl to reinforce any areas of weakness and to maintain the integrity of the bowel wall.

Discoid resection: In cases of more extensive disease where full-thickness invasion of the bowel wall is suspected, discoid excision may be considered. This involves anterior resection of a small segment of the bowel wall using a transanal circular stapler device. Depending on the size of the nodule, initial debulking using the 'shaving' technique may be necessary. A guide suture is then placed at the level of the nodule and a 33 mm circular stapler is inserted transanally. The device is fully opened and the area of bowel to be excised is placed in the groove between the anvil and the stapler. The guide suture also serves as an anchoring device and the surgeon using gentle traction can manipulate the nodule into the groove of the stapler. The stapler is angled upward to ensure only the anterior portion of the rectal wall is included in the stapler. The device is then closed and fired and removed from the anus, completing the anterior discoid resection. This procedure can be used for the excision of infiltrative bowel lesions up to 2–3 cm in size.

Limitation of this technique is that high lesions, >15 cm from the anal verge, are inaccessible due to the fixed length of the stapler. With concurrent stenotic lesions, it may be impossible to pass the stapling device beyond the lesion and as such should not be used in instances where there is greater than one-third obstruction of the bowel lumen. Lastly, nodules >3 cm are not suitable for resection using this technique due to the confined distance between the anvil and base of the circular stapler. For larger lesions, a double discoid technique can be utilized for the resection of nodules up to 5 cm. This involves two circular stapling lines. The first firing of the circular stapler removes part of the intestinal lesion and the second firing results in removal of the initial suture line and any remaining disease. This is a novel technique; however, using two separate stapling lines may theoretically lead to narrowing of the bowel lumen. The use of a hemorrhoid stapler has also been proposed for the surgical treatment of larger lesions up to 7 cm, but further evaluation is required.

Segmental bowel resection: Segmental resection is sometimes unavoidable specifically when the nodule is >3 cm, involves the sigmoid, where there is >50% circumferential disease or bowel stenosis, and in cases of multicentric disease (**Figure 21.4**).

Segmental resection often involves resecting all visible and detectable endometriosis; however, following histological analysis, positive disease margins have been recorded in up to 20% of cases (Meuleman et al. 2011). In terms of disease recurrence and pain symptoms, however, there was no significant difference between patients with and without positive margins (Mabrouk et al. 2012), although data is lacking. Before concluding that safety margins are not obligatory, and radical surgery should be avoided in favor of a more economic

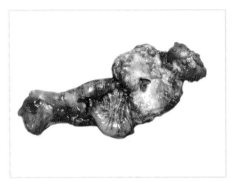

Figure 21.4
Segmental bowel resection specimen with significant stenosis.

approach more information from randomized control trials (RCTs) is required.

In order to adopt a more economical approach, the bowel is dissected at the edge of the mesentery in an attempt to preserve vasculature, lymphatics, and nerve supply, thereby minimizing associated functional complications. Laparoscopic resection and transanal anastomosis with abdominal, transvaginal, or transanal specimen extraction can be performed. For the NOSE technique, once the diseased segment has been adequately dissected, the bowel is divided caudal to the lesion using a linear stapler device. The bowel segment containing the disease is extracted through the vagina or anus. A colotomy is made at the distal part of the extracted bowel or in cases of stenosis, above the lesion. The anvil attached to a long suture is introduced using a retrograde technique and is deposited above the pathological segment of the proximal colon (see **Figure 21.1**). The diseased segment is then resected using the endoscopic linear stapler and removed transvaginally or transanally. The anvil is partially extracted using the fishing technique (see **Figure 21.2**) and a 2-0 purse string suture used to secure the anvil head in position. A circular stapler is introduced through the anus and used to perforate the rectal stump. The head of the anvil is then attached and an intracorporeal mechanical anastomosis performed completing the side to end anastomosis.

Some centers advocate the routine use of temporary defunctioning stomas for low rectal resections (<7–10 cm from the anal margin). In our experience, however, segmental resections for endometriosis can be safely performed avoiding the need for a temporary ileostomy. A conservative approach can be adopted with limited dissection of the bowel mesentery so as to preserve as much of the vasculature and nerve supply as possible. Indications for a routine protecting stoma even in cases of ultralow resections (7 cm from anal verge) should be questioned and reserved only for complex operations with suspected defective anastomosis.

Outcomes

Shaving: Low complication rates have been reported using this technique with a 1.4% risk of rectal perforation in a series of 500 patients and a recurrence rate of 7%. There was a significant improvement in pelvic pain following treatment and an overall pregnancy rate of 84% (natural conception rate of 78%).

Discoid resection: This technique has been shown to be effective in the treatment of pelvic pain with associated complication rates ranging from 0% to 12.5%. Similar studies have observed no complication rates following discoid resection. A case series by Landi et al. reported no complications of sepsis or fistulas; however, a relatively high incidence of rectal bleeding requiring transfusion was noted in 7 out of 35 patients (Landi et al. 2008). Retrospective studies have

also demonstrated high patient satisfaction with improvement in symptoms such as pelvic pain and dyspareunia (Koh et al. 2012, Moawad et al. 2013).

Segmental bowel resection: Laparoscopic excision of deeply infiltrating pelvic endometriosis within a multidisciplinary setup in a tertiary referral center appears to be safe with a low rate of significant short-term complications. Observational studies have reported complications ranging from 5% to 26%. In one study, the complication rate after excluding women with uncomplicated pyrexia was only 3.2% (Pandis et al. 2010). Similarly in a large series of 750 cases of bowel resection, the overall surgical morbidity was 9% (Ruffo et al. 2012). This included rates of anastomotic leak, rectovaginal fistula, and intra-abdominal bleeding, which were 3%, 2%, and 1%, respectively (Ruffo et al. 2012).

A recent systematic review of outcomes associated with different surgical techniques of bowel endometriosis described an overall complication rate of 13.9%. This varied from 2.8% in the shaving group to 29.6% in the resection group (Moustafa & Elnasharty 2014). Conservative surgery (i.e. shaving) may carry a lower risk of major complications, although in some studies additional surgery such as ureterolysis, uterosacral ligament resection, and hysterectomy may have had an impact (Moustafa & Elnasharty 2014).

The most appropriate surgical strategy in cases of infertility related to severe endometriosis is unclear. No RCTs have assessed whether fertility improves following radical surgery for stage 3 and 4 disease, although observational studies have shown promising results. In one study, spontaneous pregnancy rate was lower in patients found to have bowel endometriosis, and in these women improved reproductive outcome was noted if bowel resection was performed (Stepniewska et al. 2009). The place for segmental bowel resection in cases of DIE in patients whose only symptom is infertility in the absence of pain has not been determined. Bowel resection is not without its risk, and the extent to which rectovaginal endometriosis affects infertility is unclear. Patients should therefore be carefully selected and counseled regarding the specific risk of complications and uncertain benefits of surgery.

Urinary endometriosis

Urinary endometriosis can be defined as the involvement of the urinary tract by an endometriotic lesion and can include bladder, ureter, kidney, and urethra. The prevalence of urinary tract involvement in patients affected by endometriosis is rare with a reported prevalence of approximately 1%. This value is likely to be underestimated as in patient series with severe endometriosis the prevalence can rise up to 20% (Kovoor et al. 2010, Gabriel et al. 2011). The proportion of urinary tract localization in patients with urinary endometriosis is bladder (84%), ureter (10%), kidney (4%), and urethra (2%) (Chapron et al. 2006, Abrao et al. 2009). Ureteric involvement occurs less frequently than bladder endometriosis (BE); however, the proportion can differ significantly between case series depending on whether extrinsic compression of the ureter is included.

The specific symptoms of urinary endometriosis are dysuria and hematuria, although it is more commonly associated with the nonspecific symptoms such as dysmenorrhea, dyspareunia, and chronic pelvic pain.

Bladder endometriosis

BE consists of deposits of endometrial glands and stroma within the serosa muscularis, and/or mucosa of the bladder. The prevalence of BE among patients affected by DIE is close to 11% and can be associated with symptoms such as dysuria (42%), hematuria (9–15%), and recurrent urinary tract infections (18%) (Gabriel et al. 2011).

Up to 50% of patients with BE have a history of previous pelvic surgery, suggesting an iatrogenic cause, typically occurring following Cesarean section. This data should be considered in cases suggestive of BE (Comiter 2002).

Preoperative workup

Preoperative workup includes urine analysis, physical examination, TVS, MRI, and cystoscopy.

Vaginal bimanual examination is not often informative, except in cases of large nodules of the vesicovaginal septum where it is possible to palpate a thickened area, or a cystic expansion that evokes pain on pressure (Le Tohic et al. 2009).

TVS is typically the first-line investigation in cases suggestive of BE, due to its low cost and availability. The examination should be performed with a moderate amount of urine in the bladder, which provides an anechoic contrast facilitating detection of the nodule. The nodule usually appears as a heterogeneous, hyperechoic, almost spherical lesion with a small number of vessels on Power-Doppler protruding into the bladder from the posterior wall of the bladder (Chamié et al. 2011).

Nowadays, MRI is the gold standard for diagnosis of BE with a sensitivity of up to 88% and specificity of up to 99%. Even if MRI is unable to provide further information with regard to BE lesions, it is useful in detecting associated lesions such as ureteric dilatation, providing a more detailed description of the pelvis (Kumar et al. 2012) (**Figure 21.5**). Cystoscopy can also be used as a cost-effective method for diagnosis. Typically lesions appear as a nodular mass at the base or dome of the bladder with a distinctive shape and associated color change, from red-brown to blue-black. For smaller lesions, however, the findings may be equivocal due to the intraperitoneal origin of the disease. Cystoscopy can also be performed intraoperatively to further assess the mucosal involvement and distance from the ureteric orifices, in order to optimize perioperative planning (shaving vs. partial bladder resection) and consider placement of double-J stents if indicated (Wattiez et al. 2013).

Surgical technique

A minimally invasive surgical approach to BE must be tailored according to invasion and depth of the lesion of the bladder. Depending on the level of involvement of the bladder, the following procedures can be considered: shaving, mucosal skinning, and partial cystectomy (progressing from superficial to more invasive disease).

Irrespective of the surgical procedure, the first step should be to restore the anatomy. The presence of the nodule can lead to retraction of the bladder onto the anterior aspect of the uterus and anterior wall with subsequent involvement of both round ligaments (**Figure 21.6**). Once the normal anatomy is restored, the BE nodule must be isolated by opening first both paravesical fossa, medial to the umbilical artery and then the vesicovaginal septum.

The shaving technique can be applied if the nodule involves only the serosa of the bladder and suturing may not be necessary if the muscularis is not compromised. Mucosal skinning and partial cystectomy are performed in cases of more extensive disease, where the detrusor muscle is involved (**Figure 21.7**). The main difference between these two techniques is that in partial cystectomy the full thickness of the muscle is transected, whereas in mucosal skinning the urothelium is preserved.

Cystoscopy may help identify bladder lesions extending to the mucosa and can assist the surgeon in deciding between the two techniques; however, often the final decision is only made intraoperatively.

In both cases, the defect must be closed using absorbable monofilament 3/0 in a single-layer suture using either intracorporeal or extracorporeal knotting techniques. Even if there is no evidence regarding interrupted and continuous suturing techniques, in our practice the interrupted approach is preferred, causing less ischemia and improving tissue healing.

At the end of the procedure, a blue dye test must be carried out to confirm bladder integrity by filing the bladder with 150–200 mL of solution. In some instances, a suture too close to the ureteric orifice can lead to kinking of the ureter. Cystoscopy is important to evaluate the distance between the sutures and the ureteric orifices and can help determine whether ureteric stenting is required.

At the end of the procedure, a Foley catheter should be left in place for minimum of 10–14 days depending on the width of the resection and the inflammatory response. Immediately prior to removal of the catheter, a low-pressure cystography can be performed to assess

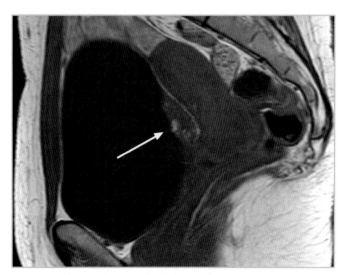

Figure 21.5 Magnetic resonance image (MRI) showing an infiltrative bladder endometriosis nodule. MRI is useful in determining presence and extent of deep infiltrating endometriosis.

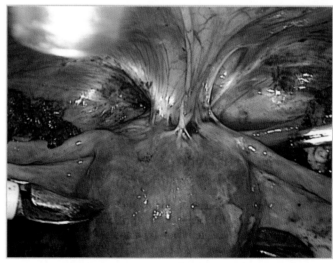

Figure 21.6 Typical laparoscopic appearance of a bladder nodule. The uterus is anteverted with bilateral retraction of both round ligaments toward the midline.

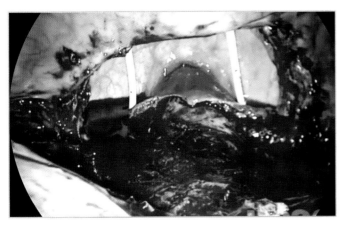

Figure 21.7 Laparoscopic view of bilateral ureteric stents following a partial cystectomy for bladder endometriosis.

integrity of the repair. If a double-J stent has been cited, and if no ureteric procedures have been performed intraoperatively, it can also be removed at the same time.

Outcomes

Following bladder resection, patients may report symptoms of urgency, describing the necessity to urinate several times per day. This sensation is temporary and normally completely resolves after a few months. Laparoscopic excision of BE leads to a significant improvement in symptoms with low recurrence rates when compared with cystoscopic resection (Kovoor et al. 2010).

Ureteral endometriosis

Ureteral endometriosis is typically unilateral and is more frequently confined to the lower third of the ureter, with a higher predisposition for the left side. Ureteral lesions are often extensions of retrocervical endometriosis and as such ureteric involvement is more commonly found in association with rectovaginal nodules and ipsilateral ueterosacral ligament involvement (Miranda-Mendoza et al. 2012).

Ureteric endometriosis can be divided into extrinsic and intrinsic disease, according to the depth of ureteral invasion occurring with a ratio of 4:1 respectively (Mereu et al. 2010). Extrinsic disease is caused by infiltration of the surrounding connective tissue and ureteral adventitia by the endometriotic nodule. Intrinsic disease, on the other hand, consists of disease infiltrating the muscularis and in some cases, the uroepithelium.

Symptoms associated with ureteral endometriosis are usually nonspecific, consisting of pelvic pain, flank pain, or renal colic and less commonly, hematuria. In up to 30% of patients, silent kidney loss can occur (Yohannes 2003).

Preoperative workup

Physical examination is not useful in predicting ureteric involvement, but it should be suspected in cases where a palpable retrocervical nodule >2 cm with uterosacral ligament involvement is present.

Ultrasound is routinely used for endometriosis screening and can be used to detect ureteral dilatation and secondary ureteral obstruction with resultant hydronephrosis. MRI can also be considered an effective diagnostic tool as it provides additional information regarding the level, extension, and degree of obstruction, in addition to a comprehensive analysis of the pelvis (Maccagnano et al. 2012). Other imaging modalities such as intravenous pyelography and ureteroscopy can be considered, although these are not commonly used in our practice.

Preoperative placement of double-J stents is not mandatory and opinions regarding its indication often differ from one expert to another. On the one hand, ureteric stents may enable easier recognition and identification of the course of the ureter, while on the other hand placement of the stent may impede dissection making it difficult to manipulate the surrounding tissue. In our practice, we do not advocate routine preoperative stent insertion, except in cases of severe obstruction, with resulting hydroureteronephrosis.

Surgical technique

Ureteral endometriosis is commonly associated with uterosacral ligament involvement and the anatomy is often distorted as a result of peritoneal inflammation caused by the disease. The first step is always to restore the normal anatomy, identify pelvic landmarks in particular the ureter in order to perform a safe ureterolysis. In some cases, identification of the ureter can be difficult, especially on the left side where it is covered by the sigmoid. To identify the ureter on the left side, the physiological attachments of the sigmoid colon should be divided and the ureter identified at the pelvic brim where it crosses the iliac vessels.

Once the ureterolysis is performed, the surgeon is able to discriminate between intrinsic and extrinsic disease. In cases of extrinsic lesions, the surgeon should be aware that fibrosis of the surrounding diseased tissue can lead to medialization of the ureter especially in its lower third. It is therefore important that the course of the ureter is followed until the ureteric channel where it crosses the parametrium.

The ureteric adventitia consists of a dense vascular network, which supplies the ureter along its course. In order to adequately resect endometriotic nodules, some of these arteries may need to be sacrificed; however, careful dissection should be performed so as to avoid complete devascularization of the ureter. If the adventitia cannot be adequately preserved as a direct result of the disease, placement of a double-J stent should be considered, to decrease the risk of fistula formation. Stent placement is also recommended in cases of persistent stenosis following removal of extrinsic lesions.

Regarding the management of intrinsic lesions, a partial ureteric resection with end-to-end anastomosis can be performed. The anastomosis can be guided by placement of a double-J stent followed by insertion of 3/4 intracorporeal stitches using 4-0 absorbable monofilament. If the lesion is located close to the bladder junction (approximately <2 cm), ureteric reimplantation should be considered. In order to perform an adequate antireflux system, a 2 cm mucosal skinning of the bladder is performed with ureteric implantation at one edge, which is then covered with the muscularis. It is important to avoid excessive tension on the anastomosis. If following resection there is inadequate ureteral length, a psoas hitch suspension of the bladder can be performed to ensure a tension-free repair.

If wide dissection of the adventitia is performed, it is recommended to leave in place a double-J stent for approximately 6–8 weeks, after which time it can be removed without the need for additional investigations. In contrast, if an end-to-end anastomosis or neoureterocystostomy is performed a urinary catheter should be left in place for a minimum of 10 days.

Outcomes

In our series of 91 women who underwent laparoscopic surgical treatment of ureteral endometriosis, we reported that in 85.7% of cases a simple ureterolysis was appropriate to treat the patients and in only 10% a resection was required (Gabriel et al. 2011). These findings are comparable with similar studies. The presence of moderate-to-severe hydronephrosis, however, can increase the risk of ureteric resection by up to 30% respectively (Mereu et al. 2010).

Surgical outcomes after 3 years of follow-up showed significant improvement in both urinary and nonspecific symptoms (Seracchioli et al. 2010).

NEW CHALLENGES

The challenge of surgical treatment of DIE is twofold: providing symptomatic relief for women often debilitated by the disease and optimizing fertility for those patients wishing to conceive immediately or in the future. The actual challenge is confounded by the fact that the disease affects younger patients who desire a later fertility. Thus, the challenge is not simply to treat infertility but to preserve future fertility.

DIE is a complex disease whose treatment has been greatly debated by experts in the field. Formerly successful surgery was dependent on aggressive excision of all the disease in a bid to remove all evidence of its presence and preserve disease-free margins. This radical approach was proposed as a means to ensure a sustainable result and reduce the risk of recurrence. With increasing awareness and understanding of endometriosis, a more individualized, patient centered approach has surfaced, with emphasis on tailoring surgery according to women's desires and expectations. This novel approach is likely to have emerged due to the increasing recognition and diagnosis of endometriosis in patients of younger age. These young women while requesting treatment of symptomatic relief also wish to safeguard their fertility, despite not choosing to conceive immediately. Surgery must therefore attempt to reconcile surgical excision with fertility preserving strategies. Disease involving the ovaries should be carefully removed to maintain ovarian reserve and a meticulous surgical approach should be adopted to minimize adhesion formation.

New challenges exist in determining which surgical technique is most favorable. Unfortunately evidence is lacking and there are few long-term follow-up studies from which any clear conclusion can be made. Further research, specifically analyzing fertility outcomes following surgical treatment of DIE, is required in order to counsel patients appropriately and recommend the most appropriate treatment of women desiring a pregnancy.

CONCLUSION

Laparoscopy has become the gold standard for the treatment of endometriosis. Image magnification using the laparoscope has made more complex procedures possible, challenging gynecologists to both develop and advance their surgical techniques. A standardized surgical approach is recommended in order to improve reproducibility, reduce operating times, and minimize complications.

REFERENCES

Abrao MS, Dias JA, Bellelis P, et al. Endometriosis of the ureter and bladder are not associated diseases. Fertil Steril 2009; 91(5):1662–1667.

Abrao MS, Gonçalves MO, Dias JA, et al. Comparison between clinical examination, transvaginal sonography and magnetic resonance imaging for the diagnosis of deep endometriosis. Hum Reprod 2007; 22(12):3092–3097.

Bazot M, Lafont C, Rouzier R, et al. Diagnostic accuracy of physical examination, transvaginal sonography, rectal endoscopic sonography, and magnetic resonance imaging to diagnose deep infiltrating endometriosis. Fertil Steril 2009; 92(6):1825–1833.

Benschop L, Farquhar C, Van Der Poel N, Heineman MJ. Interventions for women with endometrioma prior to assisted reproductive technology. Cochrane Database Syst Rev 2010; 11:CD008571.

Busacca M, Riparini J, Somigliana E, et al. Postsurgical ovarian failure after laparoscopic excision of bilateral endometriomas. Am J Obstet Gynecol 2006; 195(2):421–425.

Campagnacci R, Perretta S, Guerrieri M, et al. Laparoscopic colorectal resection for endometriosis. Surg Endosc 2005; 19(5):662–664.

Carneiro MM, Filogonia IDDS, Costa LMP, De Avila I, Fereirra MC. Accuracy of clinical signs and symptoms in the diagnosis of endometriosis. J Endometr 2010; 2(2):63–70.

Catenacci M, Sastry S, Falcone T. Laparoscopic surgery for endometriosis. Clin Obstet Gynecol 2009; 52(3):351–361.

Chamié LP, Blasbalg R, Pereira RM, Warmbrand G, Serafini PC. Findings of pelvic endometriosis at transvaginal US, MR imaging, and laparoscopy. Radiographics 2011; 31(4):E77–100.

Chapron C, Chopin N, Borghese B, et al. Deeply infiltrating endometriosis: pathogenetic implications of the anatomical distribution. Human Reproduction 2006; 21(7):1839–1845.

Chapron C, Fauconnier A, Dubuisson JB, et al. Deep infiltrating endometriosis: relation between severity of dysmenorrhoea and extent of disease. Hum Reprod 2003; 18(4):760–766.

Chapron C, Fauconnier A, Vieira M, et al. Anatomical distribution of deeply infiltrating endometriosis: surgical implications and proposition for a classification. Hum Reprod 2003; 18(1):157–161.

Comiter CV. Endometriosis of the urinary tract. Urol Clin North Am 2002; 29(3):625–635.

Dubernard G, Rouzier R, David-Montefiore E, Bazot M, Darai E. Urinary complications after surgery for posterior deep infiltrating endometriosis are related to extent of dissection and to uterosacral ligaments resection. J Minim Invasive Gynaecol 2007; 15(2):235–240.

Eriksen HL, Gunnersen KF, Sørensen JA, et al. Psychological aspects of endometriosis: differences between patients with or without pain on four psychological variables. Eur J Obstet Gynecol Reprod Biol 2008; 139(1):100–105.

Faccioli N, Foti G, Manfredi R, et al. Evaluation of colonic involvement in endometriosis: double-contrast barium enema vs. magnetic resonance imaging. Abdom Imaging 2010; 35(4):414–421.

Ferrero S, Venturini PL, Gillott DJ, Remorgida V, Leone Roberti Maggiore U. Hemostasis by bipolar coagulation versus suture after surgical stripping of bilateral ovarian endometriomas: a randomized controlled trial. J Minim Invasive Gynecol 2012; 19(6):722–730.

Gabriel B, Nassif J, Trompoukis P, Barata S, Wattiez A. Prevalence and management of urinary tract endometriosis: a clinical case series. Urology 2011; 78(6):1269–1274.

Hart RJ, Hickey M, Maouris P, Buckett W. Excisional surgery versus ablative surgery for ovarian endometriomata. Cochrane Database Syst Rev 2008; (2):CD004992.

Koh CE, Juszczyk K, Cooper MJ, Solomon MJ. Management of deeply infiltrating endometriosis involving the rectum. Dis Colon Rectum 2012; 55(9):925–931.

Kovoor E, Nassif J, Miranda-Mendoza I, Wattiez A. Endometriosis of bladder: outcomes after laparoscopic surgery. J Minim Invasive Gynecol 2010; 17(5):600–604.

Kumar S, Tiwari P, Sharma P, et al. Urinary tract endometriosis: Review of 19 cases. Urol Ann 2012; 4(1):6–12.

Landi S, Pontrelli G, Surico D, et al. Laparoscopic disk resection for bowel endometriosis using a circular stapler and a new endoscopic method to control postoperative bleeding from the stapler line. J Am Coll Surg 2008; 207(2):205–209.

Le Tohic A, Chis C, Yazbeck C, et al. Bladder endometriosis: diagnosis and treatment. A series of 24 patients. Gynecol Obstet Fertil 2009; 37(3):216–221.

Mabrouk M, Spagnolo E, Raimondo D, et al. Segmental bowel resection for colorectal endometriosis: is there a correlation between histological pattern and clinical outcomes? Hum Reprod 2012; 27(5): 1314–1319.

Maccagnano C, Pellucchi F, Rocchini L, et al. Diagnosis and treatment of bladder endometriosis: state of the art. Urol Int 2012; 89(3):249–258.

Mereu L, Gagliardi ML, Clarizia R, et al. Laparoscopic management of ureteral endometriosis in case of moderate-severe hydroureteronephrosis. Fertil Steril 2010; 93(1):46–51.

Meuleman C, Tomassetti C, D'hoore A, et al. Surgical treatment of deeply infiltrating endometriosis with colorectal involvement. Hum Reprod Update 2011; 17(3):311–326.

Miranda-Mendoza I, Kovoor E, Nassif J, Ferreira H, Wattiez A. Laparoscopic surgery for severe ureteric endometriosis. Eur J Obstet Gynecol Reprod Biol 2012; 165(2):275–279.

Moawad NS, Caplin A. Diagnosis, management, and long-term outcomes of rectovaginal endometriosis. Int J Womens Health 2013; 5:753–763.

Moustafa MM, Elnasharty MA. A systematic review of the outcome associated with different surgical technique of bowel and rectovaginal endometriosis . Gynecological Surgery 2014; 11:37-52.

Muzii L, Bellati F, Bianchi A, et al. Laparoscopic stripping of endometriomas: a randomized trial on different surgical techniques. Part II: pathological results. Hum Reprod 2005; 20(7):1987–1992.

Pandis GK, Saridogan E, Windsor AC, et al. Short-term outcome of fertility-sparing laparoscopic excision of deeply infiltrating pelvic endometriosis performed in a tertiary referral center. Fertil Steril 2010; 93(1):39–45.

Piketty M, Chopin N, Dousset B, et al. Preoperative work-up for patients with deeply infiltrating endometriosis: transvaginal ultrasonography must definitely be the first-line imaging examination. Hum Reprod 2009; 24(3):602–607.

Raffi F, Metwally M, Amer S. The impact of excision of ovarian endometrioma on ovarian reserve: a systematic review and meta-analysis. J Clin Endocrinol Metab 2012; 97(9):3146–3154.

Redwine DB. Ovarian endometriosis: a marker for more extensive pelvic and intestinal disease. Fertil Steril 1999; 72(2):310–315.

Roman H, Tarta O, Pura I, et al. Direct proportional relationship between endometrioma size and ovarian parenchyma inadvertently removed during cystectomy, and its implication on the management of enlarged endometriomas. Hum Reprod 2010; 25(6):1428–1432.

Ruffo G, Sartori A, Crippa S, et al. Laparoscopic rectal resection for severe endometriosis of the mid and low rectum: technique and operative results. Surg Endosc 2012; 26(4):1035–1040.

Seracchioli R, Mabrouk M, Montanari G, et al. Conservative laparoscopic management of urinary tract endometriosis (UTE): surgical outcome and long-term follow-up. Fertil Steril 2010; 94(3):856–861.

Stepniewska A, Pomini P, Bruni F, et al. Laparoscopic treatment of bowel endometriosis in infertile women. Hum Reprod 2009; 24(7):1619–1625.

Van Holsbeke C, Van Calster B, Guerriero S, et al. Endometriomas: their ultrasound characteristics. Ultrasound Obstet Gynecol 2010; 35(6):730–740.

Vercellini P, De Matteis S, Somigliana E, et al. Long-term adjuvant therapy for the prevention of postoperative endometrioma recurrence: a systematic review and meta-analysis. Acta Obstet Gynecol Scand 2013; 92(1):8–16.

Volpi E, Ferrero A, Sismondi P. Laparoscopic identification of pelvic nerves in patients with deep infiltrating endometriosis. Surg Endosc 2004; 18(7):1109–1112.

Wattiez A, Puga M, Albornoz J, Faller E. Surgical strategy in endometriosis. Best Pract Res Clin Obstet Gynaecol 2013; 27(3):381–392.

Yohannes P. Ureteral endometriosis. J Urol 2003; 170(1):20–25.

Chapter 22 | Management of adnexal tumors

Marco Puga, Ignacio Miranda

INTRODUCTION

The adnexa are composed of the ovary, tube, broad ligament, and the remaining embryological structures within the broad ligament. Consequently, an adnexal tumor can encompass a broad spectrum of entities from physiologic to pathologic, from benign to malignant. In addition, other intra- and retroperitoneal structures can be located in the adnexal region, making the diagnosis even more challenging (**Table 22.1**).

The overwhelming majority of these adnexal masses are benign, and the primary origin is the ovary. Ovarian parenchyma is the source of >50 different types of tumors, the most frequent being functional cysts, mature teratoma, and benign epithelial cyst or cystoadenoma. The endometrioma is also counted among the most common ovarian tumors, even if its origin is not the ovary.

Over the past decades, the use of laparoscopy has become the gold standard in the management of benign ovarian tumors (BeOT). High-level evidence demonstrates that laparoscopy significantly reduces postoperative complications, pain, days of hospitalization, and adhesions (Medeiros et al. 2009).

Several technical aspects are of paramount relevance to achieve these benefits and minimize the harm in the ovarian parenchyma during conservative surgery. In addition, strict rules should be followed when dealing with suspicious ovarian masses. The objective of this chapter is to provide the reader with an update of the best evidence of management of the benign adnexal tumors, with special emphasis on the technical aspects.

BACKGROUND

BeOT are common conditions that affect the quality of life of women worldwide and produce serious impacts on health care systems. They are associated with multiple ambulatory visits, emergency department consults, and inpatient hospitalizations (Nicholson et al. 2001, Velebil et al. 1995, Whiteman et al. 2010).

Table 22.1 Differential diagnose of adnexal tumors

	Origin	Type	Subtype
Benign	Ovarian	Non-neoplasm/functional cysts	Follicular cyst, luteal cysts, theca-luteinic cysts
		Non-neoplasm/endometriomas	
		Neoplasm/epithelial: cystadenoma	Serous, mucinous
		Neoplasm/germ cell: mature teratoma	Dermoid cyst (99%) solid mature teratoma (1%)
	Non-ovarian	Paraovarian cyst Intraligamentary myoma Hydrosalpinx, tubo-ovarian abscess Ectopic pregnancy Peritoneal pseudocysts	
	Nongynecologic	Full bladder Rectum with feces and/or gas Appendiceal abscess, mucocele Diverticulitis, abscess Pelvic kidney Retroperitoneal teratoma	Physiologic or pathologic
Malignant	Ovarian Epithelial: Cystadenocarcinoma invasive and borderline	Malignant germ cell tumor (MGCT)	Dysgerminoma, yolk sac tumor, immature teratoma, mixed MGCT
		Serous, mucinous, endometrioid, clear cells, undifferentiated, malignant Brenner tumor	
	Sex-cord/stromal tumors	Adult granulosa tumor, fibrosarcoma, lymphoma	
	Metastatic ovarian tumors	Gastrointestinal carcinoma and breast cancer with ovarian metastasis	
	Others	Colorectal carcinoma, retroperitoneal lymphoma, sarcomas, schwannomas	

According to the Royal College, up to 10% of women will undergo surgery for an ovarian tumor during their lifetime (Royal College of Obstetricians and Gynecologists 2011). In the United States, data from the Nationwide Inpatient Sample of the Healthcare Cost and Utilization Project showed that, between 1998 and 2005, there were >6 million women aged between 15 and 54 years hospitalized for a gynecologic condition as principal diagnosis. BeOT was the fourth most common etiology, accounting for almost 500,000 of these women. Seventy-three percent were submitted to some surgical procedure, ovarian surgery and hysterectomy being the two most frequent (74% and 22%, respectively). The report does not provide further information on the ovarian surgery, but, interestingly, 84% of the hysterectomies in this subset of patients were performed by laparotomy (Whiteman et al. 2010).

ETIOLOGY AND DIFFERENTIAL DIAGNOSIS

'Adnexal tumor' or 'adnexal mass' are vague terms used to denominate any increase of volume located in the adnexal region. The presence of a tumor in the adnexal region is not a guarantee of gynecologic origin or of a pathologic condition. In some cases, the tumor can correspond only to a clinical or radiological misinterpretation of normal structures, such as bowel with feces or a distended bladder. The most frequent differential diagnoses of adnexal masses are listed in **Table 22.1**.

The vast majority of these adnexal tumors are benign, and, despite the wide spectrum of etiologies, the ovary is the most frequently involved organ. BeOT can be classified as neoplastic and non-neoplastic. The former group is mainly represented by dermoid cyst and benign epithelial cyst or cystoadenoma; the latter by functional cysts and endometrioma. The Fallopian tube is not a frequent source of tumors, but it can be affected by pelvic inflammatory disease and tubal pregnancy. In the broad ligament, the two most frequent findings are paraovarian cysts and the presence of intraligamentary myomas. The most relevant aspects of BeOT are described in the following sections.

OVARIAN TUMORS
Functional cysts

During the reproductive years, incidental finding of an adnexal mass frequently corresponds to normal ovarian structures such as pre-ovulatory follicles and corpus luteum. In some instances, the spontaneous or induced ovulation process is incorrect, resulting in follicular or luteal cysts, which are called functional cysts.

Functional cysts are, in general, self-limited in size but can reach up to 10 cm, producing symptoms by compression. They are usually unilateral and present as a simple unilocular cyst with regular walls on ultrasound. Because they are associated with an altered ovulation process, menstrual disorders are frequently reported. Functional cysts often resolve spontaneously over the course of 4–6 weeks, and expectant management with ultrasound surveillance is the best alternative. The use of combined oral contraceptives in the treatment of functional cysts has been a source of conflict. A recent Cochrane review shows that treatment with combined oral contraceptives did not hasten resolution. In addition, persistent cysts tended to be pathological (e.g. cystoadenomas, endometrioma, or paraovarian cyst) and not physiological (Grimes et al. 2009).

Occasionally, functional cysts can experience internal hemorrhage, torsion, or rupture, and surgery is warranted. Laparoscopy is an ideal tool for persistent cysts and – in case of complication, because it permits both – certifying diagnosis and performing treatment.

Endometrioma

Endometriosis is a common condition affecting at least 10% of women in their reproductive years (Brown & Farquhar 2014). The ovarian involvement is identified in almost 50% of cases (Medeiros et al. 2009). Endometriomas rarely exceed 10 cm and are bilateral in half of the cases (Disaia & Creasman 2012). The lumen contains blood, mostly of dark color, that gives it a characteristic aspect (chocolate cyst). They typically remain adherent to the surrounding structures; hence, they are not prone to torsion. Pain and infertility are the two most frequent complaints of these patients (Wattiez et al. 2013). The laparoscopic treatment of endometrioma is the gold standard, and excisional surgery (cystectomy) has demonstrated better outcomes than ablative treatment (Hart et al. 2008). It is important to consider when planning the surgery that endometrioma can be associated with endometriosis elsewhere. In fact, about one-third of the cases of bilateral endometriomas coexist with deep infiltrating endometriosis (DIE). Consequently, surgeons must be prepared to perform comprehensive management of the disease and not only cyst treatment (**Figure 22.1**).

The origin of the endometrioma is not clear but probably is secondary to deposits of endometriotic tissue in the ovarian surface that produce inflammation, adherence of the ovary to the peritoneum, and progressive folding inward of the ovarian cortex. Therefore, the endometrioma corresponds to a pseudocyst (false cyst) because its wall is the inverted ovarian surface. The relevance of this goes beyond academic discussion; the removal of the endometrioma implies the removal of ovarian tissue, with potential harm to the patient's ovarian reserve (Medeiros et al. 2009).

Dermoid cyst

Dermoid cyst or cystic mature teratoma is the most frequent neoplasm of the ovary. It accounts for 27–44% of all ovarian neoplasms and 58% of benign neoplasms of the ovary (**Figure 22.2**). This tumor is frequently diagnosed during the first two decades of life; only 5% of cases affect postmenopausal women (Tavassoli & Devilee 2003). Dermoid cysts are rarely large (typically <10 cm) and are often bilateral (15–25%) (Disaia & Creasman 2012). This is a tumor frequently associated with adnexal torsion (AT); Comerci et al. (1994) reported 3.5% of patients had torsions among 517 cases of cystic teratomas (see 'Special Cases: Adnexal Torsion').

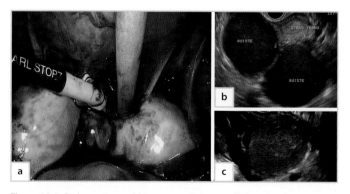

Figure 22.1 Endometriomas. (a) Laparoscopic image of bilateral endometriomas (kissing ovaries) associated with deep infiltrating endometriosis (DIE) of the rectovaginal septum. One of the cysts is opened as a result of the dissection and is draining classic chocolate-colored content. (b) Ultrasound image of bilateral endometriomas in another case of kissing ovaries associated to DIE. (c) Left endometrioma surrounded by peritoneal liquid and pelvic adhesions.

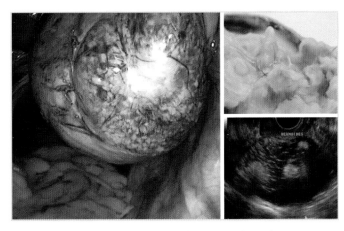

Figure 22.2 Dermoid cyst. Laparoscopic, ultrasonography, and macroscopic aspects of a dermoid cyst.

Dermoid cysts are benign tumors; however, malignant degeneration to a teratoma has been reported in 1% of cases, mainly in postmenopausal women. Among them, the most frequent are squamous carcinoma and adenocarcinoma (Disaia & Creasman 2012). The presence of immature teratoma is also possible, but rare. In addition, 15–25% of patients with malignant germ cell tumors have a teratoma in the contralateral ovary (Tavassoli & Devilee 2003).

Laparoscopic excision of the teratoma is the gold standard treatment. Special attention must be paid to avoid spilling its contents because of the risk of granulomatous peritonitis. This complication is considered rare. In a recent review of >300 cases managed by laparoscopy, only two patients (0.6%) experienced peritonitis out of 26 with intraperitoneal spillage. Interestingly, when an endoscopic bag was utilized, there were no cases of spillage and no peritonitis (Kondo et al. 2010). In our practice, prophylactic use of endoscopic bags is recommended during the entire procedure, from dissection until specimen retrieval.

Benign epithelial tumors or cystoadenomas

Epithelial tumors are the second most frequent ovarian benign neoplasm and are mainly represented by serous and mucinous cystoadenomas. Serous cystoadenomas account for 16% of all epithelial neoplasms and 25% of benign epithelial neoplasms (Bereck & Hacker 2000, Tavassoli & Devilee 2003). They affect women in the fourth to sixth decades of life. Their size fluctuates between 1 and 10 cm, although they occasionally can be larger (Tavassoli & Devilee 2003). Serous cystadenomas are bilateral in 15–20% of cases. The tumor surface is smooth, but papillary projections can exist within the internal wall. Many serous cystoadenomas are asymptomatic and are discovered incidentally during routine examination. They present usually as a simple cyst in the ultrasound, in many cases indistinguishable from a functional cyst, and they are differentiated because they persist during follow-up. Less frequently, they are multiloculated or debut with a complication such as torsion or hemorrhage (Disaia & Creasman 2012).

Mucinous cystoadenomas are the second most frequent type of this group. They present predominantly in between the third and fifth decades of life. Mucinous cystoadenomas are the largest among the ovarian neoplasms and may reach up to 20–30 cm in size. Only 2–3% are bilateral (Bereck & Hacker 2000). The surface is usually smooth, and the presence of internal papillae is rarely noted (Disaia & Creasman 2012). They are frequently multiloculated and filled with viscous mucinous material (Tavassoli & Devilee 2003).

Other adnexal tumors

Other frequent benign conditions in the differential diagnosis include inflammatory enlargement of the fallopian tubes and ovaries due to pelvic inflammatory disease (hydrosalpinx, tubo-ovarian abscess) and ectopic pregnancy (Nezhat et al. 2008). Additionally, the paraovarian cyst is a frequent differential diagnosis, distinguished from other simple cysts such as functional cysts and cystoadenomas. But BeOT are not always cysts. Fibroma and fibrothecoma are common solid tumor in postmenopausal women. Their size is variable, and they are characterized by a firm consistency. Different from malignant tumors, the vascularization is scant and they do not present areas of necrosis. The main differential diagnosis is a pedunculated or intraligamentary myoma. In some cases, fibromas can be bilateral and associated with ascites and hydrothorax in the so-called Meige's syndrome. This is a rare benign condition that can be misinterpreted as an advanced stage of ovarian carcinoma. During the two first decades of life, the presence of a solid tumor is infrequent and highly pathologic. Diagnosis of dysgerminoma must be ruled out; this is the most frequent malignancy among children and adolescents and presents as solid tumor, unilateral in 90% of the cases. Dysgerminoma is also the one of the most frequent invasive cancers diagnosed during pregnancy (Disaia & Creasman 2012).

In certain instances, the adnexal mass is the result of nongynecologic causes. Full bladder and stools in the bowel constitute a frequent differential diagnosis. Several congenital, tumoral, or inflammatory processes can affect the bowel and retroperitoneum, producing masses located in the adnexal region.

DIAGNOSIS

Regardless of the multiple possible etiologies, the most important differential diagnosis and the purpose of the study should be to rule out malignancy (**Figure 22.3**). A thorough medical history and physical examination are mandatory in the evaluation of adnexal masses. A detailed analysis of the preoperative work-up exceeds the scope of this chapter; nevertheless, some relevant issues must be discussed.

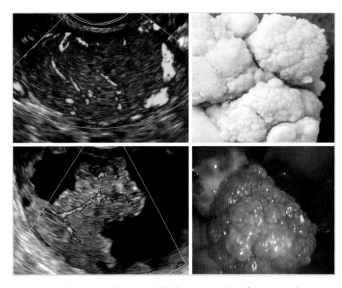

Figure 22.3 Ovarian malignancies. (a) Ultrasonography of ovarian malignant carcinoma, predominantly solid and highly vascularized. (b) Ultrasonography of a serous borderline tumor. Internal solid projection with a central vascular axis in the power Doppler study. (c) Internal surface of a serous borderline tumor. Notice the cauliflower-like papillary structures. (d) External surface of a micropapillary serous borderline tumor.

Tumor markers

CA125 is the most widely used tumor marker in the assessment of adnexal tumors. According to the American College of Obstetrics and Gynecology (ACOG), overall reported sensitivities for malignancy detection varies from 61% to 90% and specificities from 71% to 93% (ACOG 2007). The relative proportion of malignancy in the studied population, the number of postmenopausal women included, and the threshold of CA125 utilized mainly influence this wide range of variation.

In premenopausal women, CA125 is an unreliable tool to discriminate between benign and malignant disease (Royal College of Obstetricians and Gynaecologists). Lack of specificity and increased rate of false positives are associated with unnecessary invasive procedures and laparotomies. CA125 can be elevated in physiologic events such as pregnancy and menses and in numerous benign conditions frequently found during the reproductive years, such as functional cysts, endometriosis, myomas, pelvic inflammatory disease, and the like. After menopause, many of these conditions disappear, and the predictive positive value of the test improves (ACOG 2007). Nevertheless, the sensitivity of the test is limited. CA125 is elevated in 80% of epithelial carcinomas, but only in 50% of the initial stages, and it is generally normal in mucinous and non-epithelial cases. As a result, its utility is limited as screening test (ACOG 2007, Jacobs et al. 1990).

Results of CA125 should be taken cautiously and interpreted as a whole with the clinical features and image studies. For instance, the determination of CA125 can be omitted in young patient with an ultrasound diagnosis of simple cyst (Royal College of Obstetricians and Gynaecologists 2011). Alternatively, the advice of a gynecologist oncologist is recommended in premenopausal patients with adnexal masses and CA125 levels above 200 UI/L despite the low specificity of the test (ACOG 2007, Royal College of Obstetricians and Gynaecologists 2011). In postmenopausal patients, increased levels of CA125 should be considered pathologic, and this is an indication for referring patients to centers that have a gynecologist oncologist present (ACOG 2007, Im et al. 2005, Royal College of Obstetricians and Gynaecologists 2011).

Serum markers for germ cell malignancy such as α-fetoprotein (α-FP), human chorionic gonadotropin (hCG), and lactate dehydrogenase (LDH) are recommended in patients <40 years.

Ultrasound and malignancy index

Transvaginal ultrasound (TVUS) is the single most effective test in the evaluation of an adnexal mass. Several studies have shown that morphologic evaluation of a cyst is accurate in diagnosing the most frequent etiologies of BeOT (Jermy et al. 2001, Valentin 1999, Valentin et al. 2006). In addition, subjective assessment of grayscale and color Doppler ultrasound images by an experienced operator (pattern recognition) allows discrimination between malignant and benign tumors with high accuracy, >90% (Timmerman et al. 1999, Valentin 1999).

The improved quality of ultrasonography has been associated in randomized controlled trials (RCTs) with a measurable effect in the management of adnexal disease. Expert ultrasound assessment of adnexal tumor is associated with increased access to minimally invasive techniques and a reduced number of unnecessary laparotomies and reduced days of hospital stay (Yazbek et al. 2008).

The main limitation is that the results are closely related to the experience of the operator, and these abilities are not simple to transmit to younger specialists (Van Holsbeke et al. 2009). Several models and scores have been created to overcome this limitation and have achieved good results (Ameye et al. 2009, Berlanda et al. 2002, Lerner et al. 1994, Timmerman et al. 2005).However, often these models are created and validated by experts as well, and performance is reduced when they are applied by inexperienced examiners (Van Holsbeke et al. 2009).

The International Ovarian Tumor Analysis (IOTA) study group has created a two-tiered approach based on 10 ultrasound characteristics for discrimination between benign and malignant tumors, the so-called Simple Rules. They are designed to be used by less experienced operators. The Simple Rules are applicable in three-quarters of patients, with a sensitivity and specificity of 92% and 96%, respectively (Timmerman et al. 2008). If the rules do not apply, the patient should be referred for ultrasonography by an expert. This two-tiered approach yields a global sensitivity of 91% and specificity of 93% (Timmerman et al. 2010). Currently, the Royal College of Obstetrics and Gynaecologists (RCOG) integrated the use of the Simple Rules in their recommendations for the management of adnexal tumors in premenopausal women.

Two indexes for malignancy should be mentioned. First, the Risk of Ovarian Malignancy Algorithm (ROMA) is based on a combination of CA125 and HE4 (human epididymis secretory protein 4) serum markers (Moore et al. 2008). The second is the Risk Malignancy Index (RMI), an algorithm based on CA125 levels, menopausal status, and ultrasound variables (Jacobs et al. 1990). The latter is used worldwide and recommended by the National Institute for Health and Clinical Excellence (NICE) and RCOG to evaluate patient with suspected ovarian malignancy (Royal College of Obstetricians and Gynaecologists 2011, National Institute for Health and Clinical Excellence 2011). Following this recommendation, an interesting analysis comparing the ROMA, the RMI, and subjective assessment by ultrasound was published. The authors found that pattern recognition has the best ability to discriminate between benign growths and malignancy, with a sensitivity of 96.7% and specificity of 90.2%, an NPV 97.6%, a PPV 86.8%, +LR 9.84, −LR 0.04 (Van Gorp et al. 2012). In addition, the performance of the RMI and IOTA models were compared in 1938 women undergoing surgery for an ovarian mass at 21 centers. The IOTA Model was superior to the RMI in correctly diagnosing benign and malignant disease. The authors concluded that LR2 would avoid major surgery for more women with benign tumors and that more women would have been referred to a gynecological oncologist with an invasive tumor (Van Calster et al. 2012). In a recent meta-analysis and review of the literature including 19 models with external validation in 96 studies, the Simple Rules and the IOTA Logistic model were superior to all others including the RMI (Kaijser et al. 2014a).

The routine use of CT and MRI is not superior to TVUS, and they are not recommended in the initial evaluation of adnexal masses (ACOG 2007, Royal College of Obstetricians and Gynaecologists 2011). The main role of CT is to diagnose peritoneal and retroperitoneal metastasis when malignancy is suspected. MRI could be a good alternative in the 6–8% of tumors difficult to classify by TVUS, even if there is lack of consensus (Kaijser et al. 2014b).

In conclusion, the optimal assessment of adnexal masses is obtained with subjective evaluation by an expert. Alternatively, based on the evidence of recent meta-analyses, the use of the Simple Rules and LR2 can produce similar results. For the small group of tumors that are difficult to classify by experts, a second-line test is still missing. The accuracy of the expert in this subset of patients is lower (70%), and no other US-based model or algorithm has improved diagnosis. Evidence from well-designed trials using MRI could be interesting and should be encouraged. For the moment, considering the 30% risk of malignancy among this unclassified group, laparoscopic management should respect the oncologic rules of suspicious adnexal masses and guarantee adequate staging in case of malignancy.

MANAGEMENT

General

Goals

As previously mentioned, the vast majority of adnexal masses are benign, and among them the functional cysts are the most common. Consequently, the main principle underlying management in premenopausal women is to be conservative. A young woman submitted to oophorectomy for benign disease still carries a risk of 3–15% for contralateral ovarian neoplasm or torsion (Bristow et al. 2006). Utmost effort should be made to spare patients with functional cysts from surgery.

Considering the current evidence, the management of the BeOT must be laparoscopic, and laparotomy should be avoided whenever possible. The objective must be the complete resection of the tumor with minimal harm to the normal tissue to avoid impairment of the ovarian reserve. Meticulous technique cannot be overemphasized. The correct dissection in the cleavage plane is the best way to minimize the resection of normal ovarian tissue. In addition, it permits the identification of the nutrition vessels of the tumor and allows the surgeon to perform a selective coagulation in order to reduce thermic damage. In cases of emergency by acute abdomen, torsion, or hemorrhage, solid evidence also supports the role of laparoscopic management. Interestingly, the literature shows that gynecologists are 8–15 times more prone to perform conservative treatment compared with other specialists (general surgeons, pediatric surgeon) in emergency situations such as ovarian torsion. Furthermore, the use of laparoscopy in those cases was three times more frequent in the hands of gynecologists (Eskander et al. 2011).

In postmenopausal patients, BeOT usually corresponds to benign neoplasm, and general management consists of laparoscopic oophorectomy or adnexectomy. Considering recent evidence showing the tube as the origin of an important number of high-grade epithelial ovarian carcinomas, we prefer adnexectomy to oophorectomy (Anderson et al. 2013, Crum et al. 2007, Kindelberger et al. 2007, Kurman & Shih 2010). In addition, we perform prophylactic contralateral salpingectomy at the time of adnexectomy (Dietl et al. 2011). Contralateral oophorectomy in postmenopausal women with cystoadenomas can be considered. The main argument in favor is the possibility of a metachromic contralateral cystoadenoma, which is a frequent event in serous cystoadenomas, and the possibility of future ovarian malignancy (Tavassoli & Devilee 2003). If the uterus is normal, we do not routinely perform hysterectomy.

In cases of suspected malignancy, the objective of treatment is the complete resection of the tumor, avoiding rupture and spillage, and a comprehensive surgical staging if malignancy is proved. Therefore, management should be in hands of a surgeon with the competence of a gynecologist oncologist. Surgical management of ovarian tumor finally resulting in cancer by a non-oncologist is associated more frequently with incomplete staging. This is a fact independent of the use of the laparoscope. It was reported almost 30 years ago by McGowan (1985) and continues today (Grabowski et al. 2012). Increasing evidence shows the feasibility and safety of the laparoscopic management of this subset of patients, but proper knowledge and training are required to offer the best treatment to these patients. The role of laparoscopy in ovarian cancer is thoroughly analyzed in other chapters of this book.

Laparoscopy: benefits and harms

Since Semm introduced laparoscopy in the management of adnexal masses in the 1970s, substantial evidence has demonstrated its benefits over laparotomy (Semm 1980). RCTs have systematically shown reduction in pain, use of analgesics, and postoperative morbidity; shorter inpatient hospital stays; faster recovery; and fewer adhesions (Medeiros et al. 2009, Canis et al. 1994, 2002, Yuen et al. 1997). A systematic review published by Cochrane including 12 RCTs compared laparoscopy with laparotomy in the treatment of BeOT (Medeiros et al. 2009). In the analysis of postoperative pain, laparoscopy was associated with a significant reduction in visual analog scale (VAS) scores [WMD 2.25, 95% CI (–2.94,–1.56)] and an increase in patients pain-free at 24–48 hours after surgery [Peto OR 5.87, 95% CI (3.48, 9.9)]. Only two of the reports included analyzed the use of analgesics in postoperative settings; one of them found a statistically significant difference favoring laparoscopy. Although surgically related adverse effects were not frequent, laparoscopy was associated with an overall reduction in any adverse events of surgery (surgical injury, postoperative complications, and any other adverse events of surgery; [Peto OR 0.3, 95% CI (0.18,0.52)]. Hospital stay was also significantly reduced by laparoscopy, by almost 3 days [WMD –2.90, 95% CI (–3.28, –2.52)]. No conclusion can be drawn from the analysis of operative time due to the high heterogeneity of the studies and variables involved (type of tumor, size, unilateral-bilateral, technique, surgeon experience, frozen section necessity, etc.). Regarding the harms, there were no cases of readmission in any trial. Only two studies mentioned isolated recurrences in a short follow-up period, without differences between the groups. Tumoral rupture is probably the most relevant harm of the technique. Laparoscopy has been consistently associated with higher rates of tumoral rupture and secondary spillage compared with laparotomy, and this was also confirmed in the Cochrane review. The adverse effect of spillage in BeOT is mainly reserved for dermoid cysts and the possibility of granulomatous peritonitis. As previously mentioned, the incidence of this complication is low and can be safely prevented by adequate technique and use of endoscopic bags (Kondo et al. 2010). The main concerns rise when the spillage occurs during the management of a suspicious tumor. In case of malignancy, data supporting worse prognosis in patients with capsule rupture as the sole adverse factor are controversial (Bakkum-Gamez et al. 2009, Kim et al. 2013, Prat et al. 2014, Vergote et al. 2001). Regardless of the lack of consensus, ovarian cancers with capsule rupture are classified as stage IC, and chemotherapy is generally recommended (Prat et al. 2014, National Comprehensive Cancer Network 2014). Therefore, utmost effort should be paid to avoid tumoral rupture whenever possible. Technique cannot be put ahead of the welfare of the patient.

Increasing awareness has been focused recently on the detrimental effect of conservative treatments on the ovarian reserve. Ovarian parenchyma has been identified in up to 54% of the specimens of endometrioma (Muzii et al. 2002). Furthermore, 2.4% of women submitted to bilateral endometrioma resection experienced ovarian failure (Busacca et al. 2006) The harm is not exclusive to endometrioma or to laparoscopy, and it is highly related to technical aspects analyzed further in this chapter.

In addition to all the benefits, to become universally accepted, a surgical technique must be feasible to use in regular daily practice by general surgeons and not only by experts. In the past few decades, the vast majority of techniques used in laparotomy for adnexal surgery were replicated and frequently improved on with the use of the laparoscope. These techniques are, in general, simple and easy to learn; consequently, gynecologists rapidly integrate them into their practice.

Finally, cost is also a relevant issue when integrating a technique as a gold standard. Laparoscopy has been associated with a decrease in global costs due to reduction in hospital stay, rapid recovery, and labor reintegration. In the above-mentioned Cochrane review (Medeiros 2009), the cost of laparoscopic surgery was US$1000 less expensive per patient compared to laparotomy, but this conclusion is based only on one study. These analyses should be considered cautiously because many factors are involved and vary between populations and health care systems.

Indications and contraindications

Management of adnexal tumors can be expectant or surgical. In some cases, the surgical indication is obvious and cannot be postponed (e.g. when ovarian torsion is suspected). In others, the decision is not clear, and benefits and risk must be balanced and discussed with the patient. The main indications of surgery for adnexal masses are listed in **Table 22.2**.

Patients with suspicious ovarian tumors have an undoubted surgical indication. Clinical or ultrasound characteristics of malignancy warrant surgical exploration and the participation of a gynecologic oncologist on the team. CA125 values of >35 UI/L during postmenopause and >200 UI/L in premenopause are not a surgical indication by themselves, but referral to an oncologist is recommended. Patients presenting with acute abdomen, tumor rupture, active hemorrhage, or AT are unquestionable candidates for surgery, as well.

Regarding the most frequent BeOT, surgery is recommended in symptomatic endometriomas or in tumors of sizes >30 mm (Wattiez et al. 2013). Dermoid cysts have shown to grow over time, increasing the risk of pain and acute complication; consequently surgery is indicated (Royal College of Obstetricians and Gynaecologists 2011). Functional cysts and cystoadenomas present frequently as a simple cyst and, in some cases, can be impossible to differentiate with ultrasound. Surgery in these patients is based mainly on tumor size and

Table 22.2 Main indication of surgery of adnexal tumors

Suspicious tumors
Symptoms and physical examination suggesting cancer
Ultrasound: malignancy suspected (M rules, patter recognition, LR2 algorithm, RMI) and Unclassifiable tumors
CA125: >35 UI/L postmenopausal and >200 UI/L in premenopausal are indications of evaluation for a gynecologist oncologist (see section on 'Indications and contraindications')
Acute complications
Torsion (or suspicion)
Active hemorrhage
Rupture
Endometrioma >30 mm or symptomatic
Dermoid cyst
Simple cysts (see section on 'Indications and contraindications')
Size >70 mm
50–70 mm persistent in follow-up
Growth up or appearance of suspicious findings in US
Symptomatic
Differential diagnoses and management of specific pathologies
Pelvic inflammatory disease (tubo-ovarian abscess, symptomatic hydrosalpinx or previous IVF)
Intraligamentary myoma
Paraovarian symptomatic cyst
Ectopic pregnancy
RMI, risk malignancy index; US, ultrasonography; IVF, in vitro fertilization

the evolution of the cysts during follow-up. There is not an evidence-based size to indicate surgery. Generally, simple cysts of <50 mm are predominantly functional, and many guidelines and societies do not recommend further investigation (Levine et al. 2010). Simple cysts of 50–70 mm diameter that persist or increase size during follow-up are more frequently nonfunctional, and surgery is indicated. Evidently, the apparition of solid projections or other signs of malignancy during surveillance make surgery compulsory. Simple cysts >70 mm are accepted as an indication of surgery because they more possibly correspond to neoplasms and because of the risk of torsion (Royal College of Obstetricians and Gynaecologists 2011).

Contraindications of laparoscopic management of adnexal tumors are as follows:
- Anesthetic contraindications for laparoscopy (absolute)
- Inexperienced surgeon or inappropriate equipment (absolute)
- Suspicious tumors >10 cm
- Solid tumors >7 cm

Manipulation of cysts >10 cm is not simple; when this cyst corresponds to a suspicious tumor, the benefits and risk must be balanced. Laparoscopy also can be the first approach in the management of larger solid tumors when the possibility of an intraligamentary myoma cannot be ruled out. Nevertheless, if during surgery a solid tumor of the ovary is proved, oophorectomy and complete extraction is mandatory. Solid tumors >6 cm are difficult to extract through the vagina, and a laparotomy is required. This situation cannot be unexpected; it should be clearly anticipated, discussed with the patient, and the surgical route should be adapted to obtain the major benefit for the patient.

Informed consent

A careful discussion with the patient is fundamental prior to all types of surgery. The decision-making process should integrate and be adapted to the pathology and patient's goals. The pros and cons of the surgery and the route should be analyzed. Even if the conservative approach is the goal, the possibility of oophorectomy must be discussed. The risk of malignancy, the requirement of surgical staging, and the possibility of conversion should be clearly stated in patients with suspicious tumors. The benefits and harms of oophorectomy and adnexectomy should be analyzed in patients >50 years and postmenopausal.

Surgical management
Preoperative preparation

We prescribe a 5-day low-residue regimen to our patients in order to reduce intestinal peristalsis and improve the exposure of the field. In cases of endometrioma, special attention should be paid to the possibility of DIE that requires further preoperative indications (see Chapter 21, Laparoscopic treatment of endometriosis). Mechanical bowel preparation (MBP) is not recommended. In cases of suspicious ovarian tumors that could end up with a staging procedure, the only possible benefits of MBP could be improved visualization. Evidence from systematic reviews and meta-analyses of RCTs has failed to detect any benefits of MBP. Furthermore, MBP has been associated with increased risk of fistula and *Clostridium* infection (Guenaga et al. 2005, Kushnir & Diaz-Montes 2013, Slim et al. 2004).

General strategy

Surgical strategy is a key factor in the success of surgery, regardless of the complexity of the procedure. Simple details can simplify surgery and improve the surgeon's performance. In addition, the systematization of the steps makes surgery replicable and facilitates the learning process for young surgeons. Here, relevant technical aspects of the surgery of adnexal masses are analyzed.

The use of a uterine manipulator is not mandatory, but recommended. It can be helpful to improve exposure in cases of large tumors or unexpected pelvic adhesions and to assess tubal patency.

First entry should be tailored according to surgical antecedents and the size of the tumor. When adhesions are suspected, we prefer to perform a pneumoperitoneum with a Veress needle in the Palmer's point and test periumbilical adhesions with a syringe preloaded with physiologic solution (Wattiez et al. 2012). Alternatively, the open or Hasson technique can be utilized. The same alternatives are useful in cases of large tumors (>10 cm).

The use of 3 mm ancillary trocars is an interesting option in the management of BeOT. RCTs have demonstrated a reduction in pain and the use of analgesics when compared with traditional 5 mm trocars (Fagotti et al. 2011, Ghezzi et al. 2005). Surgical performance is not affected nor is the operative time. Size reduction to a 5 mm telescope could be considered in average cases because the umbilicus is a frequent source of pain. Nevertheless, the main limitation of this approach is the route for the extraction of specimens.

After the introduction of the laparoscope, the procedure starts with a thorough inspection of the cavity. The evaluation of the abdomen is not restricted to suspicious tumors. This examination permits the confirmation of the diagnosis, the real evaluation of the disease, and the adaptation of surgical strategy. Regardless of the preoperative evaluation, surgeons can face unexpected findings during surgery. If an unsuspected malignancy is found during the inspection, decision-making is based mainly on the expertise/qualification of the surgeon and the surgical alternatives discussed during the informed consent. In some cases, the best alternative consists in peritoneal cytology, peritoneal biopsy representative of the carcinomatosis, and a detailed report of the location of the implants. This approach will benefit the patient by establishing the diagnosis and permitting referral for oncologic management without any detriment to the prognosis. This is also prudent in cases when a surgeon faces an unexpected frozen pelvis or undiagnosed DIE. It is always possible to push the surgical limits providing we don't harm our patients (*Primum non nocere*).

Surgical management is pursued with adhesiolysis, if adnexal adhesions are identified. This gives mobility to the adnexa and protects the surrounding organs during the dissection. Additionally, it permits complete evaluation of the tumor surface to rule out the presence of excrescences or suspicious vascularization. During the adhesiolysis, unintended rupture of cysts can occur. This is a frequent and harmless event in the management of endometriomas. However, it is undesirable during the management of a suspicious tumor and should be avoided whenever possible. Unfortunately, malignant tumors are prone to present with heavy adhesions, and this has been associated with increased risk of intraoperative rupture (OR = 2) (Kim et al. 2013). The use of endoscopic bags is limited during this step; consequently, thorough dissection of adhesions and prudence are recommended.

Specific strategy

Puncture and aspiration, cystectomy, oophorectomy, and adnexectomy are the most frequent techniques used in the management of BeOT.

Puncture and aspiration

Laparoscopic puncture and aspiration as a sole treatment of a simple cyst is not recommended due to its high rate of recurrence (53–84%) (Royal College of Obstetricians and Gynaecologists 2011). It might be considered in cases of functional cyst that end up in surgery (e.g. in ovarian torsion). Puncture and drainage can be utilized in some cases

previous to cystectomy to facilitate manipulation. In other instances, after an oophorectomy or cystectomy with intact capsule, the tumor can be aspirated inside an endoscopic bag to reduce its size.

The procedure can be done by means of an endoscopic needle or a suction-irrigation cannula (**Figure 22.4a** and **c**). In cases of endometrioma and paraovarian cysts, we do not use an endoscopic bag. When dealing with cysts suggestive of cystadenoma, we prefer to perform the puncture inside a bag. In postmenopausal women or in patients with any risk of malignancy, the use of endoscopic bags is mandatory.

Technique

The ovary is fixed against the uterus and the surface of the ovary is grasped on the anti-mesenteric side. A small incision in the ovarian surface can make grasping the ovarian cortex easier and facilitates cannula entry. Puncture is performed between the forceps of the surgeon and the assistant. Once the cyst is drained, the incision is enlarged and the inner surface of the cyst is carefully inspected. Alternatively, the cyst can be directly perforated by means of a trocar and then the suction-irrigation introduced through this trocar (**Figure 22.4b**). The use of balloon trocars may be used for this purpose because the balloon inflated inside the cyst can block the trocar and reduce spillage (Vizza et al. 2011).

Cystectomy

The objective of cystectomy is the complete enucleation of the cyst with minimal trauma to the ovarian parenchyma. The procedure can be performed while maintaining the cyst's capsule intact or after cyst drainage. The latter might be intentional in cases of large cysts, e.g. to facilitate manipulation. Alternatively, spontaneous drainage can occur, frequently as a result of the dissection in endometriomas (**Figure 22.1a**). No matter which technique is utilized, the basic principle is to respect the cleavage plane, which facilitates the dissection, reduces bleeding, and minimizes ovarian harm.

Technique

The cystectomy with intact capsule is recommended for dermoid cysts and can be used in cases of low-risk suspicious tumors providing the manipulation is performed inside a bag. After the bag is located under the cyst, a longitudinal incision is performed in the anti-mesenteric

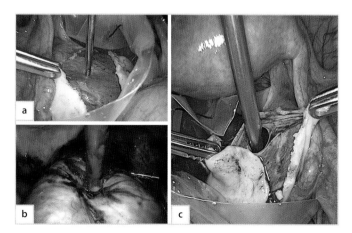

Figure 22.4 Ovarian puncture. (a) Cystoadenoma punctured in an endoscopic bag by means of an endoscopic needle. The incision in the ovarian surface facilitates grasping the ovary. (b) A 12 cm simple cyst is directly punctured with a 10 mm trocar. (c) Ovarian parenchyma is grasped with EndoCinch and atraumatic forceps (Johan), and the content of the cyst is aspirated by means of the irrigation-suction device.

border of the ovary. The borders of the ovary are held by grasping forceps. The cleavage plane is identified and dissected by the successive opening and closing of a round-tip instrument. An irrigation-suction probe can also be used for this purpose. Traction and countertraction are applied on the borders of the incision to exteriorize the cyst (**Figure 22.5**). Gentle pressure on the uterine surface can be helpful. In cases of teratoma, the weight of the cyst under gravity helps to detach it from the ovarian bed. If spillage secondary to unintended rupture of a teratoma occurs, meticulous lavage with warm fluids is recommended. The use of warm solutions avoids solidification of fat and facilitates its extraction.

In endometriomas, cystoadenomas, and paraovarian cysts, we prefer controlled puncture before the cystectomy. Afterward, the borders of the incision are examined to differentiate the ovary and the capsule. If the borders are not clear, the incision must be enlarged by means of cold scissors to obtain a sharp cut. Correct identification of the cleavage plane is the crucial point to simplify the surgery. Grasping forceps are used to exert traction and countertraction in the ovary and the capsule. While the cyst is detached from the ovarian parenchyma, small vessels along the plane can be identified and selectively coagulated. We prefer the use of grasping forceps with small teeth to exert more traction on the cyst and a blunt (nontraumatic) forceps for the ovary. In large cysts, after successive traction, sometimes the differentiation of cyst and ovary is not simple. In these cases, it is recommended that both surgeon and assistant agree who is going to handle the ovary and who the cyst during the procedure.

In endometriosis, a useful maneuver is to turn the cyst inside out by grasping the bottom of the endometrioma and pulling it out of the ovary (**Figure 22.5c**). As a result, the complete surface of the cyst is exposed. Afterward, a superficial incision is performed to divide the cyst in two. Both extremes are grasped with forceps and stripped out from the ovarian parenchyma (Wattiez et al. 2014). In cases of coexisting DIE in the posterior compartment, we leave the cystectomy for the end of the surgery. The objective is twofold: perform first the most complex steps of the surgery and avoid blood pollution of the surgical field when working.

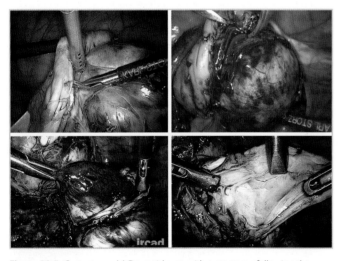

Figure 22.5 Cystectomy. (a) Dermoid cyst, with cystectomy following the cleavage plane using the irrigation-suction device. (b) Serous cysts. Cystectomy with intact capsule dissection; the cleavage plane is developed by successively opening and closing a round-tip scissors. Endometrioma is turned inside out by grabbing the bottom and pulling it out of the ovary. Endometrium is stripped out from the ovary by traction and countertraction between three graspers.

Short applications of bipolar coagulation are recommended for hemostasis of active vessels. Enthusiastic coagulation must be avoided in order to reduce thermal damage. In many cases, the time invested in rinsing the cavity or assessing the tubal patency is enough for the spontaneous resolution of small and self-limited bleeders. In addition, this allows time for the ovarian bed to shrink.

In general, the use of sutures is not required. However, when the ovarian parenchyma is widely opened and exposed to a rough area, we prefer to approximate the ovarian borders to reduce adhesion formation. A running suture on the inner surface of the cyst using 3-0 rapidly reabsorbable monofilament suture is utilized.

Oophorectomy/adnexectomy

Radical treatment is reserved for highly suspicious masses, solid tumors, and adnexal tumors in postmenopausal women. During the reproductive ages, we prefer oophorectomy, even if the role of the spared tube in the reproductive future is scant. The objective of the treatment is complete removal of the ovary while avoiding harm to surrounding structures. Hemostatic control of pedicles can be obtained by several methods such as bipolar coagulation, vessels sealing devices, ligatures, or staplers. No matter the method utilized, special attention must be paid to the close relation between the ureter and the infundibulopelvic (IP) ligament.

Technique

Exposure of the adnexa can be improved by pushing the uterus toward the contralateral side of the tumor. The ureter is identified by transparency and must be visualized during the entire procedure. When an endoscopic bag is required, it must be located under the tumor, and, when the dissection allows it, manipulation should be performed inside the bag. In oophorectomy, the procedure starts with the coagulation of the ovarian pedicle by means of bipolar instruments. Afterward, the tubo-ovarian ligament is coagulated and cut, and the meso-ovarium is progressively coagulated and divided from the uterus toward the fimbria. Special attention must be paid to minimize thermal spread toward the tube.

For adnexectomy, a linear incision in the peritoneum is performed parallel to the IP ligament. The posterior leaf of the broad ligament is fenestrated to create a safety window that maintains the ureter away from the dissection. The adnexa is maintained in tension by pulling it medially. The IP ligament is isolated, coagulated with a bipolar tool, and divided. In cases of large vascular pedicles, the use of a sealing device such as LigaSure may reduce operating time. It is recommended that the surgeon leave an adequate stump in order to safely reinforce coagulation when necessary, without risk of thermal damage to the ureter. The procedure is pursued with the coagulation and division of the tubal isthmus. Finally, the utero-ovarian ligament is coagulated and divided. Pedicles are reinspected at the end of the procedure and after intra-abdominal pressure has been lowered.

Mass extraction

Small cysts managed with puncture and cystectomy can be extracted directly through ancillary trocars. In cases of larger cysts, we prefer the extraction of pieces in a bag and through the umbilical port. This approach is associated with a shorter time of retrieval and less postoperative pain compared with using a lateral port of the same size (Royal College of Obstetricians and Gynaecologists 2011).

In cases of dermoid cyst, after cystectomy, the bag is closed and exteriorized through the umbilicus. The tumor surface is grasped with laparotomy forceps, punctured, and the liquid component can be aspirated. Solid parts of the tumor of <10 mm (hair, teeth) can be removed by means of Kelly or Kocher forceps until the reduction in size is enough to permit the complete removal of the bag. In cases of larger tumors or in the presence of large solid component such as bone or cartilage, we prefer the vaginal route for extraction. With the borders of the bag exteriorized through the vagina, a speculum is introduced into the bag and opened. The cyst is grasped, punctured, and aspirated, and the solid component can be removed by means of Pfoester (ring) clamps. The vaginal route can also be utilized in the extraction of solid tumors up to 6 cm.

ADNEXAL TORSION

Adnexal torsion (AT) is defined as the twisting of the adnexa, ovary, or tube around a central line defined by the infundibulopelvic and the utero-ovarian ligament (Huchon & Fauconnier 2010). The torsion of the pedicles produces a progressive impairment in blood flow, starting with the veins and lymphatics and continuing with the arteries. This leads to congestion, edema, and ischemia that eventually will result in an irreversible necrosis if the insult is not resolved (Oelsner & Shashar 2006).

Incidence

The real incidence of this condition is not clear due to underdiagnosis. AT is found in 2.5–7.4% of women consulting in the emergency department for acute abdominal pain (Houry & Abbott 2001, Huchon & Fauconnier 2010). Even if AT can occur at all ages, women in their reproductive years are the most affected, with 70% of the cases arising between 20 and 39 years of age (Roday et al. 2002). The incidence in children is considered lower, but still is responsible for 2.7% of the cases of acute abdomen (Aziz et al. 2004).

Etiology

Increase in the volume and weight of the adnexa is a predisposing factor in the development of the torsion. Consequently, the most common finding in these patients is the presence of an ovarian cyst. Among them, cystic teratoma and functional cysts are the most frequent (Comerci et al. 1994, Oelsner & Shashar 2006, Roday et al. 2002). Endometrioma and adnexal tumors associated with pelvic inflammatory disease are not prone to torsion, probably because of pelvic adhesions. Other increases in ovarian volume can be secondary to polycystic ovaries and to ovarian stimulation during assisted reproductive techniques. The reported rate of AT in in vitro fertilization (IVF) cycles described is low (0.8 per 1000; Huchon & Fauconnier 2010). Nevertheless, in cases of hyperstimulation, this rate can increase up to 7.5% (Mashiach et al. 1990). The fact that hyperstimulated ovaries present the highest volume probably contributes to this increment. In other cases, the increase of adnexal volume originates in a hydrosalpinx or a paraovarian cyst. Both have been associated with AT and, in more infrequent cases, pure tubal torsion (Antoniou et al. 2004, Pampal et al. 2012).

Although torsion of a normal sized ovary must be considered an infrequent event (Oelsner & Shashar 2006), several cases of idiopathic ovarian torsion have been reported, mainly in children and young adolescent girls. The explanation for these cases is not clear, and different theories suggest predisposing factors such as impaired venous flow leading to adnexal congestion, excessive mobility of adnexa secondary to a congenitally long fallopian tube, mesosalpinx, and long utero-ovarian ligaments (Celik et al. 2005, Crouch et al. 2003).

The right side is described as more frequently affected than the left. Probably the presence of the sigmoid colon reduces the space and the possibility of torsion on the left (Azia et al. 2004, Bottomley & Bourne 2009, Celik et al. 2004, Huchon & Fauconnier al. 2010).

Diagnosis

Despite advances in imaging techniques, the accuracy of the preoperative diagnosis of AT remains low. Ovarian torsion is considered in the admitting differential diagnosis in only between 40% and 60% of patients with this complication (Bar-On et al. 2010, Oelsner & Shashar 2006). The majority of patients present with pain and the presence of an adnexal mass. In a detailed analysis of symptoms by Houry et al. (Houry & Abbott 2001), the main characteristics of pain were sudden onset (59%) and a sharp or stabbing quality (70%). Nausea and vomiting are also frequently present (70%). Ultrasound scanning reveals pathological findings in approximately 90% of these cases (Bar-On et al. 2010, Houry & Abbott 2001, Hucon & Fauconnier 2010). Nevertheless, there are no pathognomonic signs of torsion. Even with the use of Doppler flow, the accuracy of detection is not high, and the recommendation is to not delay surgical exploration in cases of clinical suspicion (Bar-On et al. 2010). Computed axial tomography or MRI have not increased the diagnosis of adnexal torsion (Huchon & Fauconnier 2010).

Management

Surgery is the only certain way to establish the diagnosis, and laparoscopy is the ideal tool. Conservative treatment by untwisting the adnexa is the gold standard in premenopausal women (Aziz et al. 2004, Celik et al. 2005, Houry & Abbott 2001, Huchon & Fauconnier 2010, Oelsner & Shashar 2006, Oelsner et al. 2003, Roday et al. 2002). In the presence of a cyst, immediate treatment by means of cystectomy (or in some cases puncture) should be evaluated. However, literature reports that 7–93% of these patients are submitted to adnexectomy. The two main arguments for following this radical treatment have been the presence of a black-bluish-ischemic appearing adnexa suggestive of irreversible necrosis and the risk of embolic events after untwisting. Regarding the former, the misleading aspect of the adnexa is a result of venous and lymphatic stasis rather than gangrene (Oelsner et al. 2003). Ovarian function is preserved in 88–100% of the cases after detorsion, regardless of the aspect of the adnexa. The normalization of ovarian function has been proved by means of ultrasound, surgical second look, and oocyte retrieval in IVF cycles (Cohen et al. 1999, Oelsner & Fauconnier 2010). Normalization of ovarian flow, as assessed by ultrasound, can take 2–6 months (Celik et al. 2005). In addition, basic research using a rodent model shows complete histologic and functional recovery of the adnexa after up to 24 hours of sustained ischemia (Taskin et al. 1998). Duration of symptoms is not indicative of necrosis, and neither ultrasound nor Doppler flow can predict the remaining function of the ovary (Houry & Abbott 2001, Huchon & Fauconnier 2010, Oelsner & Shashar 2006, Roday et al. 2002). McGovern et al. (1999) reviewed the risk of embolic events reported in the literature. Among 981 patients with AT managed with detorsion versus radical treatment, the incidence of embolic events was 0.2%, with no differences between both groups.

Radical treatment should be reserved for postmenopausal women and for patients with obvious signs of adnexal disruption such as ligament detachment or ovarian tissue decomposition (Huchon & Fauconnier 2010).

The manipulation of the twisted adnexa should be performed cautiously to avoid generating more damage in the tissue. In cases of ovarian tumor of functional origin, mere puncture could be a good alternative. In the other cases, such as dermoid cyst, we prefer to perform cystectomy, but the decision should be taken according to the condition of the tissue and the experience of the surgeon. In some cases, a deferred surgery 6 weeks later, when the inflammatory process has resolved, can be a better alternative.

There is no consensus regarding the necessity of oophoropexy. The goal is to reduce the possibility of torsion without impairing both the tube's blood supply and function. The procedure is simple and consists of the fixation of the utero-ovarian ligament by its ovarian extremity to the posterior leaf of the broad ligament using non-reabsorbable suture. There are no reported complications in the literature so far (Crouch et al. 2003). Considering the simplicity of the procedure and the low rate of harm, it is recommended in cases of recurrent torsion, torsion in a single adnexa, contralateral pexy in case of adnexectomy of the twisted adnexa, and in torsion with evident enlargement of the utero-ovarian ligament or of idiopathic origin (Huchon & Fauconnier 2010, Jardon et al. 2006).

CONCLUSION

Probably the two most relevant issues in the management of adnexal masses are adequate evaluation and treatment by a trained surgeon. Considering the vast differential diagnosis, a correct evaluation is fundamental to selecting the best strategy and to reducing potential harms from the treatment. Adnexal tumors correspond frequently to functional structures that are destined to disappear, and hence mere observation and proper explanation to the patient are sufficient. When surgery is indicated, laparoscopy is the gold standard, and the surgeon's training is fundamental to achieving the best prognosis for the patient. Several techniques used in adnexal surgery are simple and can be easily integrated in the daily practice of the gynecologist, but the use of these techniques requires knowledge and training. In the same fashion that we are looking to spare patients with BeOT from laparotomy, we should seek to spare patients from unnecessary damage to the ovarian reserve as a result of an inadequate technique. Furthermore, in some cases, the adnexal tumor is just the visible part of the disease, and the surgeon can be confronted with a challenging situation in the operating theater. One of the objectives of the assessment should be to anticipate these situations to ensure that the patient is managed in the best possible way and by the appropriate surgeon.

Laparoscopic training of the gynecologic surgeon must be encouraged and should be an integral part of the curriculum of the new generation of surgeons. Management of BeOT should be considered as the starting point in the broad integration of laparoscopy in the armory of the gynecologist.

REFERENCES

ACOG Practice Bulletin. Clinical management guidelines for obstetrician-gynecologists, Number 81, May 2007. Obstet Gynecol. 2007; 109:1233–1248.

Ameye L, Valentin L, Testa AC, et al. A scoring system to differentiate malignant from benign masses in specific ultrasound-based subgroups of adnexal tumors. Ultrasound Obstet Gynecol 2009; 33:92–101.

Anderson CH, Wallace S, Guiahi M, et al. Risk-reducing salpingectomy as preventative strategy for pelvic serous cancer. Int J Gynecol Cancer 2013; 23:417–421

Antoniou N, Varras M, Akrivis C, et al. Isolated torsion of the fallopian tube: a case report and review of the literature. Clin Exp Obstet Gynecol 2004; 31:235–238.

Aziz D, Davis V, Allen L, et al. Ovarian torsion in children: is oophorectomy necessary? J Pediatr Surg 2004; 39:750–753.

Bakkum-Gamez JN, Richardson DL, Seamon LG, et al. Influence of intraoperative capsule rupture on outcomes in stage I epithelial ovarian cancer. Obstet Gynecol 2009; 113(1):11–17.

Bar-On S, Mashiach R, Stockheim D, et al. Emergency laparoscopy for suspected ovarian torsion: are we too hasty to operate? Fertil Steril 2010; 93:2012–2015.

Bereck JS, Hacker N. Practical Gynecologic Oncology, 3rd edn. Philadelphia: Lippincott Williams & Wilkins Publishers, 2000:chapter 6.

Berlanda N, Ferrari M, Mezzopane R, et al. Impact of a multiparameter, ultrasound-based triage on surgical management of adnexal masses Ultrasound Obstet Gynecol 2002; 20:181–185.

Bottomley C, Bourne T. Diagnosis and management of ovarian cyst accidents. Best Pract Res Clin Obstet Gynaecol 2009; 23:711–724.

Bristow RE, Nugent AC, Zahurak ML, et al. Impact of surgeon specialty on ovarian-conserving surgery in young females with an adnexal mass. J Adolesc Health 2006; 39:411–416.

Brown J, Farquhar C. Endometriosis: an overview of Cochrane Reviews. Cochrane Database Syst Rev 2014; 3:CD009590.

Busacca M, Riparini J, Somigliana, et al. Postsurgical ovarian failure after laparoscopic excision of bilateral endometriomas. Am J Obstet Gynecol 2006; 195:421–425.

Canis M, Mage G, Pouly JL, et al. Laparoscopic diagnosis of adnexal cysts masses: a 12-year experience with long-term follow-up. Obstet Gynecol 1994; 83:707–712.

Canis M, Rabischong B, Houlle C, et al. Laparoscopic management of adnexal masses: a gold standard? Curr Opin Obstet Gynecol 2002; 14:423–428.

Celik A, Ergün O, Aldemir H, et al. Long-term results of conservative management of adnexal torsion in children. J Pediatr Surg 2005; 40:704–708.

Cohen S, Oelsner G, Seidman D, et al. Laparoscopic detorsion allows sparing of the twisted ischemic adnexa. J Am Assoc Gynecol Laparosc 1999; 6:139–143.

Comerci JT Jr, Licciardi F, Bergh PA, et al. Mature cystic teratoma: a clinicopathologic evaluation of 517 cases and review of the literature. Obstet Gynecol 1994; 84:22–28.

Crouch NS, Gyampoh B, Cutner AS, et al. Ovarian torsion: to pex or not to pex? Case report and review of the literature. J Pediatr Adolesc Gynecol 2003; 16:381–384.

Crum CP, Drapkin R, Kindelberger D, et al. Lessons from BRCA: the tubal fimbria emerges as an origin for pelvic serous cancer. Clin Med Res 2007; 5:35Y44.

Dietl J, Wischhusen J, Hausler S. The post-reproductive Fallopian tube: better removed? Hum Reprod 2011; 26:2918–2924.

Disaia P, Creasman WT. The adnexal mass. In Clinical Gynecologic Oncology, 8th edn. New York: Saunders Elsevier, 2012:261–278.

Eskander R, Bristow R, Saenz NC, Saenz CC. A retrospective review of the effect of surgeon specialty on the management of 190 benign and malignant pediatric and adolescent adnexal masses. J Pediatr Adolesc Gynecol 2011; 24:282–285.

Fagotti A, Bottoni C, Vizzielli G, et al. Postoperative pain after conventional laparoscopy and laparoendoscopic single site surgery (LESS) for benign adnexal disease: a randomized trial. Fertil Steril 2011; 96:255–259.

Ghezzi F, Cromi A, Colombo G, et al. Minimizing ancillary ports size in gynecologic laparoscopy: a randomized trial. J Minim Invasive Gynecol 2005; 12:480–485.

Grabowski JP, Harter P, Buhrmann C, et al. Re-operation outcome in patients referred to a gynecologic oncology center with presumed ovarian cancer FIGO I-IIIA after sub-standard initial surgery. Surg Oncol 2012; 21:31–35.

Grimes DA, Jones LB, Lopez LM, et al. Oral contraceptives for functional ovarian cysts. Cochrane Database Syst Rev 2009; 2:CD006134.

Guenaga KK, Matos D, Wille-Jorgensen P. Mechanical bowel preparation for elective colorectal surgery. Cochrane Database Syst Rev 2005:CD001544.

Hart RJ, Hickey M, Maouris P, et al. Excisional surgery versus ablative surgery for ovarian endometriomata. Cochrane Database Syst Rev 2008; 2:CD004992.

Houry D, Abbott JT. Ovarian torsion: a fifteen-year review. Ann Emerg Med 2001; 38:156–159.

Huchon C, Fauconnier A. Adnexal torsion: a literature review. Eur J Obstet Gynecol Reprod Biol 2010; 150:8–12.

Im SS, Gordon AN, Buttin BM, et al. Validation of referral guidelines for women with pelvic masses. Obstet Gynecol 2005; 105:35–41.

Jacobs I, Oram D, Fairbanks J, et al. A risk of malignancy index incorporating CA 125, ultrasound and menopausal status for the accurate preoperative diagnosis of ovarian cancer. Br J Obstet Gynaecol 1990; 97:922–929.

Jardon K, Bothschorisvili R, Rabischong B, et al. How I perform an ovariopexy after adnexal torsion. Gynecol Obstet Fertil 2006; 34:529–530.

Jermy K, Luise C, Bourne T. The characterization of common ovarian cysts in premenopausal women. Ultrasound Obstet Gynecol 2001; 17:140–144.

Kaijser J, Sayasneh A, Van Hoorde K, et al. Presurgical diagnosis of adnexal tumours using mathematical models and scoring systems: a systematic review and meta-analysis. Hum Reprod Update 2014a; 20:449–462.

Kaijser J, Vandecaveye V, Deroose CM, et al. Imaging techniques for the pre-surgical diagnosis of adnexal tumours. Best Pract Res Clin Obstet Gynaecol 2014b:1–13 [Epub ahead of print]. Available at http://dx.doi.org/10.1016/j.bpobgyn. 2014.03.013

Kim HS, Ahn JH, Chung HH, et al. Impact of intraoperative rupture of the ovarian capsule on prognosis in patients with early-stage epithelial ovarian cancer: A meta-analysis. EJSO 2013; 39:279–289.

Kindelberger DW, Lee Y, Miron A, et al. Intraepithelial carcinoma of the fimbria and pelvic serous carcinoma: evidence for a causal relationship. Am J Surg Pathol 2007; 31:161–169.

Kondo W, Bourdel N, Cotte B, et al. Does prevention of intraperitoneal spillage when removing a dermoid cyst prevent granulomatous peritonitis? BJOG 2010; 117:1027–1030.

Kurman RJ, Shih I M. The origin and pathogenesis of epithelial ovarian cancer: a proposed unifying theory. Am J Surg Pathol 2010; 34:433–443.

Kushnir C, Diaz-Montes T. Perioperative care in gynecologic oncology. Curr Opin Obstet Gynecol 2013; 25:23–28.

Lerner JP, Timor-Tritsch IE, Federman A, et al. Transvaginal ultrasonographic characterization of ovarian masses with an improved, weighted scoring system. Am J Obstet Gynecol 1994; 170:81–85.

Levine D, Brown DL, Andreotti RF, et al. Management of asymptomatic ovarian and other adnexal cysts imaged at US: Society of Radiologists in Ultrasound Consensus Conference Statement. Radiology 2010; 256:943–954.

Mashiach S, Bider D, Moran O, et al. Adnexal torsion of hyperstimulated ovaries in pregnancies after gonadotropin therapy. Fertil Steril 1990; 53:76–80.

McGovern PG, Noah R, Koenigsberg R, et al. Adnexal torsion and pulmonary embolism: case report and review of the literature. Obstet Gynecol Surv 1999; 54:601.

McGowan L, Lesher LP, Norris HJ, et al. Misstaging of ovarian cancer. Obstet Gynecol 1985; 65:568–572.

Medeiros LR, Rosa DD, Bozzetti MC, et al. Laparoscopy versus laparotomy for benign ovarian tumour. Cochrane Database Syst Rev 2009; 2:CD004751.

Moore RG, Brown AK, Miller MC, et al. The use of multiple novel tumor biomarkers for the detection of ovarian carcinoma in patients with a pelvic mass. Gynecol Oncol 2008; 108:402–408.

Muzii L, Bianchi A, Crocè C, et al. Laparoscopic excision of ovarian cysts: is the stripping technique a tissue-sparing procedure? Fertil Steril 2002; 77:609–614.

National Comprehensive Cancer Network Clinical Practice Guidelines in Oncology (NCCN Guidelines). Ovarian cancer including fallopian tube cancer and peritoneal cancer (version 2) 2014. Available at http://www.nccn.org/professionals/physician_gls/pdf/ovarian.pdf. Accessed March 2014.

National Institute for Health and Clinical Excellence. Ovarian cancer: the recognition and initial management of ovarian cancer. NICE clinical guideline 122. London: NICE; 2011.

Nezhat C, Nezhat F, Nezhat CE. Management of adnexal masses. In: Nezhat's Operative Gynecologic Laparoscopy and Hysterocopy, 3rd edn. New York: Cambridge University Press;2008.

Nicholson WK, Ellison SA, Grason H, et al. Patterns of ambulatory care use for Gynecologic conditions: a national study. Am J Obstet Gynecol 2001; 184:523–530.

Oelsner G, Cohen SB, Soriano D, et al. Minimal surgery for the twisted ischaemic adnexa can preserve ovarian function. Hum Reprod 2003; 18:2599–2602.

Oelsner G, Shashar D. Adnexal torsion. Clin Obstet Gynecol 2006; 49:459–463.

Pampal A, Atac GK, Nazli ZS, et al. A rare cause of acute abdominal pain in adolescence: hydrosalpinx leading to isolated torsion of fallopian tube. J Pediatr Surg 2012; 47:e31–34.

Prat J, FIGO Committee on Gynecologic Oncology. Staging classification for cancer of the ovary, fallopian tube, and peritoneum. Int J Gynaecol Obstet 2014; 124:1–5.

Roday A, Jackish C, Klockenbusch W, et al. The conservative management of adnexal torsion—A case report and review of the literature. Eur J Obstet Gynecol Reprod Biol 2002; 101:83–86.

Royal College of Obstetricians and Gynaecologists. Management of Suspected Ovarian Masses in Premenopausal Women. Green-top Guideline No. 62 London: RCOG; November 2011.

Semm K, Mettler L. Technical progress in pelvic surgery via operative laparoscopy. Am J Obstet Gynecol 1980; 138:121–127.

Slim K, Vicaut E, Panis Y, et al. Meta-analysis of randomized clinical trials of colorectal surgery with or without mechanical bowel preparation. Br J Surg 2004; 91:1125–1130.

Taskin O, Birincioglu M, Aydin A, et al. The effects of twisted ischaemic adnexa managed by detorsion on ovarian viability and histology: an ischaemia-reperfusion rodent model. Hum Reprod 1998; 13:2823–2827.

Tavassoli, F, Devilee P , Eds. Pathology and genetics tumours of the breast and female genital organs. In IARC WHO Classification of Tumours, No. 4. Tumors of the ovary and the peritoneum. Lyon: IARC Press; 2003:113–197.

Timmerman D, Ameye L, Fischerova D, et al. Simple ultrasound rules to distinguish between benign and malignant adnexal masses before surgery: prospective validation by IOTA group. BMJ 2010; 341:c6839.

Timmerman D, Schwarzler P, Collins WP, et al. Subjective assessment of adnexal masses with the use of ultrasonography: an analysis of interobserver variability and experience. Ultrasound Obstet Gynecol 1999; 13:11–16.

Timmerman D, Testa AC, Bourne T, et al. International Ovarian Tumor Analysis Group. Logistic regression model to distinguish between the benign and malignant adnexal mass before surgery: a multicenter study by the International Ovarian Tumor Analysis Group. J Clin Oncol 2005; 23:8794–8801.

Timmerman D, Testa AC, Bourne T, et al. Simple ultrasound-based rules for the diagnosis of ovarian cancer. Ultrasound Obstet Gynecol 2008; 31:681–690.

Valentin L. Pattern recognition of pelvic masses by gray-scale ultrasound imaging: the contribution of Doppler ultrasound. Ultrasound Obstet Gynecol 1999;14:338–347.

Valentin L, Ameye L, Jurkovic D, et al. Which extrauterine pelvic masses are difficult to correctly classify as benign or malignant on the basis of ultrasound findings and is there a way of making a correct diagnosis? Ultrasound Obstet Gynecol 2006; 27:438–444

Van Calster B, Timmerman D, Valentin L, et al. Triaging women with ovarian masses for surgery: observational diagnostic study to compare RCOG guidelines with an International Ovarian Tumour Analysis (IOTA) group protocol. BJOG 2012; 119:662–671.

Van Gorp T, Veldman J, Van Calster B, et al. Subjective assessment by ultrasound is superior to the risk of malignancy index (RMI) or the risk of ovarian malignancy algorithm (ROMA) in discriminating benign from malignant adnexal masses. Eur J Cancer 2012; 48:1649–1656.

Van Holsbeke C, Daemen A, Yazbek J, et al. Ultrasound methods to distinguish between malignant and benign adnexal masses in the hands of examiners with different levels of experience. Ultrasound Obstet Gynecol 2009; 34:454–461.

Velebil P, Wingo PA, Xia Z, et al. Rate of hospitalization for gynecologic disorders among reproductive-age women in the United States. Obstet Gynecol 1995; 86:764–769.

Vergote I, De Brabanter J, Fyles A, et al. Prognostic importance of degree of differentiation and cyst rupture in stage I invasive epithelial ovarian carcinoma. Lancet 2001; 357:176–182.

Vizza E, Cutillo G, Patrizi L, et al. Use of SAND balloon catheter for laparoscopic management of extremely large ovarian cysts. J Minim Invasive Gynecol 2011; 18:779–784.

Wattiez A, Leroy J, Vázquez A, et al. Alternative ways of entry: different techniques to go into the abdominal cavity safely. Jan 2012. http://www.websurg.com/doi-vd01en3557.htm

Wattiez A, Meza Paul C, Fernandes R, et al/ Stripping of endometrioma: the inversion technique. Feb 2014. http://www.websurg.com/doi-vd01en4201.html

Wattiez A, Puga M, Albornoz J, et al. Surgical strategy in endometriosis. Best Pract Res Clin Obstet Gynaecol. 2013; 27:381–392.

Whiteman MK, Kuklina E, Jamieson DJ, et al. Inpatient hospitalization for gynecologic disorders in the United States. Am J Obstet Gynecol 2010; 202:541.e1–6.

Yazbek J, Raju SK, Ben-Nagi J, et al. Effect of quality of gynaecological ultrasonography on management of patients with suspected ovarian cancer: a randomised controlled trial. Lancet Oncol 2008; 9:124–131.

Yuen PM, Yu KM, Yip SK, et al. A randomized prospective study of laparoscopy and laparotomy in the management of benign ovarian masses. Am J Obstet Gynecol 1997; 177:109–114.

Chapter 23

Laparoscopic management and prevention of pelvic adhesions and postoperative pain

Philippe R Koninckx, Anastasia Ussia, Arnaud Wattiez, Rudy Leon De Wilde

■ INTRODUCTION

The consequences of pelvic surgery can include postoperative pain, adhesion formation, a recovery period, and postoperative fatigue.

For the same intervention, laparoscopic surgery is considered superior to laparotomy since it is associated with less pain, a faster recovery, a shorter hospitalization period, and a more aesthetic scar. Laparoscopic surgery moreover is also believed to be less adhesiogenic because the magnification of the surgical field and smaller instruments would permit a more precise surgery.

This chapter will present a mix of experimental data from animal models and observational medicine. We will emphasize the central role that acute inflammation of the peritoneal cavity plays in postoperative pain, adhesion formation, recovery, and fatigue. This should illuminate the pathophysiology of healing and recovery and thus aid in prevention of undesirable effects. In addition, this will highlight the differences between surgery by laparoscopy and by laparotomy, which requires a large incision in the abdominal wall.

The role of the peritoneal cavity might also give a glimpse of the future directions of surgery both for the patient's benefit and for the health care costs. These include both the direct costs of surgery and analgesics; and the indirect costs of recovery, fatigue, absence from work; and the costs related to adhesion formation such as chronic pain, infertility, reoperation, and possibly ovarian damage and tumor metastasis.

■ UNWANTED SIDE EFFECTS OF SURGERY

■ Postoperative pain, recovery, and fatigue

Pelvic surgery can result in both somatic pain, from the skin and wall incision(s), and visceral pain. Somatic pain results from nerve damage at the incisions site(s) and later from the inflammatory reaction that is necessary for healing.

Visceral pain is very different to somatic pain and involves specific nociceptors and specific neurotransmitters (Cervero & Laird 1999, Cervero 2009). At rest, these nociceptors are minimally reactive to a stimulus and they are more sensitive to stretch than to trauma. This explains why a full bladder can hurt more than a clean cut of a bowel. Inflammation of the pelvic cavity results in a rapid recruitment and activation of over 90% dormant nociceptors, which moreover will become much more reactive to any stimulus. Since pain results from the total firing activity while starting from a certain level of total firing activity onward, this explains why peritonitis causes even natural bowel movements to become very painful. The postoperative paralytic ileus thus could be considered a normal preventive mechanism to reduce pain, and the duration of paralytic ileus thus could be considered an indirect symptom of the severity and duration of the peritoneal inflammatory reaction.

The treatment of postoperative pain is limited to pain killers, which either reduce the inflammatory reaction or slow down the transmission of the pain stimulus to the brain. Pain killers vary from centrally acting morphine derivatives to NSAIDs and epidural anesthesia. Currently, no solution exists for the prevention of postoperative pain. The intraperitoneal administration of local anesthetics reduces pain for a limited period of time – 6 hours only (Greib et al. 2008, Park et al. 2010).

Postoperative pain, postoperative ileus, and the duration of recovery are associated with severity and duration of surgery. Duration of surgery is a predictor of duration of hospitalization and complications (Reames et al. 2014), and for the depression of the fibrinolytic system (Brokelman et al. 2009). Postoperative ileus is clinically considered to be related to the severity of surgery; however, the concept of postoperative ileus is poorly defined. Traditionally, fluid and food intake were restricted until first flatus, while bowel surgery required a bowel preparation. Recent developments cast doubt on the usefulness of a full bowel preparation and suggest early fluid and food intake in order to accelerate recovery (Mais 2014).

Postoperative fatigue (Kahokehr et al. 2011, Paddison et al. 2011, Zargar-Shoshtari & Hill 2009) following an abdominal intervention can last for up to 3 months in around 30% of patients. The mechanism is poorly understood but suggestive evidence relates postoperative fatigue to prolonged peritoneal inflammation (Paddison et al. 2008).

Although poorly understood, all evidence today points to an interrelationship between duration of surgery and postoperative complications, adhesion formation, and postoperative fatigue. It seems a logical hypothesis that postoperative pain, recovery, and fatigue have 'inflammation of the peritoneal cavity' as the common denominator.

■ Postoperative adhesions

Postoperative adhesions remain a major clinical problem. They occur in over 80% of patients and thus are the rule rather than the exception. That adhesions can cause mechanical infertility is self-evident.

It is believed that around 30% of all infertilities are the consequence of adhesions.

Adhesions are believed to be the cause of chronic abdominal pain in 30% of cases. The relationship between the severity of adhesions and abdominal pain is unclear. Some minor adhesions can cause a great deal of pain and can be painful during traction under local anesthesia, whereas women with severe adhesions can be pain-free. Adhesions may contain pain receptors, in which case the mechanism for adhesion-related pain could be understood as the activation of specific nociceptors during bowel or body movements, which are mainly stretch or traction responsive. Adhesions cause close to 100% of all small bowel obstructions.

Following surgery, some women need a reintervention. As elegantly shown in the SCAR (Bhardwaj & Parker 2007, Ellis et al. 1999, Parker 2004, Parker et al. 2005, Parker et al. 2007, Parker et al. 2004, Parker et al. 2001) study, the incidence of reinterventions increased linearly for at least 10 years. By that time, around 30% of the women studied had undergone a reintervention, of which 6% were directly related to adhesions and 29% were probably related to adhesions. Adhesions can be the cause of reinterventions and of chronic pain. Adhesions are believed to be the direct cause of infertility (30% of the time), of chronic pelvic pain (30% of the time), and of nearly all postoperative bowel obstructions.

Economic burden of adhesions (Table 23.1)

The yearly number of bowel obstructions and interventions in **Table 23.1** were extrapolated from Belgian data. An estimation of the yearly cost of reinterventions likely to be due to adhesions was extrapolated from the cost in Scotland as calculated in the SCAR study. To estimate the yearly cost of infertility due to adhesions, we assumed that 30% of all yearly in vitro fertilization costs in Belgium were due to adhesions. This figure therefore is clearly an underestimation. To estimate the yearly cost of chronic pain, specifically due to adhesions, we consider this to be about one-third of the yearly cost of endometriosis.

In any event, postoperative adhesions constitute, in addition to the personal suffering of the patient, a huge financial burden on the health care system. This figure is even more impressive if the cost of postoperative pain, recovery, hospitalization, postoperative fatigue, and absence from work are taken into account.

PATHOPHYSIOLOGY OF ADHESION FORMATION

Surgical trauma

Peritoneal injury caused by surgery induces a series of well-timed local events at the trauma site starting with an inflammatory reaction, exudation, and fibrin deposition into which white blood cells, macrophages, fibroblasts, and mesothelial cells migrate, proliferate, and/or differentiate (DiZerega 2000a, DiZerega 2000b, Diamond et al. 2010). Within a few hours, the lesion is covered by macrophages and other 'tissue repair cells' although it is still unclear what their exact precursors are. Simultaneously, a race begins between fibrinolysis with mesothelial repair and proliferation of fibroblasts invading and proliferating into the fibrin mesh. Mesothelial repair starts from multiple islands, therefore large defects heal as rapidly as small defects. The healing of a mesothelial defect, starting from multiple islands, is rapid and almost finished by postoperative day two. If fibrin however persists longer because of continued inflammation (e.g. because of suture material) or because of a lengthier depressed fibrinolysis due to more severe surgery, the proliferating fibroblasts will use the fibrin as a scaffold to invade. This will initiate an adhesion which will be covered by mesothelial cells at the outside. If inflammation persists for >5 days, angiogenesis will be initiated and the adhesions will become vascularized and severe. The role of ileus is unclear.

Peritoneum and acute inflammation of the peritoneal cavity

The peritoneal cavity is a specific microenvironment different from blood. It is lined by large and flat mesothelial cells connected by gap junctions. Fluid in this cavity results from ovarian exudation during follicular maturation (Koninckx et al. 1980). The volume of peritoneal fluid thus increases exponentially during the follicular phase up to 400 mL. Since peritoneal fluid is ovarian exudate, it is not surprising

Table 23.1 Yearly adhesion-related procedures and cost for society

	Unit	Benelux	Europe	USA
Abdominal surgery	Number	1,928,450	34,615,425	21,327,554
Laparoscopic surgery	Number	964,225	17,307,713	10,663,777
Adhesion-related infertilities (30%)	Number	628,132	11,274,877	6,946,775
Adhesion-related chronic pain (30%)	Number	1,675,018	30,066,340	18,524,732
Adhesion-related bowel obstructions (100%)	Number	41,875	751,658	463,118
Adhesion-related cost of reintervention	€ (millions)/y	39	701	432
Adhesion-related chronic pain cost	€ (millions)/y	24	416	250
Adhesion-related fertility cost	€ (millions)/y	12	208	128

Adhesion-related reintervention costs were extrapolated from the cost of the SCAR study. The adhesion-related cost of infertility is an underestimation since extrapolated from the third of the yearly cost of in vitro fertilization in Belgium (assuming that 30% was caused by adhesions).

that estrogen and also progesterone concentrations are several times higher than in plasma. Following ovulation with release of the follicular content into the peritoneal cavity, the concentrations of estrogen and of progesterone increase acutely and become around 1000 times higher than in plasma, decreasing progressively during the luteal phase (Koninckx, et al. 1980, Koninckx et al. 1980, Pattinson et al. 1981). The mesothelial cells actively regulate the transport of fluid and substances between the peritoneal cavity and the plasma. Transportation of molecules >60,000 Daltons is slow, explaining why concentrations of most plasma proteins such as lutein hormone, follicular stimulating hormone, prolactin, etc. are only 60% of the plasma concentrations, that clotting factors V and VIII are virtually absent, and that locally secreted large proteins such as CA125 and glycodelins are >100 times higher than in plasma (Koninckx et al. 1992). Also, macrophages and the immune system of the peritoneal cavity are specific, although less investigated. In women with endometriosis, natural killer cell activity is suppressed, whereas the peritoneal cavity contains more and more activated macrophages and their secretion products (Oosterlynck et al. 1992).

In addition to regulating transport of fluid, substances, and gases between the peritoneal cavity and plasma, the mesothelial cell facilitates gliding of moving organs such as bowels (and lungs and heart). Active regulation or inhibition of gas transport by the mesothelial cell is unexpected and unexplained, but it is the only hypothesis that can explain the observation that during CO_2 pneumoperitoneum in both humans and rabbits (Mynbaev et al. 2002a) the resorption of CO_2 increases progressively over time and that this increase is prevented by keeping the mesothelial layer intact through conditioning (Koninckx et al. 2013, Mynbaev et al. 2002b). In addition, intact mesothelial cells actively prevent the diffusion of nitrous oxide (N_2O) through the mesothelial layer since during N_2O anesthesia no N_2O can be measured in the pneumoperitoneum, and during pneumoperitoneum with 100% N_2O no N_2O can be measured in the lungs (Mulier & Van Acker, personal communication, 2012).

The mesothelial cell is extremely fragile and reacts very rapidly to any insult by retracting and bulging (Volz et al. 1999). This is best demonstrated by the fact that in vivo fixation in anesthetized animals is necessary to demonstrate the irritative effect of CO_2 pneumoperitoneum upon the mesothelial cell. The time to open the cavity and to take a biopsy will indeed induce severe alterations before fixation, which explains why human data on this subject is scanty and fundamentally unreliable. The retraction and bulging increase in line with the severity and duration of the insult. Additionally, within hours of insult to the mesothelial cell an acute inflammatory reaction initiates in the exposed area (Corona et al. 2011c). Repair of this mesothelial insult has not been

investigated in detail, but these insults will always be repaired without adhesion formation. Indeed in none of the mice experiments performed was de novo adhesion formation observed. It is assumed that the acute inflammation in the human reflects postoperative C-reactive protein increase and peritoneal repair, which is finalized within a few days depending on the duration and severity of the insult.

Insults to the mesothelial cells leading to acute inflammation can be very subtle (**Figure 23.1**). Minor mechanical traumas such as gently touching and moving bowels can produce this response, providing yet more evidence to support the understanding that such surgical manipulation can be harmful (Schonman et al. 2009). These cells are extremely sensitive to hypoxia as superficially induced by a CO_2 pneumoperitoneum. They start retracting and bulging within minutes and the severity of the subsequent inflammatory reaction increases with the duration and the insufflation pressure of the pneumoperitoneum, at least up to 2 hours (Molinas & Koninckx 2000). They are equally sensitive to reactive oxygen species (ROS) as caused by exposure to >10% of oxygen or a partial oxygen pressure of >75 mmHg, the normal pressure in vivo being around 25 mmHg (Binda et al. 2007, Elkelani et al. 2004). Minor desiccation (Binda et al. 2006) rapidly causes ciliary beating to stop and more severe desiccation enhances the inflammatory reaction. Although not investigated in animal models or in the human, saline is known to cause rapidly cellular retraction of monolayer cultures (Polubinska et al. 2006). Also blood, both the plasma and to a lesser extent the red blood cells, strongly increases the inflammatory reaction in a dose-dependent manner (Corona et al. 2013).

The ultimate mesothelial cell trauma and the subsequent inflammatory reaction are the sum of all detrimental and beneficial factors. The trauma is moreover strongly temperature- or metabolism-dependent; temperatures >37°C exponentially increase the inflammatory reaction, whereas at temperatures <30°C the inflammatory reaction decreases by 50% (Binda et al. 2004).

Peritoneal acute inflammation: main factor in adhesion formation

From animal models, especially the mouse model, it became clear that adhesion formation following a surgical trauma was minimal without associated acute inflammation of the peritoneal cavity. Although a surgical trauma is necessary to initiate adhesion formation, the severity of the ultimate adhesion formation mainly depends on the severity of the acute inflammation in the entire peritoneal cavity (Corona et al. 2011c).

The adhesion enhancement at the local injury site has to be mediated by substances in peritoneal fluid, since manipulation of bowels

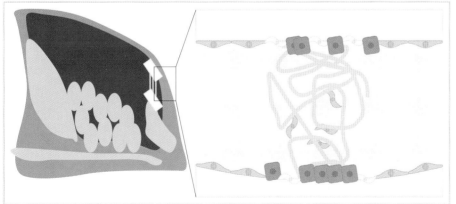

Figure 23.1 Insults of the mesothelial cells leading to retraction, bulging, and acute inflammation, and later to pain, CO_2 resorption, longer recovery, adhesion formation, fatigue, and probably tumor metastasis.

in the upper abdomen can increase adhesions at surgical trauma sites in the lower abdomen (Schonman et al. 2009).

In humans, we only have indirect evidence that the same mechanisms occur. The relative importance of each factor in human surgery, however, remains to be established. Differences between animal models and human surgery are obvious: the duration of human surgery can be much longer, the surgical trauma much greater, the bleeding can be severe, and the rinsing of the abdomen varies widely in volume, temperature, and in composition of rinsing fluid.

■ PREVENTION OF ADHESION FORMATION

Gentle tissue handling with little bleeding

Gentle tissue handling was a paradigm of microsurgery. Gentle tissue handling seems logical, but in practice this was to prove difficult in humans. Animal models have shown that increased manipulation increases postoperative adhesions. Indirect evidence for the role of manipulation is derived from adhesion formation during learning curves: when performing identical interventions, expertise results in less adhesion formation (Corona et al. 2011a).

The adhesiogenic (Corona et al. 2013) effect of blood has been known for some time. The quantitatively important adhesiogenic effect of even 0.1 mL of blood, however, came as a surprise – as demonstrated in mice models. That plasma is more adhesiogenic than red blood cells points to the effect of fibrin and the resulting inflammatory reaction. This suggests that the use of some heparin in the rinsing fluid should result in a reduction of fibrin deposits. The effectiveness of heparin however has never been demonstrated, neither experimentally nor clinically.

Prevention of acute inflammation

Prevention of acute inflammation obviously consists of avoiding all factors that are recognized as harmful for the mesothelial cell and therefore cause retraction, bulging, and acute inflammation.

- The duration and quality of surgery are important. It has been demonstrated in animal experiments that adhesion formation increases with the duration of pneumoperitoneum – the duration of surgery in humans has also been recognized as an important cofactor (Trew et al. 2011). In humans the duration of surgery is dictated by the type and complexity of the intervention, so the expertise of the surgeon becomes a key factor in adhesion formation by decreasing manipulation and operating time.
- It is important to maintain a normal physiologic partial O_2 pressure of the mesothelial cell. The addition of 4% O_2 to the CO_2 pneumoperitoneum results in a partial oxygen pressure of 28 mmHg. The same holds true for open surgery where the addition of 4% of O_2 to either CO_2 or a neutral gas such as N_2 will prevent ROS production because of the oxygen concentration, which is 20%.
- Desiccation should be avoided by humidification of the gas.
- The temperature of the peritoneal cavity should be kept <32°C so that it achieves 80% of the beneficial cooling effect. However, the peritoneal cavity can be cooled to some 25°C, which in the absence of desiccation will not affect core body temperature (Corona et al. 2011b). Cooling of the peritoneal cavity obviously has to be done with a third means, and cannot be done with the gas used for the pneumoperitoneum. Insufflating humidified but cool gas will result in desiccation since the water content of cold gas is much less, and

also this gas will be heated in the peritoneal cavity by the body.

The single most effective factor, however, is the addition of >5% of N_2O to the pneumoperitoneum. In animal models, N_2O has a half maximal effect at a concentration of 2.5% and a full effect from 5% onward as demonstrated for 100% N_2O (Corona et al. 2013, Koninckx et al. 2014). This points to an unknown drug-like effect of N_2O, although the mechanism of action is unknown.

Dexamethasone, 5 mg after surgery, has been used for many years but results were inconsistent. In animal models, however, after full conditioning, i.e. elimination of detrimental factors for the mesothelial cells, dexamethasone is highly effective in decreasing the remaining adhesion formation by 30%. The mechanism is unclear but could be the prevention of a proliferation of fibroblasts or a decrease in inflammatory reactions (Binda & Koninckx 2009).

In this context, it is important to recognize that in animal models anti-inflammatory drugs such as antitumor necrosis factor-α, and Cox I or Cox II inhibitors do not affect adhesion formation. A series of other factors slightly decrease adhesion formation in animal models but they are without direct application to the human. These comprise ROS inhibitors and vitamin C, calcium channel blockers, and antiangionetic factors as monoclonals against VEGF (vascular endothelial growth factor) or against PlGF (placental growth factor).

Barriers

Adhesion formation has been considered a rapid and local process between two opposing lesions (**Figure 23.2**). Prevention of adhesions therefore was based on the principle of keeping two opposing lesions separated for at least 5 days with resorbable solid or semisolid barriers such as Interceed or Intercoat of Johnson & Johnson, Spray-shield of Covidien or Hyalobarrier gel of Nordic, or with flotation agents such as Adept of Baxter. All "of these" ? substances are chemically hydrolysable polysugars with a minimal local inflammatory reaction. Since they are hypertonic, they all induce some local edema. The major technical problem is to keep these semisolid gels in place after application. The efficacy of these products ranges between a 40% and 50% reduction in adhesions, as demonstrated after minor interventions such as ovarian surgery or myomectomies. The variability in final adhesion formation is high, but this is probably due to the interindividual variability in sensitivity to adhesion formation.

None of these products are FDA approved, apart from Interceed and Adept. In Europe, these products were licensed to be marketed based upon (limited) safety data and the absence of serious side effects.

■ Quantitative efficacy of adhesion prevention

Efficacy in animal models

The efficacy of each individual factor could obviously only be investigated in animal models for ethical reasons. Adhesion formation after a well-performed laparoscopic surgery with humidified CO_2 is taken as a point of reference to compare the effect of the different factors affecting adhesion formation. Adhesions can be increased at least 2- to 10-fold by traumatic manipulation, excessive desiccation, and by blood.

The addition of >5% of N_2O to the CO_2 pneumoperitoneum will decrease adhesion formation by 60–70%. Although the addition of a few percent of O_2 has some beneficial effect when used alone, an additive effect when used together with N_2O could not be demonstrated. If the peritoneal cavity is cooled further to around 30°C, adhesion formation

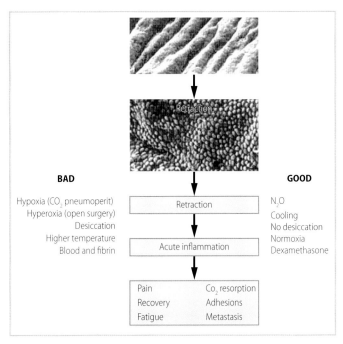

Figure 23.2 The classic model of adhesion formation between opposing lesions. Fibrin and fibrinolysis have a crucial role.

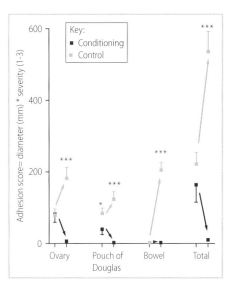

Figure 23.3 Adhesion score before surgery and at repeat laparoscopy in the full conditioning and in the control group, around the ovaries, in the pouch of Douglas (between uterus, rectum, and rectosigmoid), between bowels and side wall together with the total score (mean and standard error of the mean). Reproduced with permission from Koninckx et al. (2013). *, P<0.05; ***, P<0.001.

will further decrease to 85–90%. If, in addition to N₂O and cooling, a barrier is added, adhesion formation will be prevented by virtually 100%.

Efficacy in humans

First of all, it should be emphasized that all trials in adhesion prevention have been done by surgeons who were aware of the problem of adhesions, and thus the first assumption of good surgery by experienced surgeons has always been met.

After minor interventions such as ovarian surgery or myomectomies, barriers have an efficacy between 40% and 50%. Comparative trials between barriers to the best of our knowledge have not been performed. The interindividual variability in final adhesion formation is high, but this is probably due to the individual variability in sensitivity to adhesion formation.

In a randomized-controlled trial in severe deep endometriosis surgery, a protocol including: the addition of 10% N₂O to the pneumoperitoneum, together with cooling the abdominal cavity to 30°C without desiccation, 5 mg of dexamethasone, and a barrier (Hyalobarrier gel) at the end of surgery, was close to 100% effective. In the control group, adhesions were high (Koninckx et al. 2013) (**Figure 23.3**).

Unfortunately, because of the difficulty of performing repeat surgery to assess adhesion formation, all series on this subject are small. There are no data that demonstrate safety after bowel surgery, efficacy after severe interventions or that demonstrate a reduction in clinically important end points such as reoperation rate, chronic pain, or fertility.

LAPAROSCOPIC MANAGEMENT OF ADHESIONS

Laparoscopic adhesiolysis is not different from adhesiolysis during open surgery. The technical difficulty varies from easy velamentous adhesions to difficult dense adhesions, and the risk of bowel lesions can become real. During surgery, the surgeon therefore has to balance

the difficulty and the risk of an adhesiolysis with the expected benefits of an adhesiolysis. An adhesiolysis can be necessary to gain access to the pelvis or an adhesiolysis can be useful to relieve pain.

The creation of a pneumoperitoneum (Tulandi et al. 2011) in women suspected of adhesions can be difficult. If periumbilical adhesions are expected, Palmer's point should be used. A detailed discussion of entry technique is beyond the scope of this article. Ultrasonographic evaluation of adhesions to the anterior abdominal wall, especially the umbilicus, seems promising. Unfortunately the efficacy has not yet been demonstrated adequately.

Adhesiolysis of adhesions between the anterior abdominal wall and bowels or omentum can be technically difficult mainly because of limited access. Personal experience has demonstrated that a CO₂ laser used through an operative laparoscope has a clear advantage due to visibility, manipulation, and angle of cutting. The major challenge of managing adhesiolysis remains the prevention of adhesion reformation. Unfortunately, few studies have specifically addressed this, and the overall recommendation is the same as for general prevention of adhesion formation.

ADHESIONS, THE LARGER PICTURE AND CONCLUSIONS

Peritoneal repair and adhesion formation can be considered as a race between mesothelial repair and fibroblast growth over the course of a few days, with the duration of persistence of fibrin and fibrinous attachment between organs and the inflammatory reaction in the peritoneal cavity as important modulating players. Many aspects however remain unclear (De Wilde et al. 2014).

Genetics and fibroblasts

In mice and in humans (Tulandi et al. 2011), the genetic constitution has an important role in adhesion formation. Some strains of mice, such as BALBc mice, are highly adhesiogenic and are therefore used for research in adhesion formation. The reason why it is hard to induce adhesions in other strains is unknown. When strains of mice that are strongly adhesiogenic, are bred with mice that are much less adhesiogenic, the offspring has an adhesiogenicity that is roughly the mean of both parents. This strongly suggests underlying genetic differences. Women with keloid formation have more adhesions. It can only be speculated whether this is caused by genetic differences in fibrinolysis, fibroblast proliferation, or inflammatory reaction, and cytokines or stem cells for repair. The mice model is the perfect model to identify differences at the level of the genome, and further investigation of this could lead to new methods of adhesion prevention in the future.

A series of experiments by M Diamond (Ambler et al. 2012, Diamond et al. 2011, Shavell et al. 2012) in animal models and in humans clearly demonstrates that fibroblasts from adhesions are different from normal fibroblasts, leading to the concept of dedifferentiation of fibroblasts in adhesions. This concept could have important clinical implications. It could explain why adhesion reformation after adhesiolysis is so important, and why adhesion reformation increases with repetitive adhesiolysis. Unless the underlying mechanisms are understood, the clinical message is that repetitive adhesiolysis should not be performed (or at least should be considered carefully), and that adhesion excision with removal of the 'bad' fibroblast would be preferable to adhesiolysis.

Duration of surgery

The duration of surgery increases the infection risk, duration of hospitalization, and complications for identical interventions in bariatric laparoscopic surgery (Reames et al. 2014) and adhesion formation. A combination of the effects of learning curves, and the concept of peritoneal inflammation that increases with duration of CO_2 pneumoperitoneum, led to the duration of surgery being one of the significant covariables in the GENEVA trial (Trew et al. 2011).

Inflammation of the peritoneal cavity as a key mechanism

The peritoneal fluid has a specific microenvironment, and the role of fibroblasts as active regulators of the homeostasis of the peritoneal cavity that modulate not only the transport of liquid, ions, proteins, gases, and cells but also macrophages and natural killer cells has been well documented. The peritoneum, with its huge area of over $10\,m^2$ and the peritoneal cavity should be considered as a specific organ that serves specific functions. The mesothelial cells help the gliding of moving bowels with the help of phospholipids. It should be realized that the hormonal and immunologic environment of regurgitated endometrial cells and superficial endometriosis is not plasma but the peritoneal fluid with much higher steroid concentrations and different cytokines. The cavity reacts to infection by isolating the infection through ileus and adhesions in order to prevent a generalized peritonitis.

Only recently we realized the speed of retraction of the mesothelial cells in response to different injuries. The quantitative relationship between the severity and duration of injury and the duration and severity of the subsequent acute inflammatory reaction and of the subsequent changes in composition of the peritoneal fluid is poorly understood today.

In the process of injury repair versus adhesion formation, the peritoneal fluid has an important role. An injury without associated acute inflammation of the peritoneal cavity causes little or no adhesions. The severity of the acute inflammation of the peritoneal will enhance adhesion formation at a trauma site and is quantitatively the most important factor in adhesion formation. This is not that surprising considering the physiologic protective survival mechanism of isolating an infection in order to prevent a dangerous generalized peritonitis. It is unclear to what extent the postoperative decreased bowel movements will contribute to adhesion formation, and whether earlier postoperative bowel movements are protective against adhesion formation.

Endometriosis is associated with a chronic low-grade inflammation with more and more activated macrophages, often with few symptoms. This probably explains pain, chronic fatigue, and discomfort. Similarly, it is postulated that a more prolonged acute inflammatory reaction of the entire cavity could explain postoperative pain, chronic pain, and fatigue (Wang et al. 2012).

Prevention of acute inflammation through conditioning

We are only at the beginning of identifying the surgical insults to the mesothelial cells. CO_2 pneumoperitoneum increases the severity of acute inflammation and this effect is duration- and pressure-dependent through a mechanism of superficial cellular hypoxia and less through pH changes. Besides ROS and a partial oxygen pressure of >75 mmHg (>10%), desiccation and absence of blood are important.

Prevention of acute inflammation thus begins with an experienced surgeon combining a shorter duration, minimal manipulation, and little bleeding. During surgery, the addition of a little N_2O, possibly O_2, cooling without desiccation and dexamethasone are important. Interestingly preoperative dexamethasone accelerates recovery and postoperative fatigue following cholecystectomy (Murphy et al. 2011, Zargar-Shoshtari & Hill 2009).

Prevention of acute inflammation strongly reduces pain during surgery, reduces CO_2 adsorption and metabolic acidosis, and reduces adhesions by about 85%. It is expected that this also will reduce postoperative fatigue (Kahokehr et al. 2011), tumor cell implantation (Binda et al. 2014), ovarian damage, and leaks after bowel surgery. It is unclear to what extent the faster recovery of bowel movements and metabolism plays a role.

If together with conditioning, a barrier is also used, surgery becomes virtually adhesion-free. This indirectly confirms that adhesions are formed as a local process, which is modulated by substances from the peritoneal cavity.

Barriers are important as an additive

It is logical to offer barriers that keep opposing surfaces separate. Tissue repair and adhesion formation is a rapid process and experimental data has shown that 5 days is considered to be sufficient for the process of adhesion formation to be completed. In humans, the efficacy of adhesion barriers ranges from between 40% and 50%. It is unknown whether the mechanism of action is purely mechanical or if these barriers also restrict contact between the surgical surfaces and peritoneal fluid.

Flotation agents

Flotation agents have been useful in adhesion prevention in humans for some time. In mice models, a slight but significant improvement in adhesion prevention could be demonstrated by Ringer's lactate. It has been suggested that this agent keeps surfaces separated, but the mechanism could equally be a dilution of peritoneal fluid with a decreased effect in adhesion enhancement.

The role of Adept as a flotation agent is unclear. The clinical efficacy is limited, which is not surprising with recent data on the retention time. The resorption is exponential and the retention time is only slightly higher than that of Ringer's lactate following use.

Acknowledgment

Dr Jan Mulier, Brugge, and Professor Bernard Van Acker, UZ Gasthuisberg Leuven are thanked for information on the diffusion of N_2O into the peritoneal cavity.

REFERENCES

Ambler DR, Golden AM, Gell JS, et al. Microarray expression profiling in adhesion and normal peritoneal tissues. Fertil Steril 2012; 97:1158–1164.

Bhardwaj R, Parker MC. Impact of adhesions in colorectal surgery. Colorectal Dis 2007; 9 Suppl 2:45–53.

Binda MM, Molinas CR, Hansen P, Koninckx PR. Effect of desiccation and temperature during laparoscopy on adhesion formation in mice. Fertil Steril 2006; 86:166–175.

Binda MM, Corona R, Amant F, Koninckx PR. Conditioning of the abdominal cavity reduces tumor implantation in a laparoscopic mouse model. Surg Today 2014; 44:1328–1335.

Binda MM, Koninckx PR. Prevention of adhesion formation in a laparoscopic mouse model should combine local treatment with peritoneal cavity conditioning. Hum Reprod 2009; 24:1473–1479.

Binda MM, Molinas CR, Bastidas A, Koninckx PR. Effect of reactive oxygen species scavengers, anti-inflammatory drugs, and calcium-channel blockers on carbon dioxide pneumoperitoneum-enhanced adhesions in a laparoscopic mouse model. Surg Endosc 2007; 21:1826–1834.

Binda MM, Molinas CR, Mailova K, Koninckx PR. Effect of temperature upon adhesion formation in a laparoscopic mouse model. Hum Reprod 2004; 19:2626–2632.

Brokelman WJA, Holmdahl L, Janssen IMC, et al. Decreased peritoneal tissue plasminogen activator during prolonged laparoscopic surgery. J Surg Res 2009; 151:89–93.

Cervero F. Visceral versus somatic pain: similarities and differences. Dig Dis 2009; 27 Suppl1:3–10.

Cervero F, Laird JM. Visceral pain. Lancet. 1999; 353:2145–2148.

Corona R, Binda MM, Mailova K, Verguts J, Koninckx PR. Addition of nitrous oxide to the carbon dioxide pneumoperitoneum strongly decreases adhesion formation and the dose-dependent adhesiogenic effect of blood in a laparoscopic mouse model. Fertil Steril 2013; 100:1777–1783.

Corona R, Verguts J, Binda MM, et al. The impact of the learning curve on adhesion formation in a laparoscopic mouse model. Fertil Steril 2011a; 96:193–197.

Corona R, Verguts J, Koninckx R, et al. Intraperitoneal temperature and desiccation during endoscopic surgery. Intraoperative humidification and cooling of the peritoneal cavity can reduce adhesions. Am J Obstet Gynecol 2011b; 205:392–397.

Corona R, Verguts J, Schonman R, et al. Postoperative inflammation in the abdominal cavity increases adhesion formation in a laparoscopic mouse model. Fertil Steril 2011c; 95:1224–1228.

De Wilde RL, Bakkum EA, Brolmann H, et al. Consensus recommendations on adhesions (version 2014) for the ESGE Adhesions Research Working Group (European Society for Gynecological Endoscopy): an expert opinion. Arch Gynecol Obstet. 2014; 290:581–582.

Diamond MP, Wexner SD, DiZerega GS, et al. Adhesion prevention and reduction: current status and future recommendations of a multinational interdisciplinary consensus conference. Surgical Innovation 2010; 17;183-188.

Diamond MP, Korell M, Martinez S, Kurman E, Kamar M. A prospective, controlled, randomized, multicenter, exploratory pilot study evaluating the safety and potential trends in efficacy of Adhexil. Fertil Steril 2011; 95:1086–1090.

DiZerega GS, ed. Peritoneal surgery. New York: Springer, 2010.

DiZerega GS. Peritoneum, peritoneal healing and adhesion formation. In: DiZerega GS (ed), Peritoneal surgery. New York: Springer, 2000b:3–38.

Elkelani O, Binda MM, Molinelli BM, Koninckx PR. Effect of adding more than 3% oxygen to carbon dioxide pneumoperitoneum on adhesion formation in a laparoscopic mouse model. Fertil Steril 2004; 82:1616–1622.

Ellis H, Moran BJ, Thompson JN, et al. Adhesion-related hospital readmissions after abdominal and pelvic surgery: a retrospective cohort study. Lancet 1999; 353:1476–1480.

Greib N, Schlotterbeck H, Dow WA, et al. An evaluation of gas humidifying devices as a means of intraperitoneal local anesthetic administration for laparoscopic surgery. Anesth Analg 2008; 107:549–551.

Kahokehr A, Sammour T, Shoshtari KZ, Taylor M, Hill AG. Intraperitoneal local anesthetic improves recovery after colon resection: A double-blinded randomized controlled trial. Ann Surg 2011; 254:28–38.

Kahokehr AA, Zargar-Shoshtari K, Sammour T, Srinivasa S, Hill AG. Postoperative fatigue: Fact or fiction? Praticien en Anesthesie Reanimation 2011; 15:35–39.

Koninckx PR, Corona R, Timmerman D, Verguts J, Adamyan L . Peritoneal full-conditioning reduces postoperative adhesions and pain: a randomised controlled trial in deep endometriosis surgery. J Ovarian Res 2013; 6:90.

Koninckx PR, De Moor P, Brosens IA. Diagnosis of the luteinized unruptured follicle syndrome by steroid hormone assays on peritoneal fluid. Br J Obstet Gynaecol 1980; 87:929–934.

Koninckx PR, Heyns W, Verhoeven G, et al. Biochemical characterization of peritoneal fluid in women during the menstrual cycle. J Clin Endocrinol Metab 1980; 51:1239–1244.

Koninckx PR, Renaer M, Brosens IA. Origin of peritoneal fluid in women: an ovarian exudation product. Br J Obstet Gynaecol 1980; 87:177–183.

Koninckx PR, Riittinen L, Seppala M, Cornillie FJ. CA-125 and placental protein 14 concentrations in plasma and peritoneal fluid of women with deeply infiltrating pelvic endometriosis. Fertil Steril 1992; 57:523–530.

Koninckx PR, Verguts J, Corona R, Adamyan L, Brosens I. A mixture of 86% of CO_2, 10% of N_2O, and 4% of oxygen permits laparoscopy under local anesthesia: a pilot study. Gynecol Surg 2015;12:57-60.

Mais V. Peritoneal adhesions after laparoscopic gastrointestinal surgery. World J Gastroenterol. 2014; 20:4917–4925.

Molinas CR, Koninckx PR. Hypoxaemia induced by CO2 or helium pneumoperitoneum is a co-factor in adhesion formation in rabbits. Hum Reprod 2000; 15:1758–1763.

Murphy GS, Szokol JW, Greenberg SB, et al. Preoperative dexamethasone enhances quality of recovery after laparoscopic cholecystectomy: Effect on in-hospital and postdischarge recovery outcomes. 2011; 114:882–890.

Mynbaev OA, Molinas CR, Adamyan LV, Vanacker B, Koninckx PR. Pathogenesis of CO_2 pneumoperitoneum-induced metabolic hypoxemia in a rabbit model. J Am Assoc Gynecol Laparosc 2002a; 9:306–314.

Mynbaev OA, Molinas CR, Adamyan LV, Vanacker B, Koninckx PR. Reduction of CO2-pneumoperitoneum-induced metabolic hypoxaemia by the addition of small amounts of O2 to the CO2 in a rabbit ventilated model. A preliminary study. Hum Reprod 2002b; 17:1623–1629.

Oosterlynck DJ, Meuleman C, Waer M, Vandeputte M, Koninckx PR. The natural killer activity of peritoneal fluid lymphocytes is decreased in women with endometriosis. Fertil Steril 1992; 58:290–295.

Paddison JS, Booth RJ, Fuchs D, Hill AG. Peritoneal inflammation and fatigue experiences following colorectal surgery: A pilot study. Psychoneuroendocrinology 2008; 33:446–454.

Paddison JS, Sammour T, Kahokehr A, Zargar-Shoshtari K, Hill AG. Development and validation of the surgical recovery scale (SRS). J Surg Res 2011; 167:e85–e91.

Park YH, Kang H, Woo YC, et al. The effect of intraperitoneal ropivacaine on pain after laparoscopic colectomy: a prospective randomized controlled trial. J Surg Res 2011; 171:94-100.

Parker MC. Epidemiology of adhesions: the burden. Hosp Med 2004; 65:330–336.

Parker MC, Ellis H, Moran BJ, et al. Postoperative adhesions: ten-year follow-up of 12,584 patients undergoing lower abdominal surgery. Dis Colon Rectum 2001; 44:822–829.

Parker MC, Wilson MS, Menzies D, et al. The SCAR-3 study: 5-year adhesion-related readmission risk following lower abdominal surgical procedures. Colorectal Dis 2005; 7:551–558.

Parker MC, Wilson MS, Menzies D, et al. Colorectal surgery: the risk and burden of adhesion-related complications. Colorectal Dis 2004; 6:506–511.

Parker MC, Wilson MS, van Goor H, et al. Adhesions and colorectal surgery—call for action. Colorectal Dis 2007; 9 Suppl 2:66–72.

Pattinson HA, Koninckx PR, Brosens IA, Vermylen J. Clotting and fibrinolytic activities in peritoneal fluid. Br J Obstet Gynaecol 1981; 88:160–166.

Polubinska A, Winckiewicz M, Staniszewski R, Breborowicz A, and Oreopoulos DG. Time to reconsider saline as the ideal rinsing solution during abdominal surgery. Am J Surg 2006; 192:281–285.

Reames BN, Bacal D, Krell RW,et al. Influence of median surgeon operative duration on adverse outcomes in bariatric surgery. Surg Obes Relat Dis 2015: 11:207-13.

Schonman R, Corona R, Bastidas A, De CC, Koninckx PR. Effect of upper abdomen tissue manipulation on adhesion formation between injured areas in a laparoscopic mouse model. J Minim Invasive Gynecol 2009; 16:307–312.

Shavell VI, Fletcher NM, Jiang ZL, Saed GM, Diamond MP. Uncoupling oxidative phosphorylation with 2,4-dinitrophenol promotes development of the adhesion phenotype. Fertil Steril 2012; 97:729–733.

Trew G, Pistofidis G, Pados G, et al. Gynaecological endoscopic evaluation of 4% icodextrin solution: a European, multicentre, double-blind, randomized study of the efficacy and safety in the reduction of de novo adhesions after laparoscopic gynaecological surgery. Hum Reprod 2011; 26:2015–2027.

Tulandi T, Al-Sannan B, Akbar G, Ziegler C, Miner L. Prospective study of intraabdominal adhesions among women of different races with or without keloids. Am J Obstet Gynecol 2011; 204:132–134.

Volz J, Koster S, Spacek Z, Paweletz N. Characteristic alterations of the peritoneum after carbon dioxide pneumoperitoneum. Surg Endosc 1999; 13:611–614.

Wang Q, Du LD, Chen BC, et al. Effect of perioperative use of fish oil on 'postoperative fatigue' of rat. Chin J Clin Nutr 2012; 20:153–157.

Zargar-Shoshtari K and Hill AG. Postoperative fatigue: A review. World J Surg 2009; 33:738–745.

Chapter 24 Laparoscopic appendectomy

Didier Mutter

INTRODUCTION

Acute appendicitis results from appendiceal stump obstruction, which turns into progressive infection. This obstruction can be caused by fecaliths, foreign bodies, parasites, or tumors. It leads to the progressive increase in luminal distension, ulceration, and infection of the appendix. This is induced by a compromised epithelial mucosal barrier that can be further complicated by injury and perforation accountable for abscesses and peritonitis. Since 1894 and the definition of surgical appendectomy by McBurney, the surgical removal of the diseased appendix through a right iliac fossa incision has been considered to be the treatment of choice for acute appendicitis. The development of laparoscopy led to many debates concerning the choice of the surgical approach, namely between conventional appendectomy and laparoscopic appendectomy (LA) (Guller et al. 2004). The limited number of randomized prospective studies (Mutter et al. 1996) as well as equipment availability or inadequate cost evaluation contributed to the debate. Recent studies, however, have reported the possibilities of early medical treatment using antibiotics for noncomplicated appendicitis, which could be considered an acceptable alternative strategy (Mason 2011, Vons et al. 2011, Hansson et al. 2012).

Despite the alternative treatments available, we consider the laparoscopic approach to be the gold standard for appendectomy as it allows ideal abdominal exploration as well as a simple and standardized resection of the appendix. This approach leads to less postoperative pain, shorter hospital stay, and faster recovery. It now represents a standard of care to perform appendectomies.

PATIENT SET-UP AND INSTRUMENTATION

To perform conventional LA, the patient is usually positioned as for an open appendectomy (OA). The patient lies in supine position, legs together, and stretched out. The right arm can be placed at an angle to make it accessible for the anesthesiologist. The left arm has to be alongside the body. After installation, the operating table is slightly tilted to the left and the patient is placed in a Trendelenburg position. To perform the procedure, the surgeon and their assistant both stand to the patient's left. The operative monitor is placed on the patient's right. A standard instrumentation requires a basic set-up for laparoscopy. It includes a 0° laparoscope with an HD camera, scissors, atraumatic fenestrated grasping forceps, monopolar and bipolar cauterizing graspers, clip applicator if necessary, electrocautery hook, suction irrigation device as well as surgical loops (Surgitie ligating loop, Covidien). Finally, an extraction bag is required for the safe removal

of the infected appendix. Stapling devices (EndoGIA linear staplers, Covidien) as well as suturing material may be required.

The surgical procedure is performed using three trocars, one 10–12 mm trocar considered as the optical trocar, and two 5 mm operating trocars.

KEY STEPS OF THE PROCEDURE

Position of trocars

The 10 mm optical trocar is placed in the umbilicus through an open approach. Two 5 mm trocars are placed in the suprapubic area and in the left iliac fossa, respectively (**Figure 24.1**). These three trocars allow for a good exploration of the abdominal cavity and for the management of any local or generalized peritonitis.

Exploration of the abdomen

The first step of the procedure is to confirm the diagnosis of acute appendicitis or to determine whether another diagnosis should be established. The exploration particularly concerns the distal small bowel to search for a Meckel's diverticulum, which may be complicated or uncomplicated. In women, particularly during reproductive age, the right and left adnexa should be explored as adnexal diseases

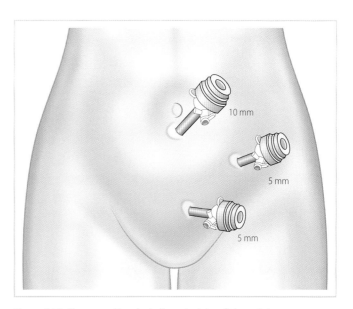

Figure 24.1 Trocars position, including principles of triangulation.

could be involved in the etiology of right iliac fossa pain in 30–40% of cases. This includes ovarian cysts, hemorrhagic cysts, and adnexal infections.

Dissection of the appendix and vascular control

When the diagnosis of acute appendicitis has been established, dissection is very standardized. The first step is the exposure of the appendix with freeing of all surrounding adhesions related to local inflammation. The second step is the management of the mesentery of the appendix. Although many techniques have been described using monopolar, bipolar cautery, vessel-sealing device (LigaSure, Covidien), stapling, or suturing of the appendicular artery, our standard technique, which is quick and effective, is the application of bipolar cautery to the appendicular artery at its origin (**Figure 24.2**). This allows for a quick control of the appendiceal stump.

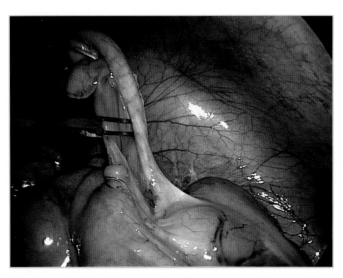

Figure 24.2 Exposure of the appendix and bipolar cautery of the artery.

Division of the appendix

The appendiceal stump is prepared and controlled by the application of surgical sutures (**Figure 24.3**). An intracorporeal suture or a pre-formed loop (Surgitie ligating loop, Covidien) can be performed. Ideally, two loops are placed, one on the side of the cecum and the second one on the side of the appendix. The appendix can then be divided between these two loops (**Figure 24.4**).

Extraction of the appendix

A surgical bag is placed into the abdomen and the appendix is immediately inserted into the bag to avoid contamination of the abdomen. The bag is pushed into the optical trocar and extracted through the umbilicus in order to prevent any further incision or enlargement of the 5 mm incisions. This allows for an ideal cosmetic result.

There is no more debate as to whether the stump should be inverted in the cecum or not. Some surgical teams prefer to coagulate the mucosa of the stump of the appendix in order to prevent secretion into the abdomen. It should be noted that the use of monopolar cautery is not recommended as the current can be concentrated at the level of the loop and can be associated with necrosis and postoperative fistula. When the mucosa has been coagulated, it should only be performed using bipolar cautery to prevent diffusion of electricity.

Abdominal lavage

There has long been debate over the necessity and efficacy of peritoneal irrigation or lavage in the setting of peritonitis. Peritoneal lavage was advocated in literature as early as 1907. Publications supporting the usefulness of peritoneal irrigation during appendectomy for perforated appendicitis began to appear in literature more than three decades ago (St Peter et al. 2012). However, the literature on this matter originates from the open surgery era, and there have been no prospective trials demonstrating any potential benefit of this approach (St Peter et al. 2012). Currently, most experts deny the benefits of this practice, and consider that, during LA, a pragmatic approach should be adopted. Focused irrigation should be used only in situations when significant contamination is present. Otherwise, a suction-only approach should be used (Vohra 2014).

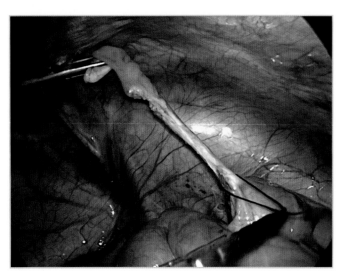

Figure 24.3 Application of a suture on the stump of the appendix.

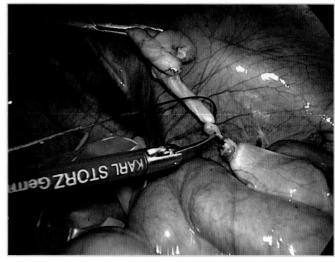

Figure 24.4 Section of the appendix close to the cecum.

APPENDICEAL STAPLING

Several studies have demonstrated the possibility of performing a stapled appendectomy. This technique is feasible. However, the cost of the stapler as compared to conventional suturing and coagulation techniques has a direct impact on team practice. Indeed, most teams have very selective stapling indications. The stapling of the appendiceal stump usually partially includes the distal part of the cecum. It is an indication in case of gangrenous appendicitis, severe inflammation of the cecum, and significant abscess, perforation or peritonitis.

In a retrospective study performed in our unit in a consecutive series of 262 patients, stapled appendectomy was performed in 55 cases of LAs (**Figure 24.5**). Indications for stapling were decided upon by the operating surgeon and were reported in the case of severe inflammation, questionable viability, or necrosis of the base of the appendix (**Figure 24.6**).

Additionally, application of the EndoGIA linear stapler is sometimes not feasible when local inflammation renders the application of the linear stapler impossible due to the thickening of the tissue. Dissection completed by hand suturing or ileocecal resection may be necessary in such extreme cases.

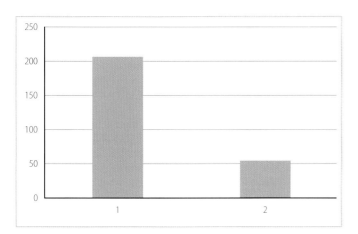

Figure 24.5 Laparoscopic surgical technique: use of a stapler to control and divide the appendix. (1) Endoloop in viable base of the appendix (n=207). (2) Caecal stapling (n=55).

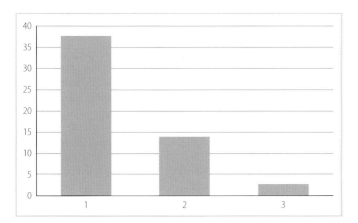

Figure 24.6 Indications for appendiceal stapling. (1) Severe inflammation of the base of the appendix (n=38). (2) Questionable viability of the base of the appendix (n =14. (3) Necrosis of the base of the appendix (n=3).

LAPAROTOMY: MCBURNEY'S INCISION

The conventional approach is currently represented by a right iliac fossa McBurney's incision, which is considered to be a standard, and allows regular appendectomies to be performed very easily. This approach has many limitations compared to the laparoscopic approach, including lack of abdominal exploration, and adnexal exploration that cannot be performed optimally in young female patients. Additionally, this approach frequently entails a significantly oversized final incision.

The ability to perform conventional laparotomy exploration through a median incision of the abdomen is still necessary in the case of severe intra-abdominal complications related to complicated appendicitis. Such complications occur very rarely since the quality of preoperative imaging allows for their early diagnosis and for their optimal management, which includes medical therapy, radiological intervention, and conservative treatment in specific cases of unrelated infections.

INTERVENTIONAL RADIOLOGY

Interventional radiology may be considered a therapeutical first-line approach in selected cases. Perforation complicates appendicitis in 23–73% of cases, and perforation with abscess formation is present in 10–13% (Brown et al. 2012). Although most periappendiceal abscesses are located in the pelvis, they may occur anywhere in the peritoneal cavity and retroperitoneum. Patients with uncomplicated appendicitis benefit from immediate appendectomy. When a periappendiceal abscess exists, early surgery is associated with an increased risk of hemorrhage, wound infection, and fistula or adhesion formation. In these cases, interventional radiology is an alternative to a surgical approach. In stable patients, intravenous antibiotics and image-guided catheter drainage must be considered as a first-stage treatment. Elective appendectomy can be delayed and performed at a later date. Technical and clinical success rates for radiological abscess drainage range from 80% to 90%. The complication rate of nonoperative management, reported as 0–15%, compares favorably with reported complication rates of 26–58% for early operations. Additionally, length of hospital stay and costs are lower in patients treated with radiological drainage and elective appendectomy as compared to patients who undergo early surgery. However, as failure of nonoperative management is associated with a high complication rate, it is essential to make an early decision about appendectomy when necessary. Persistence of pain or fever after 24 hours of treatment, as well as biological data indicating a high inflammation state (white blood cell count, polymerase chain reaction), represent signs that the management strategy must be changed and surgical appendectomy should be envisaged.

MEDICAL TREATMENT

Managing acute appendicitis can be achieved through the conventional surgical approach. However, it is worth noting that diagnosis of appendicitis is not confirmed clinically or pathologically in about 15% of surgical cases, although the use of imaging appears to have reduced the rate of negative appendectomy (i.e. appendectomy in which the diagnosis of appendicitis is not confirmed by a postoperative pathology examination) to <10% (SCOAP Collaborative et al. 2008). Several studies have demonstrated that a significant number of patients may respond favorably to antibiotics and painkillers. This was demonstrated in trials performed by Vons et al. including a series of 243 patients (mean age: 33 years) with uncomplicated appendicitis. All cases were documented by preoperative CT scan. The patients were randomly assigned to medical therapy alone with amoxicillin plus clavulanic acid for 8–15 days or to a surgical appendectomy (Vons et al. 2011). Surprisingly, 22% of the patients randomly assigned to appendectomy had complicated appendicitis at the time of surgery. In addition, postoperative peritonitis was significantly more frequent in patients treated with antibiotics as compared to those surgically managed (8% vs. 2%), and 14 patients (12%) treated medically underwent an appendectomy within 30 days of treatment. Finally, 30 patients underwent an appendectomy within the year following antibiotic therapy, 26% of whom had confirmed acute appendicitis. This study concluded that amoxicillin plus clavulanic acid was not inferior to emergency appendectomy for the treatment of acute appendicitis and pointed out that the identification of predictive markers on a CT scan might improve the targeting of antibiotic treatment. This was also confirmed by other more recent studies (Varadhan et al. 2012) stressing the need to precisely diagnose uncomplicated acute appendicitis. In this case, medical treatment appears effective even though the optimal therapeutic duration has not been certified, although a period comprised between 14 and 21 days has been evoked. Selection of these non-complicated cases appears sometimes difficult in the emergency setting and appendectomy remains the preferred option in the management of complicated or questionable cases.

CONTRAINDICATIONS TO THE MINIMALLY INVASIVE APPROACH

There are currently few limitations to performing laparoscopy in emergency settings, particularly for acute appendectomy. Age, obesity, or cardiac and pulmonary limitations are no longer considered contraindications. The laparoscopic approach to acute abdomen is associated with some limitations that are especially due to peritonitis. In cases of related obstruction, bowel manipulation for exploration purposes may be difficult or risky. It can be associated with a recommended conversion into laparotomy. Such a failure ranges between 2% and 5% (Navez et al. 2001, Kapischke et al. 2004, Sakpal et al. 2012). Sometimes, when the surgical team is not used to performing a laparoscopic approach in acute abdomen cases on a regular basis, laparoscopy may be ineffective.

SUMMARY OF EVIDENCE

The choice of a surgical technique is related to its potential advantages as compared to other ones. For the management of acute appendicitis, the results of LA have to be compared to the ones of OA. The first criterion that should be evaluated for this benign and routinely performed surgical procedure is its safety. The laparoscopic management of acute appendicitis is associated with related complications in exceptional instances. In our experience, over the last 10 years, its conversion rate has been very scarce. It ranges from between 0% and 5% (Kapischke et al. 2004, Sakpal et al. 2012), and is mainly related to associated small bowel functional obstruction or adhesions due to previous surgical procedures, and more rarely to morbidity directly linked to the laparoscopic approach. Complications appear to be significantly lower compared to OA. In addition, the onset of wound complications after a laparoscopic approach is much rarer than after a conventional McBurney's incision with a rate estimated between 0% and 8% (Guller et al. 2004, Hansson et al. 2012).

There are many advantages for surgeons routinely performing emergency surgery by laparoscopy. Although the possibilities of abdominal cavity exploration are limited through a conventional McBurney's incision, laparoscopy allows for extensive control of the whole abdomen. It provides a magnified view, thanks to the high-quality vision when HD cameras are used, hence allowing for an optimal diagnosis of the pathology or of any other abnormal abdominal findings. The differentiation between sheer appendicitis and other inflammatory diseases in the abdomen is easily identified. Additionally, the management of a purulent general peritonitis can be performed through the same incision with optimized cleansing of the abdomen.

Most recent studies have demonstrated advantages or similar results for LA compared to OA. Postoperative pain is usually lower following LA, whereas return to normal food intake and bowel habits (obtained after 12–84 hours) and length of hospital stay are similar or improved after LA versus OA (Mutter et al. 1996, Sauerland et al. 2010, Wilms et al. 2011, Hansson et al. 2012).

During the 1980s and 1990s, the main drawback to the laparoscopic approach was a longer operating time (Heikkinen et al. 1998, Hellberg et al. 1999). However, greater experience of surgeons and the availability of improved high-quality laparoscopic equipment in emergency settings since 2000 has resulted in LA duration being cut to between 35 and 40 minutes (Ghezzi et al. 2003, Kapischke et al. 2004).

AUTHOR'S EXPERIENCE

In our experience over 20 years, laparoscopy has been the standard approach for right iliac fossa pain management. Laparoscopic exploration provides a high-quality exploration of the whole abdomen in almost all patients. The most frequent alternative diagnostic finding in women is pelvic inflammation. Laparoscopy has also allowed identification of very early acute appendicitis, which is the torsion of an epiploic appendix, usually attached to the colon. Epiploic appendices are small, fat-filled sacs, or finger-like projections that may become acutely inflamed as a result of torsion. Diagnoses are more often made on CT scan imaging, but laparoscopic exploration remains useful in uncertain circumstances, allowing a differential diagnosis (Hwang et al. 2013, Savage et al. 2013).

Other cases, such as right-sided acute diverticulitis, may also be identified as an important differential diagnosis since medical therapy is the first management option for this disease.

CONCLUSION

The diagnosis of acute appendicitis is clinical, and imaging studies, mainly CT scan, allow identification of complex cases for which alternatives to surgery may be considered. The laparoscopic approach for acute appendectomy is the standard management option for acute right iliac fossa pain in all patients. Laparoscopy allows the surgeon to effectively explore the abdomen, to clearly establish alternative diagnostic findings, and to perform appendectomy in most cases. Laparoscopy, in expert hands, can also include ileocaecal resection. The minimally invasive approach offers patients excellent postoperative outcomes. Although a Cochrane review (Wilms et al. 2011) considers that appendectomy remains the standard treatment for acute appendicitis, the place of antibiotic treatment is still under evaluation in case of uncomplicated appendicitis. Likewise, interventional radiology has several indications in selected cases. These non-operative management strategies may preclude primary surgery and reduce local septic complications in complicated cases. Many studies have demonstrated that such treatment options are not inferior to appendectomy in terms of postoperative outcome (Hansson et al. 2012). Further studies should be able to determine the influence and impact of each approach and identify patients in which conservative management involves a high risk of failure. The laparoscopic approach should be considered the primary and standard approach for the management of acute and complicated appendicitis.

■ REFERENCES

Brown C, Kang L, Kim ST. Percutaneous drainage of abdominal and pelvic abscesses in children. Semin Intervent Radiol 2012; 29:286–294.

Ghezzi F, Raio L, Mueller MD, Franchi M. Laparoscopic appendectomy: a gynecological approach. Surg Laparosc Endosc Percutan Tech 2003; 13:257–260.

Guller U, Hervey S, Purves H, et al. Laparoscopic versus open appendectomy. Outcomes comparison based on a large administrative database. Ann Surg 2004; 239:43–52.

Hansson J, Körner U, Ludwigs K, et al. Antibiotics as first-line therapy for acute appendicitis: evidence for a change in clinical practice. World J Surg 2012 May 9; 36:2028-2036.

Heikkinen TJ, Haukipuro K, Hulkko A. Cost-effective appendectomy. Open or laparoscopic? A prospective randomized study. Surg Endosc 1998; 12:1204–1208.

Hellberg A, Rudberg C, Kullman E, et al. Prospective randomized multicenter study of laparoscopic versus open appendicectomy. Br J Surg 1999; 86:48–53.

Hwang JA, Kim SM, Song HJ, et al. Differential diagnosis of left-sided abdominal pain: primary epiploic appendagitis vs colonic diverticulitis. World J Gastroenterol 2013; 19:6842–6848

Kapischke M, Tepel J, Bley K. Laparoscopic appendicectomy is associated with a lower complication rate even during the introductory phase. Langenbecks Arch Surg 2004; 389:517–523.

Mason RJ. Appendicitis: is surgery the best option? The Lancet 2011; 377:1545–1546.

Mutter D, Vix M, Bui A, et al. Laparoscopy not recommended for routine appendectomy in men: results of a prospective randomized study. Surgery 1996; 120:71–74.

Mutter D, Marescaux J. Appendicitis/diverticulitis: minimally invasive surgery. Dig Dis 2013; 31:76–82.

Navez B, Delgadillo X, Cambier E, Richir C, Guiot P. Laparoscopic approach for acute appendicular peritonitis: efficacy and safety: a report of 96 consecutive cases. Surg Laparosc Endosc Percutan Tech 2001; 11:313–316.

Sakpal SV, Bindra SS, Chamberlain RS. Laparoscopic appendectomy conversion rates two decades later: an analysis of surgeon and patient-specific factors resulting in open conversion. J Surg Res 2012; 176:42–49

Sauerland S, Jaschinski T, Neugebauer EA. Laparoscopic versus open surgery for suspected appendicitis. Cochrane Database Syst Rev 2010; 10:1-136; CD001546.

Savage L, Gosling J, Suliman I, Klein M. Epiploic appendagitis with acute appendicitis. BMJ Case Rep. 2013 Jul 29;2013. pii: bcr2013010333.

SCOAP Collaborative, Cuschieri J, Florence M, et al. Negative appendectomy and imaging accuracy in the Washington State Surgical Care and Outcomes Assessment Program. Ann Surg 2008; 248:557.

St Peter SD, Adibe OO, Iqbal CW, et al. Irrigation versus suction alone during laparoscopic appendectomy for perforated appendicitis: a prospective randomized trial. Ann Surg 2012; 256:581–585.

Varadhan KK, Neal KR, Lobo DN. Safety and efficacy of antibiotics compared with appendicectomy for treatment of uncomplicated acute appendicitis: meta-analysis of randomised controlled trials. BMJ 2012; 5:344.

Vohra RS. Irrigation versus suction alone during laparoscopic appendectomy for perforated appendicitis: a prospective randomized trial. Ann Surg 2014 Feb 6. [Epub ahead of print] PMID 24509196

Vons C, Barry C, Maitre S, et al. Amoxicillin plus clavulanic acid versus appendicectomy for treatment of acute uncomplicated appendicitis: an open-label, non-inferiority, randomised controlled trial. Lancet 2011; 377:1573–1579.

Wilms IMHA, de Hoog DENM, de Visser DC, Janzing HMJ. Appendectomy versus antibiotic treatment for acute appendicitis. Reprint of a Cochrane Review, published by John Wiley & Sons, Ltd, in The Cochrane Library 2011; Issue 11:1–35.

Chapter 25 Robotic instrumentation and room set-up

Ali Ghomi

INTRODUCTION

Robotic-assisted surgery in its current form is the latest innovation in pursuit of minimally invasive surgery. There has been a widespread adoption of robotic-assisted surgery in gynecologic subspecialties since da Vinci surgical system (Intuitive Surgical, Inc., Sunnyvale, California) received Food and Drug Administration approval in 2005 for gynecologic indications. The advantages of robotic-assisted surgery compared to conventional laparoscopy include a three-dimensional, magnified, stable camera vision; superior instrumentation achieved by EndoWrist (Intuitive Surgical, Inc., Sunnyvale, California) technology; and unmatched surgical precision. Furthermore, ergonomics of seated surgical environment afforded by the da Vinci surgeon console reduces surgeon fatigue. Intimate knowledge of the da Vinci surgical system components, operating room set-up, and robotic instrumentation is paramount to successful completion of a robotic surgical procedure (Ghomi et al. 2012).

OPERATING ROOM SET-UP

The operating room should be spacious enough to accommodate all components of da Vinci surgical systems and auxiliary laparoscopic towers. There should be an unobstructed view of the patient from the surgeon console. Cable connections should be tension-free and away from the high traffic areas. Furthermore, spatial geometry of the room should allow robot docking from different angles depending on the surgical procedure being performed and surgeon's preference (Higuchi & Gettman 2011) (**Figure 25.1**).

The da Vinci robotic system

The da Vinci surgical system is a sophisticated robotic platform composed of three main components: the surgeon console, the patient cart, and the vision cart (**Figure 25.2**). The Si model is the latest platform of

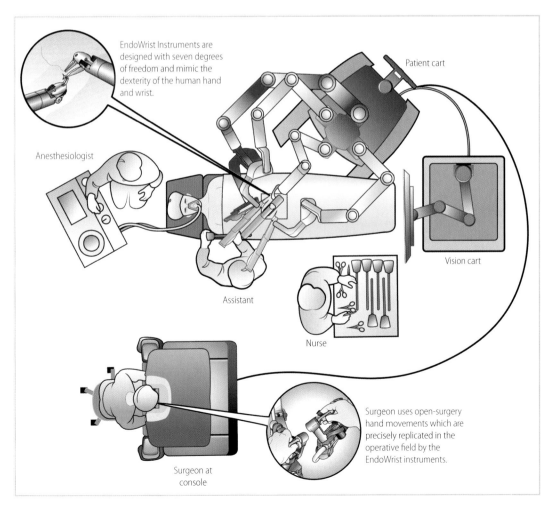

EndoWrist Instruments are designed with seven degrees of freedom and mimic the dexterity of the human hand and wrist.

Anesthesiologist

Patient cart

Vision cart

Assistant

Nurse

Surgeon at console

Surgeon uses open-surgery hand movements which are precisely replicated in the operative field by the EndoWrist instruments.

Figure 25.1 Schematic of operating room set-up for the da Vinci surgery. Reproduced with permission from Intuitive Surgical, Inc., Sunnyvale, California.

da Vinci surgical system, replacing Intuitive Surgical da Vinci system and da Vinci S system. The contents of this chapter are mainly applicable to the latest version of the da Vinci Si surgical system.

Surgeon console

The surgeon console is the main control center of the da Vinci surgical system (**Figure 25.3**). The user interface at the surgeon console consists of a pair of master controllers, the footswitch panel, and the stereo viewer displaying the surgical field. The surgeon sits at the surgeon console away from the surgical field to operate the da Vinci surgical system using hands and feet by means of two master controllers and foot pedals. The design of the surgeon console and the master controllers is intended to mirror the hand–eye coordination of open surgery (**Figure 25.4**). The tips of robotic instruments at the surgical field are perceived to be aligned with an extension of the master controllers for optimum hand–eye coordination. Each master controller is operated by the surgeon's ipsilateral index (or middle) finger and the thumb. The movements of master controllers are precisely replicated in real time at the surgical field via the robotic instruments.

The stereo viewer displays high-quality, three-dimensional video to the operator at the surgeon console via a pair of oculars. When the dual-channel robotic endoscope is activated at the patient bedside, combined right and left visual inputs at the stereo viewer recreate the depth of perception, thereby extending the surgeon's vision into the surgical field. In addition to displaying video of the surgical field, the stereo viewer ergonomically houses and supports the surgeon's head. The screen also displays messages and icons to convey operational status of the system and instruments.

The footswitch panel is located directly beneath the surgeon's feet, and is used in conjunction with the master controllers to drive the surgery (**Figure 25.5**). The footswitch panel features two groups of pedals located on either side of the panel. The left group consists of three black pedals, which control system functions (camera control, arm swap, and master clutch); the surgeon's left foot operates these pedals. The right group consists of two side-by-side pairs of lower blue

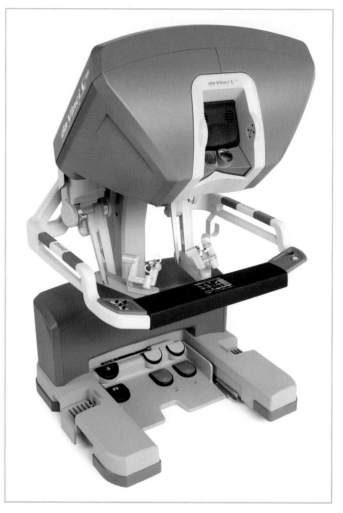

Figure 25.3 The da Vinci Si surgeon console. Reproduced with permission from Intuitive Surgical, Inc., Sunnyvale, California.

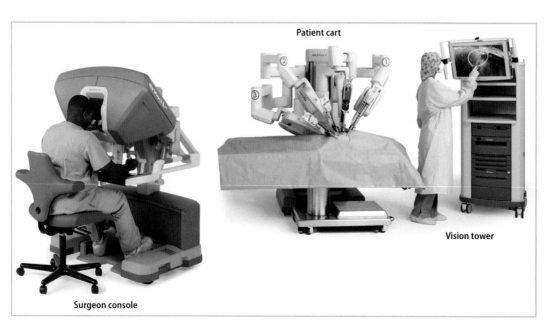

Figure 25.2 Three components of da Vinci surgical system. Reproduced with permission from Intuitive Surgical, Inc., Sunnyvale, California.

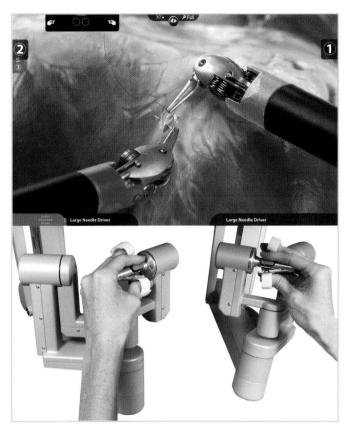

Figure 25.4 The da Vinci instruments are perceived to be an extension of surgeon hands by means of the master controllers. Reproduced with permission from Intuitive Surgical, Inc., Sunnyvale, California.

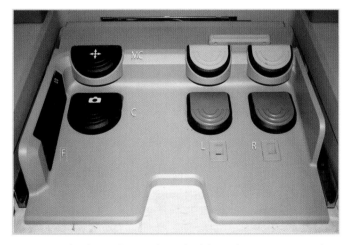

Figure 25.5 The da Vinci footswitch panel. L, left; R, right; C, camera control pedal, MC, master clutch pedal; F, arm swap pedal. Reproduced with permission from Intuitive Surgical, Inc., Sunnyvale, California.

and upper yellow pedals, which mainly control energy activation and mode of the armed instruments (e.g. on/off switch and cut current vs. coagulation); the surgeon's right foot operates these pedals. The pair of energy pedals to the right always controls the activation and energy mode of the instrument controlled by the right master controller, and vice versa.

The camera control pedal (**Figure 25.5**) on the left of the footswitch panel allows the surgeon to reposition and zoom the robotic endoscope in the surgical field. Upon pressing the camera control pedal, the master controllers disengage from instrument control mode and switch to camera control mode. Simultaneous parallel movements of the master controllers translate into endoscopic camera movements. For example, to zoom in the scope the controllers are simultaneously pulled toward the operator's eyes.

The master clutch pedal is located above the camera control pedal on the left side of the footswitch panel (**Figure 25.5**). When the master clutch pedal is pressed, all instruments are decoupled from the master controllers. This feature allows the surgeon to reposition one or both master controllers for ergonomic comfort and optimum spatial maneuvering.

The arm swap pedal is positioned upright on the left aspect of the footswitch panel (**Figure 25.5**). When tapped by the surgeon's left foot, the control between two instrument arms associated with the same master controller is swapped.

The touch pad is located in the middle of the surgeon console armrest and provides a means for the surgeon to make system adjustments (brightness, digital zoom, and movement scaling), perform camera set-up, and manually reconfigure instrument assignment to any controller with a maximum of two instruments per side. To the left of the armrest there are ergonomic controls, which allow for ergonomic adjustments of the stereo viewer height, armrest height, and footswitch panel depth (**Figure 25.3**).

Patient cart

The patient cart comprises the operational component of the da Vinci surgical system and houses three instrument arms (marked 1, 2, 3) and one camera arm (**Figure 25.6**). Each so-called robotic arm has two main components referred to as the 'set-up joint' and the 'instrument arm' (**Figure 25.7**). The 'instrument arm' has a wide range of motion and connects to the patient cart center column via the 'set-up joint'. Set-up joints are designed with limited gross vertical and horizontal movements. The instrument arm transitions to a telescopic axis end for instrument attachment. The telescopic insertion axis is designed to provide greater access into the patient anatomy and reduce external arm collision.

Vision cart

The da Vinci vision cart functions as the system's central processing unit and houses the high-definition (HD) vision system and the illuminator. The vision cart connects to the surgeon console and patient cart via fiberoptic cables. All system, auxiliary equipment, and audio/video connections are routed to the vision cart core. Energy generator and gas insufflation equipment do not come standard with the vision cart.

The da Vinci HD vision system comprises the da Vinci stereo dual channel endoscope, the HD stereo camera head with two optic channels, and the vision cart illuminator. The produced video images are high quality, three dimensional and 6–10 times magnified. The right and left video images of the surgical field captured by the endoscope are transmitted to the corresponding optic channels of the camera head. The camera head is connected to the vision cart via a bifurcated fiberoptic cable. The digital input to the camera unit is integrated in the surgeon console to create a three-dimensional view of the surgical field. The endoscope is available in 12 mm and 8.5 mm diameters, featuring both straight (0°) and angled (30°) configurations (**Figure 25.8**). The 12 mm endoscope measures 464 mm in length, whereas the 8.5 mm endoscope measures 387 mm in length.

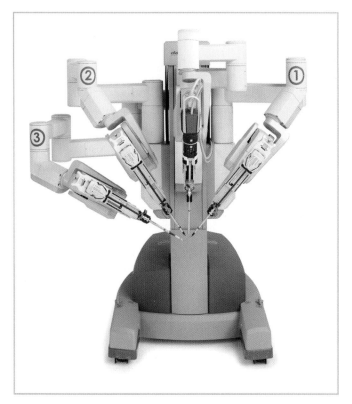

Figure 25.6 The da Vinci patient cart shown with cannulae and instruments installed. Reproduced with permission from Intuitive Surgical, Inc., Sunnyvale, California.

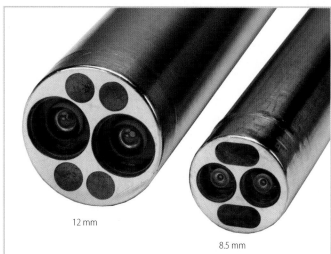

12 mm

8.5 mm

Figure 25.8 The da Vinci high definition dual channel endoscopes. Reproduced with permission from Intuitive Surgical, Inc., Sunnyvale, California.

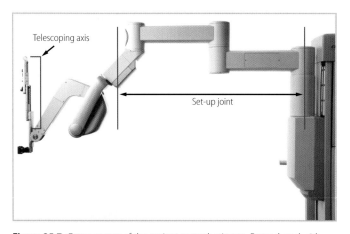

Telescoping axis

Set-up joint

Figure 25.7 Components of the patient cart robotic arm. Reproduced with permission from Intuitive Surgical, Inc., Sunnyvale, California.

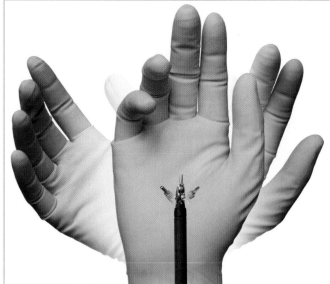

Figure 25.9 Illustration comparing surgeon wrist movement to EndoWrist. Reproduced with permission from Intuitive Surgical, Inc., Sunnyvale, California.

▮ The da Vinci instruments

The da Vinci robotic instruments are grouped into EndoWrist instruments and nonarticulating, semi-rigid instruments designed for Single-Site da Vinci surgery.

EndoWrist instruments

EndoWrist technology allows for 180° of articulation, 7° of freedom, and 540° of rotation mimicking human hand and wrist movements (**Figure 25.9**). EndoWrist instruments consist of four main components: the instruments housing (blue in color) with attached release levers, the instrument shaft, the wrist, and a wide selection of instrument tips. EndoWrist instruments are available in 5 mm and 8 mm diameter shafts, and approximately measure 55–57 cm in total length. Each instrument has a predetermined number of uses before expiring, typically 1–10 lives. EndoWrist instruments include monopolar cautery instruments, bipolar cautery instruments, scissors, graspers, scalpels, needle drivers, clip appliers, the suction/irrigator, the stapler, and specialty instruments (**Figure 25.10**). The articulating 8 mm Vessel Sealer (single use) and the nonwristed Harmonic Ace curved shears (single use) are the latest additions to the da Vinci energized instrument list. The 8 mm and 5 mm instruments differ in their EndoWrist design. The 8 mm instruments operate on an 'angled joint', as opposed to 'snake joint' design of 5 mm instruments. The 'angle joint' design allows the tip to articulate with a shorter radius (Higuchi & Gettman 2011).

Single-Site instruments

Single-Site instruments are designed specifically for da Vinci Si surgical system. Similar to the EndoWrist instruments, Single-Site instruments have predetermined number of uses before expiring, typically 1–5. The Single-Site instruments have 5 mm diameter semi-rigid shafts, which consist of four parts: the release levers, the instrument housing (light green color), the semi-rigid instruments shaft, and the instrument tip. The Single-Site instruments are flexible enough to pass through the Single-Site curved cannulae, and rigid enough to provide effective tissue handing. Due to their flexible design, 'wristed' Single-Site instruments are currently not available. It is important to note that the instrument tip of the Single-Site instruments can rotate 360° by the means of master controllers. However, the 'wristed' features of the master controllers are deactivated in the Single-Site mode. The Single-Site instruments include monopolar cautery instruments, bipolar cautery instruments, scissors, graspers, dissectors, needle drivers, the suction irrigator, and the clip applier.

■ Cannulae, obturators, and accessories

This section provides a description of cannulae, obturators, and accessories needed in multiport and Single-Site da Vinci Surgery. These devices function as a port of entry for endoscopes, da Vinci, and other compatible instruments. There are notable design differences among Single-Site and multiport cannulae, obturators, and accessories.

Cannulae

The Intuitive Surgical cannulae are stainless steel reusable components composed of a hollow bowel and a straight or curved shaft.

The straight cannulae are designed for EndoWrist instruments and the curved cannulae are exclusively designed for Single-Site da Vinci surgery. The straight cannulae are available in 5 mm diameter for 5 mm EndoWrist instruments, 8 mm for 8 mm EndoWrist instruments, 8.5 mm and 12 mm for corresponding da Vinci endoscopes, and 13 mm for the da Vinci stapler. The 8 mm straight cannulae come in regular (166 mm) and long (215 mm) lengths.

The Single-Site curved cannulae are 5 mm in diameter, and available in 250 mm and 300 mm lengths. There are also 5 mm, 8.5 mm, and 10 mm straight cannulae designed for accessory ports in Single-Site da Vinci surgery. Each cannula is attached to a disposable end piece seal featuring an attachable 5 mm reducer valve.

Obturators

The obturators insert into the cannulae and facilitate entry into the peritoneal cavity. The obturators are blunt-tipped, rigid or flexible devices available in different diameters and lengths to accommodate the corresponding cannulae. The obturators compatible with curved cannulae of Single-Site da Vinci surgery are semi-rigid. Rigid obturators are utilized for all other types of da Vinci cannulae.

Single-Site port

The Single-Site port is a single-use device designed by Intuitive Surgical to allow da Vinci robotic surgery to be performed through a 2.5 cm umbilical incision. The port is made of a pliable material with gel-like consistency that houses four cutout lumens for cannula insertion and a fifth lumen to support insufflation adaptor. The port accommodates the 8.5 mm da Vinci endoscope cannula, two curved Single-Site cannulae, and an accessory 5 mm or 10 mm straight cannula (**Figure 25.11**).

■ DRAPING PROCEDURES

Draping the patient cart instrument and camera arms is essential to maintaining a sterile surgical field. The draping procedures should be completed prior to moving the patient cart up to the operating table and connecting the patient cart arms to the cannulae – a process referred to as docking the robot. To drape the da Vinci Si, there are three similar instrument arm drapes, a camera arm drape, and a camera head drape.

■ Instrument arm draping

To drape the instrument arm, the instrument drape is opened in a sterile fashion and lowered over the instrument arm insertion axis (**Figure 25.12a**). The base of the sterile adaptor of the drape is then

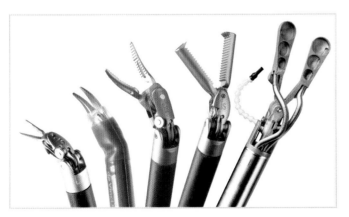

Figure 25.10 A selection of da Vinci EndoWrist instruments. Reproduced with permission from Intuitive Surgical, Inc., Sunnyvale, California.

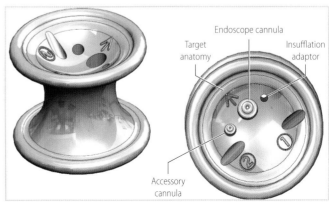

Figure 25.11 The da Vinci Single-Site port. Reproduced with permission from Intuitive Surgical, Inc., Sunnyvale, California.

inserted into the black molded piece of the instrument arm. The sterile adaptor is clicked into place by pressing the upper corners against the instrument arm (**Figure 25.12b**). The four wheels on the sterile adaptor will spin and three beeps are heard, indicating correct recognition of the sterile adaptor by the system. Using the cuff of the drape, the entire length of the instrument arm is then covered by stretching the folded drape along the arm. The cannula molding is placed into the mount molding of the instrument arm (Strother et al. 2009).

Camera arm draping

The camera arm drape features a sterile camera arm adaptor as opposed to sterile instrument adaptor piece on the arm drape. Draping of the camera arm follows similar steps as instrument arm draping with one exception: once the camera drape is lowered over the insertion axis of the camera arm, the sterile camera adaptor is firmly pushed into carriage of the camera arm to assume a secure position (**Figure 25.13a**). The entire camera arm set-up joint is then covered by stretching the drape over the length of the arm. The cannula mount of the camera arm is snuggly covered by the cannula mount molding of the drape (Strother et al. 2009).

Camera head draping

The process of draping the camera head requires collaboration of a sterile person (scrub nurse, for example) and a nonsterile assistant (circulating nurse, for example) for handling the nonsterile camera head. The sterile camera head drape features a camera head adaptor that locks into the camera head. The nonsterile person delivers the camera head into the camera adaptor of the drape. The sterile person firmly holds the opposite side of the sterile camera adaptor while having his/her hand inserted into the open end of the drape (**Figure 25.13b**). Once the camera head and camera head sterile adaptor are properly aligned, they are locked into place by pushing and turning of the camera head ring-nut. The drape is then inverted over the camera head and pulled along to cover the attached cable lines.

PATIENT POSITIONING

Proper patient positioning during surgery is essential for achieving optimal surgical exposure and for prevention of neuromuscular injuries to the patient. Patient positioning in robotic surgery is even more critical since position adjustment is not feasible once the robot is docked. The patient is placed on the operating table in modified dorsal lithotomy on an antiskid padded mattress that is attached to the bed to avoid downward sliding. Both arms are positioned alongside the torso and tucked using sheets or padded arm sleds. The legs are placed in Allen stirrups (Allen Medical Systems, Acton, Massachusetts), similar to conventional laparoscopy. Principles of adequate padding of pressure points, avoidance of extreme flexion, extension, and abduction are strictly adhered to (Ghomi et al. 2012).

Special attention should be given to protecting the patient from ocular, facial, and muscular injuries as result of external compression and direct contact caused by robotic arms, especially the camera arm. Robotic surgery poses a unique risk of inadvertent mechanical injury to the patient's face and extremities. The robotic surgeon is unaware of the surgical environment surrounding the patient while seated at the surgeon console. The members of the surgical team can easily lose sight of task of injury prevention while focusing on surgical steps. Furthermore, the patient's face is typically out of view in Trendelenburg and covered by surgical drape. In order to prevent such injuries, it is crucial for the members of the surgical team to maintain constant awareness of robotic arm movements and positions in relation to the patient's face and extremities. Instituting safeguards such as application of a face shield plate, foam wraps, and eye shields may be considered for injury prevention.

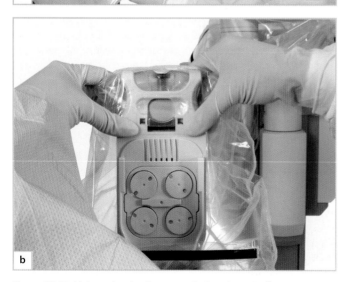

Figure 25.12 (a), Lowering the drape over the insertion axis of instrument arm 1;(b) installing the sterile adaptor of the drape by pressing the upper corners of the sterile adaptor. Reproduced with permission from Intuitive Surgical, Inc., Sunnyvale, California.

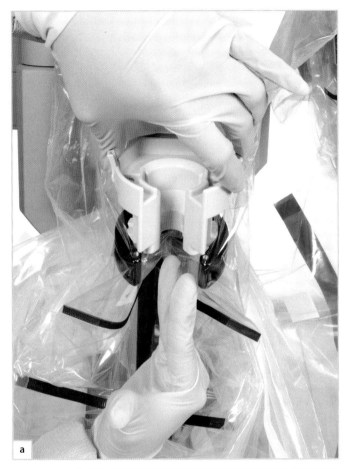

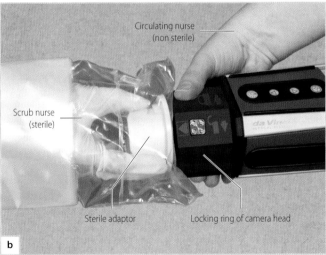

Figure 25.13 (a) Installing the camera drape sterile adaptor; (b) connecting the sterile adaptor of the camera head. Reproduced with permission from Intuitive Surgical, Inc., Sunnyvale, California.

Trendelenburg position is routinely needed in robotic gynecologic surgery to obtain adequate intraoperative exposure of the pelvic structures. However, demand for steep degree of Trendelenburg is seldom needed in benign gynecologic robotic surgery (Ghomi et al. 2012, Gould et al. 2012), and should be avoided to prevent downward sliding of the patient on the operating table. This is of particular concern in the obese patient who is more susceptible to downward sliding and potential ensuing neuromuscular injuries. Few steps have been

found to be helpful to prevent a patient in steep Trendelenburg—when necessary—from sliding while on the operating table. Utilization of an antiskid padded mattress, securely attached to the surgical bed, is a safe and reproducible strategy to avoid downward sliding (Klauschie et al. 2010). Commonly used antiskid materials include egg-crate foams (Tyco Health-care/Kendall, Mansfield, Massachusetts) and memory pads (The Pink Pad, Xodus Medical, Inc., Pittsburgh, Pennsylvania). Surgical gel pads, against the patient's bare skin, when placed on the surgical bed mattress can also serve as an effective antiskid material. There are also patient positioning stabilizing devices, such as the Beanbag Positioner (AliMed Inc., Dedham, Massachusetts), designed to stabilize and provide adequate padding during robotic surgery in steep Trendelenburg (Ghomi et al. 2012).

Some of the previously proposed strategies to stabilize the patient's position in steep Trendelenburg have been shown to contribute to neuromuscular injuries. Therefore, such position-stabilizing strategies including the use of shoulder straps, body restraints, or head/shoulder rests are discouraged secondary to potential associated morbidities (Ghomi et al. 2012).

PATIENT CART DOCKING

Once abdominal access is obtained, robotic cannulae are inserted and the required degree of Trendelenburg is placed, the docking process can begin. Docking the robot is the process of maneuvering the patient cart next to the patient's table and attaching the robotic camera and instrument arms to the corresponding robotic cannulae. Intimate knowledge of ergonomics and different techniques of docking is essential to making the process efficient and reproducible. More importantly, suboptimal docking can result in decreased range of motion of robotic instruments as a result of collision of robotic arms – an unforgiving occurrence that can necessitate redocking.

The patient cart was originally intended for center docking between the patient's legs in gynecologic surgery. Center docking is a relatively simplistic and reproducible process. However, a major limitation of center docking is restriction of vaginal access, which can pose a challenge for the gynecologic surgeon. Vaginal access can be an integral part of the gynecologic surgery by means of allowing for uterine manipulation and specimen retrieval. To overcome the challenges of center docking as it pertains to vaginal access, a novel alternative approach has recently been proposed – and widely embraced – that is referred to as side docking. In side docking, the patient cart is docked at a 45° angle leaving the vaginal access unobstructed (Einarsson et al. 2011). What follows is a description of the steps involved in center docking, side docking, and docking for Single-Site da Vinci surgery.

Center docking

Once the robotic cannulae are inserted and needed degree of Trendelenburg is achieved, the process of moving the patient cart up to the operating table and connecting the robotic arms to the cannulae is initiated. It is very important to keep the tower of the patient cart aligned with the camera cannula and the target anatomy in a straight line as the patient cart is maneuvered toward the patient, either via the motor drive on the cart or manual drive (**Figure 25.14**). Communication is critical during the docking process. Only one person should give directions to the nonsterile person who is driving the patient cart to warn of potential collisions and to direct adjustments needed for proper alignment. Once the camera cannula mount of the camera arm reaches above the camera cannula, the patient cart has reached an appropriate distance from patient. It is important to ensure the camera arm remote center is sufficiently away from the patient cart tower to facilitate optimum range of motion of the patient cart arms. This is commonly referred to as setting the 'sweet spot'. The 'sweet spot' is indicated by a blue line and a corresponding arrow located in middle of the camera arm set-up joint. To set the 'sweet spot', the camera arm is moved so that the blue arrow lines up within the boundaries of the blue line. Setting the 'sweet spot' enables the patient cart arms to have maximum reach and range of motion in the surgical field.

The camera arm should be attached first after positioning the patient cart. The patient cart camera arm is aligned with the camera cannula, target anatomy, and the cart tower using the camera arm clutch button. The camera cannula is brought into camera mount of the camera arm and is locked in place by applying the latches located on the camera mount. Pressing the camera arm clutch button during the mounting process allows for the camera arm mount to conform to the angle of camera cannula with more ease. The camera arm set-up joint is swung on the opposite side of arm 3 to maximize the range of motion of the arms (**Figure 25.14**).

After connecting the camera arm, instrument arms are positioned in place with the arm number marking and sterile adaptor facing forward. The instruments arms can be connected concurrently or sequentially in any order. Instrument arm 3 is connected last to avoid spatial crowding. To connect the instrument arm, the cannula mount is aligned with the cannula by using the instrument arm clutch. It is important to ensure the drape boot is properly aligned with the cannula mount. While stabilizing the cannula with one hand, the cannula mount is lowered toward and connected to the cannula using the latches located on the cannula mount. Once the instrument arms are all connected, attention is given to ensure maximum separation of the set-up joints to minimize collision. Once optimally positioned, set-up joint number markings should all be facing forward forming approximately a 90° angle at the second set-up joint (**Figure 25.14**). It is worth mentioning that the set-up joint of arm 3 can swing 180° on either side of the patient cart tower to connect on the patient's right or left side, depending on the surgical procedure and the surgeon's preference.

■ Side docking

Side-docking technique of the patient cart is an attractive alternative to center docking for gynecologic procedures since it provides unobstructed vaginal access (Einarsson et al. 2011). In side-docking method, the patient cart is docked at an approximately 45° angle to the patient's torso (**Figure 25.15a**). Providing precise directions to the person driving the patient cart is pivotal to proper alignment of the reference points and successful docking.

The camera cannula, the stirrup mounting clamp, the patient cart tower, and the patient's opposite shoulder can be used as reference points during side docking to create a 45° axis to the patient's torso. Patient positioning is similar to the center docking method. The stirrup clamps are mounted at the most inferior position on the operating table rail. The camera arm set-up joint is positioned on the opposite side of instrument arm 3. The patient cart tower is aligned with the camera port along an axis that crosses over the stirrup-mounting clamp. This axis should approximately cross over the patient's opposite shoulder as well, forming a 45° angle with the patient's lower torso and the operating table (**Figure 25.15**). When anatomy necessitates cephalad port placement, the roll up angle should be increased to 60° following the same basic rule of alignment (**Figure 25.15a**). The patient cart can be side-docked on either side of the patient depending on the surgeon's preference and the procedure.

The patient cart is positioned just short of contacting the outer border of the stirrup, leaving enough clearance for vertical movement of the set-up joints. It is advised to connect the robotic arm on

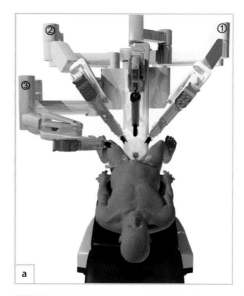

a

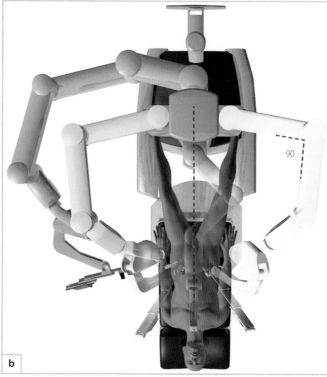

b

Figure 25.14 Illustration of center docking. (a) Front view. (b) Top view. The straight dotted red line signifies alignment of patient cart tower, camera cannula, and target anatomy; camera set-up joint (blue) is on the opposite side of arm 3 (pink), once docked all arm numbers should be facing forward; arms 1, 2 middle set-up joints form 90° angles. Reproduced with permission from Intuitive Surgical, Inc., Sunnyvale, California.

the opposite side of docking first (e.g. arm 1 is connected first when side docking on the left), as it has to extend the farthest to reach the corresponding cannula. Connecting the cannula to the instrument arm cannula mount is similar to center docking. Once connected, the number marking located on the set-up joint should face sideways – in contrast to center docking where it would face forward. The angle of the second set-up joint should be fully extended to avoid colliding with the camera arm (**Figure 25.16**).

Next, the camera arm is connected. The 'sweet spot' is set. The camera mount is aligned with the patient cart tower and the first

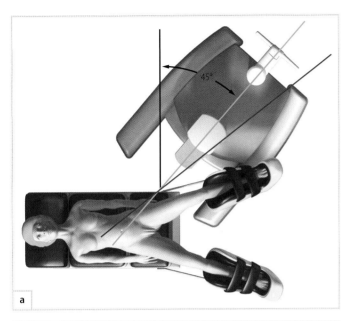

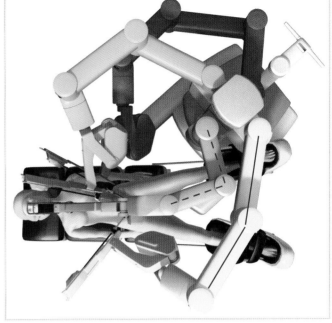

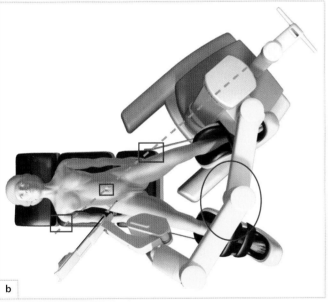

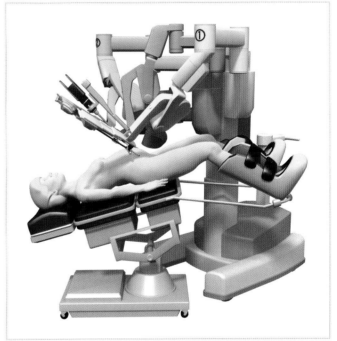

Figure 25.15 (a) Illustration of side docking at 45° angle (green line); red line signifies 60° angle in cephalad port placement; (b) alignments of reference points (red squares): tower, stirrup mount, umbilical port, and shoulder; red circle signifies the extended angle of arm 1 set-up joint. Reproduced with permission from Intuitive Surgical, Inc., Sunnyvale, California.

Figure 25.16 Overhead and side views of side docking with all arms connected; dotted red line shows the acute angle of camera arm set-up joint; solid redline shows the fully extended angle of arm 1 set-up joint. Reproduced with permission from Intuitive Surgical, Inc., Sunnyvale, California.

set-up joint of the camera arm is aligned along the midline axis of the patient. This creates a sharp angle at the second set-up joint of the camera arm (**Figure 25.16**). The camera mount is attached to the camera cannula. Arms number 2 and 3 are connected next in a similar manner. While stabilizing robotic arm cannulae, the angles of second set-up joints are adjusted by pivoting the arms 2 and 3 inward or outward to maximize spacing between all instrument arms. Range of motion of the instrument arms is checked to ensure proper positioning of the set-up joints.

Single-Site docking

Docking steps for a Single-Site procedure differ significantly from center docking and side docking. In contract to center and side docking – where cannula insertion and docking are independent steps – cannula insertion and docking take place concurrently and in a specific order in the Single-Site approach. The camera cannula is inserted and connected first. The curved cannulae 2 and 1 are then inserted and connected sequentially under endoscopic visualization.

The semi-rigid Single-Site instruments cross over each other and the camera cannula at an exact point referred to as the remote center (**Figure 25.17**). This configuration enables triangulation at the surgical site while minimizing external collision. Unlike multiport da Vinci surgery, each curved cannula is designed specifically for use with either instrument arm 1 or 2, and marked accordingly. Another unique feature of the curved cannula is the orientation tab, which is a metal piece located on the hollow base of the cannula, designed to guide the mounting process in a specific orientation (**Figure 25.18**). For example, for a hysterectomy procedure, the tabs must face the upper abdomen and slightly turned toward each other.

Patient positioning is similar to multiport da Vinci surgery. Single-Site port is inserted through a 2.5 cm umbilical fascial incision, while being folded using Kelly forceps. The curve of the clamp should lie above the lower rim of the folded port. An assistant is providing countertraction on the abdominal wall using Army–Navy retractors. Once inserted, the arrow marking on the port is pointed toward the target anatomy. The insufflation adaptor is then connected to establish pneumoperitoneum. The 8.5 mm camera cannula is inserted through the designated Single-Site port lumen, just passed the first black marking. The patient is placed in sufficient degree of Trendelenburg.

The following prepositioning of the arms minimizes adjustments needed during cannulae connection (**Figure 25.19a**). Robotic arm 3 is positioned out of view since it is not used. The camera arm and robotic arms 1 and 2 are raised high enough to clear the patient. For

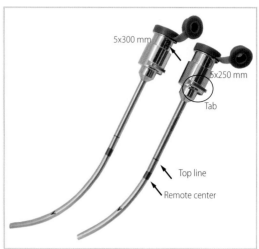

Figure 25.18 Curved cannulae for Single-Site surgery. Reproduced with permission from Intuitive Surgical, Inc., Sunnyvale, California, 2009.

arms 1 and 2, the set-up joints are aligned in a straight line and angled outward. The third set-up joint (closest to the instrument arm) is rotated inward 90° and angled toward the camera arm. This position facilitates maximum range of motion for arms 1 and 2 during Single-Site surgery. It is checked to confirm the camera arm is in the 'sweet spot'. The patient cart is moved in between the patient's legs similar to center docking until the camera cannula mount is directly above the camera cannula (**Figure 25.19b**). The camera cannula is connected to the cannula mount similar to center docking. The camera head and the endoscope are inserted next in preparation for insertion of the curved cannulae. It is helpful to use a 30° endoscope, angled up, during the next steps for better visualization of the curved cannula tips.

Each cannula must be inserted on the side corresponding with the same number instrument arm. The curved cannulae are mirror images of each other and therefore not interchangeable. The da Vinci Si system recognizes when Single-Site instruments are installed and automatically assigns the master controllers so that the instrument arm 2 is controlled by the right hand, and vice versa.

The camera head is rotated 45° toward arm 2, and positioned in a vertical axis, in preparation of visualizing the obturator tip as it enters the visual field. The curved cannula 2 is inserted in the designated Single-Site port lumen with the obturator tip pointing toward the pelvis. The cannula is advanced until the top black marking is aligned with the top of the port. The cannula is gently rotated counter clockwise to appear in view. The Dock Assist Tool is installed to collapse the insertion axis of arm 2 to create more space around the arm. While stabilizing the cannula, the cannula mount is connected to the cannula following standard docking techniques of center docking (**Figure 25.20**). It is very important to maintain visualization of the cannula tip throughout the docking steps to prevent inadvertent internal injury. Similarly, curved cannula 1 is inserted and docked.

CONCLUSION

Robotic-assisted gynecologic surgery has gained tremendous popularity over the past decade. In-depth knowledge of robotic instrumentation, proper patient positioning, and operating room set-up is critical to successful completion of a robotic surgical procedure and favorable patient outcome.

ACKNOWLEDGMENT

Some of the key technical information in this chapter is based on da Vinci Si Surgical System User Manual and reproduced with permission of Intuitive Surgical, Inc.

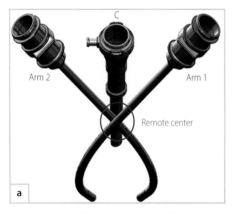

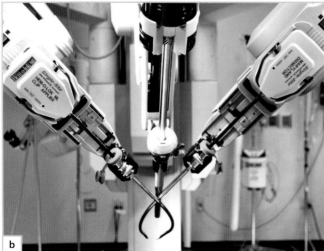

Figure 25.17 Schematic and picture of the Single-Site triangulation with cannulae and instruments installed. C, camera cannula. Reproduced with permission from Intuitive Surgical, Inc., Sunnyvale, California.

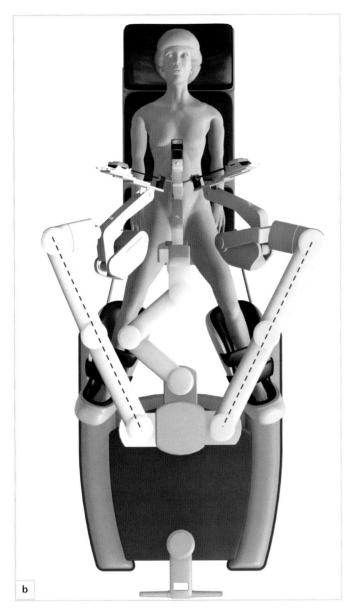

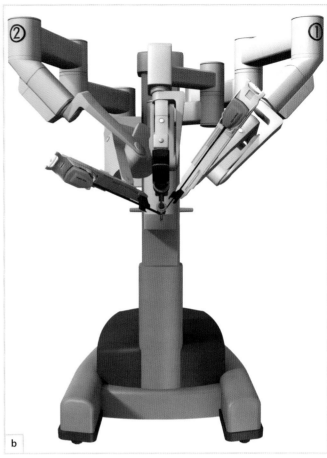

b

Figure 25.19 (a) Prepositioning the arms for Single-Site docking; (b) arms connected; red dotted lines show extended angle of the set-up joints of arms 1 and 2. Reproduced with permission from Intuitive Surgical, Inc., Sunnyvale, California.

Figure 25.20 Cannula connections in Single-Site surgery. Reproduced with permission from Intuitive Surgical, Inc., Sunnyvale, California.

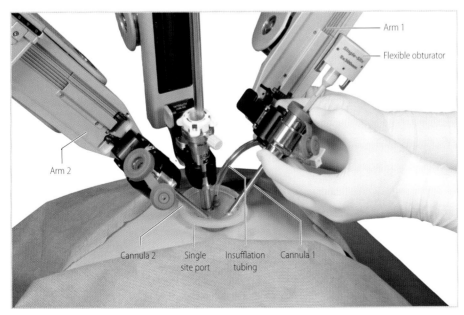

REFERENCES

Einarsson JI, Hibner M, Advincula AP. Side docking: an alternative docking method for gynecologic robotic surgery. Rev Obstet Gynecol 2011; 4(3-4):123–125.

Ghomi A, Kramer C, Askari R, Chavan NR, Einarsson JI. Trendelenburg position in gynecologic robotic-assisted surgery. J Minim Invasive Gynecol 2012; 19(4):485–489.

Gould C, Cull T, Wu YX, Osmundsen B. Blinded measure of Trendelenburg angle in pelvic robotic surgery. J Minim Invasive Gynecol 2012; 19(4):465–468

Higuchi TT, Gettman MT. Robotic instrumentation, personnel and operating room setup. In: Li-Ming Su (ed), Atlas of robotic urologic surgery, current clinical urology. New York: Springer Science and Business Media, 2011:15–30

Klauschie J1, Wechter ME, Jacob K, et al. Use of anti-skid material and patient-positioning to prevent patient shifting during robotic-assisted gynecologic procedures. J Minim Invasive Gynecol 2010; 17(4):504–507.

Strother E, Najam F, Gharagozloo F, et al. Operating room setup and robot preparation. In: Gharagozloo F, Najam F (eds), Robotic surgery. New York: The McGraw-Hill Companies, 2009:14–30

Chapter 26 | Robotic hysterectomy

Karen C Wang, Mobolaji O Ajao

INTRODUCTION

Neurosurgeons were the first to utilize robotic technology for precise stereotactic brain biopsies, followed by preoperative mapping for transurethral prostatectomy in urology and orthopedic assistance in performing hip arthroplasty. Penetration of robotic technology into the field of gynecology came as evidence for the benefits of a minimally invasive approach to surgery grew, while the limitations and difficulties of acquiring advanced laparoscopic skills were recognized since the first laparoscopic hysterectomy performed in 1988 (Reich et al. 1989). Conventional laparoscopy has been slow to gain popularity due to the two-dimensional view, counterintuitive movement of the instruments, absent articulation of the instruments, and restricted ergonomics with associated surgeon fatigue. Robotic surgical platforms became a solution to overcome these problems.

Computer Motion, Inc. (Galeta, California) has been at the forefront of robot-assisted surgery. In collaboration with the Department of Defense, the initial goal was to develop a surgical platform for providing medical care to wounded soldiers on the battlefield from a remote location. Computer Motion, Inc. developed several prototypes before arising to the current and only FDA approved surgical system known as the da Vinci surgical system (see Chapter 25), which is manufactured by Intuitive Surgical, Inc., Sunnyvale, California. The surgical systems predating the current platform of da Vinci surgical systems include AESOP (Automated Endoscopic System for Optimal Positioning), which involved a robotic arm controlled by voice activation that was based on a platform named HERMES. With the addition of two robotic arms to the robotic endoscope arm with a remote console for surgeon control, the AESOP/HERMES platform evolved into ZEUS. This allowed for the surgeon to sit at a station away from the patient with dual joysticks controlling the robotic arms while viewing a screen wearing three-dimensional (3D) glasses. With Intuitive Surgical's acquisition of Computer Motion in 2003, the ZEUS system was gradually replaced by the current da Vinci system that exists today. The technology allowed for 3D viewing, wristed instruments that could articulate, tremor filtration, and stabilized endoscope under direct control of the surgeon.

Application in gynecologic surgery was explored early on in the development of robotic surgery. The ZEUS system was used for tubal reanastomosis surgery by Falcone et al. in 2000 where the magnification, articulating instruments to facilitate suturing, and tremor filtration provided by the robotic platform allowed for the procedure that was traditionally performed by laparotomy to be accomplished laparoscopically. Diaz-Arrastia et al. reported the first series of robotic-assisted hysterectomy in 2002. In 2005, the FDA approved the da Vinci system for use in gynecologic surgery. Feasibility of using the robotic platform for total laparoscopic hysterectomy was first reported by Reynolds and Advincula in 2006. Since then, the utility and applications for which the robotic platform is used in gynecology for both benign and malignant conditions have greatly expanded.

THE DA VINCI SURGICAL SYSTEM

The da Vinci surgical system has gone through its own evolution since introduction almost two decades ago, to the current third-generation model (Intuitive Surgical, Inc. Sunnyvale, California) (**Figure 26.1**). The first generation of the da Vinci robotic system (Standard) appeared in 1999. Like all following da Vinci models, it consisted of a surgeon console, a patient-side cart, and the In-site vision system. Compared to conventional laparoscopy, this system offered 3D-imagery; 10-fold magnification, motion scaling, tremor reduction, and wristed

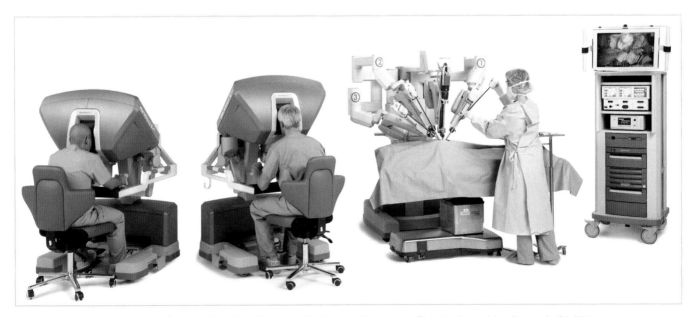

Figure 26.1 da Vinci Si system with dual console, patient side cart, and Insite tower. By courtesy of Intuitive Surgical, Inc., Sunnyvale, CA, 2014.

instrumentation (EndoWrist) simulating human-type range of motion. This initial model was manufactured with three arms, with a fourth arm added in 2003. In 2006, the second generation of da Vinci robotic system (S) was introduced. It added high-definition viewing, wider range of motion, and broader selection of instruments. An integrated touch screen monitor on the vision cart was added, which allowed for scope configuration. A TilePro function was added that allows for overlaying of patient's radiological imaging or other preoperative tests. The patient cart was less bulky, lighter, and motorized to facilitate movement in the operating room. In 2009, the third generation and current model (Si) was introduced. Dual console capability was added, which facilitated training and surgeon collaboration. More options were added to the foot pedals and the instrument selection was further expanded.

Components
Surgeon console

The surgeon sits and performs the procedure at the surgeon console located away from the patient and operating table. The newest da Vinci Si model allows for control of audio, video, setting controls, and ergonomic control. A stereoscopic viewer displays high-definition 3D image from the camera. The height of this viewer can be adjusted to surgeon's preference. A sensor-mediated safety measure disables the instruments in use when the surgeon's head is withdrawn from the viewer. The master controllers control the endoscopic instruments. Movement of each controller allows for a direct translation of movement of each instrument similar to open surgery.

Patient cart

The patient cart houses the robotic arms holding the camera and the endoscopic instruments. There is a designated arm for the camera and three other arms for the EndoWrist instruments. These instruments have seven degrees of motion, which is greater than what the human wrist can perform. Movements of the surgeon's hand in the master control of the surgeon's console are translated and scaled to the endoscopic instruments. This allows for tremor filtration to allow for fine movements. The cart is motorized and allows for quicker docking process. The patient cart can be docked midline, side, or parallel to the patient depending on the surgeon's preference. The robotic arms from the patient cart are then individually attached to special cannulas/trocars placed in procedure-specific port sites.

Vision cart

The vision cart contains the central processing unit and the illuminator that supplies the light for the endoscope. It also contains the camera assembly, which provides a 3D image translated from the two parallel endoscopes housed in the robotic camera (12 mm) to the surgeon console monitor, and the camera processing unit, which manages the image coming from the endoscope. There is an attached interactive touch screen monitor that allows for audio and video control patient-side.

INDICATIONS FOR ROBOTIC HYSTERECTOMY

Indications for robotic hysterectomy as well as the procedural steps would adhere to the normal practice of the surgeon. The sequence of these steps, as well as preferred instrumentation, is determined by the surgeon. Benign indications for robot-assisted laparoscopic hysterectomy include:

- Abnormal uterine bleeding
- Adenomyosis
- Fibroids
- Pelvic pain
- Pelvic organ prolapse
- Pelvic inflammatory disease/tube-ovarian abscess

Robotic hysterectomy is also utilized for premalignant and malignant conditions (endometrial cancer and early stage cervical and ovarian cancer).

PATIENT PREPARATION

A thorough history and physical is completed by the surgeon along with any indicated pre-operative testing (cervical cancer screening, endometrial sampling, imaging, laboratory testing, and medical clearance). Medical and surgical options are discussed with the patient. If the patient is a candidate for surgical management, the surgeon will determine which approach would be advised (vaginal, laparoscopic, or open) based on all the information as well as the patient's preference. Once the patient has been determined to be an appropriate candidate for a robotic hysterectomy approach informed consent is obtained. A thorough discussion about removal or retention of the cervix (total laparoscopic hysterectomy versus laparoscopic supra-cervical hysterectomy) as well as concomitant removal of adnexa (ovaries and/or fallopian tubes) is completed while obtaining consent. Risks, benefits, and alternatives to surgery are also discussed in detail in usual fashion. Post-operative expectations and instructions are also provided.

PATIENT POSITIONING, PORT PLACEMENT, AND DOCKING

Once taken to the operating room, the patient is positioned supine on the operating table over antiskid material to minimize sliding during Trendelenburg positioning during the procedure. Arms are tucked to the patient's side bilaterally with padding utilizing sleds or toboggans to avoid nerve injury. Legs are positioned in Allen or Yellofins stirrups with care to avoid neuropathy. Once the patient is prepped and draped, Foley catheter and uterine manipulator of the surgeon's choice are placed.

Abdominal access is then obtained by surgeon's preference (closed, open, or direct trocar entry technique and alternative left upper quadrant entry in appropriate cases with concern for intra-abdominal adhesions or large pathology extending above the umbilicus) and the abdomen is insufflated in routine fashion. The 12 mm endoscopic trocar is placed at the umbilicus for normal sized uteri or above for larger pathology for adequate visualization. For enlarged uteri, a good rule of thumb is to place the endoscopic trocar at least 8–10 cm above the fundus of the uterus while pushing up the uterus cephalad with the manipulator. Depending on surgeon's preference, two to three additional robotic 8 mm trocars are placed under direct visualization in the right lower and upper quadrants with at least 8–10 cm distance between each trocar to avoid collision of instruments and obstructed visualization. An assistant port (5, 8, or 12 mm) is also placed as per surgeon's preference in the right or left upper or lower quadrant to facilitate tissue retraction, suction, and irrigation, and introduction and removal of suture. Once the trocars are in place, the patient is placed in Trendelenburg position as much as required. A descriptive study demonstrated that the amount of Trendelenburg required to complete robot-assisted laparoscopic procedures was much less than expected or traditionally performed (mean 16.4°) (Ghomi et al. 2012).

Docking is the process of attaching the arms of the patient cart to the special robotic cannulae in the patient's abdominal wall. Docking of the patient cart takes into account the pathology as well as requirement for vaginal access. With midline docking, the center column of the patient cart, the camera arm, and endoscope should line up with the target anatomy. The patient cart is docked between the patient's legs. This does obstruct vaginal access and makes uterine manipulation difficult. Side or parallel docking is feasible without compromising movement of the robotic arms or access to the pelvis. With this approach, the patient cart is docked adjacent to the patient's hip (at 45° angle to patient vertical access or parallel to patient), and the center column is aimed toward the contralateral shoulder (Einarsson et al. 2011).

For more detail, please refer to Chapter 25, Robotic instrumentation and room setup.

HYSTERECTOMY PROCEDURE

Steps of the procedure and electrosurgical devices used are determined based on surgeon's training and preference. Simplified outline:

1. Division of gonadal vessels (infundibulopelvic ligament or utero-ovarian ligament depending on whether the adnexa are being removed or retained)
2. Division of round ligament
3. Separation of vesicouterine peritoneum, development of bladder flap
4. Skeletonization and division of the uterine vessels
5. Separation of cardinal and uterosacral ligaments for total laparoscopic hysterectomy
6. Colpotomy for total laparoscopic hysterectomy
7. Vaginal cuff repair for total laparoscopic hysterectomy
8. Amputation of uterus from cervix for laparoscopic supracervical hysterectomy
9. Cystoscopy if indicated

SINGLE PORT PLATFORM

While robotic surgery enables performance of major procedures with a minimally invasive approach, there is a minimum requirement of three ports to complete the procedure, and oftentimes five ports are used in total (**Figures 26.2** and **26.3**). Single port surgery was designed to further improve on the benefits of laparoscopy by using a single multichannel port for the procedures. The first single incision laparoscopic hysterectomy was reported in 1991 (Pelosi & Pelosi 1991). There was hesitation to uptake of this adaptation to laparoscopic surgery due to some technical challenges including crowding and clashing of instruments. The loss of triangulation created by instruments in close approximation has led to modification of instruments in attempts to overcome this. Smaller shaft instruments (5 mm) decrease the occurrence of instrument clashing and articulating instruments were developed, increasing the angles of approach to the surgical field. All these factors contribute greater technical difficulty in single incision laparoscopy especially with large pathology or complex disease (endometriosis, adhesions), thereby limiting widespread physician uptake.

With adoption of robotics in gynecology, the crossover of single incision surgery in this new realm was just a matter of time. Feasibility of single incision robotic hysterectomy was evaluated with positive results (Escobar et al. 2010, Nam et al. 2011). The steps of the hysterectomy remained the same and the robotic platform was able to overcome the extreme limitations of single incision surgery and absent triangulation that is essential to adhering to minimally invasive techniques. Since benefits of single incision surgery besides improved cosmesis have yet to be proven, adoption of this platform still lags significantly behind multi-incision robotic surgery. Further advances will need to be made to make single-site robotic surgery mainstream (Kroh et al. 2011, Iavazzo & Gkegkes 2013, Vizza et al. 2013, Sendag et al. 2014).

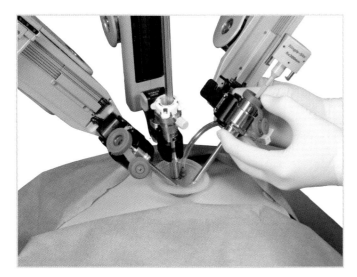

Figure 26.2 Single port platform docked. By courtesy of Intuitive Surgical, Inc., Sunnyvale, CA, 2014.

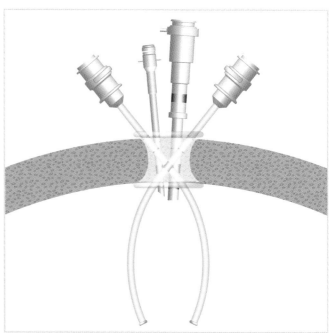

Figure 26.3 Schematic of single port platform at the umbilicus with instruments through the abdominal wall. By courtesy of Intuitive Surgical, Inc., Sunnyvale, CA, 2014.

EVIDENCE IN ROBOTIC HYSTERECTOMY

As in the case of any new medical device or technique, studies have been conducted to evaluate the advantages and benefits of new technology in order to determine their role in the gynecologist's armamentarium. The feasibility of performing laparoscopic hysterectomy with robot assistance has been clearly demonstrated (Diaz Arrastia et al. 2002, Advincula & Wang 2009). Unfortunately, there is a paucity of randomized control trials involving benign hysterectomy. A Cochrane Review published in 2012 concluded that robotic surgery is comparable to laparoscopy with regard to intraoperative complications, quality of life, length of hospital stay, and rate of conversion to laparotomy (Liu et al. 2012).

The recent systematic review of the literature was performed by the Society of Gynecologic Surgeons (SGS) comparing robotic versus nonrobotic surgical approaches for the treatment of both benign and malignant gynecologic indications. Specifically, surgical- and patient-centered outcomes, costs, and adverse events were examined in the literature (Gala et al. 2014). The literature review completed by the SGS involved assessing 97 articles of which 30 comparative studies met eligibility criteria. Only three involved hysterectomy for benign disease. The largest study published by Landeen et al. examined 569 women who underwent robotic hysterectomy compared to 230 laparoscopic hysterectomies and found that blood loss and length of stay were less in the robotic group while there was no significant difference in operative time (Landeen et al. 2011). In contrast, a study by Sarlos et al. found that laparoscopic surgery took less time compared to robotic surgery (108.9 min vs. 82.9 min, P <0.05) (Sarlos et al. 2010). Clear benefits of robotic surgery over traditional laparotomy with regard to reduced length of stay (1.5 days compared to 3.5 days, P <0.001) and less blood loss (82.3 mL vs. 430 mL, P <0.001) were demonstrated. The group concluded that the available literature does not demonstrate a difference in outcomes between robotic and laparoscopic techniques; however, compelling evidence of the benefits of robotic surgery over open technique exists.

ADVANTAGES OF THE ROBOTIC APPROACH

Beyond the purported advantages of robotic surgery with regard to improved visualization, articulation of EndoWrist instruments to facilitate suturing, tremor filtration, which allows for fine dissection and management of delicate tissue, the robotic surgical platform has been shown to reduce the learning curve for performing laparoscopic procedures compared to conventional laparoscopy. Two studies determined that between 50 and 91 robotic cases were required to achieve proficiency in robot-assisted laparoscopic surgery as defined by a stable operative time (Lenihan et al. 2008, Woelk et al. 2013).

In a case series of 200 consecutive hysterectomies (first 100 performed by conventional laparoscopy with the subsequent 100 performed with robot assistance), operative time improved after performing 75 robotic cases and resulted in shorter operative time compared to the laparoscopic approach (78.7 min vs. 92.4 min, P = 0.03). Mean blood loss was two times greater in the laparoscopic cohort compared to the robotic cohort (113 mL vs. 61.1 mL, P <0.0001) and the mean length of stay was a half-day longer in the laparoscopic cohort. Most notable in the retrospective chart review was the reduction in conversion to laparotomy from 11% in the laparoscopic cohort to 0% once the robotic device was utilized (Payne & Dauterive 2008).

LIMITATIONS OF THE ROBOTIC PLATFORM

Despite the advantages conferred by the robotic surgical platforms, some limitations do exist and most notorious is the associated cost of the robotic platform including the initial upfront cost, annual maintenance fees, and disposable instruments that can be used for 10 cases. An economic analysis comparing laparoscopic and robotic hysterectomy for benign disease showed an additional cost of $2,189 with the robotic approach (Wright et al. 2013).

Another limitation of robotic surgery in the current platform is the absence of tactile feedback from the instruments at the surgeon's console. There is no evidence that the lack of haptics adversely affects surgical outcomes and supporters of robotic surgery contend that the enhanced visualization (magnification and 3D viewing) compensates for that limitation.

CONCLUSION

Robotic surgery has undoubtedly made a significant impact on the field of gynecology. The rate at which robotic surgery has been adopted since FDA approval for gynecologic surgery in 2005 has rapidly surpassed the rate at which conventional laparoscopy gained interest since the first reported laparoscopic hysterectomy performed in 1988. Features of the robotic platform provide a mechanism to overcome the limitations of conventional laparoscopy, which can facilitate successfully completion of complex laparoscopic procedures. There is a dearth of evidence demonstrating an advantage of the robotic approach compared to conventional laparoscopy for benign hysterectomy and additional randomized control trials are needed for high-quality data evaluating patient based outcomes and cost-effectiveness. In the meantime, the robotic platform is recognized as enabling technology to facilitate converting cases traditionally done by laparotomy to a laparoscopic approach and is utilized based on surgeon preference (ACOG Committee Opinion No. 444 2009, Barbash & Glied 2010, Sarlos et al. 2010, Liu et al. 2012, AAGL Position Statement 2013).

REFERENCES

AAGL Position Statement. Robotic-assisted laparoscopic surgery in benign gynecology AAGL Advancing Minimally Invasive Gynecology Worldwide. J Minim Invas Gyn 2013; 20:2–9.

ACOG Committee Opinion No. 444. Choosing the route of hysterectomy for benign disease. Obstet Gynecol 2009; 114:1156–1158. 1110.1097/AOG.1150b1013e3181c1133c1172.

Advincula AP, Wang K. Evolving role and current state of robotics in minimally invasive gynecologic surgery. J Minim Invasive Gynecol 2009; 16:291–301.

Barbash G, Glied S. New technology and health care costs—the case of robot-assisted surgery. N Engl J Med 2010; 363:701–704.

Diaz-Arrastia C, Jurnalov C, Gomez G, Townsend C, Jr. Laparoscopic hysterectomy using a computer-enhanced surgical robot. Surg Endosc 2002; 16:1271–1273.

Einarsson JI, Hibner M, Advincula AP. Side docking: an alternative docking method for gynecologic robotic surgery. Rev Obstet Gynecol 2011; 4:123–125.

Escobar P, Starks D, Fader A, et al. Single-port risk-reducing salpingo-oophorectomy with and without hysterectomy: surgical outcomes and learning curve analysis. Gynecol Oncol 2010; 119:43–47.

Falcone T, Goldberg JM, Margossian H, Stevens L. Robotic-assisted laparoscopic microsurgical tubal anastomosis: a human pilot study. Fertil Steril 2000; 73:1040–1042.

Gala RB, Margulies R, Steinberg A, et al. Society of Gynecologic Surgeons Systematic Review Group. Systematic review of robotic surgery in gynecology: robotic techniques compared with laparoscopy and laparotomy. J Minim Invasive Gynecol 2014; 21:353–361.

Ghomi A, Kramer C, Askari R, et al. Trendelenburg position in gynecologic robotic-assisted surgery. J Minim Invasive Gynecol 2012; 19:485–489.

Iavazzo C, Gkegkes I. Single-site port robotic-assisted hysterectomy: a systematic review. Arch Gynecol Obstet 2014; 289:725–731.

Kroh M, El-Hayek K, Rosenblatt S, et al. First human surgery with a novel single-port robotic system: cholecystectomy using the da Vinci Single-Site platform. Surg Endosc 2011; 25:3566–3573.

Landeen LB, Bell MC, Hubert HB, et al. Clinical and cost comparisons for hysterectomy via abdominal, standard laparoscopic, vaginal, and robot-assisted approaches. S D Med 2011; 64:197–199.

Lenihan J Jr, Kovanda C, Seshadri-Kreaden U. What is the learning curve for robotic assisted gynecologic surgery? J Minim Invasive Gynecol 2008; 15:589–594.

Liu H, Lu D, Wang L, et al.. Robotic surgery for benign gynecological disease. Cochrane Database Syst Rev 2012; 2:CD008978. doi: 10.1002/14651858.

Nam E, Kim S, Lee M, et al. Robotic single-port transumbilical total hysterectomy: a pilot study. J Gynecol Oncol 2011; 22:120–126.

Payne TN, Dauterive FR. A comparison of total laparoscopic hysterectomy to robotically assisted hysterectomy: surgical outcomes in a community practice. J Minim Invasive Gynecol 2008; 15:286–291.

Pelosi M, Pelosi M, 3rd. Laparoscopic hysterectomy with bilateral salpingo-oophorectomy using a single umbilical puncture. N J Med 1991; 88:721–726.

Reich H, Decaprio J, Mcglynn F. Laparoscopic Hysterectomy. J Gynecol Surg 1989; 5:213–216.

Reynolds RK, Advincula AP. Robot-assisted laparoscopic hysterectomy: technique and initial experience. Am J Surg 2006; 191:555–560.

Sarlos D, Kots L, Stevanovic N, Schaer G. Robotic hysterectomy versus conventional laparoscopic hysterectomy: Outcome and cost analyses of a matched case-control study. Eur J Obstet Gyn Reprod Biol 2010; 150:92–96.

Sendag F, Akdemir A, Oztekin M. Robotic single-incision transumbilical total hysterectomy using a single-site robotic platform: initial report and technique. J Minim Invas Gyn 2014; 21:147–151.

Vizza E, Corrado G, Mancini E, et al. Robotic single-site hysterectomy in low risk endometrial cancer: a pilot study. Ann Surg Oncol 2013; 20:2759–2764.

Woelk J, Casiano E, Weaver AL, et al. The learning curve of robotic hysterectomy. Obstet Gynecol 2013; 121:87–95.

Wright J, Ananth C, Lewin S, et al. Robotically assisted vs. laparoscopic hysterectomy among women with benign gynecologic disease. JAMA 2013; 309:689–698.

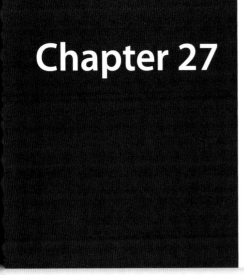

Chapter 27

A decade of robot-assisted laparoscopic myomectomy: reflections on the present and future

Antonio R Gargiulo

▉ INTRODUCTION

Advances in assisted human reproduction have significantly limited the indications for reproductive surgery. However, a functional uterus is still essential for both natural and artificial reproduction, and myomectomy remains one of the most commonly performed operations in gynecology.

Because of the highly specialized and irreplaceable nature of the tissues involved, myomectomy must be planned and executed according to reproductive priorities, and must adhere to the principles of microsurgery. Complete myometrial and endometrial preservation, thorough hemostasis, precise tissue apposition, reconstruction in layers, and the absence of exposed suture are essential. Scientific observations justify such fastidious attention to hysterotomy repair. A recent second-look laparoscopy study performed adhesion scoring 6 months after laparoscopic myomectomy (LM) to define the role of wound closure technique on healing quality. The study included 108 patients, all of whom received the same adhesion prevention agent and excluded patients with any concomitant surgery. The quality of uterine repair was directly associated with the chance of finding adhesions at the time of second-look laparoscopy. The authors concluded that adhesion formation depends on uterine wound appearance immediately after LM; a protruding wound was associated with over 2.5 times the risk of adhesions compared to a nonprotruding wound (Kumakiri et al. 2012).

Wound protrusion is associated with the technique of single-layer closure that bunches up the deep and superficial tissue layers. Indeed, single-layer hysterotomy closure is not described for classic open myomectomy. However, a recent study suggests that it represents the prevailing type of repair in conventional LM (in contrast to two- and three-layer closures prevalent in robotic myomectomy; Pluchino et al. 2014). This is most likely due to the fact that suturing in layers is the most technically challenging and time-consuming step of myomectomy, and the time consumed in the repair is directly related to blood loss. This may induce surgeons with less experience of intracorporeal laparoscopic suturing to opt for a mass closure. However, a multilayer closure remains the standard of care in myomectomy, and surgical double standards should not be accepted. There is only one myomectomy; the essential features of this operation cannot depend on access modality. Surgeons are held to the same operative standards whether or not they open the abdominal wall.

Minimally invasive myomectomy offers superior clinical and reproductive outcomes compared to abdominal myomectomy (AM). In particular, the minimally invasive route is associated with less blood loss and postoperative pain, shorter hospital stay, quicker return to normal activities, and fewer complications (Jin et al. 2009).

In terms of obstetrical risk, the incidence of uterine rupture seems to be lower after minimally invasive myomectomy (0–1.1%; Parker et al. 2010, Pitter et al. 2013, Seracchioli et al. 2006, Sizzi et al. 2007) than after open myomectomy (0.0–4%; Garnet 1964, Spong et al. 2007).

In terms of postoperative adhesion formation, the prevalence of adhesions at second-look laparoscopy has been reported to be between 55% and 94% after open myomectomy (Tulandi et al. 1993) and between 29% and 35% following LM (Dubuisson et al. 1998, Takeuchi & Kinoshita 2002).

As a consequence of the evidence accumulated on this topic, the American Society of Reproductive Medicine currently recommends the use of minimally invasive myomectomy techniques and adhesion barriers to minimize adhesions following myomectomy (Practice Committee of the American Society of Reproductive Medicine 2007).

A single study stands out as the exception to the broad evidence that points to a higher rate of adhesion following open myomectomy. In a multicenter retrospective study, Tinelli et al. identified 546 women who underwent an AM or LM and then a repeat abdominal surgery within 6 years. Patients were divided in four groups (Pfannenstiel laparotomy vs. multiport laparoscopy, either with or without the use of oxidized regenerated cellulose). The study was blinded as to the use of adhesion barriers. A statistically higher incidence of adhesions was found in the AM group without adhesion barrier (28.1%), and the lowest incidence in the LM group with adhesion barrier (15.9%). However, no statistical significance was found between groups where barriers were not employed, pointing to the importance of the use of barriers as the primary modality to prevent adhesions in this particular study. The study was limited by the lack of analysis of all those patients who did not need reoperation within 6 years of the myomectomy, and by the fact that it was performed at a time when it was considered ethical for closure of the hysterotomy to be technically different in the open and laparoscopic approaches (see above; Tinelli et al. 2011).

Second-look laparoscopy studies are available which assess adhesion formation following robot-assisted laparoscopic myomectomy (RM). A recent multicenter study reported that only 11% of women who had undergone computer-assisted LM were found to have any adhesions at the time of their subsequent cesarean section (Pitter et al. 2013).

Considering all of the above, our technique preference is for the minimally invasive myomectomy modality whenever this is safely feasible.

The avoidance of AM introduces the concept of 'laparotomy threshold' and the related concept of conversion rate. Once it is accepted that it is no longer ethical for myomectomy to be performed by surgeons who are not well versed in advanced laparoscopy, one must recognize that a personal threshold of technical complexity exists for even the most advanced laparoscopic surgeons, above which it becomes prudent to resort to laparotomy. This personal threshold is based on surgical aptitude, training opportunities, and personal ethics. However, hard evidence points to the fact that the laparotomy threshold is generally very low for myomectomy. A recent survey of Canadian gynecologists reported that only 12.7% of the surgeons who offered myomectomy in their practice used LM more often than AM (Liu et al. 2010). Stated differently, in the population studied, a woman consulting a gynecologic surgeon for a myomectomy has a one in eight chance of meeting a provider that is likely to offer her a minimally invasive myomectomy. As it has already been shown for hysterectomy (Wright et al. 2013), it is expected that the diffusion of RM will improve access to minimally invasive surgery for many more women requiring myomectomy.

However, there are other ways to raise one's own laparotomy threshold; advanced laparoscopic training and an adequately high case load may be enough for some surgeons. In fact, in the largest head-to-head comparison study to date, RM and LM both had zero conversion to open surgery, in spite of comparable tumor loads (Gargiulo et al. 2012). In other studies in gynecologic surgery robotic assistance has been shown to have a lower conversion rate than conventional laparoscopy. It must, therefore, be considered as one of the practical solutions to raise the laparotomy threshold (Lim et al. 2011, Patzkowsky et al. 2013).

Of course, no studies have ever been specifically designed to prospectively compare the effect of computer assistance on the surgeons' laparotomy threshold for specific surgical operations. The objective difficulty of designing and carrying out such a study should not distract us from using what we've learned from our own experience. To explain the concept in tangible terms, I have decided to share my personal AM threshold, with and without robot assistance. A table has been compiled on the basis of my actual experience as an independent surgeon at Brigham and Women's Hospital since 1998, and also on a conversion rate of 0%. In other words, the table illustrates the conditions within which I consider a conversion to be an unforeseen event (**Table 27.1**). It is my strong belief that, in the age of patient-centered medicine and medical research (Frank et al. 2014), whenever we propose LM to a patient, a conversion to the abdominal route should be an unforeseen event. In this perspective, a conversion is considered an acceptable failure, but not truly an expected outcome. After all, a conversion is a double operation caused by poor patient selection.

In conclusion, hysteroscopic resection aside, there is only one type of myomectomy operation; there are no shortcuts in reproductive surgery. The patient-centered approach to this operation is that it should be performed in a minimally invasive fashion whenever possible, and that a change of plan (conversion to open surgery) should be an unforeseen event. Robot assistance is one of the demonstrated practical strategies to achieve the above goals, particularly in the hands of trained laparoscopic teams.

Table 27.1. Understanding one's personal laparotomy threshold for myomectomy is essential in order to decide if robotic-assistance is needed. The overarching goal is the reasonable elimination of open myomectomy (Frank et al. 2014)

Surgical scenario	LM	RM	Open
Max diameter tumor: 5 cm	✓	✓	✓
Max diameter tumor: 10 cm	✓	✓	✓
Max diameter tumor: 15 cm		✓	✓
Max diameter tumor: 20 cm			✓
Max diameter tumor: > 20 cm			✓
Max number: 5		✓	✓
Max number: 10		✓	✓
Max number: 15		✓	✓
Max number: 20			✓
Max number: > 20			✓
Frozen pelvis		✓	✓
Cervical myoma		✓	✓
Intraligamentary myoma		✓	✓
Adenomyosis		✓	✓
Large submucous component		✓	✓
Cosmetic port placement		✓	✓
Max BMI: 30	✓	✓	✓
Max BMI: 40	✓	✓	✓
Max BMI: 50		✓	✓
Max BMI: ≥ 60		✓	✓

ROBOT-ASSISTED LAPAROSCOPIC MYOMECTOMY

History and current techniques

Arnold Advincula et al. are credited with the development and the early experimental clinical applications of RM that lead to the US Food and Drug Administration (FDA) approval of the da Vinci Surgical System for gynecologic surgery in 2005 (Advincula et al. 2004).

The safety and efficacy of this procedure are now well established, with perioperative outcomes that mirror those of LM, and excellent long-term reproductive and symptomatic outcomes have been demonstrated (Bedient et al. 2009, Gargiulo et al. 2012, Nezhat et al. 2009, Pitter et al. 2015).

In keeping with the LM literature, case-matched comparisons between patients undergoing AM or RM show lower blood loss, fewer complications, and shorter hospital stays for the minimally invasive procedure (Advincula et al. 2007, Barakat et al. 2011).

In the study by Barakat et al., perioperative outcomes of 393 AMs, 93 LMs, and 89 RMs were analyzed. No significant differences were found for LMs and RMs in terms of blood loss, operative time, or hospital stay, in spite of a larger tumor load in the RM group. RM required a significantly longer operative time compared to AM; however, blood loss, hemoglobin drop, and hospital stay were all significantly reduced, despite comparable tumor load (Barakat et al. 2011).

In a previously mentioned study, comparing short-term outcomes of 174 RMs and 115 LMs with similar tumor load, perioperative outcomes were excellent for both techniques; however, operative time was significantly longer for RMs (191 vs. 115 minutes; Gargiulo et al. 2012).

A limitation of that study was that barbed suture was used in the majority of LM cases but only in 5% of RM cases. Indeed, while the study was in progress, definitive evidence became available demonstrating that barbed suture use in LM significantly shortens operative time and decreases blood loss (Alessandri et al. 2010, Angioli et al. 2012).

In any case, the general trend that emerges from an objective analysis of the scientific literature is that RM takes longer than AM and costs more than LM. This conclusion underlines the importance of my introductory paragraph to explain that the main value of the surgical robot in myomectomy resides in the elimination of AM, rather than in supplanting LM where this modality is available to cover the community's needs. At this time, 20 years following its introduction, an uncompromised LM remains beyond practical reach for most gynecologists; by raising the laparotomy threshold, RM may represent a practical alternative to AM.

One of the advantages of writing a 'decade in review' chapter on robotic myomectomy is that one no longer needs to spend much time on the basic features of robotic surgical platforms. Current surgical robots employed for laparoscopy are teleoperators with virtual reality simulation capability. These two characteristics assist surgeons in different ways. The teleoperator is the physical interface between the eyes and limbs of the surgeon. The teleoperator can effectively eliminate all of the following ergonomic challenges of laparoscopy: (1) inverted pitch and yaw of the instruments (the fulcrum effect), (2) absent pitch and yaw at the wrist, (3) loss of stereoscopic view, (4) visual disconnect (the operator looks away from the field), and (5) postural strain. There are studies demonstrating the enabling nature of teleoperators (Gargiulo 2014).

Limitations

However, contrary to industry-driven marketing, teleoperators are not easy to use, and present the surgeon with new challenges. This is where virtual reality simulation closes the safety loop. Due to the fact that this type of surgery is performed at a console, simulation is uniquely effective; the working conditions are identical to those found during the real operation. In conclusion, the teleoperator makes laparoscopy ergonomic, while the simulator helps the surgeon become one with the teleoperator and achieve a consistent performance (Culligan et al. 2014). One technological limitation with RM is the impact of the absence of haptic feedback on the quality of the operation. A recent and small retrospective study of 16 RM cases has attempted to answer this question (Griffin et al. 2013). Unfortunately, this study enrolled an average of only one patient per month within a large group of private gynecologists, over a period of 14 months. The total number of RMs performed by the entire group over the study period was 23, suggesting an extremely small yearly case load per surgeon. This may explain the 100% increase in operating room time of RM compared with AM, which is inconsistent with the findings of larger studies (Barakat et al. 2011), as well as the findings of a five times greater residual fibroid burden observed 12 weeks after RM, compared to AM. The authors point out that the limited robotic experience of the operators makes the results of this study more applicable to surgeons in the community than in large referral centers. Regardless of the major limitations of this study, this evidence highlights the importance of high-resolution preoperative imaging for laparoscopic (and particularly robotic) excision of uterine fibroids. When dealing with large uteri, this means obtaining a magnetic resonance imaging (MRI) of the pelvis. MRI's ability to detect and accurately locate smaller fibroids is superior to ultrasound, and so is its accuracy in ruling out adenomyosis (Moghadam et al. 2006, Shwayder & Sakhel 2014). Approaching a large laparoscopic or robotic myomectomy without the advantage of radiologic myoma mapping is likely to result in a higher residual fibroid burden compared with the open approach. No comparisons exist to date between residual myoma burden in robotic and LM. Whether the removal of all fibroids represents an advantage or a disadvantage of AM is likewise unclear. Removal of clinically insignificant fibroids increases the number of uterine incisions and may negatively impact future reproductive function. To date, there is no evidence of an increased risk of reoperation for minimally invasive myomectomy compared to AM (Bhave Chittawar et al. 2014).

Looking ahead

Newly available robotic technology may eventually provide some imaging-independent advantage in the identification of smaller intramural tumors by reintroducing some degree of haptic feedback into robot-assisted laparoscopy. The Telelap-ALF X is a promising robotic surgical platform whose experimental human use has been successfully completed in Italy, and mostly in gynecology (Stark et al. 2015). Among other innovations, including multiple independent single-arm teleoperators, completely reusable instrumentation, and an eye-tracking camera, the Telelap offers simulated haptic feedback. The system obtained the European Commission's approval in 2011 and has been commercialized in Europe since 2015.

However, there is evidence to suggest that even the highest degree of tactile feedback – that which is allowed by open surgery – cannot compete with the ability of radiologic imaging to detect residual leiomyomas (Angioli et al. 2010). From this perspective, the importance of haptic feedback in myomectomy may be overstated in light of the advantages provided by preoperative and intraoperative imaging. That is to say that myoma mapping is likely to have more clinical relevance than tactile feedback in myomectomy and the definitive technological solution in RM may eventually reside in real-time image fusion, rather than haptic feedback.

Robotic myomectomy and gynecologic robotic surgery, in general, have also been criticized for imposing a higher cosmetic burden on our patients. Several recent studies have polled patients planning gynecologic surgery, asking them to rank drawings of scars in order of their cosmetic preference. Multiple upper abdominal scars were described as associated with robot-assisted surgery (likely based on old port-placement protocols). As a result, 'robotic-surgery scar patterns' were ranked consistently low by prospective patients, even when compared to laparotomy by Pfannestiel incision (Bush et al. 2011, Goebel & Goldberg 2014, Yeung et al. 2013). I disagree with the argument that robotic myomectomy necessarily results in a less cosmetically desirable scar pattern compared to standard laparoscopy (**Figures 27.1** and **27.2**). Our team employs two general approaches to laparoscopic port placement in robotic myomectomy: a standard approach for myomata greater than 8 cm in largest diameter and a cosmetic approach for myomata less than 8 cm in diameter. In the standard approach, the primary port (the camera port) is at the umbilicus or in the midline above the umbilicus. The target organ in myomectomy is the most cephalad myoma (as opposed to the hysterectomy where the target organs are the ovarian and uterine vascular pedicles). Therefore, the location of the primary port depends on the pathology at hand, and does not change between standard robotic and standard laparoscopic approaches; the resulting scar will be either

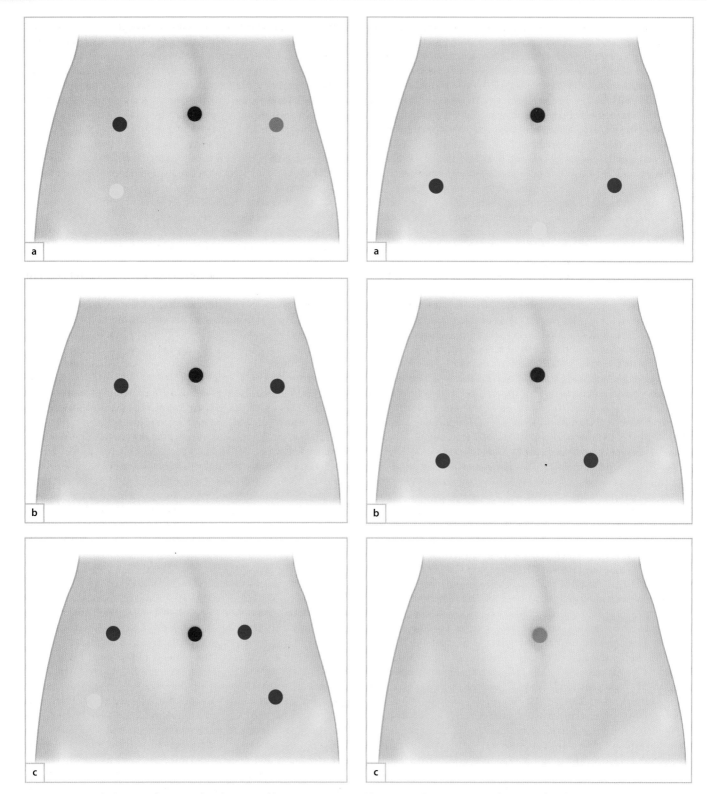

Figure 27.1 Standard port configurations for robot-assisted laparoscopic myomectomy, currently employed in our program when the largest fibroid exceeds 8 cm in maximum diameter. (a) Classic. (b) Solo. (c) All four. These standard configurations allows (1) ideal triangulation of the robotic instruments; (2) possibility to operate in the 'vertical zone' during conventional laparoscopic portion of the procedure; (3) the use of a third robotic instrument for complex cases ('all four,' refers to the fact that the three instrument arms plus the camera arm are used at the same time). The 'solo' version forgoes the use of an assistant port and necessitates expert assistance at bedside. Blue, robotic cannulas; Red, primary port; Yellow, assistant port.

Figure 27.2 Cosmetic port configurations for robot-assisted laparoscopic myomectomy with no visible scars above the anterior superior iliac spines; currently employed in our program when the largest fibroid is <8 cm in maximum diameter. (a) Cosmetic. (b) Cosmetic solo. (c) Single port. These cosmetic configurations allow superior cosmetic results at the cost of significantly more challenging techniques. MRI or three-dimensional ultrasound is essential for case selection.
Blue, robotic cannulas; Purple, single-site device; Red, primary port; Yellow, assistant port.

hidden within the umbilicus or visible above it. The assistant port for our standard robotic approach is placed in the lower quadrant, on the side of the main surgeon (usually the patient's right side), just above the anterior–superior iliac spine (ASIS). This incision is created on a distended abdomen and later recedes below the ASIS once the abdomen is deflated. Aside from this obvious cosmetic advantage, other advantages of a low assistant port in robotic myomectomy are: (1) it allows the transit of needles to occur in full view; (2) it represents the caudal component of an 'ultralateral' trocar placement, described by Koh et al., and can be used to operate in the 'vertical zone' when required (Koh & Janik 2003); (3) it makes the surgical assistant move closer to the pelvis, so that they can simultaneously handle the uterine manipulator and a laparoscopic instrument (provided that an assistant monitor is correctly placed at the head of the operating table so that the assistant can face toward the patient's head).

The right side robotic cannula is placed about 8–10 cm to the right of the camera port; this represents the cephalad component of the 'vertical zone,' as mentioned above. The left robotic cannula is placed 8–10 cm to the left of the camera port. Note that this port is the only one that is unique to robotic myomectomy. All other ports, including that for a possible third robotic cannula (placed in the left lower quadrant), are also used in conventional LM. Hence, the whole discussion about a possible decreased cosmesis of robotic laparoscopy is based on a single 8 mm extra port above the bikini line (i.e. the left robotic cannula port in this description).

Women undergoing myomectomy are generally of reproductive age and many are concerned with the cosmetic issue. Because of this objective, patient-centered consideration, we routinely employ one of three fully cosmetic port placement configurations in all robotic myomectomy cases, with the largest myoma under 8 cm. In all these cases, the camera port is consistently placed within the umbilical scar, and no ports are placed above the level of the ASIS. Depending on the complexity of the case, and the skills of the surgeon and bedside assistant, a dedicated assistant port is not always necessary. Such fully cosmetic approaches are very difficult to achieve with conventional LM, unless the surgeon is willing to put the patient's health at significant risk by operating outside the 'vertical zone' and reaching across the midline. Even then, surgeon's fatigue may hamper the quality of microsurgical repair. The majority of RMs performed in our practice can be accomplished with a fully cosmetic port placement that would be hard or impossible to achieve with conventional laparoscopy. In particular, one of the most interesting developments of robotic assistance in myomectomy is the new field of single-site robotic myomectomy. This technique was pioneered at Brigham and Women's Hospital and has recently gained particular momentum due to the uncertain future of intracorporeal morcellation (see below); the main appeal of this technique is the larger access point similar to an open laparoscopy access, which allows adequate space for effective extracorporeal tissue extraction in most patients. Our team has described two very different approaches to this ultraminimally invasive technique. The earlier reported version involves a coaxial technique performed with standard rigid robotic instruments inserted through a GelPoint device. This technique gives excellent cosmetic results in women with high body mass index, where the depth of the umbilicus allows a 4 cm incision to be made and repaired with minimal cosmetic disruption (Gargiulo et al. 2013).

The recent availability of a dedicated USFDA-approved single-site platform for the da Vinci Si Surgical System (a multi-lumen port, curved cannulas, and semi-rigid single-site 5 mm robotic instruments, including Wristed Needle Drivers) has brought about a significant miniaturization of this approach. We recently published the world's first series of myomectomies performed through a 2.5 cm umbilical incision, resulting in no noticeable scar (Lewis et al. 2015). Implicit in single-incision surgery and in any utilization of the umbilicus as a point of entry or of specimen extraction is the concept that not every umbilicus can accept a 2.5 cm long incision. In cases where significant cosmetic disruption is likely, we recommend a small suprapubic minilaparotomy for specimen extraction to our patients.

The achievement of a reproducible technique of RM through a single incision is an important step toward the emancipation of robot-assisted surgery toward a technology that is not only generally enabling, but allows results which would be virtually unattainable with conventional laparoscopy.

Indeed, conventional laparoendoscopic single-site myomectomy, reported by a group based in Asia, involves specialized suturing techniques (i.e. it does not meet the myomectomy criteria discussed earlier), is extremely hard to reproduce, and is not available in the great majority of medical centers in the world (Choi et al. 2014).

Figures 27.3–27.5 describe the main technical aspects of standard, cosmetic, and single-site RM.

Tissue extraction from the abdominal cavity following RM has never been accomplished robotically, and is currently performed with conventional laparoscopic or minilaparotomy techniques that are covered elsewhere in this volume (Srouji et al. 2015). In 2014, following a surge in patient-initiated legal actions – related to cases of inadvertent intraperitoneal dispersion of unexpected uterine malignancies by open laparoscopic electromechanical morcellation – the USFDA released statements that aimed at severely limiting the use of this technology (U.S. Food and Drugs Administration 2014). In response to this USFDA initiative, several professional societies have openly addressed the pros and cons of laparoscopic electromechanical morcellation of uterine tissue, defending its use in low-risk patients. I strongly advise surgeons to familiarize themselves with all proposed arguments when choosing their preferred technique of uterine tissue extraction and when documenting their patients' informed consents (AAGL Advancing Minimally Invasive Gynecology Worldwide 2014, American College of Obstetricians and Gynecologists 2014, Brown 2014).

At the time of this publication, the USFDA has explicitly labeled electromechanical morcellation devices as contraindicated for use in uterine tissue and uterine tumor extraction in menopausal and perimenopausal women. Such a broad statement on this highly technical surgical topic has left many questions unanswered. For example, no definition of perimenopause was provided in the USFDA statement, so this will be left to the free interpretation of providers (and lawyers), adding to confusion. Moreover, the agency's statements were solely based on data from hysterectomy, not myomectomy. Therefore, they gave very high rates of unexpected cancer found at morcellation of uterine tissue; this may unnecessarily steer surgeons and patients toward choosing a much riskier option of open myomectomy. Procedure-specific data have recently appeared, confirming the general understanding that the risk of unexpected cancer in LM is much lower than that reported for laparoscopic hysterectomy. These new data include the risk of unexpected endometrial carcinoma, which should be easily ruled out before myomectomy through a simple endometrial biopsy. Once endometrial carcinoma is excluded, the prevalence of unexpected uterine neoplasia at LM is truly a rare event (Wright et al. 2015).

The largest published meta-analysis looking at the clinical outcome of incidental morcellation of leiomyosarcoma found no evidence that this modality of tissue extraction may have a negative effect on patient survival (Parker et al. 2015).

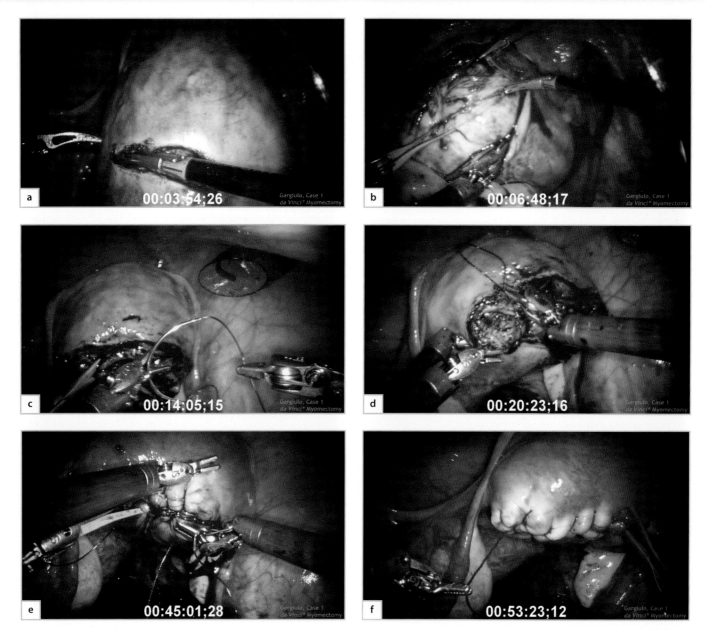

Figure 27.3 Multiport robot-assisted laparoscopic myomectomy: standard 'all-Four' configuration. Robotic instruments employed are Harmonic ACE, Fenestrated Maryland Bipolar and Tenaculum (for enucleating), and Mega Needle Driver, Large Needle Driver, and Tenaculum (for suturing). (a) Large posterior myoma enucleated with elliptical incision using the Harmonic ACE as the primary energy form and the Fenestrated Maryland Bipolar as a dissector and possible emergency coagulator. Monopolar energy is not currently employed in our reproductive surgery techniques, due to its higher thermal spread and the chance of delayed thermal injury to reproductive tissues. (b) The basic enucleating technique in robotic surgery; the Tenaculum immobilizes the myoma, the assistant immobilizes the uterus (with an Allis grasper, in this case), and the console operator works on developing the intrafascial plane of dissection. (c) One of the advantages of a lower quadrant assistant port: needles are passed in and out in front of the camera. (d–f) The many advantages of a third instrument arm. Note how the Tenaculum lifts the uterus up, immobilizes the suture line, and always 'presents' the target to instruments 1 and 2.

Surgeons in the United States (and possibly beyond) must come to terms with limitations of their surgical armamentarium until data on the potentially negative effects of the USFDA ban of morcellation on patients (in terms of unnecessary morbidity from open surgery) accumulates over the forthcoming years. Given the wealth of literature describing many reasons to avoid laparotomy for myomectomy, it seems logical that alternative techniques of morcellation in a secure containment system, or extracorporeal tissue extraction, will be adopted by many. In parallel, more attention is likely to be paid to the imaging of uterine masses. We have long maintained that investing

in a high-resolution, operator-independent, preoperative imaging of the pelvis is essential for careful preoperative planning (Lipskind & Gargiulo 2013).

MRI with and without gadolinium enhancement is an essential feature of the modern preoperative planning for myomectomy (with the exception of some cases with a few small myomata, where three-dimensional ultrasound performed by the surgeon constitutes a valid alternative). Aside from aiding in myoma mapping and in recognizing adenomyosis (as discussed above), MRI could also help lower the threshold of suspicion for leiomyosarcoma, albeit its negative and

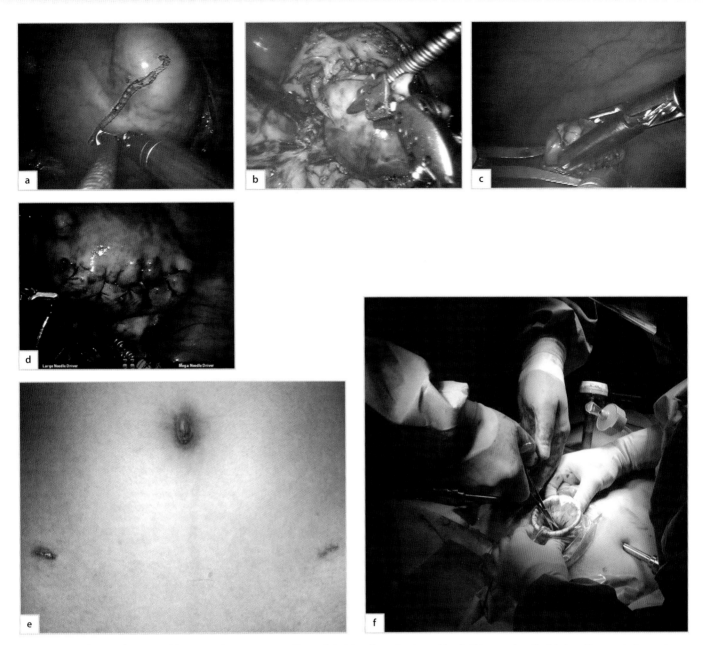

Figure 27.4 Multiport robot-assisted laparoscopic myomectomy: Cosmetic 'solo' configuration. Large Needle Driver carries a flexible laser fiber, our instrument of choice for all cosmetic and minimal impact surgeries. Monopolar Curved Shears can be substituted for this, depending on surgeon's preference. A Tenaculum acts, as also seen in Figure 27.3, to immobilize the uterus or the myoma during dissection. Mega Needle Driver and Large Needle Driver are employed for suturing. (a) A uterine incision is performed with flexible CO2 laser fiber (BeamPath Robotic, OmniGuide). (b) The endometrium can be seen bulging (intact) at chromopertubation. (c) A conventional laparoscopic instrument can be employed to extract tissue as well as to provide suction/irrigation. (d) Uncompromised reconstruction in layers is achieved, even with the lower angle of approach of the cosmetic setup. (e) The patient's abdomen 2 weeks after surgery. (f) Occasionally, patient's preference (e.g. small size of the umbilicus) will dictate the use of a minute suprapubic incision for extraction in a bag; extracorporeal tissue extraction is performed by grasping the tissue with towel clips and carefully coring it with a sharp scalpel blade, just as one does with an umbilical approach, using a conventional laparoscopic single-site port (Gelpoint Mini, Applied Medical) and an endoscopic specimen pouch.

positive predictive values in the latter application depend on the prevalence of the condition, which is clearly very low in the LM population (Moghadam et al. 2006, Sato et al. 2014, Shwayder & Sakhel 2014).

In conclusion, at 10 years from the introduction of the first USFDA-approved teleoperator for gynecologic surgery, robotic myomectomy has come of age as a reproducible, standardized, yet multifaceted, complementary laparoscopic technique, whose main role is to avoid overutilization of AM. Virtual reality simulation can shorten the technical learning curve of the teleoperator; as such, it is probably destined to become an integral and distinctive feature of robotic surgery training (Gargiulo et al. 2015). Some gynecologic surgeons can reliably offer LM without the assistance of the teleoperator; for those who can, this technology is unlikely to provide significant advantages in its present form. One notable exception may be the field of single-incision laparoscopy, where a true uncompromised myomectomy is not a practical option without robotic assistance. Single-channel surgical robotics will likely to continue to be a focal point of industry innovation for the foreseeable future.

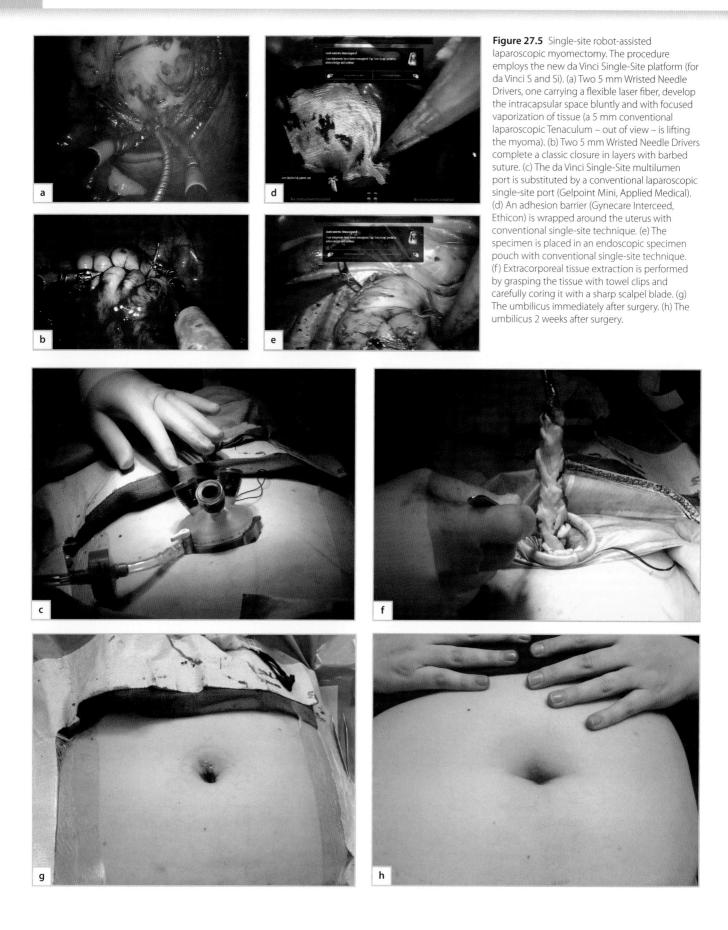

Figure 27.5 Single-site robot-assisted laparoscopic myomectomy. The procedure employs the new da Vinci Single-Site platform (for da Vinci S and Si). (a) Two 5 mm Wristed Needle Drivers, one carrying a flexible laser fiber, develop the intracapsular space bluntly and with focused vaporization of tissue (a 5 mm conventional laparoscopic Tenaculum – out of view – is lifting the myoma). (b) Two 5 mm Wristed Needle Drivers complete a classic closure in layers with barbed suture. (c) The da Vinci Single-Site multilumen port is substituted by a conventional laparoscopic single-site port (Gelpoint Mini, Applied Medical). (d) An adhesion barrier (Gynecare Interceed, Ethicon) is wrapped around the uterus with conventional single-site technique. (e) The specimen is placed in an endoscopic specimen pouch with conventional single-site technique. (f) Extracorporeal tissue extraction is performed by grasping the tissue with towel clips and carefully coring it with a sharp scalpel blade. (g) The umbilicus immediately after surgery. (h) The umbilicus 2 weeks after surgery.

REFERENCES

AAGL Advancing Minimally Invasive Gynecology Worldwide. AAGL practice report: Morcellation during uterine tissue extraction. J Minim Invasive Gynecol 2014; 21:517–530.

Advincula AP, Song A, Burke W, Reynolds RK. Preliminary experience with robot-assisted laparoscopic myomectomy. J Am Assoc Gynecol Laparosc 2004; 11:511–518.

Advincula AP, Xu X, Goudeau St, Ransom SB. Robot-assisted laparoscopic myomectomy versus abdominal myomectomy: a comparison of short-term surgical outcomes and immediate costs. J Minim Invasive Gynecol 2007; 14:698–705.

Alessandri F, Remorgida V, Venturini PL, Ferrero S. Unidirectional barbed suture versus continuous suture with intracorporeal knots in laparoscopic myomectomy: a randomized study. J Minim Invasive Gynecol 2010; 17:725–729.

American College of Obstetricians and Gynecologists. ACOG special report: power morcellation and occult malignancy in gynecologic surgery. Washington, DC: American Congress of Obstetricians and Gynecologists. http://www.acog.org/Resources-And-Publications/Task-Force-and-Work-Group-Reports/Power-Morcellation-and-Occult-Malignancy-in-Gynecologic-Surgery, 2014.

Angioli R, Battista C, Terranova C, et al. Intraoperative contact ultrasonography during open myomectomy for uterine fibroids. Fertil Steril 2010; 94:1487–1490.

Angioli R, Plotti F, Montera R, et al. A new type of absorbable barbed suture for use in laparoscopic myomectomy. Int J Gynaecol Obstet 2012; 117:220–223.

Barakat EE, Bedaiwy MA, Zimberg S, et al. Robotic-assisted,laparoscopic, and abdominal myomectomy: a comparison of surgical outcomes. Obstet Gynecol 2011; 117:256–265.

Bedient CE, Magrina JF, Noble BN, Kho RM. Comparison of robotic and laparoscopic myomectomy. Am J Obstet Gynecol 2009; 201:566 e1–566 e5.

Bhave Chittawar P, Franik S, Pouwer AW, Farquhar C. Minimally invasive surgical techniques versus open myomectomy for uterine fibroids. Cochrane Database Syst Rev 2014; 10:CD004638.

Brown J. AAGL advancing minimally invasive gynecology worldwide: statement to the FDA on power morcellation. J Minim Invasive Gynecol 2014; 21:970–971.

Bush AJ, Morris SN, Millham FH, Isaacson KB. Women's preferences for minimally invasive incisions. J Minim Invasive Gynecol 2011; 18:640–643.

Choi CH, Kim TH, Kim SH, et al. Surgical outcomes of a new approach to laparoscopic myomectomy: single-port and modified suture technique. J Minim Invasive Gynecol 2014; 21:580–585.

Culligan P, Gurshumov E, Lewis C, et al. Predictive validity of a training protocol using a robotic surgery simulator. Female Pelvic Med Reconstr Surg 2014; 20:48–51.

Dubuisson JB, Fauconnier A, Chapron C, Kreiker G, Nörgaard C. Second look after laparoscopic myomectomy. Hum Reprod 1998; 13:2102–2106.

Frank L, Basch E, Selby JV, Patient-Centered Outcomes Research Institute. The PCORI perspective on patient-centered outcomes research. JAMA 2014; 312:1513–1514.

Gargiulo A, Bailey A, Srouji S. Robot-assisted single-incision laparoscopic myomectomy: initial report and technique. J Robotic Surg 2013; 7:137–142.

Gargiulo AR. Computer-assisted reproductive surgery: why it matters to reproductive endocrinology and infertility subspecialists. Fertil Steril 2014; 102:911–921.

Gargiulo AR, Srouji SS, Missmer SA, et al. Robot-assisted laparoscopic myomectomy compared with standard laparoscopic myomectomy. Obstet Gynecol 2012; 120:284–291.

Gargiulo AR. Will computer-assisted surgery shake the foundations of surgical ethics in the age of patient-centered medicine? Innovations in patient safety for women's health: Minimally invasive gynecologic surgery. OBG Management 2015 (Suppl. pp20-24).

Garnet JD. Uterine rupture during pregnancy. An analysis of 133 patients. Obstet Gynecol 1964; 23:898–905.

Goebel K, Goldberg JM. Women's preference of cosmetic results after gynecologic surgery. J Minim Invasive Gynecol 2014; 21:64–67.

Griffin L, Feinglass J, Garrett A, et al. Postoperative outcomes after robotic versus abdominal myomectomy. JSLS 2013; 17:407–413.

Jin C, Hu Y, Chen XC, et al. Laparoscopic versus open myomectomy—a meta-analysis of randomized controlled trials. Eur J Obstet Gynecol Reprod Biol 2009; 145:14–21.

Koh C, Janik G. Laparoscopic myomectomy: the current status. Cur Opin Obstet Gynecol 2003; 15:295–301.

Kumakiri J, Kikuchi I, Kitade M, et al. Association between uterine repair at laparoscopic myomectomy and postoperative adhesions. Acta Obstet Gynecol Scand 2012; 91:331–337.

Lewis EI, Srouji SS, Gargiulo AR. Robotic single-site myomectomy: initial report and technique. Fertil Steril 2015; 103:1370-1377.e1.

Lim PC, Kang E, Park do H. A comparative detail analysis of the learning curve and surgical outcome for robotic hysterectomy with lymphadenectomy versus laparoscopic hysterectomy with lymphadenectomy in treatment of endometrial cancer: a case-matched controlled study of the first one hundred twenty two patients. Gynecol Oncol 2011; 120:413–418.

Lipskind ST, Gargiulo AR. Computer-assisted laparoscopy in fertility preservation and reproductive surgery. J Minim Invasive Gynecol 2013; 20:435–445.

Liu G, Zolis L, Kung R, et al. The laparoscopic myomectomy: a survey of Canadian gynaecologists. J Obstet Gynaecol Can 2010; 32:139–148.

Moghadam R, Lathi RB, Shahmohamady B, et al. Predictive value of magnetic resonance imaging in differentiating between leiomyoma and adenomyosis. JSLS 2006; 10:216–219.

Nezhat C, Lavie O, Hsu S, et al. Robotic-assisted laparoscopic myomectomy compared with standard laparoscopic myomectomy-a retrospective matched control study. Fertil Steril 2009; 91:556–559.

Parker W, Pritts E, Olive D. Risk of Morcellation of uterine leiomyosarcomas in laparoscopic supracervical hysterectomy and laparoscopic myomectomy, a retrospective trial including 4791 women. J Minim Invasive Gynecol 2015; 22:696–697.

Parker WH, Einarsson J, Istre O, Dubuisson JB. Risk factors for uterine rupture after laparoscopic myomectomy. J Minim Invasive Gynecol 2010; 17:551–554.

Patzkowsky KE, As-Sanie S, Smorgick N, Song AH, Advincula AP. Perioperative outcomes of robotic versus laparoscopic hysterectomy for benign disease. JSLS 2013; 17:100–106.

Pitter M, Srouji S, Gargiulo A, et al. Fertility and symptom relief following robot-assisted laparoscopic myomectomy. Obstet Gynecol International 2015; 2015:967568.

Pitter MC, Gargiulo AR, Bonaventura LM, Lehman JS, Srouji SS. Pregnancy outcomes following robot-assisted myomectomy. Hum Reprod 2013; 28:99–108.

Pluchino N, Litta P, Freschi L, et al. Comparison of the initial surgical experience with robotic and laparoscopic myomectomy. Int J Med Robot 2014; 10:208–212.

Practice Committee of the American Society for Reproductive Medicine in collaboration with Society of Reproductive Surgeons. Pathogenesis, consequences, and control of peritoneal adhesions in gynecologic surgery. Fertil Steril 2007; 88:21–26.

Sato K, Yuasa N, Fujita M, Fukushima Y. Clinical application of diffusion-weighted imaging for preoperative differentiation between uterine leiomyoma and leiomyosarcoma. Am J Obstet Gynecol 2014; 210:368.

Seracchioli R, Manuzzi L, Vianello F, et al. Obstetric and delivery outcome of pregnancies achieved after laparoscopic myomectomy. Fertil steril 2006; 86:159–165.

Shwayder J, Sakhel K. Imaging for uterine myomas and adenomyosis. J Minim Invasive Gynecol 2014; 21:362–376.

Sizzi O, Rossetti A, Malzoni M, et al. Italian multicenter study on complications of laparoscopic myomectomy. J Minim Invasive Gynecol 2007; 14:453–462.

Spong CY, Landon MB, Gilbert S, et al. Risk of uterine rupture and adverse perinatal outcome at term after cesarean delivery. Obstet Gynecol 2007; 110:801–807.

Srouji SS, Kaser DJ, Gargiulo AR. Techniques for contained morcellation in gynecologic surgery. Fertil Steril 2015; 103:e34.

Stark M, Pomati S, D'Ambrosio A, Giraudi F, Gidaro S. A new telesurgical platform —preliminary clinical results. Minim Invasive Ther Allied Technol 2015;24:31–36.

Takeuchi H, Kinoshita K. Evaluation of adhesion formation after laparoscopic myomectomy by systematic second-look microlaparoscopy. J Am Assoc Gynecol Laparosc 2002; 9:442–446.

Tinelli A, Malvasi A, Guido M, et al. Adhesion formation after intracapsular myomectomy with or without adhesion barrier. Fertil Steril 2011; 95:1780–1785.

Tulandi T, Murray C, Guralnick M. Adhesion formation and reproductive outcome after myomectomy and second-look laparoscopy. Obstet Gynecol 1993; 82:213–215.

U.S. Food and Drug Administration. Updated laparoscopic uterine power morcellation in hysterectomy and myomectomy: FDA Safety Communication, 2014. US Department of Health and Human Services, Washington DC. www.fda.gov/MedicalDevices/Safety/AlertsandNotices/ucm424443.htm. Last accessed November 24, 2014.

Wright JD, Ananth CV, Lewin SN, et al. Robotically assisted vs laparoscopic hysterectomy among women with benign gynecologic disease. JAMA 2013; 20;309:689–698.

Wright JD, Tergas AI, Cui R, et al. Use of electric power morcellation and prevalence of underlying cancer in women who undergo myomectomy. JAMA Oncol 2015; 1:69–77..

Yeung PP Jr, Bolden CR, Westreich D, et al. Patient preferences of cosmesis for abdominal incisions in gynecologic surgery. J Minim Invasive Gynecol 2013; 20:79–78.

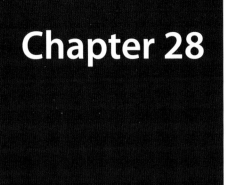

Chapter 28

Robotic management of pelvic organ prolapse and incontinence

Cecile A Unger, Marie Fidela R Paraiso

INTRODUCTION

Pelvic floor disorders such as uterovaginal prolapse, posthysterectomy vaginal apex prolapse, and urinary incontinence are common conditions that can negatively impact a woman's quality of life and are sometimes associated with significant morbidity (Hendrix et al. 2002, Jelovsek & Barber 2006). Surgical options to treat symptomatic pelvic floor disorders include vaginal and abdominal approaches. Over the last two decades, minimally invasive abdominal surgery has increasingly been utilized to treat pelvic organ prolapse and stress urinary incontinence. The minimally invasive approach is considered advantageous as it has been associated with a shorter length of hospital stay, faster recovery and return to baseline functioning, less intraoperative blood loss, and less postoperative pain (Bandera & Magrina 2009, Barbash & Glied 2010, Kehoe et al. 2007). This approach serves as an alternative to the open abdominal approach and aims at bridging the gap between the benefits of vaginal surgery with the surgical success rates of open abdominal procedures.

In 2005, the US Food and Drug Administration formally approved the use of the da Vinci Robotic Surgical System (Intuitive Surgical, Inc., Sunnyvale, California) for gynecologic procedures. The robotic platform continues to be marketed as a tool to assist with laparoscopy by offering three-dimensional visualization and a superior level of dexterity when compared to conventional laparoscopic surgery as well as a much faster learning curve for surgeons (Payne & Dauterive 2008). As a result, the use of robotic-assisted laparoscopic surgery has substantially increased in gynecology over the last decade (Schiavone et al. 2012), and has been used for the surgical treatment of pelvic organ prolapse and urinary incontinence.

The adoption of the robotic platform in reconstructive pelvic surgery has allowed many surgeons to offer a minimally invasive approach for the treatment of pelvic floor disorders. The objective of this chapter is to describe the procedures currently performed with the assistance of robotic technology, to review the important considerations related to these procedures, and to provide an overview of the literature that currently exists on the robotic-assisted laparoscopic management of pelvic floor disorders.

INDICATIONS

The indications for robotic-assisted laparoscopic repair of pelvic organ prolapse (uterovaginal prolapse, posthysterectomy vaginal apex prolapse, paravaginal defect, enterocele, perineocele, and rectal prolapse) as well as stress urinary incontinence are similar to those for the vaginal, open abdominal, and conventional laparoscopic approaches. The choice of route is determined by several factors including surgeon's and patient's preferences, the surgeon's surgical skill set,

and equipment availability. Patient-specific considerations include the history of previous pelvic or incontinence surgery, previously failed transvaginal prolapse surgery, known abdominopelvic adhesions, patient's age and weight, and need for concomitant pelvic surgery (Tarr & Paraiso 2014).

Additional important considerations include the patient's ability to undergo general anesthesia, the effects of pneumoperitoneum and Trendelenburg position, and the patient's comorbid conditions. For example, patients with known pulmonary or cardiac conditions such as chronic obstructive pulmonary disease, pulmonary hypertension, and congestive heart failure may not tolerate the effects of intra-abdominal CO_2 insufflation or steep Trendelenburg position, both of which are necessary for robotic surgery (Danic et al. 2007, Tekelioglu et al. 2013). The pneumoperitoneum needed during these cases causes important systemic changes in the body that may become more severe in the setting of Trendelenburg position. These changes include decreased venous return, increased systemic and pulmonary vascular pressures, and increased ventilation pressures (Baltayian 2008, Danic et al. 2007, Makai & Isaacson 2009, Ogunnaik et al. 2002). Robotic surgery may, therefore, be contraindicated in patients with pulmonary, cardiac, and renal conditions that may be worsened by these physiologic changes. Appropriate preoperative tests, such as chest X-ray, pulmonary function tests, electrocardiogram, and echocardiogram, may be necessary in patients with suspected comorbidities.

PERIOPERATIVE CONSIDERATIONS

Adequate visualization of the pelvis up to the level of the sacrum is important for urogynecologic procedures, and one of the most critical factors for successful robotic surgery is patient positioning. As in any gynecologic procedure, patients are positioned in the dorsal lithotomy position, allowing access to the vagina. We recommend using Allen or Yellowfin (Allen Medical Systems, Acton, Massachusetts) stirrups for proper patient positioning with the legs positioned such that they are not hyperflexed or extended at the hip or knee, with adequate padding at all bony prominences, especially the lateral knee, to prevent nerve compression injuries. The patient should be positioned so that the buttocks are slightly beyond the end of the table, which helps facilitate placement of vaginal and rectal manipulators. Patients should be secured to the table so that they may be placed in steep Trendelenburg position without slipping towards the head of the bed. This can be achieved by placing egg crate foam, a gel pad (AliGel or Overlay Pad, AliMed, Inc., Dehdam, Massachusetts), or a surgical bean bag (Olympic Vac-Pac Marlin Medical, Bayswater North, VIC, Australia) between the patient and the table. A padded strap (Alistrap, AliMed, Inc.) or silk tape with foam placed beneath at the level of the patient's chest can be used to further secure the patient's upper body to the table. Securement should be tight enough to prevent the patient from slipping on the surgical table, but should not compromise ventilation, and proper securement should be confirmed with the anesthesia team. The arms should be tucked at the patient's side, using an underlying draw sheet with or without sled arm boards, and this must be done with care to avoid upper extremity nerve injury. This is accomplished by ensuring that the arms remain in anatomic neutral position with adequate padding around the ulnar prominence at the elbow and at the level of the wrist. A Foley catheter should be placed under sterile conditions at the start of any gynecologic procedure. For procedures where bladder dissection is necessary and/or for patients who have a history of cesarean section or prior abdominal or vaginal surgery, a three-way Foley catheter should be placed to allow for retrograde fill of the bladder and better delineation of the dissection plane. In challenging cases, hydrodissection may also be performed in addition to retrograde fill of the bladder. This is done by injecting normal saline transvaginally or laparoscopically into the vesicovaginal space to help with dissection.

Patients undergoing robotic urogynecologic procedures should receive intravenous prophylactic antibiotics within 1 hour of incision to reduce the risk of surgical infection. The antibiotic of choice in all gynecologic surgery is a first-generation cephalosporin, usually cefazolin, or an alternative combination regimen such as ciprofloxacin and metronidazole if a patient has a documented penicillin allergy (ACOG Committee on Practice Bulletins – Gynecology 2009). We do not recommend routine use of preoperative mechanical bowel preparation prior to robotic urogynecologic procedures. There is currently very little evidence that supports the use of mechanical bowel preparation for the prevention of infectious complications related to bowel surgery or injury at the time of any gynecologic procedure (Güenaga et al. 2011).

Without additional risk factors, all patients undergoing prolapse and/or anti-incontinence surgery are at moderate risk of venous thromboembolic events (VTEs) and require perioperative prophylaxis. Therefore, routine use of intermittent pneumatic compression devices to the lower extremities before induction of anesthesia is recommended (Rahn et al. 2011). Patients who are at higher risk of VTE (those with significant comorbidities, personal cancer history, morbid obesity, or history of prior VTE) should have low-dose unfractionated heparin or low-molecular-weight heparin administered before surgery in addition to pneumatic compression devices (Guyatt et al. 2012).

■ TROCAR PLACEMENT AND ROBOT DOCKING

Proper trocar placement is instrumental for facilitating robotic-assisted laparoscopic procedures performed for pelvic organ prolapse and incontinence. Proper positioning and angulation of each trocar allow the laparoscopic instruments to reach from the deep pelvis to the level of the sacrum and ensure adequate articulation for suturing and knot tying. Additionally, sufficient distance between trocars is necessary to prevent the robotic arms from colliding with each other. For surgeries such as laparoscopic sacral colpopexy, which involves dissection over the sacrum and lower pelvis as well as extensive suturing of graft material to both regions, placement of at least five ports is usually necessary. Multiple-port configurations are described in the literature and we recommend placement of trocars in a shallow 'W' configuration on the abdomen (**Figure 28.1**). Placement of a 12 mm trocar is necessary in the umbilicus for the robotic laparoscope. When placing this port, the table should be leveled to avoid injury to the greater vessels and entry should be gained in the manner with which the surgeon is most comfortable. If the patient has a history of midline laparotomy or adhesions are expected, a left upper quadrant approach or an open laparoscope technique at the umbilicus is recommended. After the umbilical port is placed and the upper abdomen is inspected, the patient should be placed in steep Trendelenburg to move the bowels cephalad for good visualization of the pelvis and for the placement of the subsequent trocars. Two 8 mm robotic ports are placed 9–10 cm lateral and inferior to the umbilicus. A third 8 mm robotic port is placed in the midaxillary line on the left side and an 8 mm or 10 mm assist port is placed 9–10 cm lateral and either inferior or superior to the right-sided robotic port. If an 8 mm assist port is used, small half-circle (SH) needles can be introduced and used for suturing, and the port does not require fascial closure at the completion of the procedure. A 10 mm port allows for the passage of larger needles but requires a fascial closure. Avoiding need for fascial closure, by using only 8 mm ancillary ports, may safeguard a patient against postoperative musculofascial abdominal pain and reduce the risk of hernia if proper closure is not achieved. Another optional location for ancillary port placement is the dilated cervix if supracervical hysterectomy is performed at the time of sacrocolpopexy. The inferior epigastric vessels are the most commonly injured vessels at the time of lateral trocar placement (Makai & Isaacson 2009); therefore, placing

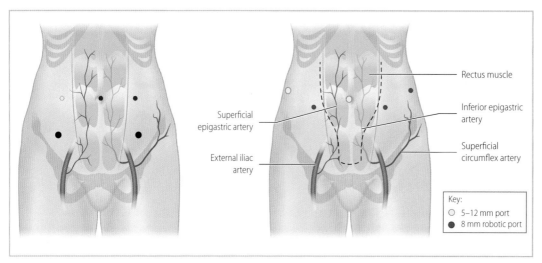

Figure 28.1 Robotic port placement.

Rectus muscle

Inferior epigastric artery

Superficial circumflex artery

Superficial epigastric artery

External iliac artery

Key:
○ 5–12 mm port
● 8 mm robotic port

the ports lateral to the rectus abdominis muscles usually ensures their avoidance. All trocars should be placed under direct visualization to avoid vascular and visceral injuries.

Once all of the ports are properly placed, the robot is then docked to the patient (**Figure 28.2**). The four-armed da Vinci and the da Vinci SI can be used to perform any gynecologic procedure. Three components make up the da Vinci Surgical System (**Figure 28.3**): Patient Cart (operative robot), Surgeon Console, and the Vision Cart. Several

approaches to robotic docking are mentioned in the literature. For the purposes of pelvic organ prolapse and anti-incontinence surgery, we recommend side docking either in a parallel fashion or at a 45° angle to the table on the patient's left side, which will decrease the risk of robotic arm collision (**Figure 28.4**). The camera arm is affixed first followed by the other robotic arms. Great care must be taken to position the arms in such a way that they triangulate well with each other and do not collide. The fourth robotic arm, which is the most lateral arm on the patient's left side, should be affixed last as it should be angled in a horizontal plane in relation to the patient (**Figure 28.5**). All arms should be positioned such that there is at least a 30° angle between the camera and the instrument arms with 45° angles being the most ideal.

The monopolar scissors are usually placed in arm 1 while a bipolar instrument is placed in arm 2, and a Prograsp in arm 3. These instruments allow for hysterectomy and peritoneal dissection at the time of sacrocolpopexy or Burch colposuspension. When suturing is necessary, a SutureCut needle driver is placed in arm 1, a need driver in arm 2, and the Prograsp remains in arm 3. Eight-inch sutures are typically used for suturing and sutures are tied with intracorporeal knots.

■ SACRAL COLPOPEXY

Abdominal sacral colpopexy is considered the gold standard for vault prolapse, and has demonstrated superior anatomic outcomes compared to transvaginal suspension procedures (Ganatra et al. 2009); however, like all open abdominal surgeries, the operation is associated with higher morbidity. As a result, laparoscopic and robotic-assisted laparoscopic sacral colpopexy have become good alternatives to the open abdominal approach.

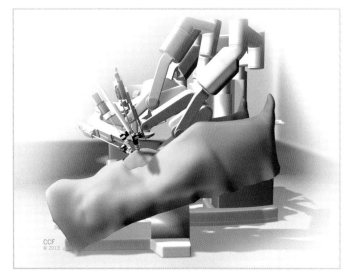

Figure 28.2 Robotic docking and Trendelenburg position. Reprinted with permission from Cleveland Clinic Center for Medical Art & Photography 2007-2013. All Rights Reserved.

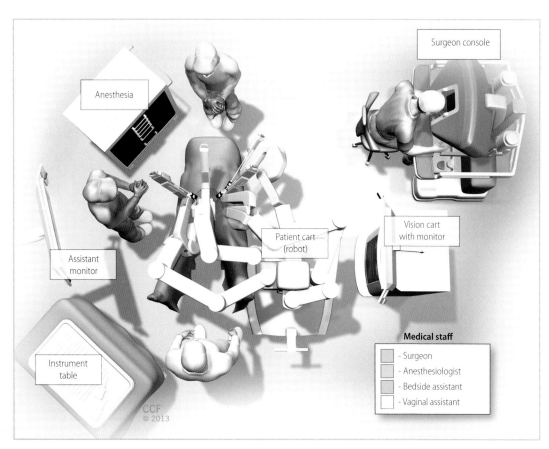

Figure 28.3 Robotic room setup. Reprinted with permission from Cleveland Clinic Center for Medical Art & Photography 2007-2013. All Rights Reserved.

Surgeon console

Anesthesia

Assistant monitor

Patient cart (robot)

Vision cart with monitor

Instrument table

Medical staff

- Surgeon
- Anesthesiologist
- Bedside assistant
- Vaginal assistant

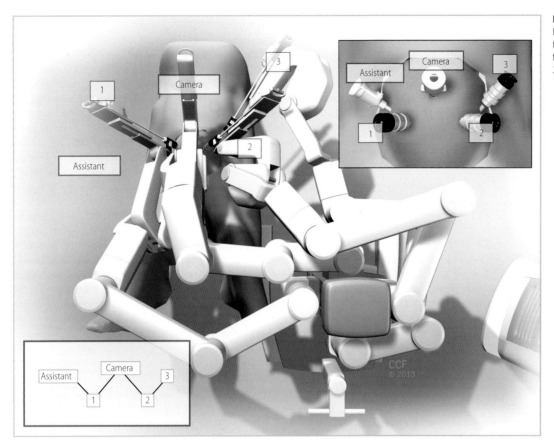

Figure 28.4 Parallel docking. Reprinted with permission from Cleveland Clinic Center for Medical Art & Photography 2007-2013. All Rights Reserved.

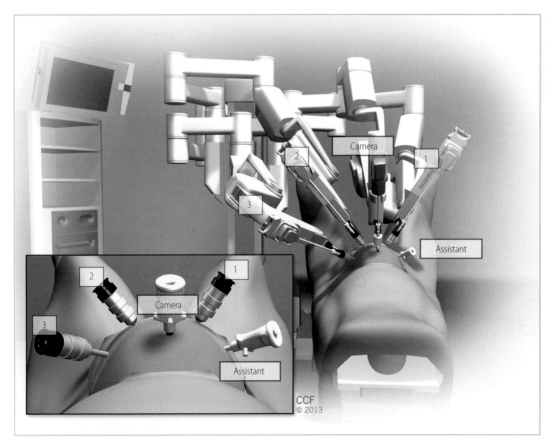

Figure 28.5 Robotic positioning to avoid collision of the arms. Reprinted with permission from Cleveland Clinic Center for Medical Art & Photography 2007-2013. All Rights Reserved.

The operation involves suspension of the vaginal apex to the anterior longitudinal ligament of the sacrum at S1 using a graft made of either synthetic or biologic material (**Figure 28.6**). If synthetic mesh is used, we recommend use of a large-pore polypropylene mesh, which has been associated with the least amount of mesh-related complications due to its advantageous synthetic properties (Walters & Ridgeway 2013). After intraperitoneal access is confirmed and the robotic trocars are placed, steep Trendelenburg will help place the small bowel into the upper abdomen, and the sigmoid colon should be retracted to the left pelvis as much as possible. For a redundant sigmoid colon, or one that is difficult to retract manually, a temporary suture can be placed through the epiploica of the colon and passed through either a trocar on the patient's left side or through a 2 mm incision in the patient's skin using the Carter Thomason endofascial closure device. This suture is clamped to the drapes and removed at the end of the case. Once anatomy is restored, the bowels are retracted, and all necessary adhesions are lysed, the robot is docked. It is helpful to have two knowledgeable assistants for this operation; one for assistance at the patient side, working intra-abdominally using the assist port, and another working vaginally to manipulate the vagina and rectum to optimize dissection and graft placement. Alternatively, the RUMI uterine manipulator can be used with the Uterine Positioning System (CooperSurgical, Inc., Trumbull, Connecticut), which frees assistants to perform other tasks.

All pertinent anatomy should be identified at the start of the procedure. The ureters are visualized bilaterally, and particular attention should be paid to the right ureter throughout the case. Because there is a lack of tactile feedback using the robot, correct identification of the sacral promontory is sometimes difficult; therefore, the promontory should be palpated with a laparoscopic instrument through the assist port before the dissection is started. The important landmarks of the presacral space include the aortic bifurcation superiorly, the common and internal iliac vessels, the ureter on the patient's right, and the sigmoid colon on the left (**Figure 28.7**). The most structures at risk, susceptible to injury during this procedure, include the left common iliac (located medial to the iliac artery), the internal iliac vessels, the right ureter, and the middle sacral artery. Once all structures are visualized, a peritoneal incision is made over the sacral promontory and

careful dissection is performed to expose the bony prominence of S1 as well as the overlying anterior longitudinal ligament, the attachment point for the graft. Approximately 3–4 cm of exposure is necessary and this can be achieved by using blunt dissection or electrocauterization to clear off the overlying subperitoneal fat. Caution should be taken to avoid the presacral venous plexus as well as the middle sacral vein and artery, which are often encountered during this portion of the dissection. Once the sacral promontory is cleared off and adequate for graft attachment, the dissection is extended caudally through the peritoneum and subperitoneal fat down to the posterior cul-de-sac. It is important to keep the rectum and right ureter in view during this part of the surgery, as the course of the dissection is located between these two structures.

An end-to-end anastomosis (EEA) sizer should be placed in the vagina and the rectum to allow for proper dissection of the vagina. The vaginal EEA sizer is elevated cephalad, and gentle pressure is applied so that the peritoneum overlying the apex of the vagina can be incised in a transverse fashion to facilitate sharp dissection of the bladder off of the anterior vagina. Retrograde filling of the bladder can be done to better delineate the planes to avoid injury to the bladder at the time of dissection. This is particularly important in the case of adhesive disease and prior pelvic

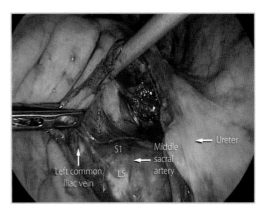

Figure 28.7 Anatomic landmarks for sacral colpopexy.

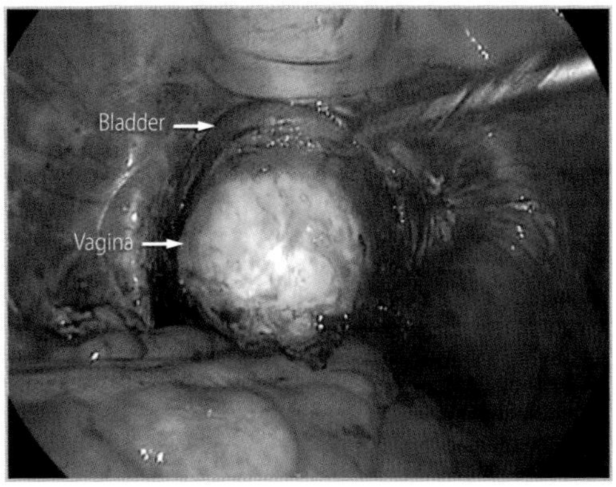

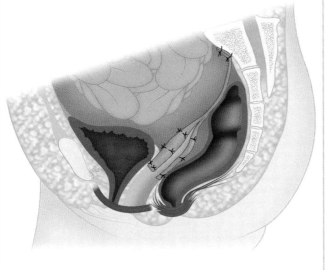

Figure 28.8 Anterior dissection for sacral colpopexy.

Figure 28.6 Placement of sacral colpopexy graft.

surgery. A 4–5 cm pocket should be created anteriorly to allow for adequate graft placement (**Figure 28.8**). The vaginal and rectal EEA sizers are positioned to allow for good identification of the rectovaginal septum. Staying as close to the posterior vagina as possible, the peritoneum is incised transversely and dissection is carried down to the posterior-cul-de-sac, creating a 4–5 cm pocket posteriorly unless the dissection is carried down to the perineum and bilateral levator ani muscles if sacrocolpoperineopexy is performed. A lightweight, macroporous polypropylene mesh or biologic graft (if indicated) is then secured to the vagina. If two separate pieces of material are used, it is fashioned into two arms that are approximately 4 ´ 15 cm in size. Some mesh grafts are manufactured in a pre-set 'Y' configuration to facilitate placement; these arms can be trimmed to the correct size as determined by the surgeon after dissection is complete. The graft is attached to either the posterior or the anterior vaginal wall first, depending on the surgeon's preference.

Attachment is accomplished using 4–6 permanent or delayed-absorbable No. 0 or 2-0 sutures, in an interrupted fashion, 1.5–2 cm apart from each other. Sutures are placed through the fibromuscular tissue of the vagina but not through the underlying epithelium. Delayed absorbable sutures should be used for the most distal stitches close to the bladder to avoid suture erosion or fistula formation into the bladder. When the posterior arm is secured first, it is easiest to place the apical posterior sutures first. Next, the posterior most distal sutures are placed, which keeps the graft from bunching along the posterior vagina and minimizes the amount of sutures required for graft attachment. When a Y mesh is used, it is easier to secure the anterior arm first, which retracts the cephalad portion of the mesh anteriorly out of the visual field so that the posterior mesh may be secured with ease. It is important to place the most apical stitch first while simulating desired suspension and maintaining the correct anatomic axis of the vagina in order to avoid the need for readjustment. Once the graft is secured to the vagina, the EEA sizer is used to place the vagina into the right pararectal space toward the sacral promontory. The graft is trimmed to the appropriate length and then secured to anterior longitudinal ligament using two No. 0 or 2-0 monofilament permanent sutures (**Figure 28.9**). Great care is taken to avoid placement of the suture through the intervertebral disk or the periosteum of the vertebra rather than the anterior longitudinal ligament of the S1 vertebra as cases of osteomyelitis have been reported after robotic sacral colpopexy (Propst et al. 2014). The peritoneum is then closed over the exposed graft with an absorbable suture (**Figure 28.10**). Mobilization of the peritoneum during initial dissection facilitates reperitonealization after graft attachment. A cystoscopy is performed to confirm no injury to the bladder and patency of the ureters bilaterally. A vaginal examination should be performed at the completion

of the procedure to ensure adequate suspension (without tension) of the vagina, and to determine if a posterior colporrhaphy and/or perineorrhaphy are necessary.

As an aside, if a hysterectomy is planned prior to sacral colpopexy, a supracervical hysterectomy should be considered as preservation of the cervix and avoidance of amputation at the level of the vagina may decrease the risk of future mesh erosions (Osmundsen et al. 2012, Tan-Kim et al. 2011, Warner et al. 2012). If total vaginal hysterectomy is indicated, we recommend performing a vaginal hysterectomy with a double-layered closure of the vaginal cuff prior to the minimally invasive abdominal repair. In addition, care should be taken to avoid suturing the mesh to the vaginal apex suture line in order to minimize the risk of mesh erosion into the vagina. From a cost-efficiency perspective, conventional laparoscopy may be more appropriate following a vaginal hysterectomy; however, indications for robotic sacral colpopexy may still be present. Total laparoscopic or robotic-assisted hysterectomy is another option; however, electrosurgical current spread to the vaginal apex tissues may predispose patients to mesh erosion.

The objective success rate for abdominal sacral colpopexy, as defined by the lack of vaginal apex prolapse postoperatively, is reported to range from 78% to 100% (Nygaard et al. 2004). The most up-to-date Cochrane review on the surgical management of pelvic organ prolapse reported that abdominal sacral colpopexy had lower rates of recurrent vaginal apex prolapse [3.5% vs. 15%; relative ratio (RR) 0.23, 95% confidence interval (CI) 0.07–0.77], reduced grade of residual prolapse (5.7% vs. 20%; RR, 95% CI 0.09–0.97), and less dyspareunia (16% vs. 36%; RR 0.39, 95% CI 0.18–0.86), when compared with vaginal sacrospinous colpopexy. However, sacral colpopexy was significantly associated with a longer operative time, longer time to recovery and was more costly than transvaginal colpopexy. The only long-term (5–7 years) prospective study that has been published on abdominal sacral colpopexy is the recently published long-term follow-up of the randomized, masked Colpopexy and Urinary Reduction Efforts trial (Nygaard et al. 2013), which reported estimated probabilities of treatment failure using parametric survival modeling. The estimated probabilities of treatment failure for symptomatic pelvic organ prolapse for open sacral colpopexy with concomitant urethropexy compared with no urethropexy were 0.29 vs. 0.24 (treatment difference of 0.049; 95% CI 0.060–0.16). Additionally, the calculated sacral colpopexy mesh erosion rate at 7 years was determined to be 10.5% (95% CI 6.8–16.1%), leading the authors to conclude that mesh-related complications continue to occur over time. All sacral colpopexy procedures in this trial were performed via the open approach; therefore, we can only extrapolate what the long-term outcomes after minimally invasive sacral colpopexy may be.

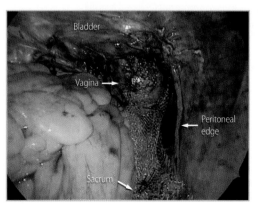

Figure 28.9
Suspension of the vagina to the sacrum using mesh.

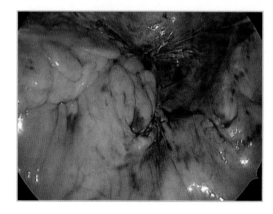

Figure 28.10
Peritoneal closure over mesh after sacral colpopexy is complete.

Most of the literature has been focused on abdominal sacral colpopexy, but there are also data on outcomes after the laparoscopic and robotic-assisted approach as well. Ganatra et al. (2009) published a large review looking at over 1000 patients in 11 series who underwent laparoscopic sacral colpopexy. They found that the conversion rates and the operative time using this modality decreased significantly with increased surgeon experience. The mean follow-up for these studies was 24.6 months; average patient satisfaction rate was 94.4%; and prolapse reoperation rate was 6.2%. The authors concluded that outcomes after laparoscopic sacral colpopexy reflected those of open abdominal sacral colpopexy making the laparoscopic approach a good minimally invasive option for patients with vaginal apex prolapse. A large multicenter retrospective cohort study by Nosti et al. (2014) compared peri- and postoperative outcomes after open abdominal and minimally invasive (laparoscopic and robotic) abdominal sacral colpopexy in 831 subjects who were operated in between 1999 and 2009. With anatomic failure defined as pelvic organ prolapse quantification (POP-Q) $\geq$ stage 2, the authors found that anatomic failures were higher in the open abdominal group than the minimally invasive group (24.1% vs. 14.3%, $P < 0.01$), with most recurrences found in the posterior compartment. Additionally, open abdominal sacral colpopexy was associated with higher operative blood loss, longer hospital stay, and longer operative times.

Randomized controlled trials have also reported on the outcomes after minimally invasive sacral colpopexy. Freeman et al. (2013) compared abdominal sacral colpopexy with laparoscopic sacral colpopexy in a multicenter randomized equivalence trial for treatment of posthysterectomy vaginal apex prolapse. Based on their primary outcomes of POP-Q C point and Patient Global Impression-Index scores at 12 months, they found the two procedures to be equivalent. Paraiso et al. (2011) randomized women with stage 2–4 pelvic organ prolapse to either conventional laparoscopic or robotic-assisted laparoscopic sacral colpopexy. The primary outcome in this study was operative time, and secondary outcomes looked at postoperative vaginal support, postoperative pain, functional activity, postoperative bowel and bladder symptoms, quality of life, and cost. The authors found that operative time was significantly longer with the robotic approach (227 ± 47 vs. 162 ± 47 minutes, $P < 0.001$), and postoperative pain was worse in the robotic group when compared to the laparoscopic group. At 6- and 12-month follow-up, anatomic and quality-of-life outcomes did not differ between the two groups. In a recent study, Anger et al. (2014) compared laparoscopic and robotic sacral colpopexy in patients with symptomatic stage 2 pelvic organ prolapse or greater. Cost was the primary outcome of this study, and the authors found that when costs of the robot and maintenance were considered, the robotic group had higher initial hospital costs ($19,616 vs. $11,573, $P < 0.001$) and over 6 weeks, hospital costs remained higher for robotic cases ($20,898 vs. $12,170, $P < 0.001$). When costs of robot purchase and maintenance were excluded, there were no statistical differences in initial day of surgery costs for the robotic group compared to the laparoscopic group ($12,586 vs. $11,573, $P = 0.16$) or hospital costs over 6 weeks ($13,867 vs. $12,170, $P = 0.060$). They also found that the robotic group had longer operating room times (202.8 vs. 178.4 minutes, $P = 0.03$) and higher pain scores 1 week after surgery compared to the laparoscopic cases.

In their large retrospective study, Nosti et al. (2014) also compared conventional and robotic sacral colpopexy and reported that the robotic group had fewer anatomic failures (5.9% vs. 18.9%, $P < 0.01$), despite more advanced preoperative prolapse. The remaining studies that compare robotic and laparoscopic sacral colpopexy are small retrospective cohorts from either one or two institutions. Measured outcomes in these studies as well as the length of follow-up are variable, and findings differ among the studies, making it hard to draw generalized conclusions about the two different minimally invasive modes.

SACRAL COLPOPERINEOPEXY

If the patient has concomitant defecatory dysfunction or perineal descent, a sacral colpoperineopexy is performed and the posterior vaginal dissection is carried down to the level of the perineal body. A T-shaped mesh is used posteriorly, and is attached to the perineum and medial aspect of the pubococcygeus and iliococcygeus muscles in addition to the posterior vagina. If rectal prolapse is present, a colorectal surgeon can perform concomitant ventral rectopexy. While there are no data to support this, we feel that the robotic platform is especially useful for sacral colpoperineopexy as the visualization and the improvement in dexterity provided helps the surgeon to reduce the difficulty that is sometimes encountered with the perineal and levator muscle dissection as well as the suturing into the deep pelvis that is necessary to accomplish the operation.

In 1997, Cundiff et al. described the first approach to sacral colpoperineopexy that involved a combined abdominal and vaginal approach (Cundiff et al. 1997). McDermott et al. (2011) described a laparoscopic approach to sacral colpoperineopexy using a polypropylene mesh. In this small retrospective study ($N = 68$), the authors compared the abdominal versus vaginal introduction of the mesh, which was then attached to the perineal body and rectovaginal septum either laparoscopically or transvaginally followed by laparoscopic attachment of a second mesh to the anterior vagina with laparoscopic securement of both mesh arms to the sacrum. At 6 months, there were no significant differences in objective anatomic outcomes. Data on the mesh erosion rate after sacral colpoperineopexy are sparse but have been estimated to be approximately 6% with sacral colpoperineopexy (Nosti et al. 2009).

VENTRAL RECTOPEXY

Rectal prolapse can coexist with pelvic organ prolapse and can be associated with significant morbidity and decreased quality of life. Mellgren et al. (1994) reported that rectal prolapse was diagnosed on defecography in 38% of cases with symptomatic pelvic organ prolapse. Patients with coexisting rectal prolapse should be referred to a colorectal surgeon for management at the time of pelvic organ prolapse repair. If minimally invasive abdominal sacral colpopexy is planned, concomitant ventral rectopexy may also be an appropriate choice for some patients (Cullen et al. 2012). The procedure is often performed with sacral colpoperineopexy and takes advantage of the extensive perineal dissection that is performed. Trocar placement remains the same for this procedure, and the colorectal surgeon usually performs his or her dissection either before or after the vaginal and presacral dissections. A polypropylene mesh or biologic graft tailored to the dimensions of the patient's pelvis and suspension needs (approximately 7 ´ 20 cm) is introduced into the abdomen and 2-0 monofilament delayed absorbable sutures are used to secure the mesh to the lateral pelvic floor muscles (**Figure 28.11**). Six to eight sutures of the same material are used to secure the mesh to the anterior serosal–muscular layer of the rectum. Care should be taken to avoid full-thickness bites into the lumen of the rectum as this will lower the risk of postoperative abscess and may reduce the rarer risk of osteomyelitis. The mesh or graft is then secured in a tension-free fashion to the anterior longitudinal ligament of the sacrum using a

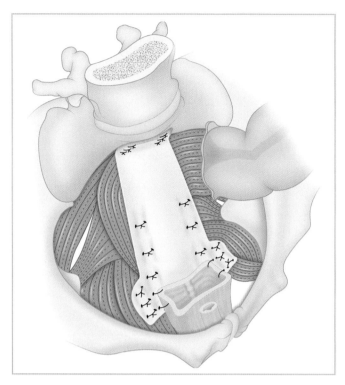

Figure 28.11 Securement of rectopexy graft.

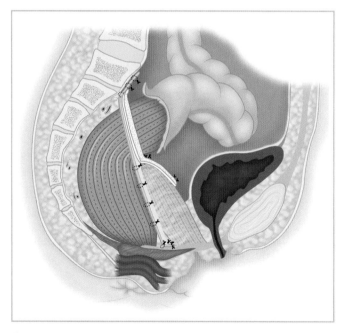

Figure 28.12 Posterior ventral rectopexy.

No. 0 or 2–0 monofilament permanent suture. Separate mesh from the sacrocolpopexy can be used to perform the rectopexy, or the posterior arm of the sacral colpopexy mesh may be used to suspend the rectum as well. Once the sacral colpopexy is completed, the peritoneum is closed over the sacral colpopexy and rectopexy mesh (**Figure 28.12**).

There are limited data on the efficacy of ventral rectopexy, and the literature specific to robotic-assisted laparoscopic rectopexy is even

sparser. A systematic review by Samaranayake et al. (2009) looking at ventral rectopexy for rectal prolapse and rectal intussusception included 12 case series with a total of 728 patients and found that the mean percentage decrease in fecal incontinence was 45%, and mean decrease in constipation was 24% with recurrent rates of rectal prolapse ranging from 0% to 15.4%. A retrospective cohort study of 110 women who underwent laparoscopic sacrocolpopexy with rectopexy for management of pelvic organ and rectal prolapse found that constipation, fecal incontinence, and overall quality-of-life symptoms improved significantly postoperatively and was associated with low overall morbidity (Watadani et al. 2013). A few comparison studies between laparoscopic and robotic-assisted laparoscopic rectopexy exist. Wong et al. (2011) compared these two cohorts and found that with regard to conversion rate, length of hospital stay, and recurrence, the robotic approach was as safe as the laparoscopic approach, with similar favorable short-term outcomes. Other studies have also compared operative, clinical, and cost outcomes between laparoscopic and robotic ventral rectopexy and have reported no difference in perioperative complications; however, operative time and cost were significantly higher in robotic cases (de Hoog et al. 2009, Heemskerk et al. 2001). A cohort study examining the long-term outcomes of robotic rectopexy for rectal prolapse followed 77 subjects for a mean follow-up time of 52.5 (12–115) months and found that constipation was resolved in 50% of subjects and the recurrence rate was 12.8%. The authors of that study concluded that the long-term results of robotic-assisted laparoscopic rectopexy were favorable (Perrenot et al. 2013).

■ UTEROSACRAL LIGAMENT COLPOPEXY

Robotic-assisted laparoscopic uterosacral ligament colpopexy can be performed at the time of hysterectomy for treatment of vaginal vault prolapse. In this procedure, the vaginal apex is affixed to the proximal portion of the uterosacral ligament, which restores the apical support of the vagina. In order to suspend the vaginal apex to the uterosacral ligaments, the pubocervical and rectovaginal fascia must first be well delineated. Next, an Allis clamp can be used to elevate the vaginal cuff to enhance visualization of the uterosacral ligaments. Alternatively, a vaginal probe can be used to elevate the vagina, demarcating the uterosacral ligaments. A No. 0 nonabsorbable suture or delayed absorbable suture should be used to suture the full thickness of the uterosacral ligament at its midportion (at the level of the ischial spine) in a lateral-to-medial fashion. A releasing peritoneal incision between the ligament and the ureter can be made in order to reduce peritoneal tension and subsequent ureteral kinking and injury from suture placement. The uterosacral ligament is then affixed to the vaginal apex, incorporating the full thickness of the vagina in the stitch as well as a portion of the nearby rectovaginal fascia (**Figure 28.13**). This stitch is tied intracorporeally, and the opposite uterosacral ligament is reattached in the same fashion. One to two additional stitches are taken more proximally on the uterosacral ligaments on each side to reattach them to the vagina and rectovaginal fascia (**Figure 28.14**). Placement of these sutures also facilitates closure of the vaginal cuff (**Figure 28.15**). We do not recommend plication of the uterosacral ligaments. If concomitant enterocele repair is performed, the uterosacral ligaments are tagged prior to dissection of the posterior vagina and rectovaginal septum. This allows the uterosacral ligaments to be easily identified for subsequent suspension.

Robotic-assisted laparoscopic uterosacral colpopexy is not a commonly performed procedure but may be very useful at the time of

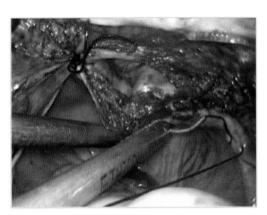

Figure 28.13
Placement of uterosacral suspension suture.

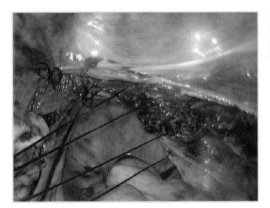

Figure 28.14
Uterosacral suspension sutures.

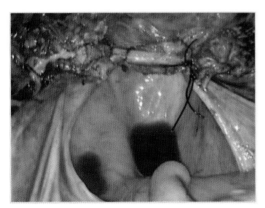

Figure 28.15
Closure of vaginal cuff after uterosacral suspension suture placement.

and found that vaginal apical support was significantly better in the laparoscopic uterosacral uterine suspension group compared with the vaginal surgery group (point c −9 vs. 7.6, P = 0.002). This study also determined that blood loss and length of hospital stay were significantly less in the laparoscopic group.

HYSTEROPEXY

Hysterectomy is commonly done at the time of surgical repair for uterine and uterovaginal prolapse. However, uterine preservation surgery can also be done in women with uterovaginal prolapse who desire future fertility, who are concerned about early-onset menopause as a result of hysterectomy, or who feel that the uterus remains important for issues related to sexuality, body image, and cultural norms (Walters & Ridgeway 2013). While the rate of occult pathology remains low in asymptomatic women (Frick et al. 2010), it is important to ensure that patients are appropriate candidates for uterine-sparing procedures. For example, women with a history of cervical dysplasia, dysfunctional uterine bleeding, postmenopausal bleeding, and risk factors for endometrial carcinoma should not be offered uterine-sparing surgeries. Women who do choose to undergo uterine-preserving surgery should be thoroughly counseled about the need for routine cancer surveillance as well as the potential complications associated with future pregnancy (Burgess & Elliott 2012).

Minimally invasive abdominal repair of uterovaginal prolapse with uterine preservation can be achieved with either laparoscopic uterosacral ligament suspension or laparoscopic sacral hysteropexy. Laparoscopic uterosacral ligament suspension can be done via conventional laparoscopy or with the assistance of the robot. The uterus is suspended to a portion of the ligament on each side, preferably using a permanent suture. For additional support, the uterosacral ligaments can be shortened with sutures. The main advantage of this approach is that it restores normal anatomy and is associated with minimal risk of future pregnancy and delivery. There are very little data that report on outcomes after minimally invasive abdominal hysteropexy with uterosacral ligament suspension. Diwan et al. (2006) published a retrospective cohort study comparing laparoscopic hysteropexy with uterosacral ligament suspension with transvaginal uterosacral ligament suspension at the time of vaginal hysterectomy. Fifty subjects were included in this study, and the authors reported that the hysteropexy patients had better postoperative anatomic outcomes and experienced fewer failures as measured by reoperation rates when compared to the transvaginal group.

Laparoscopic sacral hysteropexy has been described using varying techniques but is essentially performed using a technique similar to the one used for sacral colpopexy. A mesh or graft is sutured anteriorly and/or posteriorly, usually on the cervix, and sometimes a portion of the proximal vagina. The graft is then suspended to the anterior longitudinal ligament of the sacrum using permanent sutures. If an anterior mesh is applied, windows are created through the broad ligament to allow the graft to pass through for its attachment to the sacrum (**Figures 28.16** to **28.19**). Anterior mesh placement should be avoided in patients desiring future fertility, and solitary posterior mesh placement is sufficient in these patients. Outcome data are also sparse for this procedure; however, studies looking at open abdominal sacral hysteropexy have shown similar high success rates when compared to open abdominal hysterectomy with concomitant sacral colpopexy (Costantini et al. 2005). These favorable outcomes support the use of minimally invasive sacral hysteropexy as a good option for women desiring uterine conservation at the time of uterovaginal prolapse repair.

concomitant robotic-assisted laparoscopic hysterectomy, especially if additional transvaginal reconstruction is not necessary. An advantage of robotic suspension compared to the transvaginal approach is that the risk of rectal and ureteral injuries at the time of placement of the suspension sutures may be reduced, as these structures are more easily delineated with robotic surgery (Rardin et al. 2009). There are no substantial data on the outcomes after uterosacral ligament suspension performed via a minimally invasive abdominal route; however, cure rates are reported to range from 76% to 90% (Behnia-Willison et al. 2007, Lin et al. 2005, Seman et al. 2003). Comparison studies have been done looking at laparoscopic uterosacral ligament colpopexy and transvaginal suspension. Diwan et al. (2006) retrospectively compared laparoscopic uterosacral uterine suspension to vaginal hysterectomy with either vaginal uterosacral or sacrospinous ligament suspension

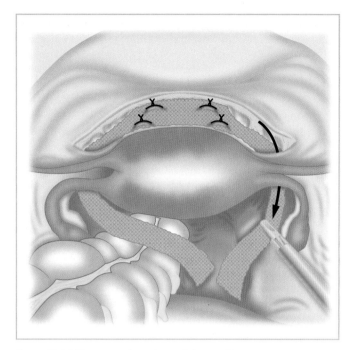

Figure 28.16 Placement of anterior mesh for sacral hysteropexy.

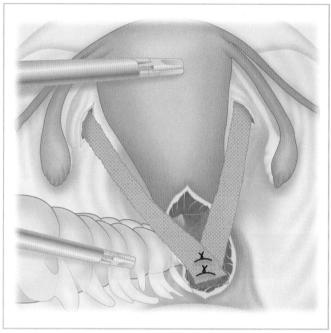

Figure 28.18 Sacral hysteropexy using anterior and posterior mesh.

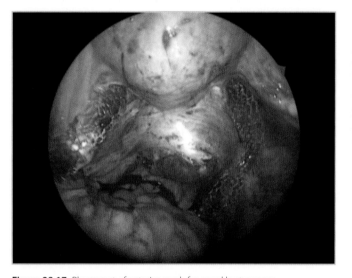

Figure 28.17 Placement of anterior mesh for sacral hysteropexy.

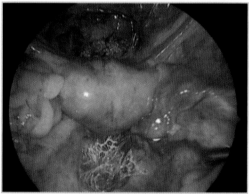

Figure 28.19
Sacral hysteropexy
using anterior and
posterior mesh.

▍ RETROPUBIC PROCEDURES
▍ Burch colposuspension

Surgery for stress incontinence is recommended when conservative treatments fail. Over the last decade, the midurethral sling has become the most commonly performed procedure for the surgical management of stress urinary incontinence. However, prior to the evolution of the midurethral sling, the open Burch colposuspension was referred to as the gold standard for surgical management of stress urinary incontinence with a reported cure rate >80% (Carey et al. 2006). The procedure remains an important technique for management of stress urinary incontinence in patients who have failed treatment with the midurethral sling, who decline synthetic mesh placement, or who are undergoing concomitant laparoscopic or robotic prolapse repair surgery and would prefer to have an abdominal approach for their incontinence procedure. Many modifications of this procedure exist without any evidence of improvement in outcomes; therefore, the recommendation is to perform this procedure in the same fashion as the open abdominal technique using suture only. Many surgeons who have not adopted laparoscopic Burch due to a prolonged learning curve to achieve proficiency have found that robotic assistance is sometimes helpful for the challenging dissection and the suturing that are necessary to perform the procedure.

The procedure can be performed using either an extraperitoneal or an intraperitoneal approach depending on the surgeon's preference, if concomitant intraperitoneal procedures are to be performed, and if the patient has had previous retropubic surgery. We recommend the intraperitoneal approach because it allows for a larger dissection, creating a larger operating space that makes it easier and safer to suture. Additional advantages of the intraperitoneal approach is that it is safer in patients who have undergone prior retropubic surgery, and it allows for concomitant culdoplasty or paravaginal defect repair to be performed. For the purposes of this chapter, we will describe the intraperitoneal approach to the Burch colposuspension since the extraperitoneal approach is neither commonly performed nor taught.

To perform the intraperitoneal technique, a three-way Foley catheter should be in place, and the bladder should be retrograde filled at the start of the procedure in order to help assist in visualizing the superior border of the bladder edge. The space of Retzius is first entered by creating a 2 cm transverse incision approximately 2 cm above the bladder reflection between the medial borders of the right and left obliterated umbilical ligaments. The proper plan is created when the loose areolar tissue is encountered and the pubic rami are visualized. To minimize the risk of bladder injury, both blunt and sharp dissections are done aiming toward the posterior–superior aspect of the pubic symphysis. Furthermore, blunt dissection is done bilaterally until the pubic symphysis, Cooper's ligaments, and the bladder neck are visualized. Cadaveric studies have shown that obturator canal is located approximately 5.4 cm (range 4.5–6.1) lateral to the pubic symphysis and 1.7 cm (1.5–2.6 cm) inferior to the iliopectineal line (Drewes et al. 2005; **Figure 28.20**). Therefore, awareness of the proximity of the structures is necessary during the dissection of this portion. Once these landmarks are identified, the bladder is drained, and careful dissection is performed until the arcus tendinus fascia pelvis is identified. The surgeon places two fingers in the vagina and identifies the urethrovesical junction by placing gentle traction on the Foley catheter. With elevation of the vaginal fingers, blunt dissection is done along the vaginal wall lateral to the bladder neck. Care should be taken to avoid aggressive dissection within 2 cm of the bladder neck to avoid bleeding and damage to the periurethral nerve supply. With digital elevation of the vagina, permanent No. 0 or 2-0 sutures on a double armed SH or CT-2 needle are used, first placed lateral to and at the level of the midurethra in a figure-of-eight fashion, through the fibromuscular tissue of the vagina, taking care not to incorporate the underlying epithelium. The suture is then passed through Cooper's ligament on the ipsilateral side. A second suture is then placed at the level of the urethrovesical junction and again through Cooper's ligament on the same side. The sutures are tied in an intracorporeal

fashion with simultaneous vaginal elevation. The goal is to elevate the vaginal wall to the level of the arcus tendineus fascia pelvis to ensure that the bladder neck is well supported by the vaginal walls; this may lead to small bilateral suture bridges, which is not uncommon, but may be result in dyspareunia especially if concomitant rectocele repair is performed (Weber & Walters 1997; **Figure 28.21**). Sutures should be tied down as they are placed to avoid suture tangling. If a double-armed suture is used, two passes are made through Cooper's ligaments and subsequently tied above the ligaments. The same procedure is repeated on the contralateral side. We recommend placement of Gelfoam (Pharmacia Upjohn, Inc., Kalamazoo, Michigan) between the vaginal wall and the obturator fascia before knot tying to promote fibrosis. A cystourethroscopy is performed after the sutures are passed to confirm ureteral patency and the absence of bladder and urethral injuries. The peritoneum may be closed on the basis of the surgeon's preference, and at the completion of the procedure, care must be taken to ensure that the surgical site is hemostatic as the abdomen is desufflated.

Paravaginal defect repair

This was once routine at the time of Burch colposuspension as lateral vaginal wall defects were thought to contribute to stress urinary incontinence symptoms (Miklos & Kohli 2000). With the increasing use of the midurethral sling for treatment of stress incontinence, the rate of Burch colposuspension began to decrease, along with the paravaginal defect repair. In addition, the presence or absence of a paravaginal defect has become very controversial in the field of urogynecology. There are data to support that the clinical examination of these support defects has poor interexaminer and intraexaminer agreement leading many providers to doubt the clinical significance of paravaginal defects (Whiteside et al. 2004). As a result of these data and less instruction in this procedure to trainees, paravaginal defect repairs are performed much less frequently than in the past. However, a Cochrane review evaluating laparoscopic Burch colposuspension reported that paravaginal repair at the time of the Burch procedure appears to be beneficial with regard to postoperative outcomes. Therefore, understanding the steps of this procedure remains important (Dean et al. 2006).

The robotic approach to the space of Retzius for the paravaginal defect repair is identical to the Burch procedure. If a Burch procedure is also performed, the paravaginal defect repair should be completed first as there will be poor exposure to the lateral defects once the Burch

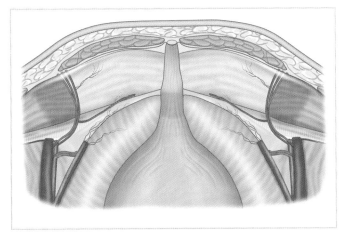

Figure 28.20 Vasculature of the retropubic space.

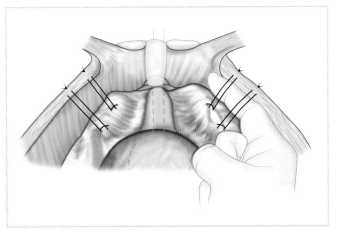

Figure 28.21 Burch colposuspension.

sutures are tied down. The dissection is carried out laterally in a blunt fashion until the obturator internus muscle, obturator foramen with neurovascular bundle, and arcus tendineus fascia pelvis are identified. The dissection is made easier with a vaginal hand elevating the vagina and medially retracting the bladder. Blunt dissection is carried out dorsally until vaginal palpation of the ischial spine is visualized laparoscopically. A No. 0 or 2-0 nonabsorbable suture on a CT-2 needle is passed through the fibromuscular layer of the vagina starting at the vaginal apex, and then through the obturator internus muscle and its fascia around the arcus tendineus at its origin, approximately 2 cm from the ischial spine (Miklos & Kohli 2000). Several sutures are placed in an interrupted fashion from the ischial spine to the proximal portion of the vesicourethral junction until there is good restoration of vaginal anatomy (**Figure 28.22**). The procedure can be done unilaterally or bilaterally depending on the extent of the defect. A cystourethroscopy is performed after the sutures are passed to confirm ureteral patency and absence of bladder and urethral injury. The peritoneum may be closed based on surgeon preference and at the completion of the procedure, care must be taken to ensure that the surgical site is hemostatic as the abdomen is desufflated.

In a randomized controlled trial, Carey et al. demonstrated that laparoscopic colposuspension was as efficacious as open colposuspension (Carey et al. 2006); however, the 2010 Cochrane review on laparoscopic Burch colposuspension reported that while women's subjective symptoms were similar for both procedures, there was evidence of poorer objective outcomes for the laparoscopic approach and the procedure was also determined to be more costly (Dean et al. 2006). A Cochrane review compared laparoscopic Burch colposuspension to the open abdominal approach for treatment of stress urinary incontinence and included 12 randomized trials (Lapitan & Cody 2012). There was significant heterogeneity in the outcome measures and designs of many of the trials. The combined estimate favored open Burch in the medium term (1–5 years), but this finding was not statistically significant. When the data were removed from one trial that showed significantly better results with open Burch col-

posuspension when mesh and staples were used in the laparoscopic cases (Ankardal et al. 2004), there were no statistical differences in stress incontinence cure rates between open and laparoscopic colposuspension (RR 0.95; 95% CI 0.80–1.11). Overall, objective outcomes for stress incontinence were not shown to be any different in these two approaches. Additionally, other perioperative outcomes have also been compared between the open abdominal and laparoscopic approaches to Burch colposuspension, and studies have found that laparoscopic colposuspension is associated with less perioperative complications, decreased hospital stay and faster return to daily activities at the expense of longer operating room time, and higher cost compared to open colposuspension (Dean et al. 2006).

An earlier Cochrane review, published in 2010, compared laparoscopic Burch colposuspension to other surgical treatments for stress urinary incontinence (Dean et al. 2006). Eight of the studies included in the review compared laparoscopic Burch colposuspension to retropubic midurethral sling placement. The subjective cure rate was not significantly different in the groups at 18 months (RR 0.91; 95% CI 0.80–1.02). A long-term follow-up study by Jelovsek et al. (2008) compared the tension-free vaginal tape (TVT) sling with the Burch colposuspension performed in patients between 1999 and 2002 and found that out of the 74% of subjects who had follow-up up to 4–8 years, there was no significant difference in the percentage of women reporting any urinary incontinence symptoms in the laparoscopic Burch (58%) and the TVT groups (48%; RR 1.19; 95% CI 0.71–2.0). Only 11% (3/28) of the laparoscopic Burch subjects and 8% (2/25) of the TVT subjects reported bothersome stress incontinence at 4–8 years (RR 1.3; 95%CI 0.24–7.4). The authors concluded that TVT had similar long-term efficacy to laparoscopic Burch for the treatment of stress incontinence. Although the literature shows that midurethral-sling procedures appear to offer greater benefits with better objective outcomes in the short term and similar subjective outcomes in the long term (Dean et al. 2006), the laparoscopic Burch procedure remains an important operation in pelvic reconstructive surgery and is appropriate for certain patients.

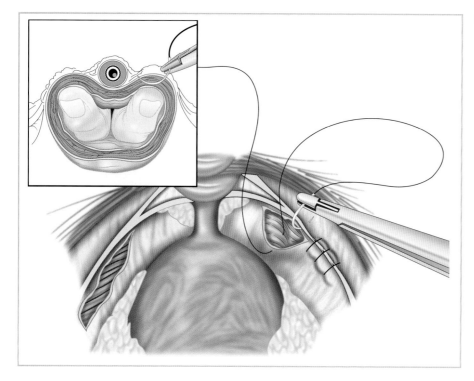

Figure 28.22 Paravaginal defect repair.

There are very little data on the use of the robotic assistance for both laparoscopic Burch colposuspension and paravaginal defect repair. Case reports exist demonstrating the feasibility of the robotic approach (Khan et al. 2007), but otherwise, the data are limited. A retrospective study by Behnia-Willison et al. (2007) reported a 76% objective cure rate in subjects undergoing bilateral paravaginal defect repair at the time of laparoscopic uterosacral ligament suspension. There are no studies evaluating outcomes after robotic-assisted paravaginal defect repair.

ENTEROCELE REPAIR

An enterocele is commonly present with uterovaginal prolapse or can develop following vaginal or abdominal hysterectomy. The repair of an enterocele is traditionally done transvaginally; however, there are times when an abdominal approach is necessary for larger enteroceles. This abdominal approach can be achieved in a minimally invasive fashion, especially when laparoscopic repair is indicated for uterovaginal prolapse (Cadeddu et al. 1996). Two different laparoscopic techniques have been described to repair an enterocele and can also be performed robotically, the Moschcowitz and Halban procedures. In both operations, a vaginal sponge stick or an EEA sizer is placed inside of the vagina for delineation of the posterior vagina, rectum, and hernia sac. The enterocele sac is dissected until the endopelvic fascial defects are identified. In the Moschcowitz procedure, the enterocele sac is obliterated by reapproximating the pelvic peritoneum between the rectum and vagina, incorporating the uterosacral ligaments with a permanent No. 0 suture in a purse-string fashion (**Figure 28.23**). The Halban culdoplasty is similar but involves placing permanent No. 0 sutures in an interrupted fashion,

starting at the posterior vagina and proceeding longitudinally over the cul-de-sac peritoneum and over the inferior serosa of the sigmoid, and the sutures are tied as they are placed, 1 cm apart (**Figure 28.24**). Visualization of the ureters is important during both of these procedures to ensure that there is no obstruction or kinking of the overlying peritoneum when the cul-de-sac is closed. The data on minimally invasive abdominal culdoplasty are very limited. The procedure is performed less frequently than it once was, and this may be because concomitant Halban or Moschcowitz culdoplasty have not been shown to improve cure or decrease recurrence of prolapse when performed concomitantly with sacral colpopexy (Nygaard et al. 2004).

ADVANTAGES OF ROBOTIC SURGERY

The use of the robotic platform provides many technical advantages to the surgeon. Such advantages include detailed three-dimensional visualization, improvement in dexterity with the use of wristed instruments, and tremor-filtered technology. These types of changes allow for easier dissection in difficult cases and facilitate intracorporeal knot tying, skills that many surgeons have found difficult to acquire by conventional laparoscopy. As a result, challenging cases such as laparoscopic sacral colpopexy and Burch colposuspension can be made more achievable with the assistance of robotic technology. Additionally, when compared to conventional laparoscopy, the learning curve for robotic surgery is less steep, and surgeons are able to learn a minimally invasive skill set at a much quicker and feasible pace (Payne & Dauterive 2008).

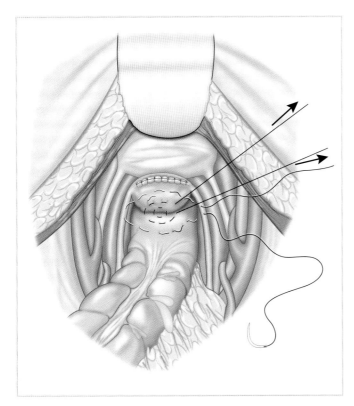

Figure 28.23 The Moschcowitz procedure.

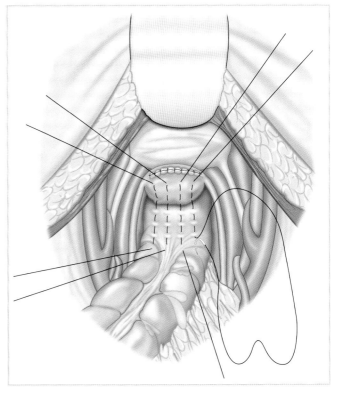

Figure 28.24 The Halban procedure.

DISADVANTAGES OF ROBOTIC SURGERY

The main disadvantages to the robotic platform are those that are inherent to the technology itself. There is no haptic feedback with the robotic system, so it is paramount that the surgeon pays close attention to visual cues when placing tension on tissues or suture. It also takes time to learn the robotic setup; successful and efficient docking requires a trained and experienced surgical team that is an investment in time and money for any institution, which adopts the platform. The surgeon must also obtain proper training to use the equipment and to become competent performing routine procedures, which also requires time and incurs certain costs. With regard to robotic setup, once the robotic system is docked, the patient's bed position cannot be changed without first removing instruments and undocking the robotic arms, which can be challenging in certain cases. Another important limitation to robotic surgery is that many functions such as the ability to clutch, exchange instruments, focus the camera, and use monopolar and bipolar energy modalities can be very different between the generations of the da Vinci Robotic Surgical Systems, and the surgical team must be able to adapt to these differences.

The most significant disadvantage associated with robotic-assisted laparoscopic procedures is the cost, and this has been well reported in the literature. There does seem to be a cost advantage in using robotic technology in lieu of the open abdominal approach for some procedures. Elliot et al. (2012) performed a retrospective cost-minimization analysis on women undergoing robotic sacral colpopexy, comparing them to women undergoing sacral colpopexy via the open abdominal approach. The authors found that the length of hospital stay after surgery was significantly longer in the open group when compared to the robotic cases (1.0 vs. 3.3 days, $P < 0.001$), which significantly increased the overall cost of the surgery. The authors of that study concluded that the number of yearly cases, length of hospital stay,

and cost of hospitalization were the largest contributing factors to the cost of surgery. In a randomized controlled trial comparing laparoscopic sacral colpopexy to robotic sacral colpopexy, Paraiso et al. (2011) looked at cost differences between the two procedures as one of their secondary outcomes. In this study, surgical cost was calculated on the basis of the actual cost of surgery, hospitalization, and all surgery-related inpatient and outpatient care through the 6-week postoperative visit. They found that the overall cost was higher in the robotic cases (mean difference +$1936 (95% CI $417–$3,454), $P = 0.008$) and was attributed to operating room costs as operating room time was significantly higher in the robotic group than the conventional group. Of note, this increase in cost did not include the cost of the robotic platform or its maintenance.

CONCLUSION

Robotic-assisted laparoscopy is a means of minimally invasive surgery that confers many benefits over conventional laparoscopy, but these advantages should continue to be weighed considerably with the cost of the technology. Procedures for the repair of pelvic organ prolapse and incontinence can be performed robotically, and sometimes are made to be less challenging with the assistance of the robot. These procedures should be performed using the same techniques employed at the time of open abdominal surgery, as we know that the open approaches to, e.g. both sacral colpopexy and Burch colposuspension are associated with high subjective and objective success rates, and are safe and effective procedures.

The data on long-term outcomes after minimally invasive abdominal procedures for the repair of pelvic organ prolapse and incontinence are sparse. Future studies should focus on comparing conventional laparoscopy and robotic-assisted laparoscopy for the treatment of pelvic floor disorders. These studies should aim to evaluate postoperative objective and subjective long-term outcomes in order to determine long-term efficacy, and to report on the associated perioperative adverse events and costs associated with these procedures.

REFERENCES

ACOG Committee on Practice Bulletins – Gynecology. ACOG practice bulletin No. 104: antibiotic prophylaxis for gynecologic procedures. Obstet Gynecol 2009; 113:1180–1189.

Anger JT, Mueller ER, Tarnay C, et al. Robotic compared with laparoscopic sacrocolpopexy: a randomized controlled trial. Obstet Gynecol 2014; 123:5–12.

Ankardal M, Ekerydh A, Crafoord K, et al. A randomized trial comparing open Burch colposuspension using sutures with laparoscopic colposuspension using mesh and staples in women with stress urinary incontinence. BJOG 2004; 111:974–981.

Baltayian S. A brief review: anesthesia for robotic prostatectomy J Robotic Surg 2008; 2:59–66.

Bandera CA, Magrina JF. Robotic surgery in gynecologic oncology. Curr Opin Obstet Gynecol 2009; 21:25–30.

Barbash GI, Glied SA. New technology and health care costs: the case of robot-assisted surgery. N Engl J Med 2010; 363:701–704.

Behnia-Willison F, Seman EI, Cook JR, O'Shea RT, Keirse MJ. Laparoscopic paravaginal repair of anterior compartment prolapse. J Minim Invasive Gynecol 2007; 14:475–480.

Burgess KL, Elliott DS. Robotic/Laparoscopic prolapse repair and the role of hysteropexy: a urology perspective. Urol Clin North Am 2012; 39:349–360.

Cadeddu JA, Micali S, Moore RG, Kavoussi LR. Laparoscopic repair of enterocele. J Endourol 1996; 10:367–369.

Carey MP, Goh JT, Rosamilia A, et al. Laparoscopic versus open Burch colposuspension: a randomised controlled trial. BJOG 2006; 113:999–1006.

Costantini E, Mearini L, Bini V, et al. Uterus preservation in surgical correction of urogenital prolapse. Eur Urol 2005; 48:642–649.

Cullen J, Rosselli JM, Gurland BH. Ventral rectopexy for recta prolapse and obstructed defecation. Clin Colon Rectal Surg 2012; 25:34–36.

Cundiff GW, Harris RL, Coates K, et al. Abdominal sacral colpoperineopexy: a new approach for correction of posterior compartment defects and perineal descent associated with vaginal vault prolapse. Am J Obstet Gynecol 1997; 177:1345–1353.

Danic MJ, Chow M, Alexander G, et al. Anesthesia considerations for robotic-assisted prostatectomy: a review of 1,500 cases. J Robotic Surg 2007; 1:11923.

Dean NM, Ellis G, Wilson PD, Herbison GP. Laparoscopic colposuspension for urinary incontinence in women. Cochrane Database Syst Rev 2006; 3:CD002239.

De Hoog DENM, Heemskerk J, Nieman FHM, et al. Recurrence and functional results after open versus conventional laparoscopic versus robot-assisted laparoscopic rectopexy for rectal prolapse: a case-control study. Int J Colorectal Dis 2009; 24:1201–1206.

Diwan A, Rardin C, Strohsnitter WC, et al. Laparoscopic uterosacral ligament uterine suspension compared with vaginal hysterectomy with vaginal vault suspension for uterovaginal prolapse. Int Urogynecol J 2006; 17:79–83.

Drewes PG, Marinis SI, Schaffer JI, et al. Vascular anatomy over the superior pubic rami in female cadavers. Am J Obstet Gynecol 2005; 193:2165–2168.

Elliot CS, Hsieh MH, Sokol ER, et al. Robot-assisted versus open sacral colpopexy: a cost minimization analysis. J Urol 2012; 187:638–643.

Freeman RM, Pantazis, Thomson A, et al. A randomised controlled trial of abdominal versus laparoscopic sacrocolpopexy for the treatment of post-hysterectomy vaginal vault prolapse: LAS study. Int Urogynecol J 2013; 24:377–378.

Frick AC, Walters MD, Larkin KS, Barber MD. Risk of unanticipated abnormal gynecologic pathology at the time of hysterectomy for uterovaginal prolapse. Am J Obstet Gynecol 2010; 202:507.e1–507.e4.

Ganatra AM, Rozet F, Sanchez-Salas R, et al. The current status of laparoscopic sacrocolpopexy: a review. Eur Urol 2009; 55:1089–1103.

Güenaga KF, Matos D, Wille-Jørgensen P. Mechanical bowel preparation for elective colorectal surgery. Cochrane Database Syst Rev 2011; 9:CD001544.

Guyatt GH, Akl EA, Crowther M, et al. Executive summary: Antithrombotic Therapy and Prevention of Thrombosis, 9th ed: American College of Chest Physicians Evidence-Based Clinical Practice Guidelines. Chest 2012; 141:7S–47S.

Heemskerk J, de Hoog DENM, van Gemert WG, et al. Robot-assisted vs conventional laparoscopic rectopexy for rectal prolapse: a comparative study on costs and time. Dis Colon Rectum 2001; 50:1825–1830.

Hendrix SL, Clark A, Nygaard I, et al. Pelvic organ prolapse in the women's health initiative: gravity and gravidity. Am J Obstet Gynecol 2002; 186:1160–1166.

Jelovsek JE, Barber MD. Women seeking treatment for advanced pelvic organ prolapse have decreased body image and quality of life. Am J Obstet Gynecol 2006; 194:1455–1461.

Jelovsek JE, Barber MD, Karram MM, et al. Randomised trial of laparoscopic Burch colposuspension versus tension-free vaginal tape: long-term follow up. BJOG 2008; 115:219–225.

Kehoe SM, Ramirez PT, Abu-Rustum NR. Innovative laparoscopic surgery in gynecologic oncology. Curr Oncol 2007; 9:472–477.

Khan MS, Challacombe B, Rose K, Dasgupta P. Robotic colposuspension: two case reports. J Endourol 2007; 21:1077–1079.

Lapitan MC, Cody JD. Open retropubic colposuspension for urinary incontinence in women. Cochrane Database Syst Rev 2012; 6:CD002912.

Lin LL, Phelps JY, Lui CY. Laparoscopic vaginal vault suspension using uterosacral ligaments: a review of 133 cases. J Minim Invasive Gynecol 2005; 12:216–220.

Makai G, Isaacson K. Complications of gynecologic laparoscopy. Clin Obstet Gynecol 2009;52:401–411.

McDermott CD, Park J, Terry CL, et al. Laparoscopic sacral colpoperineopexy: abdominal versus abdominal-vaginal posterior graft attachment. Int Urogynecol J 2011; 22:469–475.

Mellgren A, Johansson C, Dolk A, et al. Enterocele demonstrated be defecography is associated with other pelvic floor disorders. Int J Colorectal Dis 1994; 9:121–124.

Miklos JR, Kohli N. Laparoscopic paravaginal repair plus Burch colposuspension: review and descriptive technique. Urology 2000; 56:64–69.

Nosti PA, Lowman JK, Zollinger TW, et al. Risk of mesh erosion after abdominal sacral colpoperineopexy with concomitant hysterectomy. Am J Obstet Gynecol 2009; 201:541.e1-4.

Nosti PA, Umoh AU, Kane S, et al. Outcomes of abdominal and minimally invasive sacrocolpopexy: a retrospective cohort study. Female Pelvic Med Reconstr Surg 2014; 20:33–37.

Nygaard I, Brubaker L, Zyczynski HM, et al. Long-term outcomes following abdominal sacral colpopexy for pelvic organ prolapse. JAMA 2013; 309:2016–2024.

Nygaard IE, McCreery R, Brubaker L, et al. Abdominal sacrocolpopexy: a comprehensive review. Obstet Gynecol 2004; 104:805–823.

Ogunnaike BO, Jones SB, Jones DB, et al. Anesthetic considerations for bariatric surgery. Anesth Analg 2002; 95:1793–1805.

Osmundsen BC, Clark A, Goldsmith C, et al. Mesh erosion in robotic sacral colpopexy. Fem Pelvic Med Reconstr Surg 2012; 18:86–88.

Paraiso MF, Jelovsek JE, Frick A, et al. Laparoscopic compared with robotic sacral colpopexy for vaginal prolapse. Obstet Gynecol 2011; 118:1005–1013.

Payne TN, Dauterive FR. A comparison of total laparoscopic hysterectomy to robotically assisted hysterectomy: surgical outcomes in a community practice. Minim Invasive Gynecol 2008; 11:395–398.

Perrenot C, Germain A, Scherrer ML, et al. Long-term outcomes of robot-assisted laparoscopic rectopexy for rectal prolapse. Dis Colon Rectum 2013; 56:909–914.

Propst K, Tunitsky-Bitton E, Schimpf MO, Ridgeway B. Pyogenic spondylodiscitis associated with sacral colpopexy and rectopexy: report of two cases and evaluation of the literature. Int Urogynecol J 2014; 25:21–31.

Rahn DD, Mamik MM, Sanses TV, et al. Venous thromboembolism prophylaxis in gynecologic surgery: a systematic review. Obstet Gynecol 2011; 118:1111–1125.

Rardin CR, Erekson EA, Sung VW, Ward RM, Myers DL. Uterosacral colpopexy at the time of vaginal hysterectomy: comparison of laparoscopic and vaginal approaches. J Reprod Med 2009; 54:273–280.

Samaranayake CB, Luo C, Plank AW, et al. Systematic review on ventral rectopexy for rectal prolapse and intussusception. Colorectal Dis 2009; 12:504–514.

Schiavone MB, Kuo EC, Naumann RW, et al. The commercialization of robotic surgery: unsubstantiated marketing of gynecologic surgery by hospitals. Am J Obstet Gynecol 2012; 207:174.e1–174.e7.

Seman EI, Cook JR, O›Shea RT. Two-year experience with laparoscopic pelvic floor repair. J Am Assoc Gynecol Laparosc 2003; 10:38–45.

Tan-Kim J, Menefee SA, Luber KM, et al. Prevalence and risk factors for mesh erosion after laparoscopic-assisted sacral colpopexy. Int Urogynecol J 2011; 22:205–212.

Tarr ME, Paraiso MF. Minimally invasive approach to pelvic organ prolapse: a review. Minerva Ginecol 2014; 66:49–67.

Tekelioglu UY, Erdem A, Demirhan A, et al. The prolonged effect of pneumoperitoneum on cardicac autonomic functions during laparoscopic surgery: are we aware? Eur Rev Med Pharmacol Sci 2013; 17:895–902.

Walters MD, Ridgeway BM. Surgical treatment of vaginal apex prolapse. Obstet Gynecol 2013; 121:354–374.

Warner WB, Vora S, Hurtado EA, et al. Effect of operative technique on mesh exposure in laparoscopic sacral colpopexy. Female Pelvic Med Reconstr Surg 2012; 18:113–117.

Watadani Y, Vogler SA, Warshaw JS, et al. Sacrocolpopexy with rectopexy for pelvic floor prolapse improves bowel function and quality of life. Dis Colon Rectum 2013; 56:1415–1422.

Weber AM, Walters MD. Anterior vaginal prolapse: review of anatomy and techniques of surgical repair. Obstet Gynecol 1997; 89:311–318.

Whiteside JL, Barber MD, Paraiso MF, Hugney CM, Walters MD. Clinical evaluation of anterior vaginal wall support defects: interexaminer and intraexaminer reliability. Am J Obstet Gynecol 2004; 191:100–104.

Wong MT, Meurette G, Rigaud J, Regenet N, Lehur PA. Robotic versus laparoscopic rectopexy for complex rectocele: a prospective comparison of short-term outcomes. Dis Colon Rectum 2011; 54:342–346.

Chapter 29 | Laparoscopic staging of pelvic malignancies

Elisabeth Diver, David Boruta II

■ INTRODUCTION

Staging of gynecologic malignancies is a cornerstone of oncologic management. Accurate information regarding the absence or presence of metastatic disease, and its location, provides useful prognostic information and allows adjuvant treatment such as chemotherapy and/or radiation, to be prescribed appropriately. Inaccurate staging may lead to inappropriate treatment, or lack thereof, and result in compromised survival. Laparotomy for surgical staging, often utilizing a generous midline vertical abdominal incision, while allowing for a thorough survey of the abdominal cavity and its contents, is associated with significant morbidity and extended recovery. As in benign gynecologic surgery, laparoscopy has gradually replaced laparotomy as the surgical approach of choice for the completion of gynecologic oncology procedures, including staging.

While all cancers utilize a staging system, in gynecologic oncology, surgical staging is employed most commonly in uterine, ovarian, Fallopian tube, and vulvar cancers. Cervical cancer is commonly assigned the International Federation of Gynecology and Obstetrics (FIGO) stage on the basis of clinical, nonsurgical findings; however, surgical findings, including status of lymph nodal material, are often considered in treatment planning. Surgical staging of gynecologic malignancies varies according to the primary site, but may include retroperitoneal lymph nodal evaluation with biopsy, assessment of peritoneal surfaces with a collection of washings for cytology, biopsy of suspicious lesions, omental resection, and assessment and/or removal of the gynecologic organs. While other chapters will explore applications of laparoscopy in numerous disease sites in gynecologic oncology, this chapter will focus on the basics of a laparoscopic approach for completion of surgical staging within the peritoneal cavity and pelvic/para-aortic retroperitoneal spaces.

■ SET-UP AND INSTRUMENTATION

General anesthesia is administered, and orogastric drainage for stomach decompression is recommended. The patient is placed in a dorsal lithotomy position with arms tucked and padded along her sides, where the surgeon and assistant stand. During surgery in the pelvis, video monitors are positioned either centrally between the patient's legs or one laterally to each leg of the patient (**Figure 29.1a** and **b**). Depending on the direction of surgical effort, the monitors may be relocated. For example, during para-aortic lymphadenectomy, the monitors may be moved toward the patient's shoulders as surgical effort is directed toward the upper flank (**Figure 29.1c**).

Entry into the peritoneal cavity is achieved via a closed or open technique. The location and number of additional ports are patient, provider, and procedure dependent. Commonly employed positions include the umbilicus, the right and left lower quadrants, and the midline suprapubic region (**Figure 29.2a**). In lieu of a suprapubic port, additional ports can be located in either or both midclavicular lines adjacent to the umbilicus (**Figure 29.2b**). The use of two instruments from one side facilitates ergonomic contralateral dissection. Laparoendoscopic single-site surgery (LESS), which requires only a single umbilical incision, has also been described for surgical staging (Fader 2009). When multiple ports are employed, the least number and smallest diameter should be used that allow for safe completion of the procedure. Specific tools of larger diameter or the need for specimen extraction may prompt the use of larger incisions.

Although gynecologists commonly use laparoscopes with a 0° lens, an angled lens or a laparoscope with a flexible tip is useful (**Figure 29.3**). These facilitate more extensive survey within the peritoneal cavity, especially around fixed tissues and corners, such as for visualization of the diaphragmatic peritoneal surfaces cephalad to the liver.

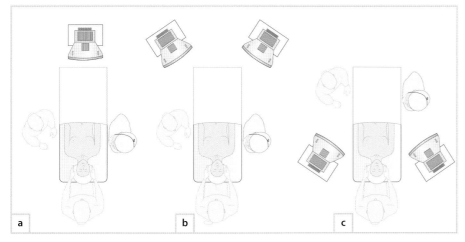

Figure 29.1 Positions of surgeons and monitors during laparoscopic surgical staging. (a and b) Monitor positioning for surgery in the pelvis. (c) Monitor positioning for surgery in the upper abdomen.

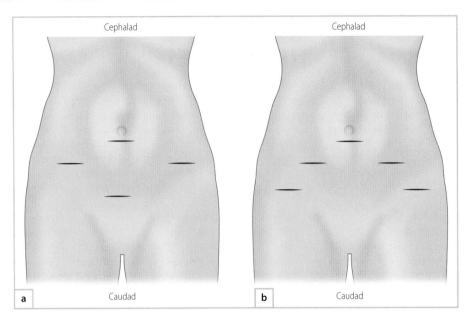

Figure 29.2 Location of incisions for laparoscopic surgical staging. Commonly employed positions include the umbilicus, the right and left lower quadrants, and the midline suprapubic region (a). Additional ports can be located in either or both midclavicular lines adjacent to the umbilicus (b).

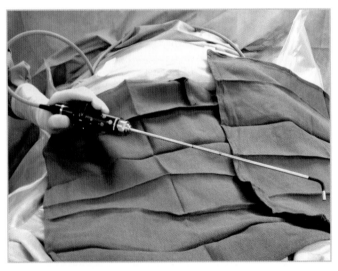

Figure 29.3 Flexible-tip laparoscope.

In addition to a laparoscope, a variety of other instruments are commonly used during surgical staging. Graspers with different tips facilitate tissue manipulation, dissection, retraction, and biopsy. Bowel forceps are useful for extensive bowel manipulation, such as when examining the length of the bowel or its mesentery. Cutting tools, often with means to maintain hemostasis, assist with the division of vasculature and connective tissues. A variety of reusable and disposable devices, including scissors with monopolar cautery, grasping forceps with bipolar cautery, or ultrasonic shears are available. Each tool has its unique advantages and disadvantages. For example, ultrasonic shears facilitate separation of relatively avascular tissue whereas the bipolar electrical energy achieves hemostasis with division of larger vessels. Suction–irrigation devices can be used to obtain abdominal pelvic washings for cytology. Laparoscopic bags are used for tissue extraction.

■ PROCEDURE

Performance of any primary procedure, such as hysterectomy or salpingo-oophorectomy, precedes surgical staging in most cases. Lysis of adhesions to allow normalization of anatomy facilitates adequate survey within the peritoneal cavity. A thorough exploration of abdominal/pelvic cavity must replicate what is accomplished at laparotomy. In addition to the use of an angled lens or flexible-tip laparoscope, tilting of the surgical table and patient to the left or right and between Trendelenburg and reverse-Trendelenburg positions helps with visualization of all four quadrants. Movement of the laparoscope and instruments used to retract and survey tissues between various ports may be advantageous. Particular care is needed to ensure adequate visualization of the peritoneal surfaces over the diaphragm, behind the liver, along the paracolic gutters, and at the root of the small bowel mesentery.

Atraumatic graspers designed for handling the bowel should be used to survey the entire length of small and large bowels. The bowel serosa and both sides of its mesentery are visualized using a hand-over-hand technique to 'run' the bowel. Biopsy of any suspicious lesions or adhesions should be performed.

Omentectomy, or at least omental biopsy, is an important part of staging in ovarian and some uterine cancers. If total omentectomy is performed, reverse-Trendelenburg may allow the omentum to fall into the pelvis allowing surgical effort to be directed in the familiar pelvic direction. If it remains primarily in the upper abdomen, movement of the video monitors to the patient's shoulders and the direction of surgical effort cephalad may be helpful.

Laparoscopic retroperitoneal exploration with lymph node biopsy or lymphadenectomy may be performed using either a transperitoneal or an extraperitoneal approach. An extraperitoneal approach to para-aortic lymphadenectomy provides exceptional exposure in heavier patients facilitating a bowel-free working space. It is also preferred when para-aortic nodal evaluation is performed in women with clinically advanced-stage cervical cancer as adhesion formation within the peritoneal cavity is minimized. This chapter will focus, however, on the more commonly performed transperitoneal approach.

■ Pelvic lymphadenectomy

The surgeon uses a cutting tool and a grasper through either a suprapubic port and a lower-quadrant port contralateral to the pelvis to be dissected or two ports in the lower quadrant. The assistant operates the laparoscope through the umbilicus and a grasper for retraction through the lower-quadrant port on the side ipsilateral to the targeted pelvis.

An incision through the posterior leaf of the broad ligament parallel to the external iliac vasculature is made if it is not already done as part of the initial gynecologic procedure. The goal is for biopsy or complete removal of the fatty/lymphatic tissues from the anatomic boundaries as described in **Table 29.1** (also see **Figure 29.4**). Thorough development of the paravesical and pararectal spaces prior to the removal of tissue facilitates safe dissection. This is primarily accomplished with blunt dissection along natural tissue planes. Discrete use of cautery or ultrasonic shears is for hemostatically transecting small vessels and connective tissue. Care must be taken to avoid injury to vasculature or nerves. Dissection proceeding from lateral to medial, up and down vasculature with effort to maintain one packet of fatty lymphatic tissue, is preferred. The specimen is then placed in an endoscopic bag and removed either vaginally or through a port-site incision. The contralateral pelvis is then dissected with the movement of the surgeon and the assistant to the opposite sides of the table.

Para-aortic lymphadenectomy

The surgeon and assistant use tools through ports as described for pelvic lymphadenectomy, but as surgical effort is directed across the patient's flank, it is helpful to move the video monitors cephalad (e.g. at patient's flank or shoulder). The assistant may find operating the camera from the side of the intended dissection awkward, with a view that is backward. Some assistants may find standing in between the patient's legs, or even adjacent to the surgeon, to be more ergonomic.

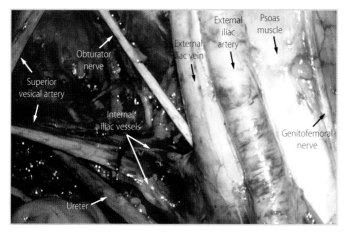

Figure 29.4 Anatomic landmarks of pelvic lymphadenectomy.

The right-side dissection is initiated with incision of the peritoneum overlying the right common iliac artery and cephalad over the aorta. Care must be taken not to injure the right ureter where it crosses the common iliac artery or the duodenum overlying the aorta. The peritoneum lateral to this incision and the ascending colon with its mesentery are elevated and mobilized laterally exposing the underlying vena cava and the right psoas muscle. The right ureter and right ovarian vasculature remain attached to the mesentery and are held elevated and lateral by the assistant's grasper. Exposure of the right para-aortic lymph nodes can be accomplished all the way to the renal vasculature, if desired. Often dissection is abbreviated and discontinued where the ovarian vasculature bifurcates off of the great vessels.

The greatest challenge of para-aortic lymphadenectomy is the maintenance of exposure over the para-aortic lymphatic chain with retraction of overlying bowel. Steep Trendelenburg and retraction of tissue by the assistant are critical. The surgeon may need to place the assistant's grasper for tissue retraction, as the surgeon will likely have the greatest command of the surgical field and desired view.

Dissection of the lymphatic tissue off of the underlying aorta and vena cava is accomplished using a combination of blunt dissection along natural tissue planes and selected use of cautery or ultrasonic shears to hemostatically transect small vessels and connective tissue. Separation of the lymphatic tissue off of the vasculature is initiated caudally near the upper limit of the pelvic lymphadenectomy and is directed cephalad to the chosen endpoint. The lymph node packet is rolled cephalad and lateral. Care must be taken not to avulse the so-called Fellow's vein that extends into the lower portion of the nodal packet from the vena cava. The anatomic boundaries of the right para-aortic lymph node dissection are described in **Table 29.1** (also see **Figure 29.5**). Once separated completely, the bundle is extracted with an endoscopic bag.

The surgeon then moves to the opposite side of the patient and directs the effort to the left side. Blunt dissection below the bifurcation of the internal mesenteric artery (IMA) is used to elevate the descending/sigmoid colon mesentery off of the aorta and expose the region of the left para-aortic lymph nodes. The left ureter is identified retroperitoneally and elevated along with the mesentery and the left ovarian vasculature by the assistant's grasper. Dissection of the lymphatic tissue is initiated caudally over the left common iliac artery. As the lymphatic tissue is elevated and separated from the artery, the bundle is rolled cephalad. Dissection of the bundle should proceed easily up to the level of the bifurcation of the internal iliac artery off of the aorta. The bundle is mobilized out of the groove between the aorta and the left psoas muscle. The lower left para-aortic lymph node bundle is often amputated at this point and removed in an endoscopic bag. Although the division of the IMA may facilitate exposure for dissection to the level of the left renal vasculature, its preservation is

Table 29.1 Anatomic borders of lymphadenectomy for surgical staging of gynecologic malignancies

Margin	Pelvic	Right para-aortic	Left para-aortic
Cephalad	Bifurcation of common iliac artery into internal and external branches	Right renal vasculature	Left renal vasculature
Caudad	External circumflex iliac vein crossing external iliac artery	Upper limit of right pelvic lymphadenectomy (bifurcation of common iliac artery)	Upper limit of left pelvic lymphadenectomy (bifurcation of common iliac artery)
Lateral	Psoas muscle	Right psoas muscle	Left psoas muscle
Medial	Internal iliac artery and superior vesical artery	Aorta	Aorta
Deep	Obturator nerve	Inferior vena cava	Vertebral bodies

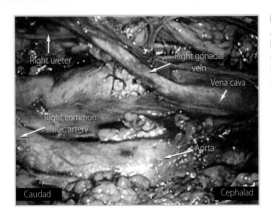

Figure 29.5 Anatomic landmarks of right para-aortic lymphadenectomy.

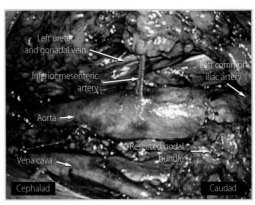

Figure 29.6 Anatomic landmarks of left para-aortic lymphadenectomy.

preferred. Further separation of the peritoneum and bowel mesentery off of the aorta above the level of the internal iliac artery, while keeping it intact, is usually feasible. Alternatively, the left para-aortic lymph node dissection can be performed from the left side of the patient with the exposure of the lymphatic bed following peritoneal incision along the left paracolic gutter and reflection of the descending colon as well as its mesentery medially. This provides similar exposure as in an extraperitoneal approach to left para-aortic dissection. Anatomic boundaries of the left para-aortic lymph node dissection are described in **Table 29.1** (also see **Figure 29.6**). Once separated completely, the bundle is extracted with an endoscopic bag.

CONTRAINDICATIONS TO A MINIMALLY INVASIVE APPROACH

In general, as surgeons become more proficient with minimally invasive techniques and technology advances, there are a few, if any, absolute contraindications to laparoscopy. Surgeon's expertise and comfort are essential for completing surgical staging via a minimally invasive approach. Patients unable to tolerate peritoneal insufflation or Trendelenburg positioning, such as those with difficult ventilatory status or elevated intracranial pressure, are poor candidates for a minimally invasive staging surgery. Barriers to adequate visualization with a laparoscope, such as acute intra-abdominal hemorrhage, large masses, or central obesity, may preclude a minimally invasive approach.

At all times, the primary goal of oncologic adequacy must be kept in mind. Inability to adequately or safely visualize the entire peritoneal cavity or perform sufficient lymphadenectomy should prompt adjustments in the approach up to and including conversion to laparotomy. Management decisions, unrelated specifically to staging procedures, may also prompt the need for conversion. Large, potentially malignant tumors, including an enlarged uterus with an underlying endometrial cancer, may not easily be removed via a natural orifice such as the vagina, let alone small port-site incisions. A laparotomy may be required for safe extraction of pathology and thus dictate a nonlaparoscopic approach to staging.

SUMMARY OF EVIDENCE

Endometrial cancer

Surgical stage of endometrial cancer is assigned following pathologic evaluation of the uterus, Fallopian tubes, ovaries, and pelvic and para-aortic lymph nodes (**Table 29.2**) (Pecorelli 2009). Patients with serous or clear cell histology also undergo omental and peritoneal

biopsies (Schorge et al. 2008). Although peritoneal cytology is no longer included in the staging of endometrial cancer according to the FIGO 2009 guidelines, washings remain predictive of patient' outcomes in some situations and are routinely obtained and reported (Garg et al. 2013).

Childers and Surwit first described laparoscopic staging for endometrial cancer including pelvic and para-aortic lymph node dissection with vaginal hysterectomy in 1992 (Childers & Surwit 1992). Controversy arose as to whether or not laparoscopy could suitably substitute laparotomy, let alone offer potential advantages. In 2009, the Gynecologic Oncology Group published initial results of the LAP 2 study (Walker et al. 2009). This prospective trial randomized >2600 women with endometrial cancer to undergo either surgical staging via laparoscopy or laparotomy. Comprehensive staging including both pelvic and para-aortic lymphadenectomy was mandated, thus requiring conversion from laparoscopy to laparotomy, if necessary. The results demonstrated the safety and feasibility of laparoscopic surgical staging for endometrial cancer as well as fewer complications and a shorter hospital stay compared to laparotomy. The conversion rate to laparotomy from laparoscopy was 26%, including 14.6% due to poor visibility, primarily related to obesity.

A second publication from the LAP 2 study described equivalent 5-year survival between the two surgical approaches for staging in

Table 29.2 The International Federation of Gynecology and Obstetrics endometrial cancer staging

I		Tumor confined to the uterine corpus
	A	Tumor invades is less than half the myometrial thickness
	B	Tumor invades is greater than or equal to half the myometrial thickness
II		Tumor invades the cervical stroma but is confined to the uterus
III		Local tumor spread outside the uterus
	A	Involves uterine serosa or adnexa
	B	Involves vagina or parametria
	C	Retroperitoneal lymph node metastasis IIIC1. Pelvic lymph node metastasis IIIC2. Para-aortic lymph node metastasis
IV		Bladder, bowel, or distant metastasis
	A	Invasion of bladder or bowel mucosa
	B	Other distant metastases

women with endometrial cancer (Walker et al. 2012). These findings have been confirmed in subsequent trials (Galaal et al. 2012, Wright et al. 2012). Early concerns regarding specific techniques utilized in minimally invasive surgical staging of endometrial cancer have been evaluated with reassuring results. For example, the use of a uterine manipulator does not increase the rate of lymphovascular space invasion or positive peritoneal cytology. Studies in patients with high-grade endometrial cancer also demonstrate the equivalent outcomes of minimally invasive staging compared to laparotomy (Fader et al. 2012).

Robotic-assisted laparoscopy is increasingly used to aid in the performance of laparoscopic surgical staging of endometrial cancer. Numerous publications suggest that this surgical approach allows for equivalent outcomes when compared to the use of traditional (nonrobotically assisted) laparoscopic equipment (Cardenas-Goicoechea et al. 2014, Escobar et al. 2012, Gaia et al. 2010 Escobar 2009). The number of lymph nodes retrieved, a proxy for staging adequacy, is equivalent, as is survival. Completion of staging procedures in obese women may be particularly facilitated with robotic assistance (Gehrig et al. 2008, Subramanian et al. 2011). Surgical staging via LESS, orifice-assisted small incision surgery (OASIS), and sentinel lymphadenectomy are areas of active investigation (Fagotti et al. 2012, Leitao et al. 2013, Pakish et al. 2014, Einarsson 2012). While surgical management of uterine sarcomas with minimally invasive techniques is less well documented, small case series have suggested it is safe and feasible (Jahns et al. 2011).

Cervical cancer

Due its prevalence in low-resource countries, cervical cancer continues to be formally staged clinically rather than surgically (Pecorelli 2009). The testing modalities approved for clinical staging include examination under anesthesia, cystoscopy, proctoscopy, and imaging and laboratory studies (Schorge et al. 2008). Laparoscopic surgery is commonly employed for cervical cancer, both for radical hysterectomy and for lymphadenectomy (Nezhat 1992, Wang 2015). A randomized trial is currently underway comparing abdominal versus minimally invasive radical hysterectomy for cervical cancer, the Laparoscopic Approach to Cervical Cancer (LACC) study (Clinicaltrials.gov). In locally advanced cervical cancer, para-aortic lymphadenectomy is often used to define the extent of metastatic disease and assist in planning adjuvant therapy. An extraperitoneal approach to para-aortic lymphadenectomy is preferred as it minimizes the risk of intraperitoneal adhesive disease that may increase the likelihood of radiation-related morbidity such as bowel obstruction (Vasilev & McGonigle 1996).

Surgical evaluation of the lymph nodes, rather than radiologic, may be preferred when these resources are available. Multiple studies have compared radiologic stage to surgical stage with the general finding that radiologic studies are less accurate than pathologic evaluation (Del Pino et al. 2013, Goff et al. 1999). Information from surgical staging leads to modification of adjuvant radiation in over 40% of women with locally advanced cervical cancer (Del Pino et al. 2013, Goff et al. 1999). Despite the change in stage and, therefore, modification in treatment, it is unclear that there is an associated change in prognosis based on surgical staging (Benedetti Panici et al. 2013). As such, a randomized controlled trial of radiographic versus radiographic and surgical staging in locally advanced cervical cancer is currently underway (Frumovitz et al. 2014). In early-stage cervical cancer patients based on clinical stage, lymph node assessment is performed at the time of surgical therapy with radical hysterectomy but is not reflected in the assigned clinical stage (Schorge et al. 2008).

Ovarian cancer

This is surgically staged on the basis of pathologic evaluation of specimens including peritoneal washings or ascites, peritoneal and omental biopsies, pelvic and para-aortic lymph nodes, Fallopian tubes, ovaries, uterus, and any other tissues suspicious for the presence of disease (Prat & FIGO Committee on Gynecologic Oncology 2014). The updated FIGO 2014 staging is detailed in **Table 29.3**. Although most women diagnosed with ovarian cancer have completed childbearing and undergo total hysterectomy and bilateral salpingo-oophorectomy during their staging procedure, in younger women in whom childbearing is desired these procedures are not required unless dictated by the need for removal of gross disease. Furthermore, the presence of bulky, gross disease in various locations may obviate the need for specific components of the staging procedure (i.e. washing for cytology in the setting of bulky omental metastases).

As surgical removal of complex ovarian masses is increasingly accomplished, the safety and feasibility of laparoscopy for surgical staging in ovarian cancer is an important consideration and a controversial topic. Given the procedures performed are similar to those in women with endometrial cancer, it may be reasonable to extrapolate the results of LAP 2 to women undergoing laparoscopic staging for ovarian cancer. A small case–control study of women with ovarian cancer who underwent staging via a laparoscopic approach demonstrated reduced blood loss and reduced hospital stay when compared to traditional laparotomy (Chi et al. 2005). The size

Table 29.3 The International Federation of Gynecology and Obstetrics ovarian cancer staging

I	Tumor confined to the ovary
A	Limited to one ovary, capsule intact without surface tumor, negative peritoneal washings
B	Tumor confined to both ovaries, otherwise as IA
C	As in stage IB and: • IC1 surgical spill • IC2 tumor present on ovarian surface or preoperative capsule rupture • IC3 positive washings
II	Pelvic extension
A	Involvement of uterus or Fallopian tubes
B	Involvement of other intraperitoneal pelvic organs
III	Spread within the peritoneal cavity outside the pelvis or to the retroperitoneal lymph nodes
A	• Positive retroperitoneal lymph nodes: • IIIA1(i) retroperitoneal lymph node metastases <10 mm only • IIIA1(ii) retroperitoneal lymph node metastases >10 mm only • IIIA2 retroperitoneal lymph node and microscopic extrapelvic peritoneal involvement
B	Macroscopic extrapelvic peritoneal involvement <2 cm
C	Macroscopic extrapelvic peritoneal involvement >2 cm
IV	Distant metastases
A	Pleural effusion with positive cytology
B	Hepatic/splenic intraparenchymal metastasis, extra-abdominal metastasis

of the omental specimen and the number of lymph nodes retrieved were similar in both laparoscopy and laparotomy, but laparoscopy required a longer operating room time (321 vs. 276 minutes, P = 0.04). Additional series have demonstrated low rates of recurrence and excellent clinical outcomes in patients who found to have stage I ovarian cancer by laparoscopic staging (Ghezzi et al. 2012, Park et al. 2008). Other publications have described laparoscopic staging for nonepithelial ovarian cancers (Shim et al. 2013). To date, there is no randomized controlled trial of laparotomy versus laparoscopy for ovarian cancer staging.

PRACTICAL TIPS

- The patient must be safely secured to the operative table to ensure the lack of movement during position changes. Table movement, including Trendelenburg and reverse-Trendelenburg positions with or without left or right lateral tilt, is helpful when examining the peritoneal cavity.
- While holding the laparoscope during para-aortic lymphadenectomy, standing adjacent to the surgeon allows the view of the surgeon and the assistant to be in sync but results in crowding. If the assistant has difficulty coordinating camera movement while standing across the table, then standing in between the patient's legs represents a useful compromise.
- The retroperitoneal spaces should be fully developed prior to initiating dissection of lymphatic tissue. Much of this can be done with blunt dissection if performed in the proper tissue plane. A thorough understanding of the pelvic and abdominal retroperitoneal anatomy is critical in the development of these spaces and in minimizing complications.
- The position of the ureters should be identified early and repetitively during retroperitoneal dissection.

- A hemostatic field should be prioritized and the use of irrigation minimized, as fluid will obscure natural planes of tissue separation and interferes with accurate dissection. A surgical sponge placed in the peritoneal cavity through a 10 mm port is helpful in maintaining a dry surgical field. It can also be used to apply pressure in the event of hemorrhage.
- When total hysterectomy is included, lymphatic and omental specimens can be retrieved transvaginally, eliminating the need for any laparoscopic port of >5 mm.
- Exposure is critical to safe dissection. Steep Trendelenburg position, gastric decompression, and use of fan retractors, marionette sutures, or internally deployed laparoscopic graspers can aid in achieving satisfactory exposure. An extraperitoneal approach to para-aortic lymphadenectomy should be considered if dissection to the renal vasculature is indicated in morbidly obese women.
- Conversion to laparotomy should be considered promptly in the event of hemorrhage requiring immediate vascular repair. Patient safety and oncologic adequacy always take precedence over completion of a minimally invasive approach.

CONCLUSION

Despite the challenging nature of surgical staging procedures for gynecologic malignancies, including the need to access and evaluate the upper abdomen and the retroperitoneum, laparoscopic surgery has been shown to be safe and feasible in comparison to laparotomy. Immediate postoperative outcomes, including reduced blood loss, infectious morbidity, and hospital stay are improved with apparent equivalent progression-free and overall survival. As there are very few absolute contraindications, the majority of women with gynecologic cancer benefit from a minimally invasive approach to surgical staging.

REFERENCES

Benedetti Panici P, Perniola G, Tomao F, et al. An update of laparoscopy in cervical cancer staging: it is a useful procedure? Oncology 2013; 85:160–105.

Cardenas-Goicoechea J, Shephard A, Momeni M, et al. Survival analysis of robotic versus traditional laparoscopic surgical staging for endometrial cancer. Am J Obstet Gynecol 2014; 210:160.e1–160.e 11.

Chi D, Abu-Rustum N, Sonoda Y. The safety and efficacy of laparoscopic surgical staging of apparent stage I ovarian and fallopian tube cancers. Am J Obstet Gynecol 2005; 192:1614–1619.

Childers J, Surwit E. Combined laparoscopic and vaginal surgery for the management of two cases of stage I endometrial cancer. Gynecol Oncol 1992; 45:46–51. Clinicaltrials.gov. Laparoscopic Approach to Cervical Cancer (LACC). https://clinicaltrials.gov/ct2/show/NCT00614211

Del Pino M, Fuste P, Pahisa J, et al. Laparoscopic lymphadenectomy in advanced cervical cancer: prognostic and therapeutic value. Int J Gynecol Cancer 2013; 23:1675–1783.

Einarsson J, Cohen S, Puntambekar S. Orifice-assisted small-incision surgery: case series in benign and oncologic gynecology. J Minim Invasive Gynecol 2012; 19:365–368.

Escobar P, Fader A, Paraiso M, et al. Robotic-assisted laparoendoscopic single-site surgery in gynecology: Initial report and technique. J Minim Invasive Gynecol 2009; 16:589–591.

Escobar P, Frumovitz M, Soliman P, et al. Comparison of single-port laparoscopy, standard laparoscopy, and robotic surgery in patients with endometrial cancer. Ann Surg Oncol 2012; 19:1583–1588.

Fader A, Escobar P. Laparoendoscopic single-site surgery (LESS) in gynecologic oncology: technique and initial report. Gynecol Oncol 2009; 114:157-161.

Fader A, Seamon L, Escobar P, et al. Minimally invasive surgery versus laparotomy in women with high grade endometrial cancer: a multi-site study performed at high volume cancer centers. Gynecol Oncol 2012; 126:180–185.

Fagotti A, Boruta D, Scambia G, et al. First 100 early endometrial cancer cases treated with laparoendoscopic single-site surgery: a multicentric retrospective study. Am J Obstet Gynecol 2012; 206:353.e1–353.e6.

Frumovitz M, Querleu D, Gil-Moreno A, et al. Lymphadenectomy in locally advanced cervical cancer study (LiLACS): Phase III clinical trial comparing surgical with radiologic staging in patients with stages IB2–IVA cervical cancer. J Minim Invasive Gynecol 2014; 21:3–8.

Gaia G, Holloway R, Santoro L, et al. Robotic-assisted hysterectomy for endometrial cancer compared with traditional laparoscopic and laparotomy approaches. Obstet Gynecol 2010; 116:1422–1431.

Galaal K, Bryant A, Fisher A, et al. Laparoscopy versus laparotomy for the management of early stage endometrial cancer. Cochrane Database Syst Rev 2012; 9:CD006655.

Garg G, Gao F, Wright J, et al. Positive peritoneal cytology is an independent risk factor in early stage endometrial cancer. Gynecol Oncol 2013; 128:77–82.

Gehrig P, Cantrell L, Shafer A, et al. What is the optimal minimally invasive surgical procedure for endometrial cancer staging in the obese and morbidly obese woman? Gynecol Oncol 2008; 111:41–45.

Ghezzi F, Malzoni M, Vizza E, et al. Laparoscopic staging of early ovarian cancer: results of a multi-institutional cohort. Ann Surg Oncol 2012; 19:1589–1594.

Goff B, Muntz H, Paley P, et al. Impact of surgical staging in women with locally advanced cervical cancer. Gynecol Oncol 1999; 74:436–342.

Jahns B, Michael N, Brunnmayr G, et al. Primary or secondary laparoscopy for staging in patients with uterine sarcomas. Eur J Obstet Gynecol Reprod Biol 2011; 154:228–234.

Lee M, Kim Y, Kim S, et al. Effects of uterine manipulation on surgical outcomes in laparoscopic management of endometrial cancer. Int J Gynecol Cancer 2013; 23:372–379.

Leitao M, Khoury-Collado F, Gardner G, et al. Impact of incorporating an algorithm that utilizes sentinel lymph node mapping during minimally invasive procedures on the detection of stage IIIC endometrial cancer. Gynecol Oncol 2013; 129:38–41.

Nezhat C, Burrell M, Nezhat F, et al. Laparoscopic radical hysterectomy with paraaortic and pelvic node dissection. Am J Obstet Gynecol 1992; 166:864–865.

Pakish J, Soliman P, Frumovitz M, et al. A comparison of extraperitoneal versus transperitoneal laparoscopic or robotic para-aortic lymphadenectomy for staging of endometrial carcinoma. Gynecol Oncol 2014; 132:366–371.

Park J, Bae J, Lim M, et al. Laparoscopic and laparotomic staging in stage I epithelial ovarian cancer: a comparison of feasibility and safety. Int J Gynecol Cancer 2008; 18:1202–1209.

Pecorelli S. Revised FIGO staging for carcinoma of the vulva, cervix, and endometrium. Int J Gynaecol Obstet 2009; 105:103–104.

Prat J, FIGO Committee on Gynecologic Oncology. Staging classification for cancer of the ovary, fallopian tube, and peritoneum. Int J Gynaecol Obstet 2014; 124:1–5.

Schorge J, Schaffer J, Halvorsen L, et al. Williams gynecology. Dallas: McGraw Medical, 2008. (Print).

Shim S, Kim D, Lee S, et al. Laparoscopic management of early-stage malignant nonepithelial ovarian tumors: surgical and survival outcomes. Int J Gynecol Cancer 2013; 23:249–255.

Subramanian A, Kim K, Bryant S, et al. A cohort study evaluating robotic versus laparotomy surgical outcomes of obese women with endometrial carcinoma. Gynecol Oncol 2011; 122:604–607.

Vasilev S, McGonigle K. Extraperitoneal laparoscopic para-aortic lymph node dissection. Gynecol Oncol 1996; 61:315–120.

Walker J, Piedmonte M, Spirtos N, et al. Laparoscopy compared with laparotomy for comprehensive surgical staging of uterine cancer: gynecologic oncology group study LAP2. J Clin Oncol 2009; 27:5331–5336.

Walker J, Piedmonte M, Spirtos N, et al. Recurrence and survival after random assignment to laparoscopy versus laparotomy for comprehensive surgical staging of uterine cancer: gynecologic oncology group LAP2 study. J Clin Oncol 2012; 30:695–700.

Wang Y, Deng L, Xu H, et al. Laparoscopy versus laparotomy for the management of early stage cervical cancer. BMC Cancer 2015; 15:928.

Wright J, Neugut A, Wilde E, et al. Use and benefits of laparoscopic hysterectomy for stage I endometrial cancer among Medicare beneficiaries. J Oncol Pract 2012; 8:e89–99.

Chapter 30

Laparoscopy and endometrial cancer

Frederic Kridelka, Eric Leblanc, Marjolein de Cuypere, Jean Doyen, Katty Delbecque, Athanassios Kakkos, Alain Thille, Frederic Goffin

■ INTRODUCTION

Endometrial cancer is the most frequent gynecological neoplasm in developed countries. The overall prognosis of patients affected by the disease is favorable, with cure rates in excess of 90% due to an early diagnosis triggered by peri-/postmenopausal bleeding. In the case of locally advanced or metastatic status, the prognosis decreases significantly, in the order of 30% 5-year disease-free survival (Jemal et al. 2009). Approximately 85% of endometrial cancers are of endometrioid (type 1) histology, whereas the remaining 15% include the more aggressive serous, clear cell, and undifferentiated (type 2) neoplasms. The central risk factor for endometrial cancer is prolonged exposure to unopposed estrogens in the context of diabetes, obesity, late menopause, estrogen replacement therapy, or use of tamoxifen (Amant et al. 2005). Results of a recent meta-analysis showed that uterine cancer was one of the cancers most strongly associated with obesity. Hence, endometrial cancer patients often present with medical comorbidities affecting their surgical risk profile as well as their short- and long-term outcome (Renehan et al. 2008).

The definitive stage of endometrial cancer is established on the basis of histological criteria defined by the International Federation of Gynecology and Obstetrics (FIGO 2009) (Pecorelli 2009). These variables are obtained at final pathology. The latter allows individualized decisions for adjuvant therapy. However, the initial treatment plan relies on the patients' medical status and on clinical and radiological information, as well as on tumor histology (histological subtype and grade) obtained at endometrial biopsy or dilatation and curettage. More than 80% of patients are then considered candidates for primary surgical management (Hacker 2009).

Most experts recommend a total hysterectomy and bilateral salpingo-oophorectomy as the standard surgical approach for patients with early-stage endometrial malignancy. Further nodal staging including pelvic and para-aortic nodes dissection may be performed with the aim of avoiding unnecessary adjuvant radiation (Lee et al. 2006), but the impact of such surgical staging on the patient's overall outcome remains unproved (ASTEC et al. 2009, Benedetti et al. 2008, Naumann 2012). Since the first laparoscopically assisted vaginal hysterectomy described by Reich in 1989, the feasibility of the total laparoscopic hysterectomy as well as regional and para-aortic nodal dissection has been reported (Köhler et al. 2004, Reich et al. 1989). To date, the surgery is recommended to be performed according to the planned staging procedure, but guidelines do not state that endoscopic surgery should be preferred to laparotomy.

Over the past two decades, as advanced laparoscopic techniques and skills have improved and as modern technologies have become more readily available, there has been a consistent increase in the uptake of minimally invasive surgery (MIS) to treat patients with endometrial neoplasms. The laparoscopic technique is presumed to bring perioperative benefits that might be of particular interest for overweight postmenopausal patients. Initial reports based on a small number of patients concluded that laparoscopy was associated with reduced hospital stay, perioperative pain, and blood loss when compared to those obtained at open surgery, whereas rates of overall and disease-specific-free survival were equivalent (Fram 2002, Magrina et al. 1999, 2004). These suggestions have been further tested in randomized controlled trials (RCTs), and more robust data from meta-analyses exist today to support an endoscopic approach in the majority of patients with endometrial cancer (Walker et al. 2009, 2012).

■ SURGICAL STAGING

From 1978, endometrial cancer was staged clinically, but this approach proved to underestimate the extent of the disease and to provide suboptimal prognostic information. The FIGO adopted a surgical staging system in 1988 (Boronow et al. 1984). The most discriminant factors that were taken into consideration were the histological grade of the disease, the depth of myometrial infiltration, a cervical extension, the nodal involvement, and the peritoneal cytology, as well as the presence of either vaginal, inguinal, or distant metastases. This staging system was further adapted in 2009 (Mariani et al. 2001). The myometrial, cervical, and cytological variables were simplified, whereas the nodal extension to either the pelvic or para-aortic region is now considered separately (respectively, FIGO stage 3C1 and 3C2).

In practice, clinicians allocate their patients to risk subgroups (low-/high-risk or low-/intermediate-/high-risk system) (Mariani et al. 2001). This risk-based approach is used to (1) evaluate the risk of extrauterine spread in order to define preoperatively the most appropriate surgical staging to be performed (Cragun et al. 2005) and (2) consider the risk of relapse based on the final pathology report and recommend individualized adjuvant therapy (Creutzberg et al. 2004, Hogberg et al. 2010).

Most oncological teams feel that patients at low risk of extrauterine extension may be appropriately treated in first intention by a simple hysterectomy and bilateral salpingo-oophorectomy (Mariani et al. 2000, Todo et al. 2010). Those at high risk of nodal and/or peritoneal spread may benefit from an extended surgical staging including pelvic +/– para-aortic nodal dissection and omentectomy (Todo et al. 2010).

Although the direct impact of nodal dissection or peritoneal staging on a patient's outcome is still debated, surgical staging is the only opportunity to define optimally the tumor extension and on which base indication for further therapies. The main benefit is for patients with disease histologically proved to be limited to the uterine corpus who can be spared adjuvant treatment and its associated potential morbidity with a reasonable degree of safety (Straughn et al. 2002). At the opposite end of the spectrum, for patients with demonstrated metastatic nodal or distant disease, the oncologist may better evaluate the risk–benefit balance of adjuvant radiation and/or chemotherapy (Zullo et al. 2009).

In this context, laparoscopy, which has demonstrated its perioperative benefits for the treatment of benign gynecological conditions, is regarded with particular interest as a minimally invasive approach with which to stage endometrial cancer patients. However, prior to implementing the endoscopic surgical staging, the technique must be carefully evaluated and demonstrate equivalence in terms of staging radicality and the absence of unfavorable impact on patients' oncological outcome.

SURGICAL RADICALITY AND ONCOLOGICAL OUTCOME

Radicality of surgical staging

The issue of laparoscopic surgical staging radicality among patients with endometrial cancer has been addressed in several key publications. The German experience was reported with >600 pelvic and periaortic lymphadenectomies performed for gynecologic neoplasms, 112 of which were endometrial cancers (Köhler et al. 2004). The learning curve period was evaluated at 20 procedures, after which a constant number of pelvic lymph nodes (16.9–21.9) were removed. The number of removed periaortic lymph nodes increased over time, from 5.5 to 18.5. Importantly, in this report, the number of harvested nodes was independent of the body mass index (BMI). Operating time for pelvic lymph node dissection was independent of BMI, but right-sided periaortic lymphadenectomy lasted significantly longer in obese patients (35 vs. 41 min, $P = 0.011$). The overall complication rate was 8.7%, with 2.9% intraoperative (vessel or bowel injury) and 5.8% postoperative complications.

An Italian group reported that laparoscopy provides equivalent lymph node staging compared with laparotomy (Zullo et al. 2009). In this study with 110 endometrial cancer patients, 55 patients (50%) were treated by laparoscopic-assisted vaginal hysterectomy (LAVH) and another 55 (50%) by total abdominal hysterectomy (TAH). All patients underwent a pelvic lymph node dissection. The mean number of lymph nodes was 17 for the LAVH group and 18.5 for the TAH group ($P = 0.294$).

In a recent meta-analysis of available RCTs addressing the issue of laparoscopic surgical staging, the number of pelvic lymph nodes harvested was also similar [mean difference (MD), 0.45; 95% confidence interval (CI) (20.41,1.32); $P = 5.30$] after open versus endoscopic surgery (Zullo et al. 2012).

Perioperative outcome, survival, and recurrence data

Nine RCTs comparing the outcome of patients surgically treated for endometrial cancer are considered of sufficient quality to be included in meta-analyses. A total of 1361 open procedures are compared to 2255 laparoscopic operations (Galaal et al. 2012, He et al. 2013).

Primary endpoints were related to overall survival and disease-specific survival variables. No statistically significant differences were noted between the laparotomy and the laparoscopy groups in terms of 3-year overall survival [odds ratio (OR), 0.91; 95% CI (0.49,1.71); $P= 5.77$], 3-year disease-free survival [OR, 0.95; 95% CI (0.29,1.80); $P = 5.89$], and recurrence rate at 3-year follow-up [OR, 1.11; 95% CI (0.60,2.06); $P = 5.74$].

Secondary endpoints concerned the perioperative outcome. The benefit of laparoscopic surgery versus laparotomy is a shorter length of hospital stay [MD, 23.42; 95% CI (23.81,23.03); $P = 0.01$] and a lower rate of postoperative complications [OR, 0.62; 95% CI (0.52,0.73); $P = 0.01$]. No statistically significant difference in intraoperative complications is noted [OR, 1.25; 95% CI (0.99,1.56); $P = 0.62$].

A disadvantage is a longer duration of the surgical procedures [MD, 32.73; 95% CI (16.34,49.13); $P = 0.01$]. This may be attributed to a longer learning curve for laparoscopy or a lack of technical skills. However, it must be noted that >75% of the patients included in the statistical analysis corresponded to the LAP2 trial in which inclusion started in 1996, at a time when surgical skills and laparoscopic material were not equal to present-day levels.

To assess long-term clinical outcomes, in particular the quality of life, more well-designed RCTs are needed (Kornblith et al. 2009).

Cost-effectiveness issues

Since the technical feasibility of laparoscopic staging in endometrial cancer is accepted and the oncological safety is demonstrated, the surgery-related cost-effectiveness becomes decisive when defining the respective role of endoscopy versus laparotomy.

Laparoscopy is considered by many as more costly than laparotomy due to the prolonged duration of surgery and the expense of disposable material, plus the incremental cost in case of conversion to laparotomy. This perception has been a central issue that has slowed the uptake of advanced laparoscopic surgery.

Although the shorter length of hospital stay appears to compensate for the increased surgery-related cost in most published series (Sculpher et al. 2004), methodological bias did not allow firm conclusions until recently.

In a properly designed randomized trial, Bijen et al. (2011) conducted an economic analysis among 279 patients treated either by laparoscopy (185) or laparotomy (96) for early-stage endometrial cancer. All costs over a period of 3 months at and after surgery were considered. The higher surgical procedure costs of laparoscopy were compensated by lower cost for hospital stay. The major complication-free rate was higher and utility scores (as defined in the EQ-SD questionnaire) were lower in the laparoscopy group. The authors concluded that laparoscopy is a preferred and cost-effective approach for the staging of early-stage endometrial cancer patients.

Although the laparoscopic technique in itself requires attention, the quality of the implementation of the laparoscopic intervention depends not only on the surgeon but also on the surgical environment, including the operating team and the peri- and postoperative care. Moreover, further development, experience, and improvement of laparoscopic equipment are to be expected when compared to the conventional approach. This advancement in laparoscopic equipment and technique, together with optimizing the efficiency of surgical teams and postoperative care, may lead to further improvements in the cost-effectiveness profile of the endoscopic approach when compared to open surgery.

SPECIFIC ISSUES
High BMI patients

The issue of overweight patients must be evaluated cautiously when considering the role of MIS in the context of endometrial cancer. Intuitively, patients with high BMI are considered to most benefit from a 'non-open' surgical approach in terms of a reduction in abdominal wall and thromboembolic complications. At the same time, these patients also represent a particular surgical challenge at laparoscopy and face an increased risk of intraoperative complications, lack of staging radicality, and conversion to laparotomy, with potential deleterious impact on oncological outcome and treatment cost.

In a retrospective study, Scribner et al. (2002) suggested that obesity is not a contraindication to laparoscopic staging. In their report, for patients with a Quetelet Index (QI) score of 28 or greater, operative time increased but hospital stay, febrile morbidity, and postoperative ileus decreased in the laparoscopy group compared with the results obtained in the laparotomy group. When the QI was >35, the capacity to achieve surgery laparoscopically decreased compared to patients with a QI of <35 (44% vs. 82%, $P = 0.004$). A prospective study of 42 obese women treated with laparoscopy reported a 7.5% conversion rate. Compared to historical controls from 2 years prior, women who underwent laparoscopy had a significantly longer operative time, more pelvic lymph nodes removed, and a shorter hospital stay (194.8 vs. 137.7 min, $P < 0.001$; 11.3 vs. 5.3, $P < 0.001$; and 2.5 vs. 5.6 days, $P < 0.001$, respectively). Provided the patient is medically fit for the procedure, obese patients with apparent early-stage endometrial cancer can be safely and effectively managed with laparoscopy. In a prospective multicenter study, investigators evaluated outcomes in 33 obese and 32 nonobese patients undergoing laparoscopy for endometrial cancer. They reported equivalent operating time, node counts, blood loss, and hospital stay. More complications occurred in the obese group (8 vs. 5), including pulmonary embolism, injury to the epigastric artery, bladder injury, bleeding, and conversion to laparotomy (Helm et al. 2011).

More recently, the LAP2 study reported that failure to successfully complete laparoscopy was greater with increasing BMI [OR = 1.11; 95% CI (1.09,1.13) for a one-unit increase in BMI; $P < 0.0001$] (Walker et al. 2009).

Due to a higher incidence of perioperative complications and an increased rate of conversion to laparotomy, a recent review concentrating on cost issues in an RCT comparing laparoscopy and open surgery for endometrial cancer patients operated on by proven skilled surgeons concluded that laparoscopy was linked to an incremental cost and was not cost-effective for patients with a BMI >35 (Bijen et al. 2011).

Incomplete staging/restaging surgery

Occasionally, the diagnosis of endometrial cancer is not established preoperatively. To define the extent of disease, some patients may benefit from completion staging. The decision of whether to pursue a second procedure is determined by factors such as the depth of myometrial invasion, histology, grade, cervical/adnexal involvement, imaging, and medical comorbidities. Laparoscopy has been used with success in this setting when there is a desire to minimize morbidity with a second operation (Childers et al. 1993). A faster recovery may also minimize delay of any adjuvant therapy that may be recommended. A recent Gynecologic Oncology Group (GOG) study of patients with incompletely staged gynecologic malignancies showed that laparoscopic staging was possible in 80% of patients, whereas 20% required laparotomy (Spirtos et al. 2005).

Trocar-site metastases

High CO_2 concentration and prolonged intra-abdominal elevated pressure have been described as potential promoters of post-laparoscopic peritoneal extension either through the abdominal cavity or in the subcutaneous tissue at the trocar site of insertion.

Approximately 80 cases have been published in the context of gynecological malignancies staged endoscopically. The global incidence appears extremely low (1–2% risk), except for advanced ovarian cancer patients who undergo diagnostic laparoscopy.

A recent review of published and unpublished data demonstrate that a total of 12 cases of port-site recurrences have been reported after laparoscopic staging of uterine cancer (Palomba et al. 2012). Four cases are considered as being isolated relapses, while the other eight remaining cases were associated with peritoneal carcinomatosis. Patients' prognosis was poor, with a single patient being alive 10 months after recurrence.

Available data do not allow us to make recommendations for the prevention or the treatment of port-site relapse after laparoscopic staging of early endometrial cancer.

Robotic surgery

Despite the evidence supporting the central role of MIS in the surgical approach of patients with endometrial cancer, several reports from Europe and the United States mention low rates of MIS for hysterectomy. It appears that laparoscopy is underused compared to laparotomy. Cited reasons are a long learning curve, complexity of procedures, and, frequently, obese and comorbid patients.

In 2005, the FDA approved the da Vinci robotic system for gynecology. The da Vinci system (Intuitive Surgical, Sunnyvale, California) is characterized by high 3D definition vision, four surgeon-controlled arms, wristed instrumentation with high motion of freedom, tremor filtration, and improved ergonomy. These advantages may help to overcome the potential drawbacks associated with laparoscopy.

Many reports compared robotics to either laparotomy or laparoscopy, and two meta-analyses of observational studies were recently published (Gaia et al. 2010, Leitao et al. 2012). Most of the studies have a retrospective design. These studies are subjected to bias, and randomized trials are eagerly awaited.

Nevertheless, available studies underline the fact that the benefits of the robot should be assessed in terms of altering the rate of laparotomy and should not be limited to a direct comparison with either laparotomy or laparoscopy. The robotic platform is merely a tool with which to perform laparoscopy. Several recent publications report a decreased rate in open surgery after the introduction of robotics, particularly in obese patients.

An important issue surrounding the use of robotic surgery is the economic viability of the technology (Lau et al. 2012, Wright et al. 2014). It has been demonstrated that a significantly decreased rate of laparotomy has a positive impact on global treatment costs. It has been argued that the best assessment of the clinical and economical impacts of robotic surgery should be to evaluate how the rate of laparotomy is altered.

Everyone caring for women with endometrial cancer understands the most important issue: MIS is superior to open procedures. Because this patient population is at increased risk of treatment-related complications and death from all causes, all efforts should be made to improve their outcomes, and MIS provides a useful tool by which this can occur. Robotic-assisted surgery may extend these benefits to a larger proportion of patients with endometrial cancer by generalizing MIS in the setting of a vulnerable and obese patient sub-population.

CONCLUSION

Over the past several decades, MIS techniques, instrumentation, and technology have improved significantly. The laparoscopic approach for endometrial cancer patients has been widely reported in single-institution experiences and, more recently, in RCTs evaluating its oncological safety and its beneficial profile in terms of perioperative morbidity. Presently, laparoscopy should be considered the 'by default' surgical option for patients with uterine malignancy. Laparoscopy provides equivalent surgical staging radicality and disease-free and overall survival rates while improving the perioperative outcome with faster recovery, decreased pain, and improved quality of life. The risk of port-site metastasis appears low and should not represent a contraindication to laparoscopy. The cost-effectiveness of laparoscopy is now accepted for most patients. High BMI patients represent a significant proportion of patients with endometrial neoplasm and need to be considered cautiously. Laparoscopy is a safe approach for surgical restaging when indicated. A robotic approach may, in parallel, increase the uptake of MIS in the context of endometrial cancer and reduce further the number of laparotomies in the subset of fragile and morbidly obese patients.

REFERENCES

Amant F, Moerman P, Neven P, et al. Endometrial cancer. Lancet 2005;366:491–505

ASTEC study group, Kitchener H, Swart AM, Qian Q, Amos C, Parmar MK. Efficacy of systematic pelvic lymphadenectomy in endometrial cancer (MRC ASTEC trial): a randomised study. Lancet 2009; 373(9658):125–136. Epub 2008 December 16.

Benedetti Panici P, Basile S, Maneschi F, et al. Systematic pelvic lymphadenectomy vs. no lymphadenectomy in early-stage endometrial carcinoma: randomized clinical trial. J Natl Cancer Inst 2008; 100:1707–1716.

Bijen CB, de Bock GH, Vermeulen KM, et al. Laparoscopic hysterectomy is preferred over laparotomy in early endometrial cancer patients, however not cost effective in the very obese. Eur J Cancer 2011; 47:2158–2165. Epub 2011 June 1.

Bijen CB, Vermeulen KM, Mourits MJ, et al. Cost effectiveness of laparoscopy versus laparotomy in early stage endometrial cancer: a randomised trial. Gynecol Oncol 2011; 121:76–82.

Boronow RC, Morrow CP, Creasman WT, et al. Surgical staging in endometrial cancer: clinical-pathologic findings of a prospective study. Obstet Gynecol 1984; 63:825–832.

Childers JM, Brzechffa PR, Hatch KD, et al. Laparoscopically assisted surgical staging (LASS) of endometrial cancer. Gynecol Oncol 1993; 51:33–38.

Cragun JM, Havrilesky LJ, Calingaert B, et al. Retrospective analysis of selective lymphadenectomy in apparent early-stage endometrial cancer. J Clin Oncol 2005; 23:3668–3675.

Creutzberg CL, van Putten WL, Warlam-Rodenhuis CC, et al. Outcome of high-risk stage IC, grade 3, compared with stage I endometrial carcinoma patients: the Postoperative Radiation Therapy in Endometrial Carcinoma Trial. J Clin Oncol 2004; 22:1234–1241.

Fram KM. Laparoscopically assisted vaginal hysterectomy versus abdominal hysterectomy in stage I endometrial cancer. Int J Gynecol Cancer 2002; 12:57–61.

Gaia G, Holloway RW, Santoro L, et al. Robotic-assisted hysterectomy for endometrial cancer compared with traditional laparoscopic and laparotomy approaches: a systematic review. Obstet Gynecol 2010; 116:1422–1431.

Galaal K, Bryant A, Fisher AD, et al. Laparoscopy versus laparotomy for the management of early stage endometrial cancer. Cochrane Database Syst Rev 2012; 9:CD006655.

Hacker NF. Practical Gynecologic Oncology, 3rd ed. Philadelphia: Lippincott Williams & Wilkins, 2009.

He H, Zeng D, Ou H, et al. Laparoscopic treatment of endometrial cancer: systematic review. J Minim Invasive Gynecol 2013 ; 20:413–423.

Helm CW, Arumugam C, Gordinier ME, et al. Laparoscopic surgery for endometrial cancer: increasing body mass index does not impact postoperative complications. J Gynecol Oncol 2011; 22:168–176. Epub 2011 September 28.

Hogberg T, Signorelli M, de Oliveira CF, et al. Sequential adjuvant chemotherapy and radiotherapy in endometrial cancer results from two randomised studies. Eur J Cancer 2010; 46:2422–2431.

Jemal A, Siegel R, Ward E, et al. Cancer statistics, 2009. CA Cancer J Clin 2009; 59:225–249.

Köhler C, Klemm P, Schau A, et al. Introduction of transperitoneal lymphadenectomy in a gynecologic oncology center: analysis of 650 laparoscopic pelvic and/or paraaortic transperitoneal lymphadenectomies. Gynecol Oncol 2004; 95:52–61.

Kornblith AB, Huang HQ, Walker JL, et al. Quality of life of patients with endometrial cancer undergoing laparoscopic international federation of gynecology and obstetrics staging compared with laparotomy: a Gynecologic Oncology Group study. J Clin Oncol 2009; 10:5337–5342.

Lau S, Vaknin Z, Ramana-Kumar AV, et al. Outcomes and cost comparisons after introducing a robotics program for endometrial cancer surgery. Obstet Gynecol 2012; 119:717–724.

Lee CM, Szabo A, Shrieve DC, et al. Frequency and effect of adjuvant radiation therapy among women with stage I endometrial adenocarcinoma. JAMA 2006; 295:389–397.

Leitao MM, Briscoe G, Santos K, et al. Introduction of a computer-based surgical platform in the surgical care of patients with newly diagnosed uterine cancer: outcomes and impact on approach. Gynecol Oncol 2012; 125:394–399.

Magrina JF, Mutone NF, Weaver AL, et al. Laparoscopic lymphadenectomy and vaginal or laparoscopic hysterectomy with bilateral salpingo-oophorectomy for endometrial cancer: morbidity and survival. Am J Obstet Gynecol 1999; 181:376–381.

Magrina JF, Weaver AL. Laparoscopic treatment of endometrial cancer: five-year recurrence and survival rates. Eur J Gynaecol Oncol 2004; 25:439–441.

Mariani A, Webb MJ, Keeney GL, et al. Low-risk corpus cancer: is lymphadenectomy or radiotherapy necessary? Am J Obstet Gynecol 2000; 182:1506–1519.

Mariani A, Webb MJ, Rao SK, et al. Significance of pathologic patterns of pelvic lymph node metastases in endometrial cancer. Gynecol Oncol 2001; 80:113–120.

Naumann RW. The role of lymphadenectomy in endometrial cancer: was the ASTEC trial doomed by design and are we destined to repeat that mistake? Gynecol Oncol 2012; 126:5–11. doi: 10.1016/j.ygyno.2012.04.040. Epub 2012 April 30.

Palomba S, Falbo A, Russo T, et al. Port-site metastasis after laparoscopic surgical staging of endometrial cancer: a systematic review of the published and unpublished data. J Minim Invasive Gynecol 2012; 19:531–537.

Pecorelli S. Revised FIGO staging for carcinoma of the vulva, cervix, and endometrium. Int J Gynaecol Obstet 2009; 105:103–104

Reich H, DeCaprio J, McFlynn F. Laparoscopic hysterectomy. J Gynecol Surg 1989; 5:213–216.

Renehan AG, Tyson M, Egger M, et al. Body-mass index and incidence of cancer: a systematic review and meta-analysis of prospective observational studies. Lancet 2008; 371:569–578.

Scribner DR Jr, Walker JL, Johnson GA, et al. Laparoscopic pelvic and paraaortic lymph node dissection in the obese. Gynecol Oncol. 2002; 84:426–430.

Sculpher M, Manca A, Abbott J, et al. Cost effectiveness analysis of laparoscopic hysterectomy compared with standard hysterectomy: results from a randomised trial. BMJ 2004; 17:134.

Spirtos NM, Eisekop SM, Boike G, et al. Laparoscopic staging in patients with incompletely staged cancers of the uterus, ovary, fallopian tube, and primary peritoneum: a Gynecologic Oncology Group (GOG) study. Am J Obstet Gynecol 2005; 193:1645–1649.

Straughn JM Jr, Huh WK, Kelly FJ, et al. Conservative management of stage endometrial carcinoma after surgical staging. Gynecol Oncol 2002; 84:194–200.

Todo Y, Kato H, Kaneuchi M, et al. Survival effect of para-aortic lymphadenectomy in endometrial cancer (SEPAL study): a retrospective cohort analysis. Lancet 2010; 375:1165–1172.

Walker JL, Piedmonte MR, Spirtos NM, et al. Laparoscopy compared with laparotomy for comprehensive surgical staging of uterine cancer: Gynecologic Oncology Group Study LAP2. J Clin Oncol 2009; 27:5331–5336.

Walker JL, Piedmonte MR, Spirtos NM, et al. Recurrence and survival after random assignment to laparoscopy versus laparotomy for comprehensive surgical staging of uterine cancer: Gynecologic Oncology Group LAP2 Study. J Clin Oncol 2012; 30:695–700.

Wright JD, Ananth CV, Tergas AI, et al. An economic analysis of robotically assisted hysterectomy. Obstet Gynecol 2014; 123:1038–1048.

Zullo F, Falbo A, Palomba S. Safety of laparoscopy vs laparotomy in the surgical staging of endometrial cancer: a systematic review and metaanalysis of randomized controlled trials. Am J Obstet Gynecol 2012; 207:94–100.

Zullo F, Palomba S, Falbo A, et al. Laparoscopic surgery vs laparotomy for early stage endometrial cancer: long-term data of a randomized controlled trial. Am J Obstet Gynecol 2009; 200:296.e1–296.e9.

Chapter 31 Laparoscopic management of cervical cancer

Francesco Fanfani, Maria Lucia Gagliardi, Anna Fagotti, Giovanni Scambia

■ INTRODUCTION

Cervical cancer (CC) remains a significant cause of death and one of the most common cancers in women worldwide. Although the Papanicolaou test (Pap test) has reduced the percentage of advanced-stage disease, the incidence of CC remains at 550,000 new cases and 310,000 deaths per year, 80% of which occur in developed countries; it mainly affects sexually active women between 30 and 55 years (Thun et al. 2010).

The presence of human papilloma virus (HPV) in virtually all CCs implies the highest worldwide attributable fraction so far reported for a specific cause of any major human cancer. The extreme rarity of HPV-negative cancers reinforces the rationale for HPV testing in addition to, or even instead of, cervical cytology in routine cervical screening (Garland & Smith 2010). The most common histological type of CC is squamous (80%), but, in the recent years, adenocarcinoma represents an emerging type, whether related to HPV infection or not (Muñoz et al. 2003).

Because of these considerations, some authors argue that massive screening using the Pap test and vaccine against the most common HPV subtypes could eradicate all dysplastic lesions and reduce by 70% the invasive forms (Collins et al. 2006).

■ DIAGNOSIS AND STAGING

The suspicion of CC arises, in the most cases, through a Pap test followed by a second-level examination and colposcopy and/or biopsy. Despite the impact of the stage of disease on the treatment plan, CC staging is based on clinical assessment. Thus, the extent of the disease is evaluated by the bimanual gynecological examination under anesthesia and other tests in selected cases, such as cystoscopy and proctoscopy. Lymph node status or tumor spread within the abdominal cavity and the peritoneal surface are certainly the most difficult variables to evaluate by clinical examination with respect to a possible infiltration of the paracervix, vagina, and vesicovaginal and rectovaginal septa.

Although not recognized by the International Federation of Gynecology and Obstetrics (FIGO) (Pecorelli et al. 2009), CT and MRI are widely used for therapeutic decisions in patients with CC (Amendola et al. 2005, Choi et al. 2006). The National Comprehensive Cancer Network (NCCN) recently added the MRI evaluation for the clinical evaluation of FIGO stages higher than IB1 disease (Table 31.1). Some authors proposed a lymph node laparoscopic staging to determine the extent of the disease outside the cervix, vagina, and paracervix (Fagotti et al. 2007, Marnitz et al. 2005).

Presently, there is a general consensus among authors that dichotomizes CC into two categories: early-stage and locally advanced stage (Pecorelli et al. 2009). Early CC (ECC) is an invasive carcinoma that is strictly confined to the cervix or involves the vagina but not as far as the lower third, is no greater than 4 cm in diameter, and has no obvious paracervical involvement or spread of the growth to adjacent or distant organs (FIGO stages IA1, IA2, IB1, and IIA1, Table 31.1); locally advanced CC (LACC) is defined as every FIGO stage disease higher than IIA1 (Salicrù et al. 2013).

Table 31.1 FIGO staging for cervical cancer

Stage	Description
I	**The carcinoma is strictly confined to the cervix**
A	Invasive carcinoma that can be diagnosed only by microscopy, with deepest invasion ≤5 mm and largest extension ≤7 mm
1	Measured stromal invasion of ≤3.0 mm in depth and extension of ≤7.0 mm
2	Measured stromal invasion of >3.0 mm and 5.0 mm with an extension of not >7.0 mm
B	Clinically visible lesions limited to the cervix uteri or preclinical cancers greater than stage IA
1	Clinically visible lesion ≤4.0 cm in greatest dimension
2	Clinically visible lesion >4.0 cm in greatest dimension
II	**Cervical carcinoma invades beyond the uterus, but not to the pelvic wall or to the lower third of the vagina**
A	Without parametrial invasion
1	Clinically visible lesion ≤4.0 cm in greatest dimension
2	Clinically visible lesion >4 cm in greatest dimension
B	Obvious parametrial invasion
III	**The tumor extends to the pelvic wall and/or involves lower third of the vagina and/or causes hydronephrosis or nonfunctioning kidney**
A	Tumor involves lower third of the vagina, with no extension to the pelvic wall
B	Extension to the pelvic wall and/or hydronephrosis or nonfunctioning kidney
IV	**The carcinoma has extended beyond the true pelvis or has involved (biopsy proven) the mucosa of the bladder or rectum. A bullous edema, as such, does not permit a case to be allotted to Stage IV**
A	Spread of the growth to adjacent organs
B	Spread to distant organs

Based on Pecorelli et al. (2009)

CERVICAL CANCER AND SURGICAL MANAGEMENT

Radical hysterectomy (RH) was firstly described for CC patients at the turn of the century by Schauta (1902); it allowed for radical extirpation of the parametria using a vaginal approach without the possibility of performing lymphadenectomy [vaginal radical hysterectomy (VRH)]. Wertheim developed the abdominal radical technique (ARH) (Wertheim 1912), but because of the morbidity and mortality of surgery and with the introduction of radiation as a therapeutic modality for CC, all surgical approaches declined. In the 1940s, Meigs reintroduced ARH, combining it with a complete pelvic lymphadenectomy to improve prognosis (Meigs 1945). Antibiotics and advances in operating techniques brought complications to acceptable levels. In order to reduce morbidity and mortality while preserving the radicality, Piver described five different types of extended ARH (Piver et al. 1974). Furthermore, Dargent proposed a laparoscopic pelvic lymphadenectomy plus VRH that showed the benefits of the vaginal approach with fewer intraoperative complications, shorter operative times (OTs), and a more rapid postoperative recovery (Dargent 1987).

The crucial improvement in the modulation of surgical radicality for CC patients was twofold, coming from the contributions of European authors on the patterns of tumoral lymphatic spread and the contributions of Japanese authors on nerve-sparing hysterectomy.

Several Italian studies demonstrated a close correlation between the pathological status of lower pelvic lymph nodes and the paracervix and upper pelvic nodes in early and locally advanced CC (Benedetti Panici et al. 1996, 2009, Ercoli et al. 2009, Scambia et al. 2001). If the frozen section of the lower lymph nodes is negative, the surgeon can avoid the para-aortic lymphadenectomy. Moreover, Japanese studies, integrating old and new anatomic information about the autonomic nerves of the pelvis, focused efforts on their preservation when performing a radical hysterectomy (Fujii et al. 2007, Nakano 1981, Sakuragi et al. 2005, Sekiba 1985, Yabuki et al. 2000). The negative consequences of initial radical surgery related to damages involving lymphatic vessels and/or the sympathetic and parasympathetic branches of the pelvic autonomic nerve system (inferior hypogastric plexus), such as bladder dysfunction, anorectal mobility disorders, and sexual problems can be overcome through a nerve-sparing hysterectomy [type C1 hysterectomy (**Table 31.2**); Querleu & Morrow 2008] and a selective lymphadenectomy; these seem to be adequate for ECC cases, even though prospective and long-term studies are needed to definitively demonstrate their oncologic safety. These findings are summarized in a new classification system proposed by Querleu and Morrow in 2008 (Querleu & Morrow 2008) and developed by Cibula in 2011 (Cibula et al. 2011) that divides radical hysterectomy into four main types and reports specific anatomical limits and the margins of resection for hysterectomy and for pelvic and aortic lymphadenectomy. **Table 31.3** shows the algorithm of treatment for CC according to FIGO stage.

LAPAROSCOPIC RADICAL HYSTERECTOMY FOR ECC MANAGEMENT

In less than two decades, laparoscopy has definitely modified the management of ECC patients. After its introduction in 1990 (Canis et al. 1990, Nezhat et al. 1992), several studies have documented the safety and feasibility of laparoscopic radical hysterectomy in this population of patients (Dottino et al. 2006, Frumovitz et al. 2007, Jackson et al. 2004, Lee et al. 2002, Li et al. 2007, Malur et al. 2001,

Table 31.2 Querleu and Morrow hysterectomies*

Type of hysterectomy	Description
A	This is an extra-fascial hysterectomy, without freeing the ureters from their beds. The paracervix is transected medial to the ureter, but lateral to the cervix. The uterosacral and vesicouterine ligaments are transected close to the uterus. Vaginal resection is generally at a minimum, routinely <10 mm
B1	Partial resection of the uterosacral and vesicouterine ligaments is necessary. The ureter is unroofed and rolled laterally, permitting transection of the paracervix at the level of the ureteral tunnel. The caudal (posterior, deep) neural component of the paracervix caudal to the deep uterine vein is not resected. At least 10 mm of the vagina from the cervix or tumor is resected
B2	B1 with additional removal of the lateral paracervical lymph nodes that are medial and caudal to obturator nerve
C1	This type needs a transection of the uterosacral ligament at the rectum and vesicouterine ligament at the bladder. The ureter is mobilized completely. Vagina is resected for 15–20 mm, depending on vaginal and paracervical extent and on surgeon choice. The autonomic nerves are spared
C2	C1 without preservation of autonomic nerves and the paracervix is transected completely, including the part caudal to the deep uterine vein
D1	The resection of the entire paracervix at the pelvic sidewall along with the hypogastric vessels is necessary, exposing the roots of the sciatic nerve
D2	D1 plus resection of the entire paracervix with the hypogastric vessels and adjacent fascial or muscular structures

*Adapted from Querleu et al. (2008)

Table 31.3 Management of early cervical cancer for stage of disease*

FIGO-stage	Management
IA1 without lymphovascular space invasion	Type A radical hysterectomy
IA1 with lymphovascular space invasion	Type A radical hysterectomy plus systematic pelvic lymphadenectomy
IA2–IIA1	Type B1/C1 radical hysterectomy plus pelvic lymphadenectomy ±aortic lymphadenectomy or exclusive radiotherapy
IIA2–IVA	Exclusive radio-chemotherapy or neoadjuvant chemotherapy or chemoradiation plus type B2/C2 radical hysterectomy
IVB	Palliative treatment
IA1–IIA1	Fertility-sparing surgery, if requested

Data from Benedetti-Panici et al. 2002, Fagotti et al. 2010, Ferrandina et al. 2007, Querleu et al. 2008, Scambia et al. 2001.

Malzoni et al. 2004, Malzoni et al. 2007, Morgan et al. 2007, Nam et al. 2004, Obermaier et al. 2003, Sharma et al. 2006, Steed et al. 2004). Early in its development, laparoscopy was considered an adjunct to the radical vaginal approach (laparoscopic-assisted radical vaginal hysterectomy; LARVH), whereas more recently there is general agreement that all procedures of a radical hysterectomy can be achieved through laparoscopy (total laparoscopic radical hysterectomy, TLRH) (Koehler et al. 2012).

Following publications showing the feasibility of laparoscopic lymphadenectomy, Dargent and Querleu described LARVH and reported encouraging intra-/postoperative parameters with respect to ARH (Dargent & Mathevet 1992, Querleu et al. 1993). Recently, publications comparing LARVH with ARH showed that estimated blood loss (EBL), rate of transfusion, length of hospital stay, and time to spontaneous voiding favored LARVH over ARH (Jackson et al. 2004, Malur et al. 2001, Morgan et al. 2007, Naik et al. 2010, Nam et al. 2004, Pahisa et al. 2010, Sharma et al. 2006, Steed et al. 2004). Following early improvements in laparoscopic instrumentation and surgical skills, Canis and Nezhat (Canis et al. 1990, Nezhat et al. 1993) introduced TLRH for ECC management. The advantages of this procedure are similar to those of laparoscopy in general: shorter hospitalization, faster bowel function recovery, less postoperative pain, decreased EBL, and no difference in the mean count of pelvic and aortic lymph nodes removed, but a longer OT with overlapping oncologic outcomes (Abu-Rustum et al. 2003, Canis et al. 1995, Lee et al. 2002, Malzoni et al. 2007, Pomel et al. 1997, Spirtos et al. 1996, 2002). Recently, Wright et al. (2012) published a study comparing 1610 abdominal approaches to 217 laparoscopic approaches. They found significantly higher rates of any complication (15.8 vs. 9.2%; P < 0.04), a hospital length of stay longer than 3 days (44.3 vs. 11.1; P < 0.0001), and blood transfusions (15 vs. 5.1; P < 0.0001) in the abdominal group. Li et al. (2007) reported a retrospective study of 35 ARH and 90 TLRH and also looked at recurrence rates. The follow-up from this study (a median of 26 months) showed no differences in the rate of recurrence (12% vs. 13.7%; P > 0.05) or mortality between the two groups (8% vs. 10%; P > 0.05). Nam et al. reviewed 263 cases of TLRH matched 1:1 with ARH and found significant differences between the two groups in terms of EBL and hospital stay, without statistically significant differences in terms of 5-year overall and recurrence-free survival (Nam et al. 2012).

Several comparisons have been made between ARH and LAVRH or TLRH, but we found only one significant study on LAVRH versus TLRH (Choi et al. 2012). Although the extent of laparoscopic preparation can differ among institutions, it is reasonable that if ureter dissection and distal paracervical resection is carried out vaginally, the surgery should be classified as LARVH. The direct comparison between LAVRH and TLRH showed that EBL and return of bowel activity were significantly reduced in the second group, with a higher incidence of intraoperative complications in LAVRH procedures. The difficulty in learning the vaginal technique is one of the main drawbacks of LARVH and may explain the limited diffusion of the procedure and evidence.

In recent years, more attention has focused on the role of new endoscopic techniques aimed to further minimize the invasiveness of surgical treatment and minimize possible morbidity. In this context, mini-laparoscopy and laparoendoscopic single-site (LESS) surgery could represent an upgrade of standard laparoscopy in terms of surgical trauma, postoperative pain, and less damage to a woman's body image and privacy since both techniques produce no or invisible scars (Fagotti et al. 2011, Fanfani et al. 2012). Initial experiences are reported in the literature for both procedures (Boruta et al. 2013, Fanfani et al. 2013, Ghezzi et al. 2013 a, 2013b and 2013c), but it is too early to definitively establish their safety and/or radicality; on the other hand, these studies do report the feasibility of these two very minimally invasive approaches as applied to radical hysterectomy plus pelvic lymphadenectomy with intra-/postoperative parameters overlapping

those of TLRH or LAVRH but showing reduced postoperative pain and microscopic or absent scars.

Since the first robotic-assisted radical hysterectomy was described in 2006 (Sert & Abeler 2006), a consistent number of reports have been published. Generic advantages offered by this new technology include a 3D magnified field, tremor filtration, and 5° or 6° of instrument mobility inside the body, thus significantly reducing the ergonomic problems associated with the conventional laparoscopic approach. Specific advantages in performing robotic TLRH or LAVRH are related to uterine artery and ureter dissection, lymphadenectomy, and vaginal suturing. Another possible innovation is the application of robotics to LESS, thus overcoming its ergonomic challenges. A general drawback to robotics is the expense of robotic platforms and instruments.

The choice between LAVRH and TLRH can be made exclusively on the basis of surgeon skills because the literature states that every standard laparoscopic approach is adequate and safe for early-stage disease and shows better intra-/postoperative outcomes and quality of life, and concludes that ARH should be reserved to limited cases. Contraindications to minimally invasive surgery in ECC cases are tight vagina, conditions enabling vaginal extraction of the uterus without the need for morcellation, patient refusal, high-risk cases for which the use of a pneumoperitoneum and/or Trendelenburg position are hazardous; and severe cardiovascular insufficiency, advanced chronic obstructive bronchitis, glaucoma, blood dyscrasia, severe obesity, and neurologic diseases. For these women, surgical treatment must be delegated to traditional ARH, which has been upgraded with new knowledge about selective lymphadenectomy and nerve-sparing surgery, as explained earlier (**Figure 31.1**).

Finally, two experiences are reported on TLRH in LACC patients after neoadjuvant treatment. Vizza et al. published a prospective study on 40 LACC cases (IB2-IIB FIGO-stage disease). Four patients (10%) required conversion to laparotomy, and EBL and OT were comparable to ECC patients managed in the same surgical way (Vizza et al. 2011). More recently, Ghezzi et al. reported a multi-institutional cohort study comparing 68 ACC patients (IB2-IIB FIGO-stage disease) managed with neoadjuvant chemotherapy and submitted to TLRH

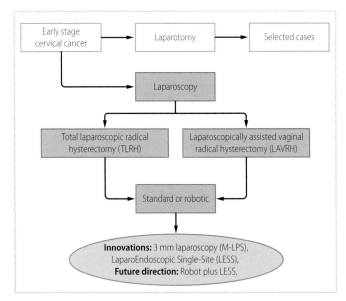

Figure 31.1 Actual application of laparoscopy to early-stage cervical cancer management. This flowchart of laparotomic and laparoscopic approaches for early-stage disease shows innovation and future directions as well.

matched with comparable clinical cases (263 women) submitted to ARH. Complication rates were similar, whereas EBL and hospital stay length were favorable in the TLRH group (Ghezzi et al. 2013). Despite the lack of conclusive evidence supporting laparoscopy in LACC patients, these preliminary studies demonstrate the feasibility of this approach; further data are needed to confirm this modality of treatment, which seems encouraging in terms of perioperative outcomes and quality of life.

LAPAROSCOPIC RADICAL HYSTERECTOMY: SETUP AND INSTRUMENTATION

The operating room setup and supply of dedicated instruments are essential for every kind of surgery but are even more important for laparoscopic radical hysterectomy. **Figure 31.2** illustrates the ideal disposition of the surgical team: the first surgeon is to the left of the patient, the first assistant to the right. The patient's legs are positioned in special stirrups that keep them flexed and abducted in order to both improve pelvis width and to mobilize them during the procedure, if necessary. A second assistant is seated between the legs in order to change the position of the uterus using a device (either a manipulator or vaginal sponge). The operating room nurse is to the left of the patient in front of the first surgeon. The anesthetist is located behind the head of the patient, and there are at least two monitors: one for the first operator and first assistant, which is situated in front of them, with the second monitor positioned behind the head of the patient. The patient is in the Trendelenburg position.

Although many new devices are available for laparoscopy, our goal in this section is to illustrate the use of basic instruments that are, in our opinion, indispensable to performing a safe, cost-effective procedure. The first essential tool is a reusable uterus manipulator; this is a very important tool in every hysterectomy but especially in radical hysterectomies because it allows the surgeon to mobilize and stretch the uterus into different positions, thus facilitating dissection, reducing bleeding, visualizing vascular structures, and increasing the internal operating space. It also allows the surgeon to maintain the pneumoperitoneum during vaginal opening and to extract the intact uterus through the vaginal canal.

The second essential device is bipolar forceps. Many different types are available, each with its own different characteristics, but a reusable bipolar forceps with a atraumatic grips capable of applying traction is sufficient. Scissors should be disposable in order to ensure consistent cutting capacity; some models can be connected to mono- or bipolar current. A dissecting forceps with atraumatic spikes is indispensable

for nerve-sparing surgery and the retroperitoneal approach. Two atraumatic forceps are used for bowel mobilization, one for the first surgeon and one for the assistant; in addition, a reusable suction-irrigation system and a reusable monopolar hook for colpotomy should be available. For uterine artery closing, either bipolar forceps or metallic clips can be used. In our opinion, clips allow the surgeon to ensure a safe closing without possible damage to the ureter and to immediately identify the ureter during surgery. Finally, for vaginal cuff closure, a set comprising a reusable needle holder, a contra-needle holder, and absorbable sutures is required.

KEY STEPS OF THE SURGICAL PROCEDURE

Table 31.4 summarizes the key steps of TLRH explained in this section. At our center, hysterectomy types B and C (as categorized by Querleu and Morrow; see **Table 31.2**) are currently performed using a reusable uterine manipulator that is emplaced before the procedure is started and after a bimanual vaginal exploration to confirm the preoperative clinical staging. In the presence of contraindications to uterine manipulator utilization, a vaginal sponge can be utilized as an alternative. We consider neoadjuvant chemoradiation and/or tumor volume of greater than 2 cm as contraindications for uterine manipulator use.

Table 31.4 Key surgical steps of radical hysterectomy. The main surgical passages for performing a radical hysterectomy

Key surgical steps of radical hysterectomy
• Coagulation and section of round ligament
• Pelvic retroperitoneum opening
• Ureter identification
• Uterine artery at the origin closing
• Latzko space opening
• Paravesical space opening
• Okabayashi space opening
• Ureter isolation
• Coagulation and section of infundibulopelvic ligament or utero-ovarian ligament
• Posterior peritoneum and rectovaginal space opening
• Uterosacral ligament section
• Vesicovaginal space opening
• Uterine artery section
• Colpotomy
• Extraction of intact uterus
• Vaginal cuff suturing

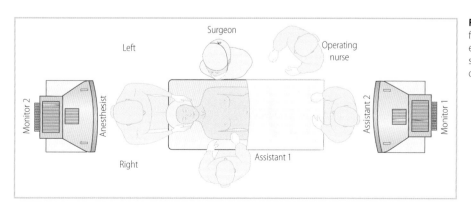

Figure 31.2 Ideal disposition of surgical team for laparoscopic hysterectomy, showing the most ergonomic colocation of each member of the surgical team and anesthetist, as well as the best disposition of monitors.

Generally, the patient's arms are blocked at her side. She is placed in a steep Trendelenburg position after pneumoperitoneum is completed. A 10 mm 0° high-definition video laparoscope is placed at the level of the umbilicus either by open technique or under direct visualization. An alternative 5 mm 0° video laparoscope can be adopted. Three additional 5 mm trocars are placed medially and cranially with respect to the iliac spines (the lateral ones) and 4 cm below the umbilicus (the medial one), all under visualization. Intra-abdominal pressure is maintained at 12 mmHg.

The small bowel is mobilized to the upper abdomen, and, if necessary, the sigmoid is fixed to the abdominal wall in order to free Douglas's pouch. The round ligaments are transected bilaterally along their lateral section. After opening the wide ligament cranially, the infundibulopelvic ligament is stretched medially to identify the ureter. The pelvic retroperitoneum opening is performed according to the following sequence: lateral pararectal space (Latzko), paravesical space, and medial pararectal space (Okabayashi). The uterine arteries are bilaterally identified at their origin from the umbilical artery or internal iliac artery and closed by metallic clips (**Figure 31.3a**). A pelvic lymphadenectomy is then performed from the level of the iliac (type I) or aortic (type II) bifurcation to the circumflex iliac vein according to tumor staging. The obturator lymph nodes are removed, with care taken to identify the obturator nerve and avoid injuring it. Para-aortic lymphadenectomy is not routinely performed unless suspicious pelvic lymph nodes are confirmed to have metastatic disease on frozen section evaluation. If a bilateral salpingo-oophorectomy is being performed, the infundibulopelvic ligament is transected. Fallopian tubes are always removed. The bladder is then mobilized inferiorly by a lateral approach to ensure adequate vaginal margins (**Figure 31.3b**). The posterior peritoneum is incised using monopolar or bipolar forceps, and the rectovaginal space is entered. Uterine arteries are transected at the origin, and the paracervix overturned (**Figure 31.3c**). The uterosacral

ligaments are identified, isolated, and transected bilaterally at different levels (following the anatomic landmarks of Querleu and Morrow's classification; see **Table 31.2**), sparing uterine vessels and nerves that remain laterally under vision. The ureters are separated from their medial attachments to the peritoneum; the paracervical tissue over the ureters is dissected, and they are unroofed. Using a monopolar hook, colpotomy is performed (**Figure 31.3d**).

The specimen is completely separated from the upper vagina and removed. The vaginal cuff is laparoscopically or vaginally sutured according to the surgeon's preference. To minimize the risk of port-site metastases, the abdominal cavity is deflated prior to removal of the ports; moreover, the vagina and all the ports sites are irrigated with 5% Povidone-iodine solution before completing the surgery. With the aim of sparing ovarian function after eventual adjuvant radiotherapy, the ovaries are transposed laterally to the paracolic gutters and fixed securely to the abdominal wall.

CONCLUSION

Minimally invasive surgical techniques in gynecologic oncology have greatly evolved since the introduction of laparoscopy to the field. The advantages of laparoscopy over laparotomy in the appropriately selected cancer patient have proven benefits to the patient both intra- and postoperatively, and produce similar outcomes.

With our current knowledge and experience, it appears that laparoscopy is the gold standard in the management of ECC, but radical hysterectomy and lymphadenectomy are complex surgeries and they require significant technical expertise and dedicated centers.

In our opinion, after an adequate learning curve is mastered, the essentials for a safe procedure are:
1. the correct setup of the surgical team and instruments
2. an excellent knowledge of anatomic landmarks

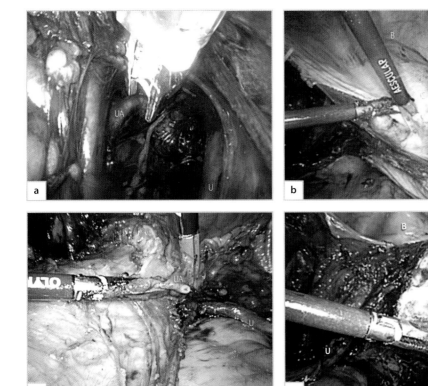

Figure 31.3 (a) Uterine artery closing, showing the uterine artery (UA) at the cross with the ureter (U) and its closing by metallic clips. (b) Vesicovaginal space opening, using a lateral approach to the vesicovaginal peritoneum, with bladder (b) caudally, cervix (c) cranially, and iliac vessels laterally. (c) Uterine artery transaction, showing the uterine artery transected (UA) with paracervix overturned and the ureter totally isolated below. (d) Circular colpotomy, guided by the uterine manipulator and after an adequate preparation, a circular colpotomy is performed using a monopolar hook. Visible are the proximal section of uterine artery (UA) and the mobilized bladder (b).

3. a continuous surveying of the literature and new devices
4. a thorough knowledge of key surgical steps
5. repeated practice of all surgical steps
6. the clear visualization of structures to safeguard during surgery, and
7. the capacity to quickly refer to a more experienced surgeon in case of doubt.

The long-term oncologic data remain to be determined with these procedures but are unlikely to differ greatly from the laparoscopic outcome data that we currently have. As we continue to develop new surgical techniques, we may be able to even further decrease the risk of postoperative complications and improve patient satisfaction in the laparoscopic management of CC.

With every new advance and novel technology or technique, it will be prudent for the gynecologic oncology field as a whole to carefully evaluate the risks and benefits. Randomized studies and long-term follow-up studies are needed to confirm the superiority of the laparoscopic approach over the abdominal one in the management of CC.

■ REFERENCES

Abu-Rustum NR, Gemignani ML, Moore K, et al. Total laparoscopic radical hysterectomy with pelvic lymphadenectomy using the argon-beam coagulator: pilot data and comparison to laparotomy. Gynecol Oncol 2003; 91:402–409.

Amendola MA, Hricak H, Mitchell DG, et al. Utilization of diagnostic studies in the pretreatment evaluation of invasive cervical cancer in the United States: results of intergroup protocol ACRIN 6651/GOG 183. J Clin Oncol 2005; 23:7454–7459.

Benedetti-Panici P, Basile S, Angioli R. Pelvic and aortic lymphadenectomy in cervical cancer: the standardization of surgical procedure and its clinical impact. Gynecol Oncol 2009; 113:284–290.

Benedetti-Panici P, Maneschi F, Scambia G, et al. Lymphatic spread of cervical cancer: an anatomical and pathological study based on 225 radical hysterectomies with systematic pelvic and aortic lymphadenectomy. Gynecol Oncol 1996; 62:19–24.

Boruta DM, Fagotti A, Bradford LS, et al. Laparoendoscopic single-site radical hysterectomy with pelvic lymphadenectomy: initial multi-institutional experience for treatment of invasive cervical cancer. J Min Invas Gynecol 2013; doi: 10.1016/j.jmig.2013.10.005. [Epub ahead of print].

Canis M, Mage G, Pouly JL, et al. Laparoscopic radical hysterectomy for cervical cancer. Baillieres Clin Obstet Gynaecol 1995; 9:675–689.

Canis M, Mage G, Wattiez A, et al. Does endoscopic surgery have a role in radical surgery of cancer of the cervix uteri? J Gynecol Obstet Biol Reprod 1990; 19:921.

Choi CH, Lee JW, Lee YY, et al. Comparison of laparoscopic-assisted radical vaginal hysterectomy and laparoscopic radical hysterectomy in the treatment of cervical cancer. Ann Surg Oncol 2012; 19:3839-3848.

Choi HJ, Roh JW, Seo SS, et al. Comparison of the accuracy of magnetic resonance imaging and positron emission tomography/computed tomography in the presurgical detection of lymph node metastases in patients with uterine cervical carcinoma. Cancer 2006; 106:914–922.

Cibula D, Abu-Rustum NR, Benedetti-Panici P, et al. New classification system of radical hysterectomy: emphasis on a three-dimensional anatomic template for parametrial resection. Gynecol Oncol 2011; 122:264–268.

Collins Y, Einstein MH, Gostout BS, et al. Cervical prevention in the era of prophylactic vaccines: a preview for gynecologic oncologists. Gynecol Oncol 2006; 102:552–556.

Dargent D. A new future for Schauta's hysterectomy through pre-surgical retroperitoneal pelviscopy. Eur J Gynecol Oncol 1987; 8:292–295.

Dargent D, Mathevet P. Radical laparoscopic vaginal hysterectomy. J Gynecol Obstet Biol Reprod 1992; 21:709–710.

Dottino PS, Segna RA, Zakashansky K, et al. A case controlled study of radical vaginal hysterectomy with laparoscopic lymphadenectomy versus radical abdominal hysterectomy for the treatment of early stage cervical cancer. Gynecol Oncol 2006; 101:18.

Ercoli A, Iannone V, Legge F, et al. Advances in surgical management of cervical cancer. Minerva Gynecol 2009; 61:227–237.

Fagotti A, Boruta DM 2nd, Scambia G, et al. First 100 early endometrial cancer cases treated with laparoendoscopic single-site surgery: a multicentric retrospective study. Am J Obstet Gynecol 2012; 206:353.e1–e6.

Fagotti A, Fanfani F, Longo R, et al. Which role for pretreatment laparoscopic staging? Gynecol Oncol 2007; 107:S101–105.

Fagotti A, Gagliardi ML, Moruzzi C, et al. Excisional cone as fertility sparing treatment in early stage cervical cancer. Fert Steril. 2011; 95:1009–1012.

Fanfani F, Gallotta V, Fagotti A, et al. Total microlaparoscopic radical hysterectomy in early cervical cancer. JSLS 2013; 17:111–115.

Fanfani F, Rossitto C, Gagliardi ML, et al. Total laparoendoscopic single-site surgery (LESS) hysterectomy in low-risk early endometrial cancer: a pilot study. Surg Endosc 2012; 26:41–46.

Ferrandina G, Legge F, Fagotti A, et al. Preoperative concomitant chemoradiotherapy in locally advanced cervical cancer: safety, outcome, and prognostic measures. Gynecol Oncol 2007; 107:S127–132.

Frumovitz M, dos Reis R, Sun CC, et al. Comparison of total laparoscopic and abdominal radical hysterectomy for patients with early-stage cervical cancer. Obstet Gynecol 2007; 110:96–102.

Fujii S, Takakura K, Matsumura N, et al. Anatomic identification and functional outcomes of the nerve sparing Okabayashi radical hysterectomy. Gynecol Oncol 2007; 107:4–13.

Garland SM, Smith JS. Human Papillomavirus vaccines: current status and future prospects. Drugs 2010; 70:1079–1098.

Ghezzi F, Cromi A, Ditto A, et al. Laparoscopic versus open radical hysterectomy for stage IB-IIB cervical cancer in the setting of neoadjuvant chemotherapy: a multi-institutional cohort study. Ann Surg Oncol 2013a; 20:2007–2015.

Ghezzi F, Cromi A, Uccella S, et al. Nerve-sparing minilaparoscopic versus conventional laparoscopic radical hysterectomy plus systematic pelvic lymphadenectomy in cervical cancer patients. Surg Innov 2013b; 20:493–501.

Ghezzi F, Fanfani F, Malzoni M, et al. Minilaparoscopic radical hysterectomy for cervical cancer: multi-institutional experience in comparison with conventional laparoscopy. EJSO 2013c; 39:1094–1100.

Jackson KS, Das N, Naik R, et al. Laparoscopically assisted radical vaginal hysterectomy vs. radical abdominal hysterectomy for cervical cancer: a match controlled study. Gynecol Oncol 2004; 95:655–661.

Koehler C, Gottschalk E, Chiantera V, et al. From laparoscopic assisted radical vaginal hysterectomy to vaginal assisted laparoscopic radical hysterectomy. BJOG 2012; 119:254–262.

Lee CL, Huang KG, Jain S, et al. Comparison of laparoscopic and conventional surgery in the treatment of early cervical cancer. J Am Assoc Gynecol Laparosc 2002; 9:481–487.

Li G, Yan X, Shang H, et al. A comparison of laparoscopic radical hysterectomy and pelvic lymphadenectomy and laparotomy in the treatment of IB-IIA cervical cancer. Gynecol Oncol 2007; 105:176–180.

Malur S, Possover M, Schneider A. Laparoscopically assisted radical vaginal versus radical abdominal hysterectomy type II in patients with cervical cancer. Surg Endosc 2001; 15:289–292.

Malzoni M, Malzoni C, Perone C, et al. Total laparoscopic radical hysterectomy (type III) and pelvic lymphadenectomy. Eur J Gynaecol Oncol 2004; 25:525–527.

Malzoni M, Tinelli R, Cosentino F, et al. Feasibility, morbidity, and safety of total laparoscopic radical hysterectomy with lymphadenectomy: our experience. J Minim Invasive Gynecol 2007; 14:584–590.

Marnitz S, Kohler C, Roth C, et al. Is there a benefit of pretreatment laparoscopic transperitoneal surgical staging in patients with advanced cervical cancer? Gynecol Oncol 2005; 99:536–544.

Meigs J. The Wertheim operation for carcinoma of the cervix. Am J Obstet Gynecol 1945; 40:542–543.

Morgan DJ, Hunter DC, McCracken G, et al. Is laparoscopically assisted radical vaginal hysterectomy for cervical carcinoma safe? A case control study with follow up. BJOG 2007; 114:537–542.

Muñoz N, Bosch FX, de Sanjose S, et al. Epidemiologic classification of human papillomavirus types associated with cervical cancer. N Engl J Med 2003; 348:518–527.

Naik R, Jackson KS, Lopes A, et al. Laparoscopic assisted radical vaginal hysterectomy versus radical abdominal hysterectomy–a randomized phase II trial: perioperative outcomes and surgicopathological measurements. BJOG 2010; 117:746–751.

Nakano R. Abdominal radical hysterectomy and bilateral pelvic lymph node dissections for cancer of the cervix. The Okabayashi operation its modification. Gynecol Obstet Invest 1981; 12:281–293.

Nam JH, Kim JH, Kim DY, et al. Comparative study of laparoscopic-vaginal radical hysterectomy and abdominal radical hysterectomy in patients with early cervical cancer. Gynecol Oncol 2004; 92:277–283.

Nam JH, Park JY, Kim DY, et al. Laparoscopic versus open radical hysterectomy in early stage long-term survival outcomes in a matched cohort study. Ann Oncol. 2012; 23:903–911.

Nezhat CR, Burrell MO, Nezhat FR, et al. Laparoscopic radical hysterectomy with para-aortic and pelvic node dissection. Am J Obstet Gynecol 1992; 166:864–865.

Obermair A, Ginbey P, McCartney AJ. Feasibility and safety of total laparoscopic radical hysterectomy. J Am Assoc Gynecol Laparosc 2003; 10:345–349.

Pahisa J, Martinez-Roman S, Torne A, et al. Comparative study of laparoscopically assisted radical vaginal hysterectomy and open Wertheim-Meigs in patients with early-stage cervical cancer: eleven years of experience. Int J Gynecol Cancer 2010; 20:173–178.

Pecorelli S, Zigliani L, Odicino F. Revised FIGO staging for carcinoma of the cervix. Int J Gynecol Obstet 2009; 109:107–108.

Piver MS, Rutledge F, Smith JP. Five classes of extended hysterectomy for women with cervical cancer. Obstet Gynecol 1974; 44:265–272.

Pomel C, Canis M, Mage G, et al. Laparoscopically extended hysterectomy for cervix cancer: technique, indications and results. A propos of a series of 41 cases in Clermont. Chirurgie 1997; 122:133–136.

Querleu D. Laparoscopically assisted radical vaginal hysterectomy. Gynecol Oncol 1993; 51:248–254.

Querleu D, Morrow CP. Classification of radical hysterectomy. Lancet Oncol 2008; 9:297–303.

Sakuragi N, Todo Y, Kudo M, et al. A systematic nerve-sparing radical hysterectomy technique in invasive cervical cancer for preserving postsurgical bladder function. Int J Gynecol Cancer 2005; 15:389–397.

Salicrù SB, de la Torre JFV, Gil-Moreno A. The surgical management of early stage cervical cancer. Curr Opin Obstet Gynecol 2013; 25:312–319.

Scambia G, Ferrandina G, Di Stefano M, et al. Is there a place for a less extensive radical surgery in locally advanced cervical cancer patients? Gynecol Oncol 2001; 83:319–324.

Schauta F. Die operation des gebaermutterkrebs mitteldes schuchardtschen paravaginal schnittes. Monatsschr Geburtshiffe Gynaekol 1902; 15:133–152.

Sekiba K. Radical hysterectomy for cancer of the uterine cervix. Semin Surg Oncol. 1985; 1:95–104.

Sert BM, Abeler VM. Robotic-assisted laparoscopic radical hysterectomy (Piver type III) with pelvic node dissection–case report. Eur J Gynaecol Oncol 2006; 27:531–533.

Sharma R, Bailey J, Anderson R, Murdoch J. Laparoscopically assisted radical vaginal hysterectomy (Coelio-Schauta): a comparison with open Wertheim/Meigs hysterectomy. Int J Gynecol Cancer 2006; 16:1927–1932.

Spirtos NM, Eisenkop SM, Schlaerth JB, Ballon SC. Laparoscopic radical hysterectomy (type III) with aortic and pelvic lymphadenectomy in patients with stage I cervical cancer: surgical morbidity and intermediate follow-up. Am J Obstet Gynecol 2002; 187:340–348.

Spirtos NM, Schlaerth JB, Kimball RE, et al. Laparoscopic radical hysterectomy (type III) with aortic and pelvic lymphadenectomy. Am J Obstet Gynecol 1996; 174:1763–1767.

Steed H, Rosen B, Murphy J, et al. A comparison of laparoscopic-assisted radical vaginal hysterectomy and radical abdominal hysterectomy in the treatment of cervical cancer. Gynecol Oncol 2004; 93:588–593.

Thun MJ, DeLancey JO, Center MM, et al. The global burden of cancer: priorities for prevention. Carcinogenesis 2010; 31:100–110.

Wertheim E. The extended abdominal operation for carcinoma uteri. Am J Obstet Gynecol 1912; 6:169–232.

Vizza E, Pellegrino A, Milani R, et al. Total laparoscopic radical hysterectomy and pelvic lymphadenectomy in locally advanced stage IB2-IIB cervical cancer patients after neoadjuvant chemotherapy. EJSO 2011; 37:364–369.

Wright JD, Herzog TJ, Neugut AI, et al. Comparative effectiveness of minimally invasive and abdominal radical hysterectomy for cervical cancer. Gynecol Oncol 2012; 127:11–17.

Yabuki Y, Asamoto A, Hoshiba T, et al. Radical hysterectomy: an anatomic evaluation of parametrial dissection. Gynecol Oncol 2000; 77:155–163.

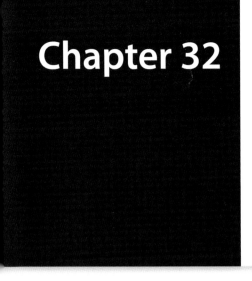

Chapter 32

Laparoscopic management of adnexal tumors

Eric Leblanc, Frédéric Kridelka, Fabrice Narducci, Lucie Bresson, Delphine Hudry, Athanassios Kakkos, Claudia Andrade, Marco Puga, Audrey Tsunoda, Sophie Taieb

■ INTRODUCTION

Surgery is the cornerstone of management of any adnexal tumor. It is necessary at any stage of the disease: diagnosis, staging, treatment, and, sometimes, in palliative indications.

Laparoscopic surgery has long been used for the diagnosis of suspicious adnexal tumors. Thanks to experience in nodal dissections, its application field has been extended to staging and beyond – to the full treatment of selected early malignant ovarian tumors.

In advanced-stage disease, laparoscopy is quasi exclusively used as a diagnostic tool. Indeed, not all carcinomatoses in women are of adnexal origin, and biopsy under laparoscopy may avoid inadequate management. Although this indication is more controversial, laparoscopy seems an essential tool to assess the extent of peritoneal disease in order to better select suitable patients for up-front maximal cytoreduction. More recently, minimally invasive surgery is being explored in cytoreductive surgeries.

All these aspects are addressed in this chapter while highlighting the advantages and limits of this approach according to current standards of management.

■ LAPAROSCOPIC DIAGNOSIS OF A SUSPICIOUS ORGANIC MASS

The first goal for a surgeon faced with an organic ovarian mass is to obtain an accurate pathological diagnosis. The second objective, in the case of a confirmed malignancy, is to adequately assess the macro- and microscopic extent of the disease to indicate and adapt the adjuvant treatment.

Apart from some rare tumors expressing specific blood markers that usually assessed in a special clinical context [such as malignant ovarian germ cell tumors (MOGCT) in young women or sex cord tumors with clinical endocrine disorders], the definitive diagnosis of an ovarian tumor is generally obtained thanks to its complete removal followed by a thorough pathological evaluation.

Complete tumor resection can be obtained using two main procedures: ovarian cystectomy or adnexectomy. The choice of procedure will be based on both the preoperative imaging results and the intraoperative aspect of the lesion.

After having installed the optical and operative trocars, a peritoneal cytology will always be the first step of the exploration, performed prior to any dissection or adhesiolysis, in order to avoid blood contamination. It is obtained by direct aspiration, if some peritoneal fluid is present, or by peritoneal washing.

This is followed by a thorough exploration of all peritoneal surfaces of the abdominopelvic cavity by direct vision along with the mobilization of bowel and organs using instruments. In areas of difficult access in the upper abdomen, such as the posterior part of hemidiaphragms, porta hepatis, and the lesser sac, the addition of an endoscopic retractor may facilitate this exploration.

After these necessary explorative steps, the first issue to address is whether to continue with laparoscopic management. If a suspicious aspect of carcinomatosis is found out, biopsies of peritoneal implants are performed and sent for frozen section. According to results, an immediate or secondary conversion into laparotomy for a cytoreductive surgery is decided. If there is no obvious suspicious aspect, the laparoscopic procedure is continued for tumor removal. It is of paramount importance to respect the conditions of oncological safety: the tumor must be confined to ovary, of a small volume (adapted to the size of endoscopic retrieval bags), and without dense adhesions with other organs. The goal is to avoid any risk of contamination of the abdominal cavity and/or port sites by an inadvertent tumor rupture. Prognosis of this accident is controversial. In the past, the intraoperative rupture of a carcinoma has been claimed to significantly impair patient survival (Vergote et al. 2001). However, more recent but retrospective studies on larger numbers of patients seem to reduce this impact, provided this accident is immediately and adequately managed (full suction of the liquid followed by an abundant peritoneal washing) (Goudge et al. 2009, Kim et al. 2013).

If all oncologic conditions cannot be fulfilled, a small-sized laparotomy is preferable to safely resect the tumor. In the case of a rather benign tumor, a low transverse Maylard's incision is cosmetically acceptable. In the case of a highly suspicious and/or a very large tumor, a midline laparotomy seems the only reasonable access for a safe resection.

The choice of adequate technique for tumor resection will be based on preoperative imaging aspects of the tumor structure and the laparoscopic aspect of its surface, while considering the patient's age and her desire to preserve fertility as well.

In the case of a pure and nonsuspicious cyst, a cystectomy is indicated by direct dissection from the ovary or after puncture and complete suction of its content. To limit spillage from large cysts, this suction can be performed after having placed the tumor into an endoscopic bag. Then the cyst wall is opened, and a direct cystoscopy using the laparoscope is performed to check the cyst's interior aspect. The cystectomy is then performed by the gentle separation of the cyst wall from the ovarian parenchyma using atraumatic grasping forceps. Then cyst, enclosed in an endoscopic bag, is extracted from the abdomen. If at the end of the procedure, the closure of the remaining ovary is not mandatory, thorough hemostasis of its parenchyma is advocated. In case of a difficult endometriotic cyst, the excision of the cyst wall is preferable to the simple suction of its content (Hart et al. 2008). Assessment of other endometriotic lesion with their concomitant destruction is recommended if possible.

In the case of a mixed/solid tumor or if the ovary looks to be destroyed by the mass, adnexectomy is the best choice. Technically, the broad ligament is entered along the external iliac pedicle axis in order to check the ureter and to safely isolate the gonadal pedicle for a bipolar desiccation division. Adnexa is then detached from the posterior leaflet of the broad ligament, down to its uterine insertion. The utero adnexal pedicle is then thoroughly dissected and divided (care must be paid at this level to avoid any pedicle retraction, a possible source of a significant hemorrhage). As for a cyst, the specimen is systematically placed in an endoscopic bag before extraction. In the case of a large tumor, the port site may be enlarged to prevent tearing the bag and/or specimen morcellation.

In the case of a bilateral suspicious adnexal mass in a young patient wishing to preserve fertility, a unilateral adnexectomy with contralateral cystectomy is recommended if possible. Otherwise, a bilateral adnexectomy while preserving the uterus is indicated. In menopausal patients, a systematic bilateral adnexectomy will prevent contralateral abnormalities.

A frozen section of the specimen is desirable, if possible. Its reliability depends on tumor size and pathologist experience. Generally, it is possible to differentiate a benign from a malignant tumor. In a recent French study of 141 ovarian tumors removed by laparoscopy, accuracy of frozen section for diagnosis of malignancy was 89%, especially for cyst of less than 10 cm in size. Beyond this limit, results were worse, as observed in other series (Shih et al. 2011). However, in case of malignancy, a frozen section may not easily differentiate a borderline from a true invasive carcinomas (Medeiros et al. 2005), especially in the case of a mucinous subtype (Pongsuvareeyakul et al. 2012). In this situation, it seems wiser to stop the procedure and consider a two- step policy, with a possible reoperation after reception of the definitive pathological report. Patients must be informed before consenting to surgery that this may happen, as well as the possibility for a laparoconversion if laparoscopic management looks impossible or dangerous.

■ LAPAROSCOPY IN EARLY ADNEXAL CARCINOMAS

■ Laparoscopic staging/restaging

In the case of a malignant subtype, a staging procedure is required to assess the true extent of the disease and to decide further management. Technically, staging must follow the same steps already described for laparotomy (Trimbos et al. 2000). These steps may differ according to the lesion's pathological subtype.

Early ovarian carcinomas (EOC) (ovarian or tubal origin)

A complete peritoneal and retroperitoneal assessment is necessary since 33% of EOC apparently confined to ovary have residual disease at reoperation (Young 1987). This staging has a prognostic and possibly

therapeutic impact, as demonstrated in the EORTC trial ACTION. Patients with nonoptimal peritoneal and retroperitoneal staging and submitted to observation had a poorer survival rate than did those submitted to systematic chemotherapy. By contrast, the subgroup of patients with a negative comprehensive staging, followed clinically, had similar survival to those submitted to systematic chemotherapy (Trimbos et al. 2003). In addition, within the subgroup of patients submitted to surveillance, those who had a comprehensive peritoneal and retroperitoneal staging had a survival advantage over patients who had only the peritoneal and/or an incomplete retroperitoneal staging (Timmers et al. 2010).

Peritoneal staging (**Figures 32.1–32.3**) involves an infracolic omentectomy and multiple systematic random peritoneal biopsies, sampled from the Douglas cul-de-sac, the paracolic gutters up to each hemidiaphragm, and the root of mesentery (i.e. along the pathways of peritoneal fluid). Technically, this procedure is rapidly performed thanks to sealing-cutting devices such as LigaSure (Covidien, Dublin, Ireland) or Ultracision (Ethicon, Somerville, New Jersey). The patient

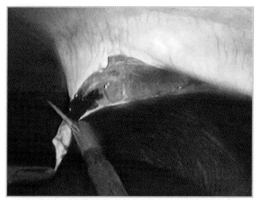

Figure 32.1 Infracolic omentectomy.

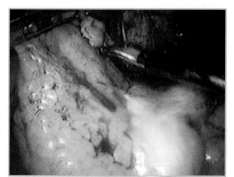

Figure 32.2 Peritoneal biopsy.

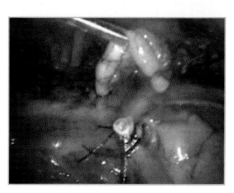

Figure 32.3 Appendectomy.

is placed in a proclive position. The surgeon stands between the patient's legs with a video monitor in front of him. The assistant holds the laparoscope to the patient's left side while grasping the omentum with an atraumatic forceps close to its insertion on the transverse colon. Using bipolar cautery-scissors (or better, a LigaSure), the omentum is detached from the transverse colon from right to left (or reverse). Care must be taken not to burn the colon by keeping the tip of the device a safe distance from the organ. In the case of a suspicious aspect, the resection can be extended to the infragastric area, with resection of the gastroepiploic pedicles. When fully detached, the omentum is packed into a large endoscopic bag before extraction. Biopsies are performed by sharp dissection, removing 4–5 cm2 of peritoneum each.

Although the yield of a systematic omentectomy and random biopsies of a visually normal peritoneum is low [3–4% in the Shroff et al. (2011) or Lee et al. series (2014)], they remain indicated in early-stage disease owing to the low morbidity of the procedure and a small but real possibility of upstaging and altered management. Furthermore, systematic peritoneal biopsies warrant the careful examination of all surfaces. There are no specific guidelines as to how much of the omentum should be removed, but pathology studies show that for the purpose of staging and detecting microscopic disease, omental biopsies are probably sufficient in a grossly normal appearing omentum (Arie et al. 2013).

Appendectomy is generally recommended in this context (Ayhan et al. 2005) as well, especially in case of mucinous tumors. The appendectomy is performed by sectioning by sectionning its basis between Endoloops (Ethicon France) after the bipolar hemostasis-division of its pedicle. However, its yield is not clear in the absence of obvious appendiceal abnormality or aspect of pseudomyxoma (Feigenberg et al. 2013, Lin et al. 2013). A complete digestive tract endoscopic exploration is usually recommended in mucinous cysts of digestive origin. Appendectomy does not protect against mucinous ovarian carcinomas, regardless of subtype (invasive or borderline) (Elias et al. 2014).

Finally, the completion of pelvic organ resection (hysterectomy, contralateral adnexectomy, etc.) is part of the peritoneal staging as well.

The retroperitoneal staging encompasses pelvic and para-aortic (PA) node dissections (**Figures 32.4–32.6**). These techniques have been extensively reported using the transperitoneal (Querleu & LeBlanc 1994) or the extraperitoneal routes (Dargent et al. 2000). Because the transperitoneal approach enables the surgeon to perform both peritoneal and retroperitoneal staging in obese patients, it can be easier to start with the ilioinfrarenal PA dissection extraperitoneally and complete the procedure transperitoneally.

Whatever the approach, node dissections must be systematic (and not elective or selective) and must lie between precise anatomic boundaries. This yield is superior to any other pattern of dissection (Maggioni et al. 2006). The parameters are the left renal vein cranially, obturator foramens caudally, and both ureters laterally (Morice et al. 2003, Powless et al. 2011). As shown in a recent comprehensive review of the literature reviewing 1347 stage I–II ovarian invasive carcinomas, node involvement is found in approximately 14% of early stages. It is more frequently observed at the PA level only (49.7%) than at the pelvic level only (20.3%) or at both levels (29.9%). In addition, node dissection must be bilateral since positive nodes can be observed contralaterally only to the tumor in 18% of cases. Finally, tumor subtype and grade play an important role as well, since node spread is more frequently observed in grade 3 tumors (20%) compared to grade 1 (4%). It ranges between 23% and 29% in serous and undifferentiated carcinomas compared to 14% in clear cell, 6% in endometrioid, and 2% in mucinous carcinomas (Kleppe et al. 2011). Given the low rate of spread for mucinous carcinomas, some suggest omitting node dissection in mucinous tumors (Morice et al. 2003). However, this decision should be restricted to mucinous carcinomas of the expansile subtype, for which node involvement is essentially nil, compared to the infiltrative subtype for which it remains significant, confirming the indication of node staging in this latter subtype (Muyldermans et al. 2013). Finally, the complete resection of gonadal pedicles is recommended to resect possible tumor cells in transit to the PA nodes.

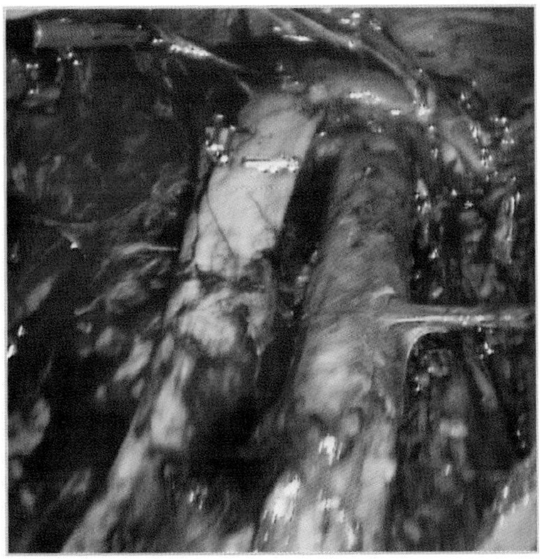

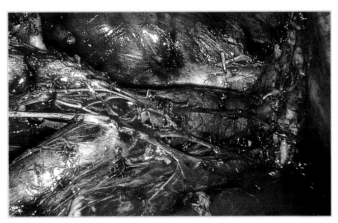

Figure 32.5 Extraperitoneal paraaortic nerve-sparing lymphadenectomy (final aspect of the upper part).

Figure 32.4 Transperitoneal oneal para-aortic lymphadenectomy (final aspect).

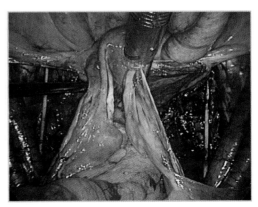

Figure 32.6 Bilateral pelvic lymphadenectomy (final aspect).

In young patients, fertility preservation can be safely considered in stage IA grade 1 EOC (du Bois et al. 2013), but discussed in stage IC grade 1 or IA grade 2, and strongly questioned in any grade 3 lesion due to too short series and follow-up studies (Morice et al. 2011, Menczer 2013). Fertility preservation should not be performed in higher stages disease (Petrillo et al. 2014). The same comprehensive staging described earlier must be performed in these young patients. However, instead of hysterectomy, a hysteroscopy-curettage is preferred to detect occult endometrial spread. To reduce the risk of adhesions leading to fertility problems, the contralateral ovary will be biopsied (or removed) only if it looks suspicious.

Borderline ovarian tumors (BOT)

Borderline tumors are tumors with an excellent prognosis (Trimble et al. 2002) and are usually managed by ovariectomy/adnexectomy, either with hysterectomy or not, according to the patient's age and her desire to preserve fertility. Due to the high risk of recurrence (Uzan et al. 2014), cystectomy only should be reserved for patients with bilateral tumors (if feasible) (Palomba et al. 2010) or in very young patients with unilateral tumors who wish to preserve fertility.

In the case of a borderline tumor, peritoneal staging only is indicated. It consists of a peritoneal cytology, infracolic omentectomy, random peritoneal biopsies. An appendectomy will be performed in mucinous BOT only if grossly abnormal (Kleppe et al. 2014b). This peritoneal staging should be systematically performed if the aspect is likely to correspond to a borderline tumor in order to avoid reoperation. This peritoneal staging removes potential sites of recurrence. For these reasons, BOT is a good indication for full laparoscopic management, provided the limits of resectability, along with a minimal staging, are respected (Querleu et al. 2003, Fauvet et al. 2005). Hysterectomy should be considered only in the presence of serosal implants and/or in the case of endometrioid borderline subtypes due to the frequent association of endometrial abnormalities (Uzan et al. 2012).

Retroperitoneal staging is not required in cases of BOT. Node involvement usually corresponds to endosalpingiosis (Fadare 2009), frequently observed in BOT of the serous type. It has no impact on patient survival (Camatte et al. 2002, Lesieur et al. 2011). Lymphadenectomy can be replaced by simple adenectomy in the case of lymphadenomegaly.

Indications for a secondary restaging procedure are rare. In fact, the yield of a restaging is questionable because results rarely impact management (unless infiltrative implants are found) or prognosis, which remains good (Camatte et al. 2002, Zapardiel et al. 2010). However, secondary restaging should be considered in selected cases, as in BOT of micropapillary serous subtype because it is frequently associated with infiltrative implants (Morice et al. 2012) and is a possible indication for systemic chemotherapy. For the mucinous subtype, appendectomy is important to consider in order not to miss an appendiceal tumor and a possible source of peritoneal pseudomyxoma (Cadron et al. 2007). In the case of inadequate surgery (such as a simple cystectomy) or of intraoperative rupture [which is more frequent after laparoscopic resection (Trillsch et al. 2013)], the question is raised of whether to undertake a restaging procedure with completion of ovariectomy/adnexectomy along with peritoneal staging due the significant risk of recurrence (Yinon et al. 2007, De Iaco et al. 2009). This restaging can be effectively performed through laparoscopy as well (Azuar et al. 2013).

A long follow-up (>10 years) is recommended because late recurrences, usually borderline as well but sometimes invasive, have been observed (Ji et al. 2010), especially in the case of micropapillary serous BOT (Silva et al. 2006, Fischerova et al. 2012).

However, despite the risk of recurrence, fertility preservation should be systematically considered in young patients (even in stage III disease) unless the peritoneal staging demonstrates the presence of invasive implants (Palomba et al. 2010, Uzan et al. 2010, Fischerova et al. 2012). A close and prolonged surveillance is therefore necessary after conservative treatment of BOT because the main factors of recurrence are cystectomy, bilateral tumors, and young age (Uzan et al. 2014).

Nonepithelial tumors

Fertility-sparing management must be systematically considered in MOGCT because they usually occur in very young patients. In these young patients, a diagnostic ovariectomy/adnexectomy is preferable as primary surgery, and the surgeon should wait for definitive pathological results before discussing a secondary operation for completion and/or a restaging procedure according to subtype. This policy can be applied even in cases of advanced disease because results are good in terms of fertility and survival, even after chemotherapy (Weinberg et al. 2011).

A thorough surgical peritoneal staging is the rule, and the node assessment should be discussed on a case-by-case basis, according to the pathological subtype (Kumar et al. 2008, Kleppe et al. 2014a). The node assessment can be advantageously replaced by a selective adenectomy of any enlarged/suspicious node (Gershenson et al. 2007).

In older women with no desire for pregnancy, a more radical treatment with total hysterectomy and bilateral salpingo-oophorectomy can be discussed, especially in the case of sex cord tumors such as granulosa cell tumors due to the frequent association of this subtype with endometrial abnormalities, especially endometrioid carcinomas (Ukah et al. 2011). As for borderline tumors, nonepithelial tumors seem to be safely managed laparoscopically by trained teams although reported series are very rare (Shim et al. 2013).

Finally, definitive pathological results of the tumor and staging specimens enable the surgeon to define the genuine FIGO stage (defined as early if IA or B) and, during a tumor board session, to decide the indication and modalities of chemotherapy (which may be omitted in true stage I grade 1 or 2 tumors), and confirm if fertility preservation will be a goal of treatment.

■ Clinical results of laparoscopic staging procedure for EOC

The different operative steps, especially lymph node dissections, have all been described through laparoscopic trans- or extraperitoneal approaches (Querleu & LeBlanc 1994, Pomel et al. 1995, Dargent et al. 2000). Recently, the technique of staging has been simplified by the use of integrated sealing -cutting devices using either bipolar current (LigaSure, Covidien, Dublin, Ireland), harmonic dissection (Ultracision, Ethicon, Somerville, New Jersey), or a combination (Thunderbeat, Olympus, Paris, France). They enable the surgeon to significantly reduce operative time and increase the safety of resections (lymphadenectomy, omentectomy, or hysterectomy).

Our pioneer experience, updated from our last publication (Leblanc et al. 2006), considers 125 restaging laparoscopies for invasive adnexal carcinoma performed between 1991 and 2011. Eighty-four cases were performed after initial adnexectomy (66 ovarian and 18 fallopian tube carcinomas). Forty-one patients had received 3-6 courses of platinum-based chemotherapy for a pathological high-risk stage 1 EOC. They were offered a secondary "restaging" procedure to complete an initially incomplete surgery. Median age and body mass index (BMI) were 50 years old (18–74) and 24.2 kg/m2 (18.1–40), respectively. All patients had a complete peritoneal and retroperitoneal staging. For PA node dissection, the approach was transperitoneal in 61 cases and extraperitoneal in 64 cases. Median operative time and hospital stay were 238 min (180–450) and 3 days (2–6), respectively. A laparoconversion was necessary in five cases due to carcinomatosis (two cases), dense adhesions (two cases), and fixed nodes (one case). Perioperative morbidity consisted in a caval and a gonadal pedicle injury, both managed laparoscopically. Three reoperations were necessary to fix a ureter injury, peritonitis, and a digestive fistula. Ten symptomatic lymphocysts and one ascites were managed by scanner-guided puncture with no complication. Three patients were left with leg edema. Fertility preservation was performed in 10 patient; three became pregnant and delivered uneventfully.

In the group of 48 chemo-naïve patients, restaging laparoscopy upstaged eight (16.6%) patients who a received postoperative chemotherapy. Seven (39%) out of 18 patients with an early fallopian tube carcinoma were upstaged.

In the subgroup of 40 stage IA ovarian cancer patients with 53-month (6–217) median follow-up, two patients (5%) recurred (one mucinous and one grade 2 serous tumor) at 3 and 7 years after laparoscopic surgery, respectively. The former developed a peritoneal carcinomatosis, the latter pulmonary metastases. Five-year survival for this group was 95.8%, similar to that observed in the literature for laparotomy (Heinz et al. 2003). Only six patients received chemotherapy due to a high-risk histopathology (clear cell or high-grade serous tumor).

In a recent review of retrospective series, Ghezzi et al. (2009) reported, for a pooled total of 241 patients, a mean operative time of 230 min (149–348) and blood loss of consistently less than 300 mL, and no death was reported. Serious complications were rare and consisted of four conversions due to vascular or ureter injuries. The mean hospital stay was 4.2 days (1.6–9.4), 4.9–23% of patients were upstaged, disease-free survival ranged from 83% to 100%, and overall survival ranged from 94% to 100%.

So far, no there is no randomized study comparing laparoscopic and open staging. The first retrospective series by Park et al. (2008b) compared 19 open versus 17 laparoscopic staging procedures for EOC. It did not show a difference in operative time, node counts, or complication rate. Blood loss, return of bowel function, and postoperative stay were significantly shorter in the laparoscopy group and significant survival results. Another study by Lee et al. (2011) compared 26 laparoscopic versus 87 open restaging procedures for early EOC. Except for operative time, which was longer in the laparoscopy group, all other results were similar to Park's study. No difference in recurrence rate was observed after 23-month mean follow-up. Laparoscopy appeared to be slightly more costly than laparotomy. In the report by Liu et al. (2014), 40 open staging procedures for EOC were compared to a similar group of 35 cases with laparoscopic staging. The same results were observed concerning the advantage of laparoscopy in terms of rapid recovery, shorter stay, and no difference in operative criteria; no data on follow-up are provided. The most recent Italian comparative experience confirmed the efficiency of laparoscopic staging with apparently no detrimental effects on long-term survival (Bogani et al. 2014).

All authors stress the importance of specific training to safely perform this surgery; it is of utmost importance to refer these patients to an expert center that concentrates both the experience and the regular practice of advanced laparoscopy. Limits for the laparoscopic approach do exist; the presence of a peritoneal carcinomatosis or dense adhesions is a clear indication for laparoconversion (Spirtos et al. 2005). However, even in this situation, the PA dissection can be performed extraperitoneally, and the reopening of initial subumbilical laparotomy will facilitate the completion of pelvic resections. Thus, the patient will be spared a large xiphopubic incision. Obesity may be a serious difficulty in completing an infrarenal PA dissection, but

the use of the extraperitoneal approach has pushed this limit. In our series of ovarian cancers, the procedure was feasible in patients of up to 40 kg/m2 BMI. Similarly, advanced age is not a strict limit in itself because we have performed this operation in patients up to 74 years old. However, comorbidities may modify the decision because the minimally invasive laparoscopic approach implies a prolonged Trendelenburg position and specific hemodynamic conditions that may be incompatible with patient's general status.

Finally, laparoscopic staging is an efficient option that should be considered whenever possible. More recently, robotically assisted laparoscopy (RAL) was reported in the management of EOC. In Nezhat's report, nine RAL restaging procedures were compared to 10 laparoscopic restaging procedures. No difference in intra- or perioperative outcomes was observed (Nezhat et al. 2014), but there are cost differences.

SOME ISSUES CONCERNING THE USE OF LAPAROSCOPY IN EOC

So far, there is no clear evidence of a relationship between the pneumoperitoneum and the development or increase of peritoneal dissemination (Azuar et al. 2009). As addressed earlier, the intraoperative rupture of an ovarian cystic tumor does not seem to dramatically impair a patient's prognosis when compared to a preoperative rupture. These patients should no longer be considered as FIGO stage IC. However, a careful handling of any ovarian tumors is required regardless of technique, and a laparoconversion must be considered if a rupture is obviously predictable.

Although the issue of port-site metastases seems to be a rare event in the large experience of MSKCC (only 1.2% of port metastases were observed after approximately 1694 laparoscopies delating with a carcinomatosis or metastasis), they can be observed in the staging of early carcinomas (Zivanovic et al. 2008). In this case, they are due to the mismanagement of the primary tumor.

Finally, the risk of recurrence in stage IA after a laparoscopic restaging, as reported in Ghezzi's review, seems no different from the results reported after an open staging (Ghezzi et al. 2009).

COMPLETE LAPAROSCOPIC MANAGEMENT OF EARLY ADNEXAL TUMORS

A comprehensive knowledge and control of laparoscopic staging procedures enables experienced surgeons to perform the complete laparoscopic management of an apparent EOC. For invasive carcinomas, the results of pioneer teams confirm the feasibility, reproducibility, and safety of this policy for selected cases. Series with important follow-up are rare; however, all confirm the feasibility of tumor resection and thorough staging through the scope. With trained teams, results (e.g. operative time, node numbers) are similar to those obtained through an open approach but with better perioperative outcomes, although the costs of the laparoscopic approach might be higher (Lee et al. 2011). Although no randomized study exists, no differences in recurrence or survival rates have been reported in true stage IA cases (Pomel et al. 1995, Leblanc et al. 2004, Park et al. 2008a, Ghezzi et al. 2009); however, study populations are small in size with a relative short follow-up. It is therefore difficult to provide definitive conclusions on this policy. Our team has performed full laparoscopic management on seven patients with ovarian carcinomas. After a 48-month follow-up, although no patient had received adjuvant treatment, none recurred so far.

As stressed earlier, strict selection criteria are required: a small-sized lesion, without adhesions to other organs, and present in a patient with no obvious difficulty to perform a thorough laparoscopic staging (Tozzi et al. 2004).

The same rules must be applied for borderline tumors. Some recurrences have been reported after laparoscopic management of stage III tumors (Kane et al. 2010), but fortunately, as discussed earlier, these tumors are of an exceptionally invasive subtype (Ji et al. 2010).

Finally, the literature is sparse regarding the laparoscopic management of nonepithelial tumors. Although there is no theoretical contraindication if conditions of oncological safety are followed, no definitive conclusions can be drawn from the very short series currently available.

Thus, great care in selection criteria and technique must be the rule to avoid damaging a likely very good prognosis through the misuse of laparoscopy. A consensus exists that potentially curable EOC be subjected to rigorous management to define candidates for fertility preservation and/or adjuvant treatment. Minimally invasive surgery, especially laparoscopy with or without robotic assistance, is part of the modern surgical armamentarium, especially in the diagnostic and staging steps and sometimes, in highly selected cases, in the full treatment of an adnexal carcinoma.

This approach seems as efficient as laparotomy; however, due to the rarity of early-stage disease, it is unlikely that a randomized trial comparing the two approaches will ever be undertaken. Nevertheless it is clear that this surgery requires real expertise in advanced laparoscopic surgery to ensure operative safety and oncological accuracy.

LAPAROSCOPY IN ADVANCED STAGES OF OVARIAN CANCER

Macroscopically complete debulking surgery by laparotomy is the current standard of care in ovarian carcinomatosis, but it is not always suitable if the tumor turns out to be larger than expected from the imaging workup. Thus, laparoscopy has traditionally been recommended as a diagnostic tool to confirm the ovarian origin (Rosenoff et al. 1975, Qu et al. 1984), as well as to assess the possibility to optimally debulk an ovarian carcinomatosis (Vergote et al. 1998). A significant proportion of carcinomatoses are not of ovarian origin and deserve specific management. By performing multiple biopsies of peritoneal implants, the diagnosis of ovarian origin is thus confirmed.

A second role of laparoscopy is the triage of patients between upfront or interval debulking surgeries. This decision is an important but controversial issue because the result will impact the patient's outcome and possibly her survival. Indeed an open-close exploratory laparotomy is useless because it delays chemotherapy. Because only laparotomy with no residual tumor (or at least with <1 cm residuum) is acceptable, laparoscopy may help to reduce the number of inadequate debulking surgeries. Fagotti et al. (2005) were the first to prospectively assess the accuracy of decisional laparoscopy in ovarian carcinomatoses. Sixty-four patients with advanced ovarian cancer were submitted to a laparoscopic exploration systematically followed by a laparotomy to confirm or rule complete operability. Overall accuracy of laparoscopy was 90%, making this technique equivalent to laparotomy. Following this study, a laparoscopic score [similar to Sugarbaker's peritoneal cancer index (PCI) for laparotomy] was created based on the assessment of carcinomatosis in five areas. A score of 8 or greater predicts suboptimal surgery in 100% of cases (Fagotti et al. 2006). A modified version of the Fagotti's score was suggested by Brun et al. (2008). Finally, the Sugarbaker's PCI, Fagotti's original, and Brun's

modified laparoscopic scores were prospectively compared to laparotomy in predicting the completeness of a cytoreduction. Finally, in this prospective nonrandomized study, the PCI and modified Fagotti scores were the most reliable (Chereau et al. 2010). In addition, the PCI score can be reproduced through laparoscopy with a good correlation with laparotomy (Gouy et al. 2013). However, the Fagotti's score can be easily implemented in the workup of advanced ovarian cancer by less experienced teams as shown in the prospective study Olympia-Mito 13 (Fagotti et al. 2013). In a recent Cochrane review on laparoscopy and resectability of ovarian carcinomatosis, the authors concluded that no firm conclusions could be drawn, due to too few studies. Only two of them confirm that thanks to criteria of inoperability, no patient was inappropriately explored (Rutten et al. 2014). Recently, the sensitization of laparoscopy by hand assistance improved the results in a prospective study (Varnoux et al. 2013). However, the decision of primary debulking or neoadjuvant chemotherapy is based not only on a laparoscopic examination, but it must also consider other imaging results, the patient's general status, and the surgeon's experience in cytoreductive surgery.

Finally, the accuracy and reliability of a diagnostic laparoscopy in advanced ovarian disease seems valuable only in trained and experienced teams in both laparoscopy and advanced ovarian cancer management statement not applicable any other situations. A trained team can be defined if it fulfils all modern and internationally recognized criteria for the management of advanced ovarian cancers (Querleu et al. 2013).

The role of laparoscopy in the field of cytoreductive surgery is very limited. Some attempted to primary cytoreduce carcinomatosis, but only 36% of patients were left with no residual disease after 2.3 hours of an only peritoneal laparoscopic surgery (Fanning et al. 2011).. According to current standards, this example seems to not be followed. Others, in selected cases with quite no residual disease after chemotherapy, were able to optimally cytoreduce the residual or recurrent disease by mini-invasive surgery (Nezhat et al. 2014). However, microscopical foci of tumors are still frequent after chemotherapy, which may be missed by laparoscopy (Hynninen et al. 2013). Other options such as HIPEC under laparoscopy are being explored as well in this context, but should be considered as investigational so far (Lygidakis & Seretis 2012).

CONCLUSION

- Despite progress in imaging technologies, the diagnosis of a suspicious mass implies to remove the tumor (cystectomy/ovariectomy, adnexectomy) while avoiding any contamination of the abdominal cavity or the abdominal wall.
- According to tumor size and aspect at imaging, laparoscopy may be a preferred approach. However, a conversion into laparotomy may be required if all conditions of a management with oncological safety are not fulfilled. This possibility must have been previously addressed with the patient.
- The intraoperative diagnosis of malignancy is not always easy, thus a two-step management is far preferable to a systematic radical treatment, especially in younger patients for which the possibility of an ovarian germ-cell tumor with their specific management as well as a fertility-preservation policy must be systematically considered.
- The adequate management of a malignant adnexal tumor is based on the precise knowledge of its extent, thanks to a thorough staging procedure. This staging operation, adapted to tumor histological subtype can be performed by laparoscopy, as soon as possible, if technical conditions are favorable, either by the initial surgeon if experienced in advanced laparoscopy, or by an expert team to which

the patient is referred in order to offer the advantage of laparoscopic surgery with no detrimental effects on oncological outcomes

- The complete management by minimally invasive techniques of an early ovarian cancer is feasible, in selected cases and by selected teams. It must follow the same rules of oncologic security of laparotomy in order not to impair a good prognosis.
- In advanced stage tumors, laparoscopic surgery is an important diagnostic tool for the characterization of a peritoneal carcinomatosis, especially when CT scan–guided biopsies are impossible or not contributive. Interesting but more controversial is the use of laparoscopy to assess the tumor extent and to assist the decision of upfront, interval, or secondary surgery. If laparoscopic debulking surgery has been suggested in selected ovarian carcinomatosis, it should be considered today as an experimental procedure and consequently not be recommended as a routine procedure.

Minimally invasive surgery (laparoscopy assisted or not by a robot) is increasingly considered in the management of adnexal tumors. It is especially indicated as a diagnostic tool for the origin and the extent of disease. Its main advantage is to spare the patient an unnecessary explorative laparotomy or an incomplete cytoreduction. By contrast, it is not really adapted to perform extensive cytoreductive surgery yet. But it is a surgery of specialized teams with a large experience in advanced laparoscopic surgery along with a regular practice, two necessary qualities to warrant efficacy and safety of this method.

REFERENCES

Arie AB, et al. The omentum and omentectomy in epithelial ovarian cancer: a reappraisal: part II–The role of omentectomy in the staging and treatment of apparent early stage epithelial ovarian cancer. Gynecol Oncol 2013; 131:784–790.

Ayhan A, et al. Routine appendectomy in epithelial ovarian carcinoma: is it necessary? Obstet Gynecol 2005; 105:719–724.

Azuar AS, et al. Impact of surgical peritoneal environment on postoperative tumor growth and dissemination in a preimplanted tumor model. Surg Endosc 2009; 23:1733–1739.

Azuar AS, et al. Laparoscopic restaging of borderline ovarian tumours (BLOT): a retrospective study of 142 cases. Eur J Obstet Gynecol Reprod Biol 2013; 168:87–91.

Bogani G, et al. Laparoscopic staging in women older than 75 years with early-stage endometrial cancer: comparison with open surgical operation. Menopause 2014; 21:945-951.

Brun JL, et al. External validation of a laparoscopic-based score to evaluate resectability of advanced ovarian cancers: clues for a simplified score. Gynecol Oncol 2008; 110:354–359.

Cadron I, et al. Management of borderline ovarian neoplasms. J Clin Oncol 2007; 25:2928–2937.

Camatte S, et al. Impact of surgical staging in patients with macroscopic "stage I" ovarian borderline tumours: analysis of a continuous series of 101 cases. Eur J Cancer 2004; 40:1842–1849.

Camatte S, et al. Lymph node disorders and prognostic value of nodal involvement in patients treated for a borderline ovarian tumor: an analysis of a series of 42 lymphadenectomies. J Am Coll Surg 2002; 195:332–338.

Chereau E, et al. Comparison of peritoneal carcinomatosis scoring methods in predicting resectability and prognosis in advanced ovarian cancer. Am J Obstet Gynecol 2010; 202:178 e1–178 e10.

Dargent D, Ansquer Y, Mathevet P. Technical development and results of left extraperitoneal laparoscopic paraaortic lymphadenectomy for cervical cancer. Gynecol Oncol 2000; 77:87–92.

De Iaco P, et al. Behaviour of ovarian tumors of low malignant potential treated with conservative surgery. Eur J Surg Oncol 2009; 35:643–648.

du Bois A, Heitz F, Harter P. Fertility-sparing surgery in ovarian cancer: a systematic review. Onkologie 2013; 36:436–443.

Elias KM, et al. Prior appendectomy does not protect against subsequent development of malignant or borderline mucinous ovarian neoplasms. Gynecol Oncol 2014; 132:328–333.

Fadare O. Recent developments on the significance and pathogenesis of lymph node involvement in ovarian serous tumors of low malignant potential (borderline tumors). Int J Gynecol Cancer 2009; 19:103–108.

Fagotti A, et al. A laparoscopy-based score to predict surgical outcome in patients with advanced ovarian carcinoma: a pilot study. Ann Surg Oncol. 2006; 13:1156–1161.

Fagotti A, et al. A multicentric trial (Olympia-MITO 13) on the accuracy of laparoscopy to assess peritoneal spread in ovarian cancer. Am J Obstet Gynecol 2013; 209:462 e1–462 e11.

Fagotti A, et al. Role of laparoscopy to assess the chance of optimal cytoreductive surgery in advanced ovarian cancer: a pilot study. Gynecol Oncol 2005; 96:729–735.

Fanning J, Yacoub E, Hojat R. Laparoscopic-assisted cytoreduction for primary advanced ovarian cancer: success, morbidity and survival. Gynecol Oncol 2011; 123:47–49.

Fauvet R, et al. Laparoscopic management of borderline ovarian tumors: results of a French multicenter study. Ann Oncol 2005; 16:403–410.

Feigenberg T, et al. Is routine appendectomy at the time of primary surgery for mucinous ovarian neoplasms beneficial? Int J Gynecol Cancer 2013; 23:1205–1209.

Fischerova D, et al. Diagnosis, treatment, and follow-up of borderline ovarian tumors. Oncologist 2012; 17:1515–1533.

Gershenson DM, et al. Reproductive and sexual function after platinum-based chemotherapy in long-term ovarian germ cell tumor survivors: a Gynecologic Oncology Group Study. J Clin Oncol 2007; 25:2792–2797.

Ghezzi F, et al. Laparoscopy staging of early ovarian cancer: our experience and review of the literature. Int J Gynecol Cancer 2009; 19 Suppl 2:S7–S13.

Goudge, CS, Li Z, Downs LS, Jr. The influence of intraoperative tumor rupture on recurrence risk in Stage Ic epithelial ovarian cancer. Eur J Gynaecol Oncol 2009; 30:25–28.

Gouy S, et al. Accuracy and reproducibility of the peritoneal cancer index in advanced ovarian cancer during laparoscopy and laparotomy. Int J Gynecol Cancer 2013; 23:1699–703.

Hart RJ, et al. Excisional surgery versus ablative surgery for ovarian endometriomata. Cochrane Database Syst Rev 2008; 2:CD004992.

Heinz A, Odicino F, Maisonneuve P. Carcinoma of the ovary. Int J Gynaecol Obstet 2003; 83:135–166.

Hynninen J, et al. Is perioperative visual estimation of intra-abdominal tumor spread reliable in ovarian cancer surgery after neoadjuvant chemotherapy? Gynecol Oncol 2013; 128:229–232.

Ji EY, et al. Can laparoscopy really complete full surgical staging? A case of early recurrence and malignant transformation of borderline ovarian tumor. Eur J Gynaecol Oncol 2010; 31:449–451.

Kane A, et al. Fertility results and outcomes after pure laparoscopic management of advanced-stage serous borderline tumors of the ovary. Fertility Steril 2010; 94:2891–2894.

Kim HS, et al. Impact of intraoperative rupture of the ovarian capsule on prognosis in patients with early-stage epithelial ovarian cancer: a meta-analysis. Eur J Surg Oncol 2013; 39:279–289.

Kleppe M, et al. Lymph node metastasis in stages I and II ovarian cancer: a review. Gynecol Oncol 2011; 123:610–614.

Kleppe M, et al. Lymph-node metastasis in stage I and II sex cord stromal and malignant germ cell tumours of the ovary: A systematic review. Gynecol Oncol 2014a; 133:124-127.

Kleppe M, et al. Mucinous borderline tumours of the ovary and the appendix: A retrospective study and overview of the literature. Gynecol Oncol ; 133:155-158.

Kumar S, et al. The prevalence and prognostic impact of lymph node metastasis in malignant germ cell tumors of the ovary. Gynecol Oncol 2008; 110:125–132.

Leblanc E, et al. Laparoscopic restaging of early stage invasive adnexal tumors: a 10-year experience. Gynecol Oncol 2004; 94:624–629.

Leblanc E, et al. Laparoscopic staging of early ovarian carcinoma. Curr Opin Obstet Gynecol 2006; 18:407–412.

Lee JY, et al. The role of omentectomy and random peritoneal biopsies as part of comprehensive surgical staging in apparent early-stage epithelial ovarian cancer. Ann Surg Oncol 2014; 21:2762–2766.

Lee M, et al. Comparisons of surgical outcomes, complications, and costs between laparotomy and laparoscopy in early-stage ovarian cancer. Int J Gynecol Cancer 2011; 21:251–256.

Lesieur B, et al. Prognostic value of lymph node involvement in ovarian serous borderline tumors. Am J Obstet Gynecol 2011; 204:438 e1–7.

Lin JE, et al. The role of appendectomy for mucinous ovarian neoplasms. Am J Obstet Gynecol 2013; 208:46 e1–4.

Liu M, et al. Comparison of laparoscopy and laparotomy in the surgical management of early- stage ovarian cancer. Int J Gynecol Cancer 2014; 24:352–357.

Lygidakis NJ, Seretis K. Laparoscopic HIPEC in the treatment of advanced ovarian cancer. Hepatogastroenterology 2012; 59:667–670.

Maggioni A, et al. Randomised study of systematic lymphadenectomy in patients with epithelial ovarian cancer macroscopically confined to the pelvis. Br J Cancer 2006; 95:699–704.

Morice P, et al. Borderline ovarian tumour: pathological diagnostic dilemma and risk factors for invasive or lethal recurrence. Lancet Oncol 2012; 13:e103–115.

Morice P, et al. Lymph node involvement in epithelial ovarian cancer: analysis of 276 pelvic and paraaortic lymphadenectomies and surgical implications. J Am Coll Surg 2003; 197:198–205.

Medeiros LR, et al. Accuracy of frozen-section analysis in the diagnosis of ovarian tumors: a systematic quantitative review. Int J Gynecol Cancer 2005; 15:192–202.

Menczer J. Conservative fertility-sparing surgical treatment of invasive epithelial ovarian cancer: when is it acceptable? Isr Med Assoc J 2013; 15:116–120.

Morice P, et al. Recommendations of the Fertility Task Force of the European Society of Gynecologic Oncology about the conservative management of ovarian malignant tumors. Int J Gynecol Cancer 2011; 21:951–963.

Muyldermans K, et al. Primary invasive mucinous ovarian carcinoma of the intestinal type: importance of the expansile versus infiltrative type in predicting recurrence and lymph node metastases. Eur J Cancer 2013; 49:1600–1608.

Nezhat FR, et al. Comparison of perioperative outcomes and complication rates between conventional versus robotic-assisted laparoscopy in the evaluation and management of early, advanced, and recurrent stage ovarian, fallopian tube, and primary peritoneal cancer. Int J Gynecol Cancer 2014; 24:600–607.

Palomba S, et al. Ultra-conservative fertility-sparing strategy for bilateral borderline ovarian tumours: an 11-year follow-up. Hum Reprod 2010; 25:1966–1972.

Park JY, et al. Comparison of laparoscopy and laparotomy in surgical staging of early-stage ovarian and fallopian tubal cancer. Ann Surg Oncol 2008a; 15:2012–2019.

Park JY, et al. Laparoscopic and laparotomic staging in stage I epithelial ovarian cancer: a comparison of feasibility and safety. Int J Gynecol Cancer 2008b; 18:1202–1209.

Petrillo M, et al. Fertility-sparing surgery in ovarian cancer extended beyond the ovaries: a case report and review of the literature. Gynecol Obstet Invest 2014; 77:1–5.

Pomel C, et al. Laparoscopic staging of early ovarian cancer. Gynecol Oncol 1995; 58:301–306.

Pongsuvareeyakul I, et al. Accuracy of frozen-section diagnosis of ovarian mucinous tumors. Int J Gynecol Cancer 2012; 22:400–406.

Powless CA, et al. Risk factors for lymph node metastasis in apparent early-stage epithelial ovarian cancer: implications for surgical staging. Gynecol Oncol 2011; 122:536–540.

Qu JY, Sun AD, Lien LC. Laparoscopy in the diagnosis and management of ovarian cancer. J Reprod Med 1984; 29:483–488.

Querleu D, LeBlanc E. Laparoscopic infrarenal paraaortic lymph node dissection for restaging of carcinoma of the ovary or fallopian tube. Cancer 1994; 73:1467–1471.

Querleu D, et al. Laparoscopic restaging of borderline ovarian tumours: results of 30 cases initially presumed as stage IA borderline ovarian tumours. BJOG 2003; 110:201–204.

Querleu D, et al. Quality indicators in ovarian cancer surgery: report from the French Society of Gynecologic Oncology (Societe Francaise d'Oncologie Gynecologique, SFOG). Ann Oncol 2013; 24:2732–2739.

Rosenoff SH, et al. Use of peritoneoscopy for initial staging and posttherapy evaluation of patients with ovarian carcinoma. Natl Cancer Inst Monogr 1975; 42:81–86.

Rutten MJ, et al. Laparoscopy for diagnosing resectability of disease in patients with advanced ovarian cancer. Cochrane Database Syst Rev 2014; 2:CD009786.

Shih KK, et al. Accuracy of frozen section diagnosis of ovarian borderline tumor. Gynecol Oncol 2011; 123:517–521.

Shim SH, et al. Laparoscopic management of early-stage malignant nonepithelial ovarian tumors: surgical and survival outcomes. Int J Gynecol Cancer 2013; 23:249–255.

Shroff R, et al. The utility of peritoneal biopsy and omentectomy in the upstaging of apparent early ovarian cancer. Int J Gynecol Cancer 2011; 21:1208–1212.

Silva EG, et al. The recurrence and the overall survival rates of ovarian serous borderline neoplasms with noninvasive implants is time dependent. Am J Surg Pathol 2006; 30:1367–1371.

Spirtos NM, et al. Laparoscopic staging in patients with incompletely staged cancers of the uterus, ovary, fallopian tube, and primary peritoneum: a Gynecologic Oncology Group (GOG) study. Am J Obstet Gynecol 2005; 193:1645–1649.

Timmers PJ, et al. Lymph node sampling and taking of blind biopsies are important elements of the surgical staging of early ovarian cancer. Int J Gynecol Cancer 2010; 20:1142–1147.

Tozzi R, et al. Laparoscopic treatment of early ovarian cancer: surgical and survival outcomes. Gynecol Oncol 2004; 93:199–203.

Trillsch F, et al. Surgical management and perioperative morbidity of patients with primary borderline ovarian tumor (BOT). J Ovarian Res 2013; 6:48.

Trimble CL, Kosary C, Trimble EL. Long-term survival and patterns of care in women with ovarian tumors of low malignant potential. Gynecol Oncol 2002; 86:34–37.

Trimbos JB. Staging of early ovarian cancer and the impact of lymph node sampling. Int J Gynecol Cancer 2000; 10:8–11.

Trimbos JB, et al. Impact of adjuvant chemotherapy and surgical staging in early-stage ovarian carcinoma: European Organisation for Research and Treatment of Cancer-Adjuvant ChemoTherapy in Ovarian Neoplasm trial. J Natl Cancer Inst 2003; 95:113–125.

Ukah CO, et al. Adult granulosa cell tumor associated with endometrial carcinoma: a case report. J Med Case Rep 2011; 5:340.

Uzan C, et al. Management and prognosis of endometrioid borderline tumors of the ovary. Surg Oncol 2012; 21178–184.

Uzan C, et al. Outcomes after conservative treatment of advanced-stage serous borderline tumors of the ovary. Ann Oncol 2010; 21:55–60.

Uzan C, et al. Prognostic factors for recurrence after conservative treatment in a series of 119 patients with stage I serous borderline tumors of the ovary. Ann Oncol 2014; 25:166–171.

Varnoux C, et al. Diagnostic accuracy of hand-assisted laparoscopy in predicting resectability of peritoneal carcinomatosis from gynecological malignancies. Eur J Surg Oncol 2013; 39(7):774–779.

Vergote I, et al. Neoadjuvant chemotherapy or primary debulking surgery in advanced ovarian carcinoma: a retrospective analysis of 285 patients. Gynecol Oncol 1998; 71:431–436.

Vergote I, et al. Prognostic importance of degree of differentiation and cyst rupture in stage I invasive epithelial ovarian carcinoma. Lancet 2001; 357:176–82.

Weinberg LE, et al. Survival and reproductive outcomes in women treated for malignant ovarian germ cell tumors. Gynecol Oncol 2011; 121:285–289.

Yinon Y, et al. Clinical outcome of cystectomy compared with unilateral salpingo-oophorectomy as fertility-sparing treatment of borderline ovarian tumors. Fertil Steril 2007; 88:479–484.

Young RC. Initial therapy for early ovarian carcinoma. Cancer 1987; 60:2042–2049.

Zapardiel I, et al. The role of restaging borderline ovarian tumors: single institution experience and review of the literature. Gynecol Oncol 2010; 119:274–277.

Zivanovic O, et al. The rate of port-site metastases after 2251 laparoscopic procedures in women with underlying malignant disease. Gynecol Oncol 2008; 111:431–437.

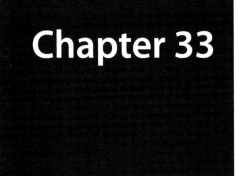

Chapter 33

Role of laparoscopy in advanced pelvic cancers

Shailesh P Puntambekar, Neha Mookim, Rahul Vashishth, Geetanjali Agarwal-Joshi, Sanjay Kumar, Saurabh N Joshi, Seema S Puntambekar

INTRODUCTION

Surgery has progressed significantly from the era of open pelvic cancer surgeries to the present-day minimally invasive approach. Gone are the days where big surgeries would translate to bigger incisions. We have entered the era where the toughest cancers can be approached through key-hole incisions and laparoscopy has become the modality for the treatment of pelvic cancers. Surgeries range from nerve-sparing radical hysterectomies to anterior exenteration, posterior exenteration, or even to total pelvic exenteration. Postradiated and advanced cancers are no longer contraindications for minimally invasive surgeries.

Pelvic exenteration is a radical procedure performed for locally advanced cancers. It involves the en-bloc resection of the pelvic organs, i.e. the internal reproductive organs along with bladder or rectosigmoid, or both (Diver et al. 2012). Brunschwich (1948) first published his series on 22 pelvic exenterations where he had 23% intraoperative deaths. In the following 10 years, he performed 430 pelvic exenterations for cervical cancers with a 5-year survival rate of 21.6%. By 1967, he had performed 925 exenterations. The evolution of surgical techniques, as well as implementation of reconstructive procedure, along with the improvement of perioperative and postoperative care has reduced the postoperative mortality to between 0–23% (the transition of pelvic exenteration from a palliative procedure to a potentially curative one in patients with advanced pelvic cancer has been established; Berek et al. 2005, Sevin & Koechli 2001).

Exenteration was subsequently established as a curative procedure for centrally located tumors (Diver et al. 2012). The indication for pelvic exenteration in recurrent cervical cancer following chemoradiation is well established now (Marnitz et al. 2009). The role of exenteration as a primary treatment of locally advanced pelvic cancers has yet to be established.

Exenteration may be offered as a primary modality for the treatment of the following cases:
- Patients with fistulas (vesicovaginal/rectovaginal)
- Stage IVa tumors

Thus these exenterations can be divided into those performed primarily and those performed following either previous surgery, chemotherapy, or radiation.

TYPES OF EXENTERATION

The exenterations are divided into three types. These are as follows:
1. Anterior exenteration. This involves the removal of the uterus, or the vaginal vault with en-bloc removal of bladder and distal urethra (Sergio Renato Pais Costa et al. 2008)
2. Posterior exenteration. This includes the removal of the uterus as well as the rectum with or without the establishment of colorectal continuity (Hafner & Petrelli 1994)
3. Total pelvic exenteration. This includes removal of the uterus, bladder, and the rectum. Supralevator pelvic exenteration is a modification of pelvic exenteration where pelvic organs are excised at the level of the levator muscles, preserving the lowest portion of the rectum and the urogenital diaphragm (Rodriguez-Bigas et al. 1994)

Literature in support of the application of laparoscopy for pelvic exenterations has shown it to be an optimal method, with results comparable to open surgery; however, we found very few studies of it (Tables 33.1-33.2).

We have reported a large case series of 248 patients of total laparoscopic radical hysterectomy (Puntambekar et al. 2007) and 16 patients of laparoscopic anterior exenteration (Puntambekar et al. 2006). The success of these procedures prompted us to perform laparoscopic pelvic exenteration for palliation in a select group of cases with advanced or recurrent central pelvic tumors involving the rectum and bladder. Literature shows that there is minimal intraoperative blood loss or complications reduced postoperative complications, shorter hospital stay, and better cosmetic result (Lavazzo et al. 2008).

The aim of the surgery can be either curative or palliative, although some argue that pelvic exenteration remains the only curative intervention in patients with recurrent or persistent pelvic cancer after prior radiation therapy. Palliative surgery is undertaken for the alleviation of local symptoms, such as foul-smelling discharge or fistulas.

The selection criteria for exenterative procedures are as follows (Stan Hope & Symmonds 1985):
1. Centrally located tumors not reaching up to the pelvic wall
2. No para-aortic lymphadenopathy
3. No peritoneal deposits
4. No pedal edema
5. No distant metastasis
6. No ascites
7. Medically fit patient

Anterior exenteration

This involves the removal of the uterus, or the vaginal vault with en-bloc removal of bladder and distal urethra (Sergio Renato Pais Costa et al. 2008). It is performed when there is pathological involvement of the bladder by the tumor. Therefore, this is the most commonly performed procedure for advanced/stage IVa cervical cancers (Figure 33.5).

The main challenge is not in the procedure but in the urinary reconstruction following the procedure.

The options for urinary reconstruction procedures are as follows:
1. Ureterosigmoidostomy: Symmonds
2. Ileocecal pouch
3. Ileal conduit
4. Ileal neobladder
5. Cutaneous ureterostomy

In patients with urethral involvement, creation of a continent neobladder cannot be performed. The main objective of a urinary diversion is to prevent damage to the upper urinary tracts. Thus, in females, the ileocecal pouch and ileal conduit remain the most commonly performed diversion. Ileocecal pouch and ileal conduit are involved in the formation of an abdominal stoma. In patients refusing abdominal stoma, ureterosigmoidostomy (**Figure 33.6**) is a viable option, though there is a risk of hyperchloremic acidosis and biochemical alterations.

Procedure

Step 1. See **Figures 33.1** and **33.2** for port position and positioning of patient, respectively. The uterus is manipulated with the help of a myoma screw. The right ureter identified under the peritoneum at the level of the sacral promontory and the peritoneum over it is incised. The ureter is medialized and the pararectal space dissection is carried parallel to the ureter. The internal iliac artery is identified. The anterior division is clipped or ligated and then cut. Uterine artery and vein are identified, clipped, and cut. The dissection is carried on to the paravesical space anteriorly and the levator ani caudally. Similar steps are repeated on the left side.

Step 2. Posterior dissection in the pouch of Douglas is carried out in a similar manner as in laparoscopic radical hysterectomy. Thus, the rectum is separated from the posterior vaginal wall. A posterior U cut (**Figure 33.3**) is taken as explained in the radical hysterectomy. The ureter is pushed medially to expose the cardinal ligaments and the uterosacrals that are cut on both sides. The caudal limit is the levator ani muscle.

Step 3. The anterior dissection is done by cutting the anterior leaf of the broad ligament and the round ligament on the right. The peritoneum medial to the obliterated hypogastric artery is cut, and the peritoneal cut is extended into the anterior abdominal wall to separate the bladder from the anterior abdominal wall (**Figure 33.4**). Similar steps are repeated on the left side.

Step 4. The bladder is then brought down from the anterior abdominal wall to enter the retropubic space, i.e. the cave of Retzius. The tissue anterior and lateral to the urethra and vagina is cut. The urethra is accessed anteriorly. The posterior urethral wall and the anterior vaginal wall are cut. A good length of vagina below the growth is exposed. The aim is to have a distal vaginal cuff of 2.5–3 cm.

Step 5. Colpotomy is performed. An Ilio-obturator nodal dissection is carried out on both sides and the tissue is put in an endobag. The

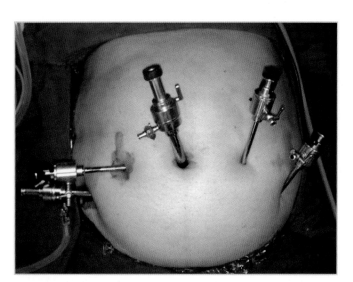

Figure 33.1 Port position.

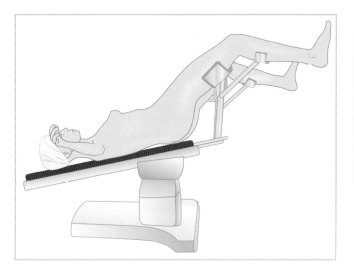

Figure 33.2 Position of patient.

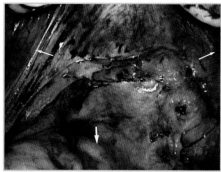

Figure 33.3 Posterior 'U' cut (fat belongs to rectum).

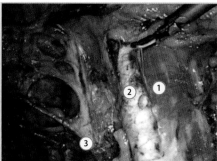

Figure 33.4 Neurovascular bundle. (1) Psoas muscle. (2) External iliac artery. (3) Hypogastric plexus.

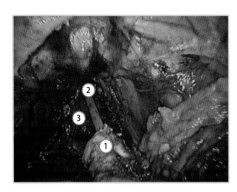

Figure 33.5 Anterior exenteration (urethra being cut). (1) Urethra. (2) Foleys catheter. (3) Pelvic floor.

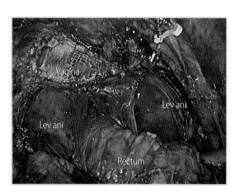

Figure 33.8 Pelvis after anterior exenteration.

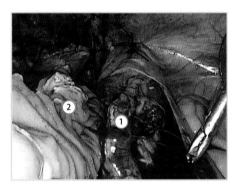

Figure 33.6 Laparoscopic ureterosigmoidestomy. (1) ureter. (2) sigmoid colon.

Criteria for laparoscopic posterior exenteration

1. Inclusion criteria

a. Ovarian cancer involving pouch of Douglas
b. Postradiation cervical cancer recurrence localized posteriorly
c. Cervical cancer with rectovaginal fistula
d. Vaginal cancer with rectal involvement

2. Exclusion criteria (Puntambekar et al. 2009)

a. Extrapelvic spread
b. Distant metastasis including para-aortic nodes
c. Peritoneal or multiple bowel involvement
d. Involvement of urinary bladder
e. Limb edema or sciatic pain
f. Patient medically unfit

Procedure

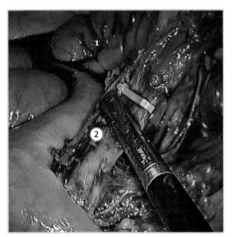

Figure 33.7 Clipping of inferior mesenteric artery in total pelvic exenteration.

Step 1. The uterus is manipulated with the help of a myoma screw. Uterus can be hitched to anterior abdominal wall with a suture that helps with manipulation instead of a myoma screw.

Step 2. The ureter is identified at the level of sacral promontory. The pararectal spaces on both sides are dissected as in a laparoscopic radical hysterectomy.

Step 3. The paravesical space anterior to the uterine artery is dissected to reach the levator ani, which is the distal limit of dissection. The uterine artery and vein are clipped or ligated. The cardinal ligaments on both sides are coagulated and cut.

Step 4. The anterior U cut is taken from one round ligament to the other as in laparoscopic hysterectomy, and the urinary bladder is separated and pushed downward.

Step 5. Remembering the dictum, fat belongs to the rectum, the dissection is carried out in the avascular presacral space between the rectum and the presacral fascia, i.e. two layers of Denonvilliers' fascia. The plane is dissected distally to the levator ani.

Step 6. The distal level of rectal involvement is one of the criteria to decide if rectal continuity can be achieved by performing a supralevator resection or an infralevator resection in case of extensive involvement of rectum with that of sphincter complex.

Step 7. A low colpotomy is performed. Following the colpotomy, the pneumoperitoneum is maintained by placing a pack in the vagina. The rectum distal to the tumor becomes visible, enabling the transaction with the endostapling device.

Step 8. The infundibulopelvic ligament on both sides are coagulated and cut.

Step 9. The inferior mesenteric artery is clipped and cut at its origin.

Step 10. The proximal descending colon and splenic flexure are then mobilized.

specimen is removed vaginally. The vagina is repacked to prevent air leakage.

Step 6. Urinary reconstruction. The type of urinary diversion plays an important role in the quality of life. The various types of urinary diversions that can be performed are ileal conduit, ureterosigmoid, orthotropic ileal neobladder, and Indiana pouch.

Step 7. The vagina is then sutured with continuous intracorporeal suturing. Hemostasis is achieved. An abdominal drain is placed through the right iliac fossa lower port. The ports are then removed under vision and closed (**Figure 33.8**).

■ Posterior exenteration

This includes the removal of the uterus, as well as the rectum with or without establishment of colorectal continuity. In our institute, we have reviewed the criteria, techniques, and outcomes for the procedure (Puntambekar et al. 2011).

Step 11. A 12 mm port about 2 cm above the pubic symphysis is inserted through which an Endo GI stapler (Echelon) is also inserted. After mobilization of the proximal colon, the stapler is fired.

Step 12. There are two methods of coloanal anastomosis. A lower midline minilaparotomy can be done for specimen extraction, proximal bowel transaction, and placement of the anvil of the EEA (end-to-end anastomosis) stapler. The other method is to retrieve the specimen vaginally and bring the proximal colon out through the anal canal, and the anvil of the stapler can be thus inserted.

Step 13. Circular stapled coloanal end-to-end anastomosis is performed.

Step 14. Bilateral ileo-obturator lymph nodes dissection is done.

Step 15. A temporary transverse colostomy is done. Abdominal drain is placed. Port sites are closed.

Total pelvic exenteration

In cases of advanced cervical cancer that spread to the bladder and the rectum, total pelvic exenteration is offered as a method of palliation, so as to improve the quality of life.

Procedure

Step 1. A 10 mm 0° telescope is introduced through the 10 mm umbilical port, and first a staging laparoscopy is done to assess the operability after analyzing the extent of the disease, the fixity of the tumor to the pelvic side walls, and the involvement of iliac vessels.

Step 2. Ureter on the right side is identified at the level of the sacral promontory, and the peritoneum over it is incised with harmonic shears. Ureter is medialized and the pararectal space is dissected. Internal iliac artery is identified, and its anterior division is clipped, or ligated and cut. Uterine artery is identified.

Step 3. Dissection is done anterior to the uterine artery and medial to the obliterated umbilical artery in the paravesical space up to the levator ani. The ureter is medialized, and the uterosacral and cardinal ligaments are coagulated and cut. The same steps are done on the left side.

Step 4. The right round ligament is cut, and the cut is extended anteriorly remaining medial to obliterated umbilical vessels. The bladder is dissected off the anterior abdominal wall and the cave of Retzius is entered. The paraurethral tissue and urethra are cut with the harmonic shears.

Step 5. Colpotomy is performed. The infundibulopelvic ligaments are cut.

Step 6. The ureters are clipped and cut. The sigmoid mesentery is opened to enter the presacral space posterior to the rectum. The inferior mesenteric vessels are ligated and cut (**Figure 33.7**). The dissection posterior to the rectosigmoid is continued until the levator ani is reached. The sigmoid colon is then dissected off the lateral pelvic wall, and the rectum distal to the tumor is stapled with linear stapler and cut. Proximally, the colon is tied at two places and cut in between the ligatures. Splenic flexure mobilization is carried out.

Step 7. An Ilio-obturator nodal dissection is performed. The specimen is placed in the endobag.

Step 8. The abdomen is opened by a small incision of 5–6 cm either midline vertical or transverse muscle cutting. The mouth of the bag is brought out at the incision and the specimen is removed piece by piece from the bag, thus avoiding any contamination.

Step 9. The vagina is then sutured intracorporeally with 2–0 Vicryl. Colorectal anastomosis (**Figure 33.9**) is done by inserting the anvil of a circular stapler in the proximal cut end of the colon, and the head of the stapler is introduced rectally into the distal stump. The ureters are brought out through this incision and are implanted into the ileum extracorporeally. A temporary transverse colostomy is performed. The ureters can also be implanted into the sigmoid colon, and a wet colostomy can also be performed instead.

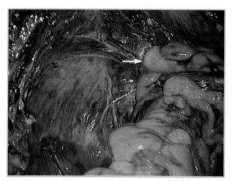

Figure 33.9 Colorectal anastomosis (with circular stapler EEA) after total pelvic exenteration (TPE).

Table 33.1 Classical pelvic exenteration (Lavazzo et al. 2008)

Author	Number of patients	Mean time of procedure	Blood loss	Complications	Follow-up (years)
Goldberg et al. (2006)	95			14% ureteral anastomotic leaks 17% wound complications 4% parastomal leak hernias 36% UTIs/pyelonephritis 11% gastrointestinal fistulas, pouch incontinence 9% small bowel obstruction 7% thromboembolic complications	48% 5-year survival
Berek et al. (2005)	75	7–7.75 hours	2.51	UTIs, wound infection, intestinal fistula, intestinal obstruction	54% 5-year survival
UTI, urinary tract infection					

Table 33.2 Laparoscopic pelvic exenteration

Author	Type of article	No. of patients	Surgical method	Mean time of procedure	Blood loss	Complications	Hospital stay	Follow-up
Ferron et al. (2006)	Case series	7	Laparoscopy-assisted pelvic exenteration: 2 patients total 3 patients anterior 2 patients posterior	6.5 hours	< 500 mL	4 patients minor complications	27 days	14 months 2 patients free of disease
Uzan et al. (2006)	Case series	5	Laparoscopic pelvic exenteration: 2 patients total 1 patient posterior 2 patients anterior Laparoscopic pelvic exenteration	4.5–9 hours	370 mL			3 patients died (three were metastatic) 2 patients alive for 11 and 15 months
Puntambekar et al (2006)	Case series	12	Laparascopic anterior pelvic exenteration	180 minutes	100–500 mL	1 pt: internal iliac artery injury 3 patients: postoperative complications 2 patients: subacute intestinal obstruction 1 pt: ureteric leakage	3 days	

Table 33.3 Open and pelvic laparoscopic pelvic exenteration series (Puntambekar et al. 2006)

Series and year	N	PE type	Type of UD	EBL (mL)	HS (day)	Postoperative complications	Mortality	Reoperation	5-year survival
Open series									
Soper et al. (1989)	69	APE 16 TPE 41 PPE 12	NS	3500 (500–2600)	26 (14–199)	38%	7.2%	29%	48%
Magrina et al. (1997)	133	APE 39 TPE 67 PPE11	NS	1812 (200–6555)	26.6 (9–118)	24%	6.7%	6.7%	41%
Laparoscopic series									
Puntambekar et al. (2006)	16	APE 13 TPE- Total pelvic exenteration 2	13 US2 wet colostomy	400 (100–500)	3.5	Two SAIO one ureteric leak	0	No	NS NED 15 months

APE, anterior pelvic exenteration; EBL, estimated blood loss; HS, median hospital stay; NED: number of evidence of disease; NS, not stated; PE, pelvic exenteration; PPE, posterior pelvic exenteration; SAIO, subacute intestinal obstruction; TPE, total pelvic exenteration; UD, urinary diversion; US: ureterosigmoidostomy

■ CONCLUSION

Studies have shown that in patients with stage IV A primary cervical cancers, and in those with persistent or recurrent tumors, primary and secondary exenterations can be offered as curative procedures (Marnitz et al. 2006). Laparoscopic total pelvic exenteration is a feasible procedure in the management of patients with advanced cervical carcinoma selected carefully. The feasibility of this procedure defines newer limits for the use of laparoscopy in gynecological cancers. Anterior exenteration in advanced pelvic tumors offers good quality of life, especially with current methods of urinary diversion. It offers cure as well in a selected group. Posterior exenteration can also be performed with palliative intent. Whether this translates into a survival benefit needs to be observed further through randomized studies.

■ REFERENCES

Berek JS, Howe C, Lagasse LD, Hacker NF. Pelvic exenteration for recurrent gynecologic malignancy: survival and morbidity analysis of the 45-year experience at UCLA. Gynecol Oncol 2005; 99:153–159.

Brunschwich A. Complete excision of pelvic viscera for advanced carcinoma; a one-stage abdominoperineal operation with end colostomy and bilateral ureteral implantation into the colon above the colostomy. Cancer 1948; 1:177–183.

Diver EJ, Rauh-Hain JA, Del Carmen MG. Total pelvic exenteration for gynecologic malignancies. Int J Surg Oncol 2012; 2012:693535.

Ferron G, Querleu D, Martel P, et al. Laparoscopy-assisted vaginal pelvic exenteration. Gynecologci Oncology 2006; 100:551-555.

Goldberg GL, Sukumvanich P, Einstein MH, et al. Total pelvic exenteration: The Albert Einstein College of Medicine/Montefiore Medical Center Experience (1987 to 2003). Gynecologic Oncology 2006; 101:261-268.

Hafner GH, Petrelli NJ. Pelvic exenteration for colorectal adenocarcinoma. In: Sugarbaker PH (ed.), Pelvic surgery and treatment for cancer. Missouri: Mosby, 1994:285–296.

Lavazzo C, Vorgias G, Akrivos T. Laparoscopic pelvic exenteration: a new option in the surgical treatment of locally advanced and recurrent cervical carcinoma, Bratisl Lek Listy 2008; 109:467–469.

Magrina JF, Stanhope CR, Weaver AL. Pelvic exenterations: supralevator, infralevator, and with vulvectomy. Gynecol Oncol 1997;64:130-135.

Marnitz S, Dowdy S, Lanowska M, et al. Exenterations 60 years after first description: results of a survey among US and German Gynecologic Oncology Centers. Int J Gynecol Cancer 2009; 19:974–977.

Marnitz S, Köhler C, Müller M, et al. Indications for primary and secondary exenterations in patients with cervical cancer. Gynecol Oncol 2006; 103:1023–1030.

Pais Costa SR, Pinto Antunes RC, Lupinacci RA, et al. Pelvic exenteration for locally advanced primary and recurrent pelvic neoplasm. Einstein 2008; 6:302–310.

Puntambekar S, Kudchadkar RJ, Gurjar AM, et al. Laparoscopic pelvic exenteration for advanced pelvic cancers: a review of 16 cases. Gynecol Oncol 2006; 102:513–516.

Puntambekar S, Rajamanickam S, Agarwal G, et al. Laparoscopic posterior exenteration in advanced gynecologic malignant disease. J Minim Invasive Gynecol. 2011; 18:59–63.

Puntambekar SP, Agarwal GA, Puntambekar SS, Sathe RM, Patil AM. Stretching the limits of laparoscopy in gynecological oncology: technical feasibility of doing a laparoscopic total pelvic exenteration for palliation in advanced cervical cancer. Int J Biomed Sci 2009; 5:17–22.

Puntambekar SP, Kurchadkar RJ, Choudari YP, et al. Role of pelvic exenteration in advanced and recurrent pelvic tumours. J Pelvic Surg 2002; 8:241–245.

Puntambekar SP, Palep RJ, Puntambekar SS, et al. Laparoscopic total radical hysterectomy by the Pune technique. Our experience of 248 cases. J Minim Invasive Gynecol 2007; 14:682–689.

Rodriguez-Bigas MA, Petrelli NJ, Lopez MJ, Petros JG. Modified pelvic exenterations. Surg Oncol Clin N Am 1994; 3:239–246.

Sevin BU, Koechli OR. Pelvic exenteration. Surg Clin North Am 2001; 81:771–779.

Soper JT1, Berchuck A, Creasman WT, Clarke-Pearson DL. Pelvic exenteration: factors associated with major surgical morbidity. Gynecol Oncol 1989; 35:93-98.

Stan Hope CR, Symmonds RE. Palliative exenteration—what, when, and why? Am J Obstet Gynecol 1985; 152:12–16.

Uzan C, Rouzier R, Castaigne D, Pomel C. Laparoscopic pelvic exenteration for cervical cancer relapse: preliminary study. J Gynecol Obstet Biol Reprod (Paris) 2006; 35:136-145.

Chapter 34 | Robotic procedures for malignant conditions

João Siufi Neto, Daniela FS Siufi, Javier F Magrina

INTRODUCTION

The treatment of gynecological tumors by minimally invasive surgery has become standard in some countries, especially with the possibility of combining radicality with less surgical morbidity. Compared to conventional laparoscopy, robot-assisted surgery offers additional benefits in terms of ergonomics, and has become the surgeon's preference over laparoscopy.

Since the advent of robotic technology, many authors have shown the benefits of this technique for the performance of complex procedures such as radical hysterectomy, pelvic and aortic lymphadenectomy, radical trachelectomy, resection of diaphragm and liver metastasis, and cytoreduction for selected patients with ovarian cancer, which has led to a major reduction in laparotomic procedures.

This chapter will focus on the application of robotic surgery for patients with endometrial, cervical, and ovarian malignancies.

ENDOMETRIAL CANCER

Endometrial adenocarcinoma is the most common malignancy of the female genital tract in North America (Jemal et al. 2010). The American Cancer Society estimates 52,630 new cases in 2014 with 8590 casualties (American Cancer Society, 2014). Among the risk factors associated with the disease, obesity is one of the most challenging ones for the surgeon and a minimally invasive approach is preferred.

It has been demonstrated in different studies that patients with endometrial cancer treated by robotics have reductions in blood loss, complications, hospital stay, and recovery time, without compromising recurrence and survival outcomes as compared to laparotomy (Cho et al. 2007, Magrina 2005, Magrina et al. 1999). In comparison with laparoscopy, robotics is associated with a lower conversion rate (3% vs. 10%), while operating time, blood loss, hospital stay, and complications are similar for both surgical approaches (Magrina et al. 2011a).

Robotic hysterectomy and pelvic and aortic lymphadenectomy

Patient position and preparation

The patient is placed in a dorsal semilithotomy position with the legs in Allen stirrups. The patient's torso is resting directly on an egg-crate mattress to prevent sliding during Trendelenburg (**Figure 34.1**). The patient's arms and legs are properly protected to avoid injuries, particularly of the neural type. A three-way Foley catheter is routinely used to allow bladder distention whenever needed during any operation.

Trocar placement and docking

The open Hasson transumbilical entry technique is routinely used. Pelvic and upper abdominal inspection is made with the robotic scope. Additional trocars are placed as follows: two 8 mm robotic trocars are placed to the right and left of the umbilicus and about 10 cm from it, respectively. One assistant 10 mm trocar is placed 3 cm cranial and equidistant in between the umbilical and the left robotic trocars; one robotic 8 mm trocar is placed at the level of the cecum in the right lower quadrant (**Figure 34.2**). The patient is placed in Trendelenburg now or before the trocar placement but always before robotic arms docking.

The robotic column is advanced to the operating table and side-docked to the patient's right leg (**Figure 34.3**). Our mean docking time is about 3 minutes (Kho et al. 2007). Being dependent on the surgeon's preference, a monopolar spatula or scissors is inserted through the right trocar and a Plasma Kinetics bipolar grasper is inserted through the left trocar. At the right lower quadrant trocar, a Prograsp forceps is inserted and used as the fourth arm for retraction. The assistant uses the left upper quadrant trocar.

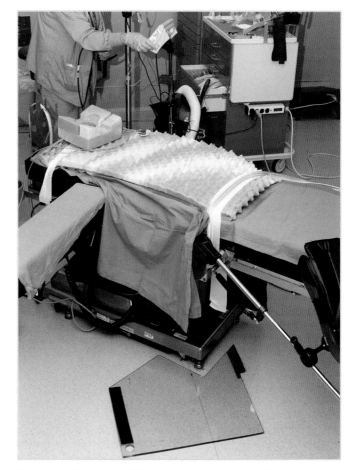

Figure 34.1 Operating table. The egg-crate mattress fastened to the table by wide tissue tape as an antisliding device. A floor template is positioned so that the robotic column is placed in the same location.

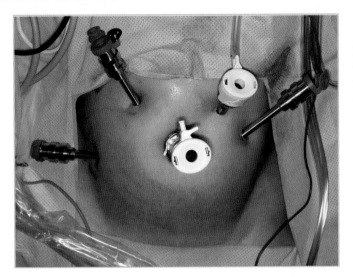

Figure 34.2 Usual trocar position for pelvic robotic gynecologic surgeries. Note the 'M' configuration of the trocars.

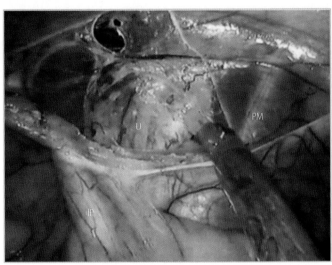

Figure 34.4 Peritoneal incision lateral to the right infundibulopelvic ligament. IP, infundibulopelvic ligament; PM, psoas muscle; U, ureter.

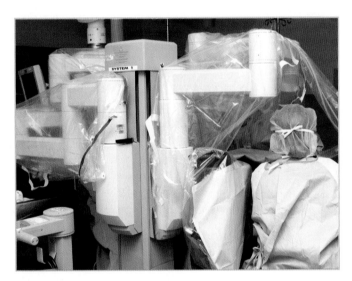

Figure 34.3 Right-side docking allowing direct access to the vagina for the assistant.

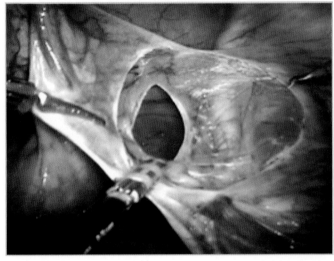

Figure 34.5 Isolation of the right ovarian vessels to prevent ureteral injury. The ureter is located dorsally to the peritoneal window. The ovarian vessels are being divided.

Technique

The lateral pelvic peritoneum is opened at the level of the pelvic brim parallel to ovarian vessels. Through this peritoneal incision, it is possible to identify the ureter (**Figure 34.4**). A peritoneal window is then created between the ovarian vessels and the ureter isolating the ovarian vessels and preventing ureteral injury (**Figure 34.5**). The broad ligament is then opened anteriorly and posteriorly by the division of the round ligament and both cardinal ligaments are sealed and divided close to the cervix (**Figure 34.6**). The bladder is pulled ventrally by the fourth arm and the vesicovaginal space is dissected. At this point, a vaginal probe or cervical cup is inserted by the scrub nurse allowing the identification of the cervicovaginal junction and the vaginal fornices. When the dissection of the vesicovaginal space is completed, a colpotomy is initiated at the 12 o'clock location and completed in a circumferential fashion (**Figure 34.7**).

The uterus and adnexa are removed through the vagina by the scrub nurse (**Figure 34.8**), and a 60h mL sterile occlusive balloon is positioned in the vagina to maintain the pneumoperitoneum until cuff

closure (**Figure 34.9**). The uterus is sent for frozen section analysis, a very important step to define the performance, or not, of the lymphadenectomy and the extension of the lymphadenectomy.

The cuff is left opened until the completion of the nodal dissection that allows their removal through the vagina with or without the use of an endobag. Once completed, the cuff is sutured with interrupted figure-of-eight sutures or continuous sutures using 2–0 polydioxanone, incorporating the uterosacral ligaments at each angle (**Figure 34.10**).

Pelvic lymphadenectomy
Indications

The uterus is sent for frozen section to provide directions for the performance of pelvic and aortic lymphadenectomy. Our criteria for pelvic lymphadenectomy include all patients with tumor types other than adenocarcinoma, and all patients with adenocarcinoma grade 2 or 3, tumor diameter ≥2 cm, myometrial invasion >50% (Mariani et al. 2008), lymphovascular invasion, and involvement of the lower uterine segment or cervix. In the absence of these factors, pelvic

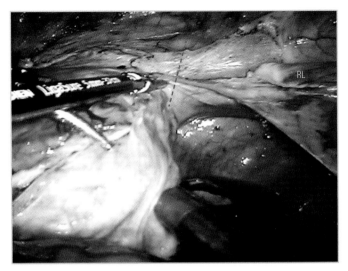

Figure 34.6 Division of right cardinal ligament close to the cervix with a vessel-sealing device (the dashed blue line). RL, round ligament transected.

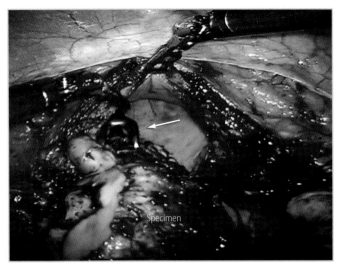

Figure 34.8 Specimen removal through the vagina. The uterus is retrieved through the open vaginal cuff by scrub technicians.

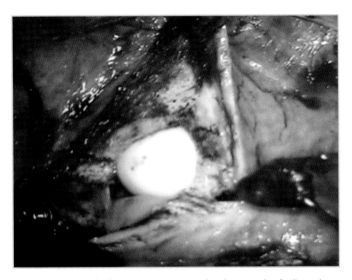

Figure 34.7 Vaginal colpotomy. A resin vaginal probe is used to facilitate the colpotomy.

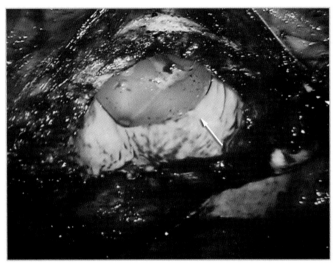

Figure 34.9 Sterile occlusive balloon (arrow) positioned in the vagina to maintain the pneumoperitoneum until cuff closure.

lymphadenectomy is omitted. The sentinel node technique for endometrial cancer appears to have merit but is not considered standard practice at present.

Technique

The paravesical and the pararectal spaces are dissected (**Figures 34.11 and 34.12**). The anatomic borders of the paravesical space are the superior vesical artery (medially), the external iliac vein (laterally), the pubic ramus (anteriorly), and the parametrium (posteriorly). The pararectal space margins are the ureter (medially), the internal iliac artery (laterally), the parametrium (anteriorly), and the sacrum (posteriorly).

The lymph nodes lateral and ventral to the external iliac vessels are removed first, followed by the superficial lateral common iliac vessels, and then the internal iliac and obturator nodes (**Figure 34.13**). All removed lymph nodes are sent for frozen section. A pelvic lymphadenectomy can be considered adequate when the common iliac artery and vein, the external and internal iliac arteries, the anterior branches of the internal iliac artery, and the obturator nerve are clearly visible.

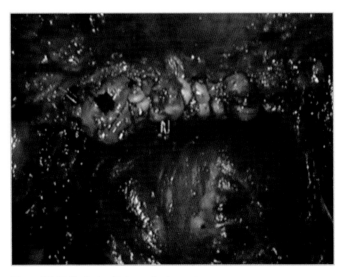

Figure 34.10 Vaginal cuff closure final aspect.

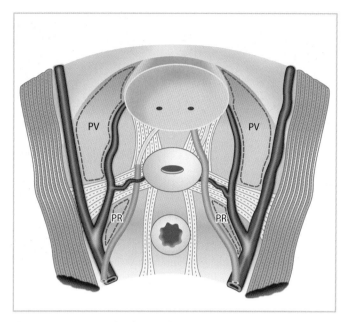

Figure 34.11 Paravesical and parectal spaces. PR, pararectal space; PV, paravesical space.

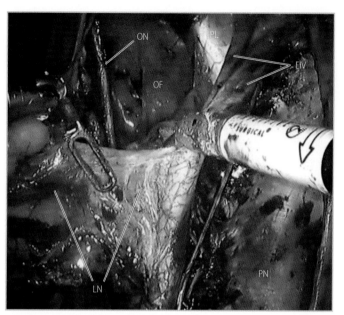

Figure 34.13 Right pelvic lymphadenectomy. Note the anatomic landmarks. EIV, external iliac vessels; LN, lymph nodes; OF, obturator fossa; ON, obturator nerve; PL, pectineal ligament; PM, psoas muscle.

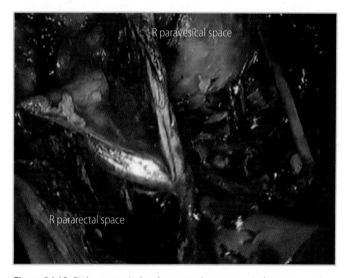

Figure 34.12 Right paravesical and pararectal spaces surgical aspect.

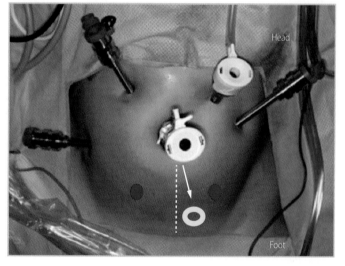

Figure 34.14 Trocar position for aortic lymphadenectomy. The yellow circle represents the new position for the optical trocar, now dislocated to the left side in relation to the midline (the dashed line) for direct vision of the aorta; the red circles show the position for the two accessory assistant ports.

Aortic lymphadenectomy

Indications

Patients with positive pelvic nodes, lymphatic invasion, and/or tumor grade 3 with 50% myometrial invasion are candidates for inframesenteric and infrarenal aortic lymphadenectomy, since aortic nodal metastases may bypass the inframesenteric nodes and be present only in the infrarenal group.

Technique

In patients requiring an aortic lymphadenectomy, it is necessary to undock the robotic column, to rotate the operating table by 180°, and to place three additional trocars in the lower pelvis. The optical 12 mm trocar is inserted suprapubically and two accessory trocars are placed 2 cm cranially and 5 cm laterally to the right and left of the optical trocar (**Figure 34.14**).

The robotic column is docked to the patient's head or side-docked to the patient's right shoulder (**Figure 34.15**). The assistant is positioned between the patient's legs and uses a fan retractor with the left hand to retract the duodenum and pancreas ventrally while the right hand is used for vessel-sealing blood vessels, suction–irrigation, and lateral retraction of the sigmoid mesentery.

The aortic lymph node dissection begins with the opening of the peritoneum overlying the midportion of the right common iliac artery up to the aortic bifurcation. The left renal vein is identified,

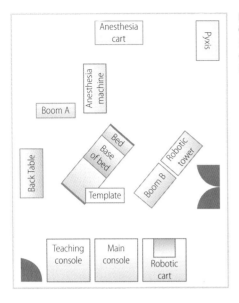

Figure 34.15
Operating room. Right shoulder docking for aortic lymphadenectomy.

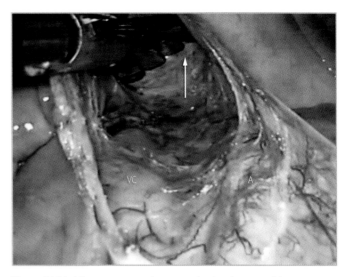

Figure 34.16 A fan retractor used to retract the duodenum and the pancreas.

and the duodenum and pancreas are retracted ventrally by the assistant with a fan retractor (**Figure 34.16**). The right aortic nodes over the vena cava and aorta are excised first, followed by the interaortic nodes (**Figure 34.17**). The dissection is extended cranially over the vena cava until no nodal tissue is visible, usually above the right gonadal vein entrance site into the vena cava. The inframesenteric left aortic nodal area is exposed by extending the initial peritoneal incision for a distance of about 5 cm starting at the aortic bifurcation and extending caudally over the left common iliac artery. The sigmoid mesentery is retracted laterally by the assistant. The left inframesenteric nodes are removed from the bifurcation of the aorta to the inferior mesenteric artery and sent separately for pathological examination (**Figure 34.18**).

The infrarenal nodal area is optimally exposed by dividing the inferior mesenteric artery with a vessel-sealing device at its origin from the aorta and by lateral retraction of the left colon mesentery by the assistant (**Figure 34.19**). The infrarenal nodes are removed from the level of the stump of the inferior mesenteric artery to the left renal vein and medial to the left ovarian vessels (**Figure 34.20**). A second lumbar vein is found crossing this nodal group in about one third of the patients, originating in the lumbar spine and draining directly to the left renal vein or, less frequently, to the left gonadal vein.

■ CERVICAL CANCER

The rate of cervical cancer incidence and death in developed countries has decreased steadily over the last decade owing to early detection and treatment. Standard surgical treatment of early-stage cervical cancer is radical hysterectomy with pelvic lymphadenectomy, and including an aortic lymphadenectomy in the presence of specific indications. Studies have demonstrated the feasibility of robotics for the surgical treatment of cervical cancer, with similar operating time but decreased blood loss and shorter hospital stay as compared to laparotomy. In comparison with laparoscopy, robotics operating time is shorter but has similar blood loss, complications, recurrence, and survival (Magrina 2007, Magrina et al. 2008).

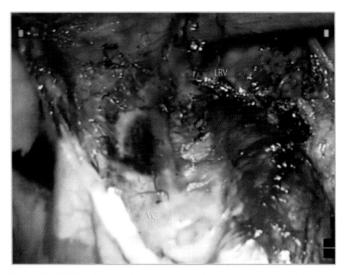

Figure 34.17 The right and the interaortic nodes have been removed. A, aorta; LRV, left renal vein; VC, vena cava.

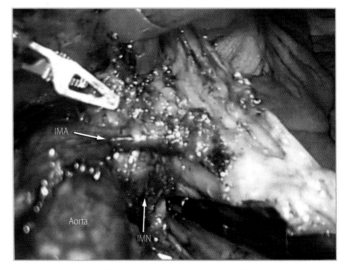

Figure 34.18 Removal of inframesenteric aortic nodes after dissection. These nodes are sent separately for pathologic evaluation. IMA, inferior mesenteric artery.

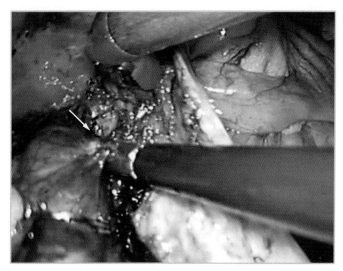

Figure 34.19 Inferior mesenteric artery (arrow) division with a vessel-sealing device.

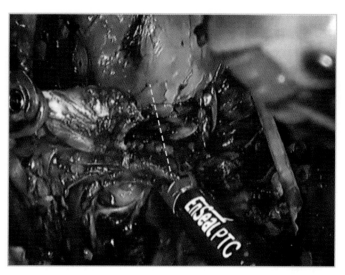

Figure 34.21 Right parametrium transection using a vessel-sealing device.

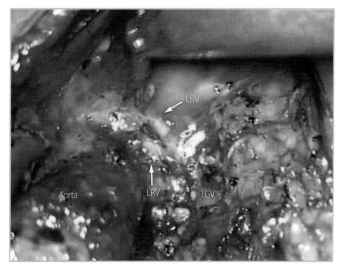

Figure 34.20 The infrarenal left nodes have been removed. The left renal artery and vein are clearly seen. LGV, left gonadal vein; LRA, left renal artery; LRV, left renal vein.

Robotic radical hysterectomy
Patient position and preparation

In robotic radical hysterectomy, patient position and preparation, equipment and robotic column, trocar placement, and docking are the same as described above for endometrial cancer patients.

Radical hysterectomy technique

The technique described here has been previously described (Magrina et al. 2009) and corresponds to type C1 according to the recently revised classification of radical hysterectomy (Querleu & Morrow 2008).

A peritoneal incision is made lateral to the infundibulopelvic ligaments for the identification of the ovarian vessels and the ureter (**Figure 34.4**). A peritoneal window is created between the ovarian vessels and the left ureter isolating the ovarian vessels and preventing ureteral injury (**Figure 34.5**). If adnexectomy is indicated, the ovarian

vessels are sealed and transected by the assistant with a vessel-sealing device. The round ligament is divided, and the broad ligament is opened anteriorly and posteriorly.

The paravesical and the pararectal spaces are dissected (**Figures 34.11** and **34.12**). The anatomic borders of the paravesical space are the superior vesical artery (medially), the external iliac vein (laterally), the pubic ramus (anteriorly), and the parametrium (posteriorly). The pararectal space margins are the ureter (medially), the internal iliac artery (laterally), the parametrium (anteriorly), and the sacrum (posteriorly).

A pelvic lymphadenectomy of levels 1 and 2 (Querleu & Morrow 2008) is now performed bilaterally, and the lymph nodes are submitted for frozen section (**Figure 34.13**). The operation may be aborted depending on the size, number, fixation, and location of positive nodes. In addition to providing information about nodal status, removal of the nodes allows for an easier identification of the retroperitoneal vessels and nerves during the radical hysterectomy.

Once the lymphadenectomy is completed, the parametrium is transected at its origin from the internal iliac artery and vein, using a vessel-sealing device (**Figure 34.21**), starting with the superior vesical and uterine arteries ventrally and extending dorsally to the deep uterine vein, joining the paravesical and pararectal spaces when the division is completed.

Next is the division of the uterosacral ligaments followed by bladder and ureteral dissection. A transverse peritoneal incision is made across the cul-de-sac, and the rectovaginal space is dissected to the midportion of the vagina (**Figure 34.22**). This provides identification of both uterosacral ligaments that are transected with a vessel-sealing device at the level of the anterior rectal wall, depending on the tumor size and tumor proximity to the posterior vaginal wall (**Figure 34.23**). Transection of the uterosacral ligament facilitates ventral displacement of the uterus.

A transverse peritoneal incision is made over the vesicouterine junction; the vesicovaginal space is dissected to the midportion of the anterior vaginal wall by ventral retraction of the bladder and with the assistance of a vaginal probe manipulated by the scrub nurse (**Figure 34.24**).

Once the bladder has been mobilized from the cervix and vagina, the entrance of the ureter into the parametrial tunnel is identified by

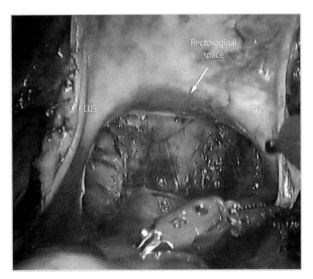

Figure 34.22 The rectovaginal space is incised (the dashed line) and dissected until the midportion of the vagina. LUS, left uterosacral ligament; RUS, right uterosacral ligament.

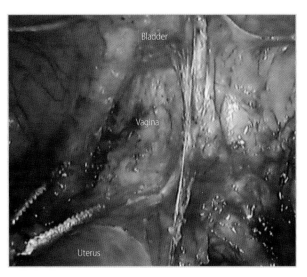

Figure 34.24 Vesicovaginal space dissected.

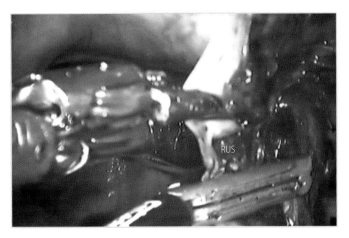

Figure 34.23 Right uterosacral ligament division with a vessel-sealing device.

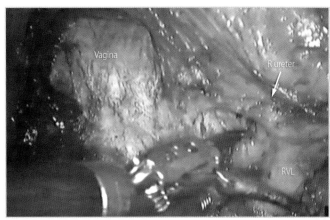

Figure 34.25 Isolation of the dorsal right vesicouterine ligament or bladder pillar for subsequent division with a vessel-sealing device.

pulling on the stump of the transected uterine artery. The avascular space located at 12 o'clock over the ureter and immediately dorsal to the crossing with the uterine artery is widened and dissected to the vesicovaginal space, isolating the ventral bladder pillar (also known as the vesicouterine ligament), which is divided preferably with a vessel-sealing device or monopolar spatula (**Figure 34.25**). The ureter is then gently mobilized laterally (rolled away), isolating the dorsal bladder pillar. The medial limit of the dorsal bladder pillar is identified by developing the avascular space located below the entrance of the ureter into the bladder following which the dorsal bladder pillar is transected. Once the ventral and dorsal bladder pillars are transected, the ureters can be lifted ventrally exposing the underlying paravaginal tissue and assuring a complete removal of the lateral parametrium (**Figure 34.26**).

The paravaginal tissue is transected with a vessel-sealing device to the lateral aspect of the vaginal wall, and ensuring the complete resection of the entire transected parametrium and uterosacral ligaments. A vaginal probe is used to assist in the identification of the cervicovaginal junction, which is used to determine the level of

transection of the vagina to obtain adequate margins. The colpotomy is performed in a circumferential fashion starting at the 12 o'clock position of the vagina (**Figure 34.7**) and proceeding to the left vaginal angle and posterior vagina, and then to the right vaginal angle. The uterus is removed through the vagina using an endobag, if necessary for easier removal. The vaginal cuff is closed with a double-layer continuous suture or interrupted figure-of-eight sutures using 2–0 polydioxanone (**Figure 34.10**).

Nerve-sparing technique

This technique follows the same steps as the conventional technique with the exception of preservation of the pelvic splanchnic nerves (PSNs), the superior- and inferior hypogastric plexuses (IHPs). The following are the additional steps over the conventional technique:

1. The PSNs are identified in the lowermost portion of the pararectal space (**Figure 34.27**). The parametria are transected at their origin from the internal iliac artery and vein up to and including the deep uterine vein.

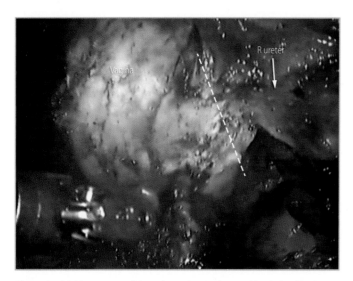

Figure 34.26 Transection of the right paravaginal tissue (the dashed line) for complete lateral parametrium resection. The ureter has been mobilized ventrally to allow complete resection of the lateral parametrium.

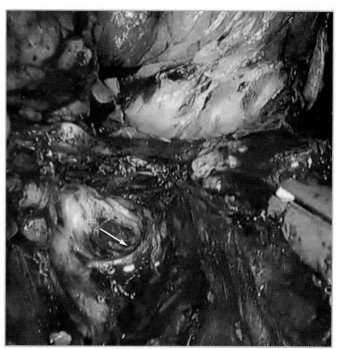

Figure 34.28 The inferior hypogastric plexus (also known as pelvic plexus) is identified immediately dorsal to the transected parametria. IHP, inferior hypogastric plexus.

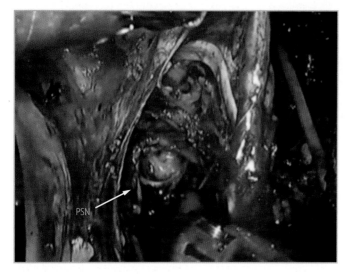

Figure 34.27 The pelvic splanchnic nerves are identified in the lowermost portion of the pararectal space.

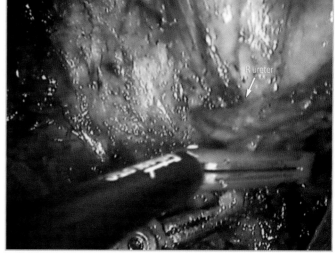

Figure 34.29 The dorsal bladder pillar is transected remaining close to the ureter, preserving the efferent branches of the inferior hypogastric plexus to the bladder.

2. The IHP (also known as pelvic plexus) is identified immediately dorsal to the transected parametria (**Figure 34.28**).
3. The superior hypogastric plexus (also known as hypogastric nerves) is identified on the lateral aspect of the uterosacral ligaments and dissected laterally from them. The uterosacral ligaments are divided but the superior hypogastric nerves are preserved (**Figure 34.23**).
4. The ureters are dissected in a similar manner but the dorsal bladder pillar is transected remaining close to the ureter, preserving the dorsal and the lateral aspect of the pillar where the efferent branches of the IHP to the bladder are present (**Figure 34.29**).

5. During the colpotomy the efferent fibers of the IHP to the bladder, identified along the lateral vaginal wall, are mobilized dorsally to the colpotomy site to prevent their transection (**Figure 34.30**).

Aortic lymphadenectomy

In the presence of positive pelvic nodes, a tumor size of >5 cm diameter, and/or enlarged aortic nodes on preoperative imaging, the pelvic lymphadenectomy is extended to an aortic lymphadenectomy, levels 3 and 4 (Querleu & Morrow 2008). The aortic lymphadenectomy must include the infrarenal nodes because pelvic nodal metastases can bypass the ipsilateral inframesenteric nodes (Gil-Moreno et al.

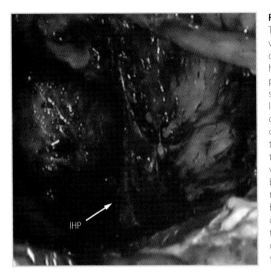

Figure 34.30
The efferent vesical fibers of the inferior hypogastric plexus (IHP) are seen coursing lateral to the open vaginal cuff toward the bladder. If the additional vagina must be removed, the fibers can be mobilized dorsally to allow their preservation during further vaginal resection.

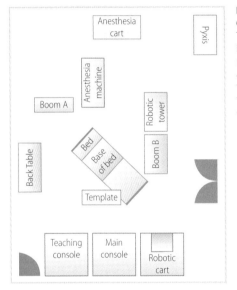

Figure 34.31
Operating room. The robotic column is positioned to the patient's right side and almost perpendicular to the operating table for robotic extraperitoneal aortic lymphadenectomy.

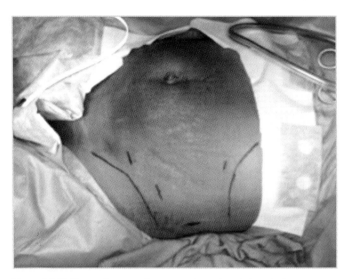

Figure 34.32 Trocar placement for extraperitoneal aortic lymphadenectomy. The optical trocar is at the lowest incision, and the two upper are for the robotic trocars. The assistant trocar is between the optical and the left robotic trocar.

subsequently reaching over the aorta, which is facilitated by instrument articulation.

■ Robotic fertility-sparing radical trachelectomy

In women with early-stage cervical cancer, who are desirous to preserve fertility, radical trachelectomy with pelvic lymphadenectomy is an option in the presence of a tumor of 2 cm or less in diameter and without lymphovascular invasion (Beiner & Covens 2007, Diaz et al. 2008). Fertility is slightly impaired due to reduced spontaneous pregnancies and increased premature labor, while recurrence and survival remain unaltered (Gizzo et al. 2013). The robotic approach is associated with lower blood loss and shorter hospital stay, with no differences in operative time or survival as compared to laparotomy (Nick et al. 2012).

Patient position and preparation

It is similar as described for patients with endometrial cancer.

Technique

The technique is similar to that described for radical hysterectomy including dissection of the lateral pelvic spaces, pelvic lymphadenectomy, uterosacral ligament division, bladder and ureteral dissection, and colpotomy. The main differences are (1) in the preservation of the uterine artery during the transection of the lateral parametrium, and (2) in the transection of the cervix at its upper third for uterine preservation. The procedure begins with the development of the paravesical and pararectal spaces. A pelvic lymphadenectomy is performed following the same steps as mentioned previously. All lymph nodes retrieved are sent for intraoperative frozen section. In the presence of positive pelvic nodes, the sparing procedure is aborted and a radical hysterectomy and an aortic lymphadenectomy are performed depending on the size, number, location, and fixation of the positive pelvic nodes. An infrarenal aortic lymphadenectomy is also performed.

The parametrium is divided at its origin from the internal iliac artery preserving the uterine artery, which is dissected from its origin to the lateral wall of the uterus. Some authors have reported division of the uterine artery at its origin apparently without any ill consequences

2012). A transperitoneal approach is used when the aortic lymphadenectomy is performed concomitant to radical hysterectomy and pelvic lymphadenectomy (Magrina et al. 2009), as described above for endometrial cancer.

The extraperitoneal approach is preferable in patients with locally advanced cervical cancer prior to chemoirradiation therapy to determine the extent of the irradiation field and improve survival by removing positive nodes that may not be sterilized with chemoirradiation (Magrina et al. 2008). For this approach, the robotic column must be positioned perpendicular to the patient's right side at the level of the midabdomen (**Figure 34.31**).

The placement of trocar sites is demonstrated in **Figure 34.32**. An incision is made laterally and cranially to the anterior iliac spine, and the extraperitoneal space is developed with CO_2 or using an inflatable balloon (Spacemaker Plus Dissector System, United States Surgical, Tyco Healthcare Group LP, Norwalk, Connecticut) and the robotic arms docked to the trocars.

The left ovarian vessels and left ureter are displaced ventrally and followed cranially until the left renal vein is identified. The left aortic nodes are removed starting at the aortic bifurcation and progressed to the left renal vein. The right aortic nodes are excised for uterine blood supply or subsequent pregnancy. The uterosacral ligaments are divided next, followed by bladder dissection and ureteral dissection. In the latter dissection, the uterine artery is lifted above the ureter and dissected medially allowing a lateral displacement of the ureter and the division of the ventral bladder pillar.

The cervix is then transected at its midportion and a frozen section is obtained to determine a 1 cm negative endocervical margin. If the margin is inadequate, an additional portion of the cervix is removed and a repeat frozen section is performed. A cervical cerclage is performed using a No. 2 polypropylene suture placed below the internal cervical os and tied over a No. 2 cervical dilator. The vagina is sutured to the future exocervix and as close as possible to the new external cervical with interrupted sutures of 3-0 Vicryl (Perrson et al. 2012; Zagnanolo & Magrina 2009).

Robotic parametrectomy

This is a surgical option for young patients with occult invasive cervical cancer and negative margins after simple hysterectomy. The safety and feasibility of robotic nerve-sparing radical parametrectomy has been demonstrated (Magrina & Magtibay 2012).

Patient position and preparation

Patient position and preparation, equipment, and robotic column, trocar placement, and docking are the same as described above for robotic radical hysterectomy.

Technique

The technique is the same as described for radical hysterectomy with the exception that the uterus has already been removed. This results in a more difficult dissection of the bladder and ureters due to the presence of scar tissue. In between simple hysterectomy and radical parametrectomy, a waiting period of at least 6 weeks is recommended.

After the lateral pelvic spaces are developed, a pelvic lymphadenectomy is performed, and the parametrium is transected. A vaginal probe is placed in the vagina and a similar one is placed in the rectum for easier identification of these two structures. The bladder is distended with 300 mL water. With the bladder, the rectum, and the vagina well identified, the vesicovaginal and rectovaginal spaces are dissected to the midportion of the vagina (**Figures 34.22** and **34.24**). The procedure continues in the same way as that for a radical hysterectomy, with transection of the uterosacral ligaments and bladder pillars followed by a colpotomy and removal of the specimen (**Figures 34.23** to **34.26**).

Nerve-sparing technique

This technique follows the same steps as described for the nerve-sparing radical hysterectomy technique above.

OVARIAN CANCER

There are only a few studies reporting on the use of robotics for ovarian cancer. The most important issue is patient selection, which is carried out preoperatively and at the time of initial laparoscopic exploration. Preoperatively, the presence of peritoneal carcinomatosis, advanced retroperitoneal disease, especially in the porta hepatis area, large-volume ascites, stage IV disease, poor nutritional status, and/or multiple comorbidities are indications for neoadjuvant chemotherapy. Patients selected for surgery are evaluated by laparoscopic exploration. Through laparoscopy, the extent of disease is evaluated to determine (1) if all disease can

be removed (complete debulking) and (2) the number of major procedures required to achieve complete tumor resection. Patients with disease requiring one or two major procedures in addition to hysterectomy, adnexectomy, and omentectomy are candidates for robotic cytoreduction. For patients requiring three or more major procedures, a laparotomic cytoreduction is preferable (Magrina et al. 2011b). Patients with limited recurrent disease may also benefit from robotic secondary cytoreduction, following the same criteria as described for primary robotic cytoreduction, and after an interval, free of disease, of 12 months or longer from completion of previous chemotherapy.

The techniques of robotic hysterectomy, adnexectomy, and lymphadenectomy are described above for patients with endometrial cancer.

Resection of diaphragmatic and hepatic metastases

Patient position and preparation

These are already described above for endometrial cancer. Reverse Trendelenburg is necessary when the lesions are in the dorsal part of the right lobe of the liver or close to the coronary ligament of the right diaphragm.

Trocar placement and docking

The robotic column is placed at the patient's head or side-docked at the right or left shoulder. The trocar placement depends on the location of the lesions. For lesions located on the anterior portion of both diaphragms or the liver, the trocar placement is as used for pelvic surgery (**Figure 34.2**). The robotic instruments are the same as used for pelvic surgery.

For lesions on the dome of the right hepatic lobe and dorsal right diaphragm, all trocars, including the optical trocar, must be supraumbilical, and the left trocar and both right trocars must be in a subcostal position. The right robotic trocar is close to the subcostal margin, and the left lateral robotic trocar is on the anterior axillary line. The assistant trocar is to the right or left of the optical trocar depending on the location of the lesion. A 30° scope is used to improve the visualization over the right hepatic lobe. A subhepatic approach is always preferable for lesions near the triangular or coronary ligament whenever possible. In that case, an additional right subcostal trocar is necessary to retract the right hepatic lobe ventrally with a fan retractor by a second assistant, while the first assistant uses a fan retractor to retract the right kidney. In the case of a suprahepatic approach, the assistant uses a fan retractor over the right hepatic lobe to provide exposure to the posterior portion of the diaphragm or liver.

Technique

Diaphragmatic lesions are excised using a monopolar spatula at a low voltage of 15 W to prevent diaphragm perforation, since the diaphragm muscle will contract when stimulated by monopolar current. A full-thickness diaphragm resection is performed if there is any involvement of the diaphragm muscle. Positive pressure ventilation prevents lung collapse once the pleural cavity is entered (**Figures 34.33** and **34.34**).

Closure of the diaphragmatic defect is performed with one or more running, locking 2-0 polydioxanone sutures, each precut to 15 cm length with a Lapra-Ty clip (Ethicon Endo-Surgery, Cincinnati, Ohio) at their distal end. Before closure is completed, remaining fluids and CO_2 in the pleural cavity are aspirated through a red Robinson catheter connected to continuous suction (**Figures 34.35** to **34.37**). Pleural leaks

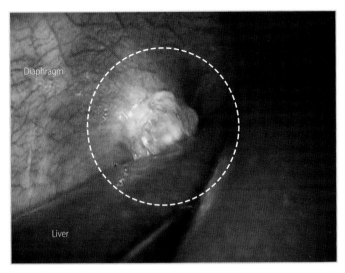

Figure 34.33 Recurrent ovarian carcinoma involving the diaphragm and the liver.

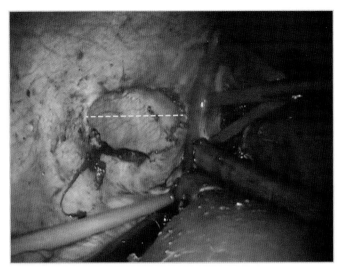

Figure 34.35 Diaphragmatic defect before closure.

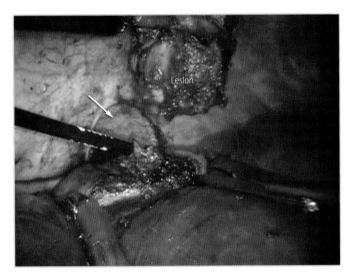

Figure 34.34 En-bloc resection of the tumor implant including liver and diaphragm margins.

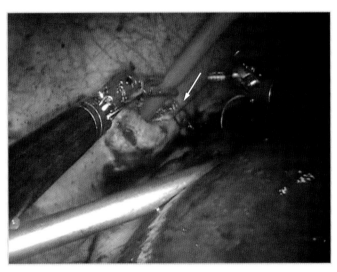

Figure 34.36 Diaphragmatic defect partially closed (arrow) with a red Robinson catheter inside the pleural cavity. The catheter is connected to a continuous suction to remove CO_2 and fluids during a Valsalva maneuver. It is then removed and the defect is closed with one pass of the running locking suture.

are checked with Valsalva under water, and a chest X-ray is obtained intraoperatively to check for residual pneumothorax.

Because most hepatic lesions are superficially invasive, they can be resected using a monopolar spatula or scissors on a co-agulating setting set at 60–80 W or using a saline bipolar device. Deeply invasive lesions into the liver parenchyma require a partial or complete segmentectomy and are performed by a liver surgeon in our institution.

■ CONCLUSION

The use of robotic technology for the treatment of gynecologic malignancies has proven to be feasible and safe. The possibility of combining the well-known benefits of laparoscopy with articulated instruments, a three-dimensional vision system, and the superior ergonomic features of the robotic technology over laparoscopy represent a step forward in minimally invasive surgery.

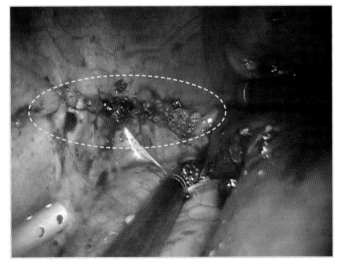

Figure 34.37 Diaphragmatic defect closure final aspect.

REFERENCES

American Cancer Society. Cancer facts and figures 2014. Atlanta, GA: American Cancer Society, 2014. Available from: www.cancer.org/acs/groups/content/@research/documents/webcontent/acspc-042151.pdf (Last accessed 31 March 2014).

Beiner ME, Covens A. Surgery insight: radical vaginal trachelectomy as a method of fertility preservation for cervical cancer. Nat Clin Pract Oncol 2007; 4:353–361.

Cho YH, Kim DY, Kim JH, et al. Laparoscopic management of early uterine cancer: 10-year experience in Asian Medical Center. Gynecol Oncol 2007; 106:585–590.

Diaz JP, Sonoda Y, Leitao MM, et al. Oncologic outcome of fertility-sparing radical trachelectomy versus radical hysterectomy for stage IB1 cervical carcinoma. Gynecol Oncol 2008; 111:255–260.

Gil-Moreno A, Magrina JF, Perez-Benavente A, et al. Location of aortic node metastases in locally advanced cervical cancer. Gynecol Oncol 2012; 125:312–314.

Gizzo S, Ancona E, Saccardi C, et al. Radical trachelectomy: the first step of fertility preservation in young women with cervical cancer (Review). Oncol Rep 2013; 30:2545–2554.

Jemal A, Siegel R, Ward E, et al. Cancer statistics, 2010. CA Cancer J Clin 2010; 60:277–300.

Kho RM, Hilger WS, Hentz JG, et al. Robotic hysterectomy: technique and initial outcomes. Am J Obstet Gynecol 2007; 197:332.

Magrina JF. Outcomes of laparoscopic treatment for endometrial cancer. Curr Opin Obstet Gynecol 2005; 17:343–346.

Magrina JF. Robotic surgery in gynecology. Eur J Gynaecol Oncol 2007; 28:77–82.

Magrina JF, Kho R, Magtibay PM. Robotic radical hysterectomy: technical aspects. Gynecol Oncol 2009; 113:28–31.

Magrina JF, Kho R, Montero RP, Magtibay PM, Pawlina W. Robotic extraperitoneal aortic lymphadenectomy: development of a technique. Gynecol Oncol 2008a; 113:32–35.

Magrina JF, Kho RM, Weaver AL, Montero RP, Magtibay PM. Robotic radical hysterectomy: comparison with laparoscopy and laparotomy. Gynecol Oncol 2008b; 109:86–91.

Magrina JF, Long JB, Kho RM, et al. Robotic transperitoneal infrarenal aortic lymphadenectomy: technique and results. Int J Gynecol Cancer 2010; 20:184–187.

Magrina JF, Magtibay PM. Robotic nerve-sparing radical parametrectomy: feasibility and technique. Int J Med Robot 2012; 8:206–209.

Magrina JF, Mutone NF, Weaver AL, et al. Laparoscopic lymphadenectomy and vaginal or laparoscopic hysterectomy with bilateral salpingo-oophorectomy for endometrial cancer: morbidity and survival. Am J Obstet Gynecol 1999; 181:376–381.

Magrina JF, Zanagnolo V, Giles D, et al. Robotic surgery for endometrial cancer: comparison of perioperative outcomes and recurrence with laparoscopy, vaginal/laparoscopy and laparotomy. Eur J Gynaecol Oncol 2011a; 32:476–480.

Magrina JF, Zanagnolo V, Noble BN, Kho RM, Magtibay P. Robotic approach for ovarian cancer: perioperative and survival results and comparison with laparoscopy and laparotomy. Gynecol Oncol 2011b; 121:100–105.

Mariani A, Dowdy SC, Cliby WA, et al. Prospective assessment of lymphatic dissemination in endometrial cancer: a paradigm shift in surgical staging. Gynecol Oncol 2008; 109:11–18.

Nick AM, Frumovitz MM, Soliman PT, Schmeler KM, Ramirez PT. Fertility sparing surgery for treatment of early-stage cervical cancer: open vs. robotic radical trachelectomy. Gynecol Oncol 2012; 124:276–280.

Persson J, Imboden S, Reynisson P, et al. Reproducibility of and accuracy of robot-assisted laparoscopic fertility sparing radical trachelectomy. Gynecol Oncol 2012; 127:484–488.

Querleu D, Morrow C. Classification of radical hysterectomy. Lancet Oncol 2008; 9: 297–303.

Zanagnolo V, Magrina JF. Robotic trachelectomy after supracervical hysterectomy for a cut-through endometrial adenocarcinoma stage IIB: a case report. J Minim Invasive Gynecol 2009; 16:655–657.

Index

Note: Page numbers in **bold** or *italic* refer to tables or figures respectively.